PERIPHERAL NERVE SURGERY: PRACTICAL APPLICATIONS IN THE UPPER EXTREMITY

PERIPHERAL NERVE SURGERY: PRACTICAL APPLICATIONS IN THE UPPER EXTREMITY

Editors

David J. Slutsky, M.D., F.R.C.S.(C)
Assistant Clinical Professor
Department of Orthopedic Surgery
UCLA School of Medicine
Los Angeles, California

Vincent R. Hentz, M.D.
Professor, Department of Surgery
Stanford University
Stanford, California

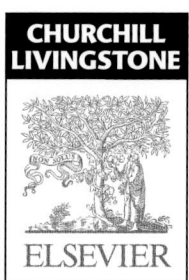

CHURCHILL LIVINGSTONE

ELSEVIER

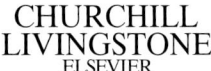

CHURCHILL
LIVINGSTONE
ELSEVIER

1600 John F. Kennedy Blvd.
Suite 1800
Philadelphia, PA 19103-2899

PERIPHERAL NERVE SURGERY: PRACTICAL APPLICATIONS   ISBN-13: 978-0-443-06667-2
IN THE UPPER EXTREMITY   ISBN-10: 0-443-06667-1

Notice

Knowledge and best practice in this field are constantly changing. As new research and experience broaden our knowledge, changes in practice, treatment and drug therapy may become necessary or appropriate. Readers are advised to check the most current information provided (i) on procedures featured or (ii) by the manufacturer of each product to be administered, to verify the recommended dose or formula, the method and duration of administration, and contraindications. It is the responsibility of the practitioner, relying on their own experience and knowledge of the patient, to make diagnoses, to determine dosages and the best treatment for each individual patient, and to take all appropriate safety precautions. To the fullest extent of the law, neither the Publisher nor the authors assumes any liability for any injury and/or damage to persons or property arising out or related to any use of the material contained in this book.

The Publisher

Library of Congress Cataloging-in-Publication Data

Peripheral nerve surgery / [edited by] David J. Slutsky, Vincent R. Hentz.–1st ed.
   p. ; cm.
   ISBN 0-443-06667-1
    1. Nerves, Peripheral–Surgery. 2. Hand–Surgery. I. Slutsky, David J. II. Hentz, Vincent R.
  [DNLM: 1. Peripheral Nerves–surgery. 2. Neurosurgical Procedures–methods. WL 500
  P4447 2006]
  RD595.P48 2006
  617.4'83–dc22

2005054901

Acquisitions Editor: Elyse O'Grady
Editorial Assistant: Boris Ginsburgs
Project Manager: Mary Stermel
Design Direction: Gene Harris

Printed in China

Last digit is the print number: 9 8 7 6 5 4 3 2 1

To Paul and Rose Slutsky; for a lifetime of sacrifice for those they love.

David Slutsky

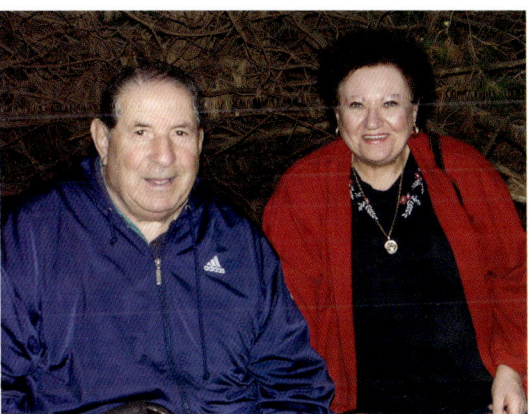

Dedicated to the masters of nerve reconstruction: Algis Narakas and Alain Gilbert and to my personal heroes, Drs. J. William Littler and Robert A. Chase who lived and live this quotation: "Imagine how much more we could accomplish if it didn't matter who got the credit."

V. R. Hentz

Christopher H. Allan, M.D.
Department of Orthopaedics, Harborview Medical Center, University of Washington, Seattle, Washington

Simon Archibald, Ph.D.
Chief Scientific Officer, Integra Neurosciences, Plainsboro, New Jersey

Robert W. Beasley, M.D.
Department of Surgery, New York University, New York, New York

Sean M. Bidic, M.D., M.F.A.
Department of Plastic Surgery, University of Texas Southwestern Medical Center, Dallas, Texas

Michael J. Botte, M.D.
Division of Orthopaedic Surgery, Scripps Clinic, La Jolla, California

Warren C. Breidenbach, M.D., F.R.C.S.(C)
Kleinert, Kutz and Associates Hand Care Center, Louisville, Kentucky

Giorgio A. Brunelli, M.D.
Department of Orthopaedics, University of Brescia, Brescia, Italy

Lars B. Dahlin, M.D., Ph.D.
Department of Hand Surgery, University Hospital Malmö, Malmö, Sweden

Nickolaos A. Darlis, M.D.
Department of Orthopaedic Surgery, University of Ioannina, Ioannina, Greece

A. Lee Dellon, M.D.
Johns Hopkins University, Baltimore, Maryland

Richard H. Gelberman, M.D.
Department of Orthopaedic Surgery, Washington University in St. Louis, St. Louis, Missouri

Vincent R. Hentz, M.D.
Professor, Department of Surgery, Stanford University, Stanford Hospital and Clinics, Robert A. Chase Center for Surgery of the Hand and Upper Limb, Stanford, California

Michael E. Jabaley, M.D., F.A.C.S.
12 Provence Boulevard, Madison, Mississippi

Rashid M. Janjua, M.D.
Department of Neurosurgery, Mayfield Clinic, University of Cincinnati Medical Center, Cincinnati, Ohio

Neil F. Jones, M.D.
UCLA Hand Center, Los Angeles, California

David G. Kline, M.D.
Department of Neurosurgery, Louisiana State University, New Orleans, Louisiana

Jason T. Koo
3250 Horace Avenue, Keller, Texas

W. P. Andrew Lee, M.D.
Division of Plastic and Reconstructive Surgery, University of Pittsburgh Medical Center, Pittsburgh, Pennsylvania

Erika G. Lumsden, M.D.
Miller Orthopaedic Clinic, Charlotte, North Carolina

Susan E. Mackinnon, M.D.
Division of Plastic and Reconstructive Surgery, Washington University School of Medicine, St. Louis, Missouri

James W. May, Jr., M.D.
Department of Surgery, Massachusetts General Hospital, Boston, Massachusetts

Hanno Millesi, M.D.
Professor, Medical University of Vienna, Vienna, Austria

George E. Omer, Jr., M.D.
316 Big Horn Ridge Road, NE, Albuquerque, New Mexico

A. Lee Osterman, M.D.
Hand Rehabilitation Foundation, Philadelphia, Pennsylvania

Tuna Ozyurekoglu, M.D.
Department of Surgery, University of Louisville, Louisville, Kentucky

Lorenzo L. Pacelli, M.D.
Division of Orthopaedic Surgery, Scripps Clinic, La Jolla, California

Debra Parisi, M.D.
Department of Orthopaedics, University of Washington Medical Center, Seattle, Washington

Ziv M. Peled, M.D.
Surgery Education Office, Brigham and Women's Hospital, Boston, Massachusetts

Martin A. Posner, M.D.
New York University School of Medicine, NYU–Hospital for Joint Diseases, New York, New York

Dean G. Sotereanos, M.D.
Allegheny General Hospital, Pittsburgh, Pennsylvania

David J. Slutsky, M.D., F.R.C.S.(C)
Assistant Clinical Professor, Department of Orthopedic Surgery, UCLA School of Medicine, Los Angeles, California

Robert M. Szabo, M.D.
Department of Orthopaedics, University of California, Davis, Sacramento, California

Gabriel C. Tender, M.D.
Charity Hospital New Orleans, New Orleans, Louisiana

Robert L. Tiel, M.D.
Department of Neurosurgery, Louisiana State University, New Orleans, Louisiana

Thomas E. Trumble, M.D.
Department of Orthopaedics, University of Washington, Seattle, Washington

James R. Urbaniak, M.D.
Department of Surgery, Division of Orthopaedic Surgery, Duke University Medical Center, Durham, North Carolina

Tedman L. Vance, M.D.
Duke University Medical Center, Durham, North Carolina

Renata V. Weber, M.D.
School of Medicine, Washington University in St. Louis, St. Louis, Missouri

Bradon J. Wilhelmi, M.D.
Department of Surgery, Division of Plastic Surgery, Southern Illinois University School of Medicine, Springfield, Illinois

Jonathan M. Winograd, M.D.
Massachusetts General Hospital, Boston, Massachusetts

Michael B. Wood, M.D.
Department of Orthopedic Surgery, Mayo Clinic School of Medicine, Jacksonville, Florida

Jeffrey Yao, M.D.
Department of Hand and Upper Extremity Surgery, Stanford University, Palo Alto, California

What an exciting time to be learning about nerve healing! Almost daily, investigators are reporting new understanding emanating from molecular and electron microscopic studies on the bench, from mechanical and chemical techniques in laboratory animals, and from clinical trials initiated in the operating room. One advance feeds on the others, and new techniques of proven clinical value steadily emerge. Even classic techniques, enduringly worthwhile, can now be understood thoroughly on microscopic and molecular levels.

Peripheral Nerve Surgery: Practical Applications in the Upper Extremity highlights this exciting era for these amazing cells that are so many thousands of times larger in one dimension than in the others. And then to think that they conduct electricity in an orderly manner and have the capacity to heal. Drs. Slutsky and Hentz have assembled a world-class list of authors to celebrate this expansion of knowledge. One specialist or one discipline cannot expect to grasp the entire breadth of the topic, and the book appropriately pays heed to the multidisciplinary excitement and cross-fertilization that this field demands.

Congratulations to all of the authors for contributing their current thinking on this rapidly expanding and important field. Undoubtedly the book will both consolidate ideas and generate new questions and additional avenues of investigation. An exciting time indeed.

Roy A. Meals, M.D.
Clinical Professor of Orthopedic Surgery
UCLA

The management of nerve injuries is in the midst of a renaissance. The treatment locus is shifting from the operating theater towards the culture tube. Although repair by suture must appear inherently crude from the nerve's standpoint, the techniques have been refined to the point of eloquence. This book is a mixture of old time-honored methods and newer procedures that work in concert with the biochemical events that accompany nerve regeneration rather than in spite of them.

Lars Dahlin starts things off with a comprehensive discussion of nerve injury and repair from a cellular level. Michael Jabaley zooms out a million-fold to share his 30 years of experience with the methods of nerve repair. Professor Hanno Millesi reprises his life-long pioneering work with nerve grafting when direct repair is not possible, accompanied by a chapter on some practical aspects of grafting. James Urbaniak and coauthors give us the basic science behind end-to-side nerve repairs. Susan Mackinnon and Renata Weber share the possible windfalls with their landmark work on nerve transfers. Michael Wood illustrates this technique using the anterior interosseous nerve for reinnervation of the distal median and ulnar motor branch. Thomas Trumble, Chris Allan, and coauthors give us a succinct summary of the experimental work with biological and manmade collagen nerve guidance channels in harnessing the regenerative capacities of injured nerve tissue, whereas Lee Dellon shares his 18-year clinical experience with PGA nerve tubes. Dean Sotereanos and Nickolaos Darlis instruct us in their method for autogenous vein wrapping of partial nerve injuries when repair is not indicated. Giorgio Brunelli summarizes his masterful technique with direct muscular neurotization when a distal nerve stump is unavailable for repair.

Soft tissue reconstruction of the hand differs from other anatomical regions by the requirement for sensibility. Jonathan Winograd, James May, and Ziv Peled detail their work with the free neurotized first web-space flap. Drs. Bradon Wilhelmi and W. P. Andrew Lee's imaginative use of a myriad of innervated free flaps complements a like-minded chapter on pedicled neurosensory flaps. When the free tissue transfer involves a toe or digit, Neil Jones and Sean Bidic show us how to reconstruct the nerve pedicle. For irreparable nerve injuries, George Omer, Jr. shares his wisdom and experience with the possible tendon transfers that may be used to improve hand function.

No book on nerve injury is complete without a discussion of compressive neuropathies. The magnificent chapter on median nerve compression by Bob Szabo and Jason Koo is followed by Michael Botte, Richard Gelberman, and Lorenzo Pacelli's comprehensive experience with distal ulnar nerve compression. Robert Beasley gives us his pearls on radial nerve compression while Lee Osterman and Jeffrey Yao sort out the challenge of treating combined neuropathies. David Kline and coauthors reprise his seminal work on the diagnosis and treatment of thoracic outlet compression.

Electrodiagnostic testing has become a gold standard in the assessment of nerve disorders. Although these tests are invaluable extensions of the physical examination, the techniques for recording the electrophysiological events in nerve and muscle carry with them a number of potential pitfalls. The methodology underlying the standard nerve conduction studies are reviewed with this in mind, as well as some of the newer techniques that have special application to hand surgeons. Tuna Ozyurekoglu and Warren Breidenbach review their experience with intraoperative nerve recordings as a guide to the treatment of nerve injuries.

It was a joy to collaborate with so many of the true pioneers in the field of peripheral nerve surgery as well as some of the up-and-coming stars. We hope the reader of this book experiences the same. We owe a debt of gratitude to Richard Lampert, formerly of Elsevier, for having the faith to proceed with this book, and to the editors Elyse O'Grady and Vera Ginsburgs for bringing the book to completion.

David J. Slutsky, M.D., F.R.C.S.(C)

Vincent R. Hentz, M.D.

CONTENTS

1

Nerve Injury and Repair: From Molecule to Man

Lars B. Dahlin

Brains first and then hard work.

EEYORE

INTRODUCTION

The human hand is a very delicate sensory organ and a working tool. The upper extremity is a unique construction with extensive range of motion in the shoulder, flexion and extension in the elbow, and pro/supination of the forearm and a wide range of motion in the wrist. Therefore, it is possible to put the hand in an optimal position in various situations, and to use it as a grip organ as well as to palpate different surfaces with the tactile surfaces of the finger pulps. The function of the human hand is dependent on a well-developed sensory system working properly on all levels, from the brain down to the delicate receptors in the skin, muscle, and joints. A nerve injury to the upper extremity, irrespective of its origin, can therefore more or less severely affect the function of the hand.[1] Such injuries belong to one of the most difficult conditions that physicians and surgeons face. After the injury the patient may not be able to return to work during a rehabilitation period, and in some cases they have to change work or even be retired. Nerve injuries can therefore cause personal tragedies and great suffering for the patients. Transection injuries of nerve trunks constitute around 3% of the hand injuries at a hand unit,[2] but such injuries are also highly costly for society. It has been calculated that the total median cost for the society of an employed person with a median nerve injury in the forearm is around 51,238 euros, where nearly 90% of the total costs is due to the loss of production, that is, sick leave.[3] The costs are even higher than those reported for patients with a flexor tendon injury.[4]

Even a minor nerve injury such as carpal tunnel syndrome (CTS) may cause socioeconomic consequences for the patient and the society. The prevalence of clinically and neurophysiologically confirmed CTS is 2% to 3%.[5] After surgical treatment of CTS, it has been reported that more than 10% of these patients permanently stop working. Given the large number of patients suffering from CTS, this condition causes a substantial socioeconomic burden.[6] Nerve-related upper extremity outpatient visits and procedures in United States have been estimated at around 2.7 million per year, which accounts for almost 13% of total outpatient visits. Of these, 90% are related to CTS, and 8% to other upper extremity nerve lesions. The number of nerve-related procedures were around 2.3 million (32% of total operations), and around 93% of procedures were related to CTS. Of the inpatient operations, CTS counted for 57% of the nervous system procedures.[7] Thus, nerve-related conditions, especially CTS, does not only cause suffering for the patients, but also consume a tremendous amount of resources in the healthcare sector. In contrast to nerve transection injuries, medical costs seem to be higher than the benefits to the injured worker in an average CTS case.[8]

There is a definitive need to improve treatment not only of severe nerve injuries, like transection or avulsion injuries, occurring all the way up to the brachial plexus level, but also of less extensive nerve injuries, such as nerve compression injuries, that are considered to be minor conditions and easy to treat. A thorough knowledge about the microanatomy, basic physiology, and various pathophysiologic events at nerve trunk level all the way up to the brain is necessary for physicians and surgeons who treat patients suffering from various nerve trunk conditions. In recent years, there has been a growing interest in the alterations that may be very rapid occurring in the brain after a peripheral nerve injury.[9] The use of brain capacity to readjust after nerve injury and repair should be considered during the rehabilitation. A large amount of data from animal experiments, investigating changes in neurons and non-neuronal cells following various types of injuries, have accumulated during the last 100 years, including the early fascinating work by Ramon y Cajal.[10] In the present chapter, selected aspects of nerve injury and repair from the neurobiological point of view will be discussed.

NEURONS, SCHWANN CELLS, AND THE MICROANATOMY OF THE PERIPHERAL NERVE TRUNK

The neuron consists of a cell body and the extension, which is the axon projecting out to the target in the periphery, that is, receptors in the skin and muscles. The cell bodies of motor neurons are located in the ventral horn of the spinal cord, and the cell bodies of the sensory neurons are located in dorsal root ganglia (DRG) positioned close to the spinal cord. Sensory neurons are pseudounipolar with a central process that projects to the spinal cord and a peripherally extended axon. In contrast to a peripheral injury, a transection or an avulsion of the central process does not induce a regenerative response in the sensory cell body.[11]

Intracellular Communication System

There is a communication system in neurons, which is extremely important for transferring information in the neuron, and for provision of cell components to the axon and the synapse. The axonal transport system occurs along the microtubules, both in an anterograde (from cell body to periphery) and in a retrograde (from axon terminal to cell body) direction. Microtubules are important both for the buildup of the cytoskeleton and for axonal transport. Microtubules are cylinders built by the protein tubulin that are symmetrically arranged, thereby making it easy to polymerize and depolymerize. The polymerization process could, for example, be inhibited by application of colchicine, and thereby axonal transport is blocked. Various molecules and organelles are transported along microtubules with "motor proteins" that transport the molecules distally (kinesins) to the axon, and axon terminal and retrogradedly (dyneins) to the nucleus. The energy-dependent transport occurs at various velocities from a few up to 400 mm/day. Neurofilaments, actin and tubulin, which are structural proteins, are transported by slow axonal transport that may be a consequence of conventional fast movement that is interrupted by extended pausing.[12–14] Actin is one of the most common proteins in cells. It forms a network close to the plasma membrane, and is also anchored to the cell membrane. In this way, actin filaments are anchored all the way up to the extracellular matrix through, among other things, the receptors for the extracellularly located fibronectin. This is important when the growth cone and its filopodia are palpating the surface on which the distal part of the axon grows after an injury. Integrins are the important receptors for the connection between the actin and the extracellular matrix substances; like fibronectin, which also binds to collagen, they consist of a family of receptors built up with various subunits (see review by van der Flier and Sonnenberg[15]; see below).

Schwann Cells

Schwann cells are located around the axons; they are related individually (myelinated axons) or to several axons (nonmyelinated axons). The size of the axon seems to determine whether a Schwann cell will form a myelin sheath, and thus whether a myelinated nerve fiber is formed. The differentiation of cells to Schwann cells and postnatal regulation of myelination can be influenced by the transcription factor Krox-20, neuregulin, and transforming growth factor β (TGF-β).[16,17] The transcription factor cAMP response element binding protein (CREB), but not c-jun, is expressed at high levels in Schwann cells during development.[18] A basal lamina surrounds the axon/Schwann cell unit, which is composed by extracellular matrix molecules such as collagen type IV, fibronectin, and laminin,[19,20] thus forming the endoneurial tube. It should be emphasized that the composition of the basal lamina is not static, as its composition changes during regeneration.[21,22]

There is a very intimate and close interaction between the neuron and its axon and the Schwann cells, not only during development and normal conditions, but particularly after injury and during regeneration.[23,24] During development, glial-lined derived neurotrophic factors (GDNF) and neurturin can control survival of motor neurons,[25] and other glial-derived signals include ciliary neurotrophic factor (CNTF) and leukemia inhibitory factor (LIF). Conversely, the axon–Schwann cell interaction regulates also expression of the immediate early gene c-jun in Schwann cells.[16,26] Above this paracrine mechanism of interaction between the neuron and its axon and the Schwann cells, there are also autocrine signals from the Schwann cells regulating themselves[16,26] (Fig. 1–1).

Bundles of axons, surrounding Schwann cells, and basal lamina form units, which are surrounded by a very distinct sheath, the perineurium, composed of flattened cells with both mechanical and diffusion properties, thereby acting as a barrier against dangerous substances reaching the axons. These units are called fascicles and a peripheral nerve trunk usually consists of a number of fascicles. At wrist level, the median nerve may be composed of 13 to 35 fascicles. Interestingly, there are signals from the Schwann cells, such as the signal molecule Desert hedgehog, which contributes to the organization of the perineurium during development.[16,27] The formation of a new perineurium at a suture line can also involve presence of specific types of macrophages.[28] The content inside the perineurial barrier, that is, the endoneurial space, consists not only of axons and Schwann cells, but also of fibroblasts, macrophages, mast cells, mucopolysaccharide ground substance, and collagen fibrils. Fascicles are embedded in a loose connective tissue, the epineurium, in which longitudinal vessels are formed into plexa. Such microvessels send branches, which traverse obliquely through the perineurial barrier forming new plexa of vessels, consisting mainly of capillaries, in the endoneurium space.[29] The vessels in the epineurium and endoneurium have different susceptibilities to trauma,[30] and the former are more vulnerable to compression.

Satellite Cells

Satellite cells are located around sensory neurons in the DRG, which respond, together with present macrophages, with proliferation to trauma.[31,32] The satellite cells have been suggested to induce noradrenergic sprouting after injury, dependent on the type of injury, and implicated in sympathetically maintained pain.[32,33]

Sensory Neurons and DRG

The DRG consists mainly of a heterogenous group of pseudounipolar sensory neurons that vary in morphology and function, with the purpose of conveying multitude of information centrally. DRG neurons are classified according to size as small, medium, and large neurons,[34] and the neurons express the tyrosine receptor kinase (trk) A, B, or C. The neurotrophins nerve growth factor (NGF), brain derived neurotrophic factor (BDNF), and neurotrophin-3 (NT-3) bind to the receptors trk A, B, and C, respectively.[35] In an adult mouse DRG, about 50% of the neurons are small trk A–positive cells that extend nonmyelinated axons to the periphery and transmit nociceptive information.[36] The trk B–positive neurons, constituting 30% to 35% of neurons, are small- and medium-sized, and transmit information from

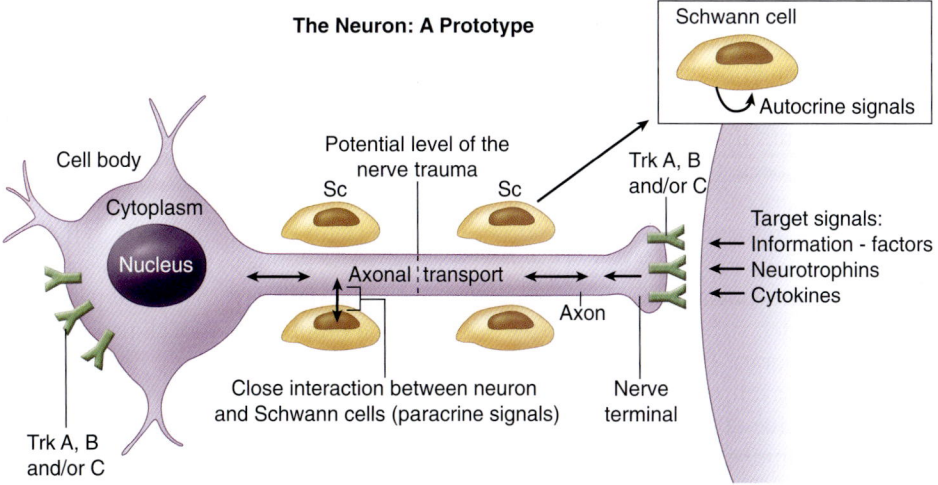

Figure 1–1 Schematic drawing showing the principle of the close interaction between the neuron and the Schwann cells surrounding the axon, and the communication between the neuron and its target. Along the neuron, information is conveyed by axonal transport, which is of crucial importance for survival and function of the neuron normally and to adapt to and relocate the production machinery after an injury. (Modified from Dahlin LB. The biology of nerve injury and repair. J Am Soc Surg Hand 2004;4:143–55,[180] with permission.)

mechanoreceptors.[37] The neurons that are propriocep-tive and contain information about position are large, and trk C–positive neurons constitute 20% of the popu-lation.[37] It should be emphasized that there is an overlap of expression of trk receptors, and that trk receptors are found on satellite cells.[38] During development, sensory neurons are dependent, sometimes synergistically, on a large number of different growth factors such as NGF, NT-3, BDNF, CNTF, TGF-β, GDNF, and LIF,[39–41] and there is a switch concerning expression of trk A, B, and C receptors in sensory neurons during embryogene-sis.[42–44] During a restricted time period, there is a pro-nounced dependence of target-derived factors for survival of the neurons, and it remains up to a week after birth in rats, a property that may be of importance in this context for the pathophysiology of nerve injury in obstetric brachial plexus injury.

NEURONAL AND NON–NEURONAL RESPONSE TO INJURY

Signals and Biochemical Changes

After transection of the axon due to an injury, the prox-imal part retracts up to a few nodes of Ranvier, and the length of retraction is related to the number of injured Schwann cells. The distal tip of the injured axon on the proximal nerve segment is sealed rapidly, which is a process that is dependent on Ca^{2+}.[45] Calcium is also important for growth cone formation and the activation of mitogen-activated protein kinase (MAP kinase; see below).[46] After a cellular injury, signals are initiated and required to start the repair process. A large amount of data has accumulated concerning such signal transduc-tion mechanisms, which includes all biological events that occur in a cell between the binding of a signaling molecule to the cell surface and the physiologic outcome of the message signified of that specific mole-cule. Some of the basic signal transduction mechanisms regarding the molecular events that occur in neurons after an axonal injury have been identified using the marine mollusc *Aplysia californica*.[47] The signal trans-duction processes take place in the neuron from the tip of the normal (axonal terminal) or the transected axon to the cell body, and in the nucleus with its gene program. In the aplysia model, it has been suggested that there are series of temporary different, but over-lapping phases, along which axon regeneration is con-ducted. The early signals arrive at the nucleus within seconds to minutes after the injury with injury-induced action potential, which can turn on genes used in the early stages of repair. Intermediate signals arrive in hours to days after injury via retrograde transported signals that are conveyed through the axon to the

nucleus with the transport informing the nucleus of the severity of axonal injury reinforcing earlier events and triggering additional changes. Signals originating from extrinsic growth factors and cytokines released by cells at the site of injury characterize the third phase; these signals reach the nucleus days to weeks after injury.

The retrogradely transported information signaling an injury may be negative or positive. The negative signals include the deprivation of retrograde transport from the target of neurotrophic factor.[48,49] Positive injury signals may constitutely be in the axoplasm or may be released from non-neuronal cells and taken up at the site of injury. For neurons, there seems to be a "prema-ture return" of conformational changed substances ret-rogradely transported back to the cell body. There is also a local uptake of injury-induced local factors at the site of injury that are retrogradely transported[47,50–53] (Fig. 1–2). The proteins that are conveyed as signals are con-sidered to contain a nuclear localization sequence that may be uncovered and modified by injury such as the particularly interesting new cysteine-histidine–rich protein (PINCH), a protein present in neurons, axons, satellite cells, and Schwann cells with a relevance for initiating and/or maintaining Schwann cell–axon attach-ment after injury.[54] Importin beta is another relevant protein that increase after nerve injury by a local trans-lation of axonal mRNA forming a complex trafficking retrogradely with the motor protein dynein.[55] In the final phase, signals from target derived growth factors arrive in the cell nucleus to stop growth. It is not only in neurons that numerous steps in signal transduction pathways are initiated after a peripheral nerve injury but the steps also occur in Schwann cells and in the targets. The signal pathways and the regulation of these processes are very complex and not completely under-stood; they are the focus of an intense research. In this chapter, only selected signal transduction events occur-ring in neurons and Schwann cells that may be of rele-vance after nerve injury are highlighted.

Receptors

When a factor or a signal binds to the cell it is attached to a receptor, that is located on the cell membrane or sit-uated intracellulary, various cellular processes are initi-ated via a number of intracellular and intranuclear steps (Fig. 1–3). Generally, many of the signals are immedi-ate through a second messenger in the cell and proteins are later activated, which can modify the cellular process and gene transcription. Essentially, there are three types of cell membrane bound receptors in cells like neurons and non-neuronal cells: enzyme-coupled (or linked) receptors (like trk), G-protein–coupled receptors and ion channels (like acetylcholine receptor), and only the

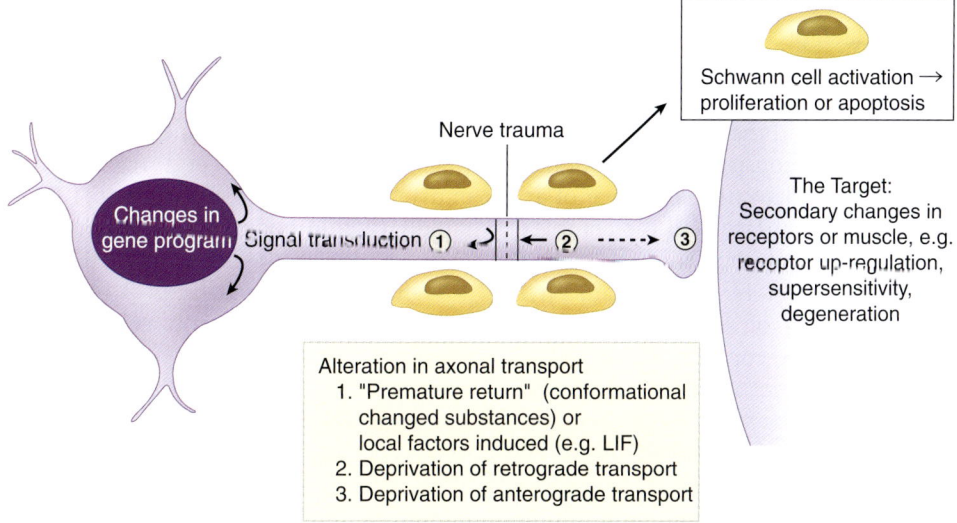

Figure 1–2 Schematic drawing of the possible signals that initiate the signal transduction steps in neurons after a nerve trauma. (Modified from Dahlin LB. The biology of nerve injury and repair. J Am Soc Surg Hand 2004;4:143–55,[180] with permission.)

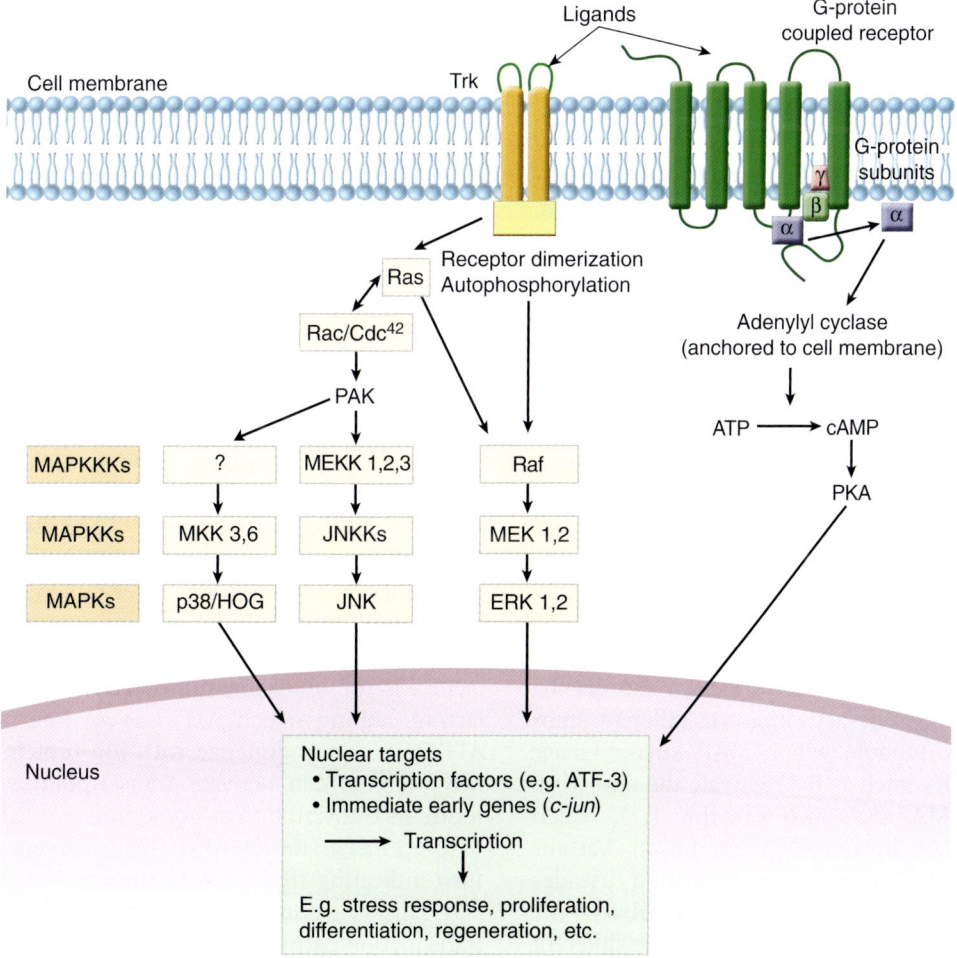

Figure 1–3 A simple schematic drawing of signal transduction steps in neurons and non-neuronal cells. Stimulation by a ligand to various membrane bound receptors in the cell membrane activates different intracellular steps, which in the MAPK module involves phosphorylation steps. The signal transduction processes leads to different changes in the nucleus with gene expression and a change in the production machinery in response to the stimulation or trauma. There are also other pathways such as PKB and PKC. See text for details.

previous two are covered here. Some signals use the G-proteins,[56] which are located on the intracellular side of the cell membrane. G-protein–coupled receptors bind to G-proteins, which work as a connection between the transmembraneous receptor and the intracellular signal chain. The G-protein complex consists of three subunits (a, β, and γ). The G-proteins detect the presence of an activated receptor on the cell surface, and the complex is usually activated via the α-subunit. The response in the cell is amplified via effectors such as adenylyl cyclase, resulting in synthesis of second messengers (e.g., cAMP).[57] Adenylyl cyclase converts ATP to cyclic AMP (cAMP) with the subsequent activation of protein kinase A. This is later followed by activation of so-called mediators such as various protein kinases.[47] Adenylyl cyclase can be activated by forskolin, which is used to improve Schwann cell proliferation in vitro when such cells are cultured with the purpose to add to acellular nerve grafts[18] (see below). Transcription factors are important substrates for protein kinase A, which can start phosphorylation of the transcription complex located in the promoter region of a gene.

There are other receptors, as pointed out previously. Enzyme-linked protein tyrosine kinase receptors located in the cell membrane consisting of 20 subfamilies, one of them tyrosine receptor kinases (trk), are very complex with a large extracellular domain, a short transmembraneous region, and an intracellular domain. When a ligand (first messenger), like a growth factor, binds to the receptor that dimerize, and there is an autophosphorylation of the receptor with a conformational change leading to phosphorylation of proteins on the amino acid tyrosine. The signal transduction pathways activated by the tyrosine receptor kinase (trk) lead to activation of enzymes like Ras (see below).

The various protein phosphorylation cascades that are present in neurons include protein kinase A (PKA), protein kinase B (PKB), protein kinase C (PKC), and mitogen-activated protein kinase (MAPK; for review see Denhardt[58,59]). The MAPK module consists of essentially three cascades: ERK/MAPkinase, JNK/SAPK and p38/HOG (Fig. 1–3). In one of the pathways, Ras, which is attached to the inner surface of the plasma membrane, continues its activation via different steps along the MAPK module where MAP kinase kinase kinases (MAPKKKs, such as Raf) activate the next MAP kinase kinases (MAPKKs, such as MEK 1,2), which phosphorylate MAP kinases (MAPKs, ERKs). Various pathways along these protein phosphorylation cascades occur (Fig. 1–3),[58–60] and there is crosstalk between the various pathways.[58] The interaction between different receptors is very complex, since trk receptors can be activated by ligands of G-protein–coupled receptors in the absence of neurotrophins like NGF and BDNF.[57] By the crosstalk interaction between two different signal transduction pathways, a specific signal from the acti-

vation of the receptor can be "adjusted." Along one of these MAPK pathways, the c-Jun N-terminal kinase (JNK) phosphorylates and activates the transcription factor c-jun, a factor that has been implicated both in neuronal stress response and subsequent apoptosis,[61] as well as in protective and regenerative events after injury.[62–64] The phosphorylation of JNK occurs very rapidly (within hours) and transiently, while the phosphorylation of c-jun and the next step, induction of the activating transcription factor-3 (ATF-3), persists. This response is associated with axonal outgrowth and not apoptosis.[64] It is also known that ATF-3 induction can occur independently of c-jun activation. Recently, it was suggested that ATF-3 induction in c-jun activated sensory neurons from superior cervical ganglia promotes HSP27, thereby acting neuroprotective and promoting neurite elongation.[65] The signal transduction pathways that are activated through protein phosphorylation performed by protein kinases—for example, MAP kinases—are stopped by protein phosphatases, which dephosphorylate the protein kinases.

Transcription is the synthesis of messenger RNA (mRNA) from DNA, while the synthesis of a protein after instruction from RNA is called translation. The formed mRNA molecules leave the nucleus and relocate to the ribosomes in the cytoplasm where the synthesis of the new proteins occurs. The transcription factors decide which genes should be read, and usually several transcription factors are acquired to bind to the same promoter region to allow transcription. Several of the transcription factors are dependent on cAMP. These belong to the CREB superfamily (cAMP-responsive elements binding protein). The CREB family of transcription factors is a superfamily, which can be activated by different signaling pathways including activation of gene protein-coupled receptors via PKA, calcium activation, and activation via tyrosine receptor kinases along, for example, the ras/ERK pathway.[58,66] The phosphorylation of CREB can interact indirectly with components of the basal transcription machinery, thereby facilitating initiation of transcription and gene expression. Another member of the CREB superfamily of transcription factors is the abovementioned activating transcription factors, among which ATF-3 is an interesting factor. ATF-3 can heterodimerize with Jun-proteins, and such heterodimers can activate transcription while ATF-3 represses transcription as homodimers.[67,68] The gene for GAP-43 has a site for AP-1 (heterodimers of ATF-3/c-Jun) indicating that GAP-43 present in injured motor and sensory neurons can be regulated by this signal transduction pathway.[69] ATF-3 is a stress-inducible gene and the induction of ATF-3 appears to correlate with neural injury in DRG and the spinal cord as well as in Schwann cells.[68,70] Interestingly, the induction of ATF-3 can be completely inhibited by N-acetyl-L-cystein (NAC) in liver cells.[71] It was recently shown that this substance can act as a neuroprotective agent by mitochondrial preservation in the nervous system thereby inhibiting sensory neuronal loss.[72] The stress signals that induce ATF-3 may involve not only the described signal pathways of JNK-mediated c-jun activation,[64] but also other pathways.[68] The rapid and profound induction of ATF-3 in sensory neurons in DRG after nerve injury can be suppressed by inhibition of RNA and protein synthesis as well as by inhibitors to JNK resulting in impaired nerve regeneration.[64] Data also indicate that adding NGF and GDNF can ameliorate ATF-3 induction in response to peripheral nerve injury in specific populations of sensory neurons in DRG.[73] The rapid up-regulation of transcription factors, such as c-jun and ATF-3 in neurons after peripheral nerve injury,[70,74,75] play a pivotal role in the redirection of gene expression in neurons (Fig. 1–4). In such conditions the injured neuron has to transform itself from the stage of maintenance at a steady state to another state of dynamic growth leading to regeneration of the transected axon.

Gene Expression After Nerve Injury

A cellular injury results in major changes in gene expression, not only in the neuron itself, but also in the surrounding satellite cells (and in Schwann cells; see below). The alterations are elicited by the abovementioned signals created by the injury. A massive induc-

tion of transcription factors in sensory neurons in DRG after nerve injury is observed already at 12 to 24 hours postinjury.[76] Of the genes that are up-regulated in sensory neurons in DRG in mice, 40% are transcription factors, and several of them, such as c-jun, ATF-3, c-Fos, and SOX-11, are found to be related to regeneration.[76,77] A careful cellular control of the transcriptional events during the regeneration process is necessary, which is observed as up-regulation of transcriptional regulators such as the transcriptional repressor NFIL3/E4BP4.[76,78] The alterations shift the neurons "from transmitting mode to growth mode."[79] The expression of substances as neuropeptides, such as NPY and its precursor,[80] galanin,[81,82] and PACAP,[83] are up-regulated after injury, while some others are down-regulated (e.g., CGRP[84]). The genes for PACAP, galanin, and NPY are expressed in mice already 24 hours post-injury, and the genes for the transcription factors c-jun and ATF3 are expressed at least within 12 hours.[76] Heat shock proteins (HSP) are stress proteins that are up-regulated in adult sensory and motor neurons after injury, and HSP27 probably has a neuroprotective role.[85,86] The capacity of sensory neurons to express HSP27 varies between neonatal and adult rats after axotomy, which could be relevant for the treatment strategies of obstetric and adult brachial plexus lesions.[85] TGF-β may have an important role for the survival of sensory neurons after injury via the receptor of GDNF, which is also up-

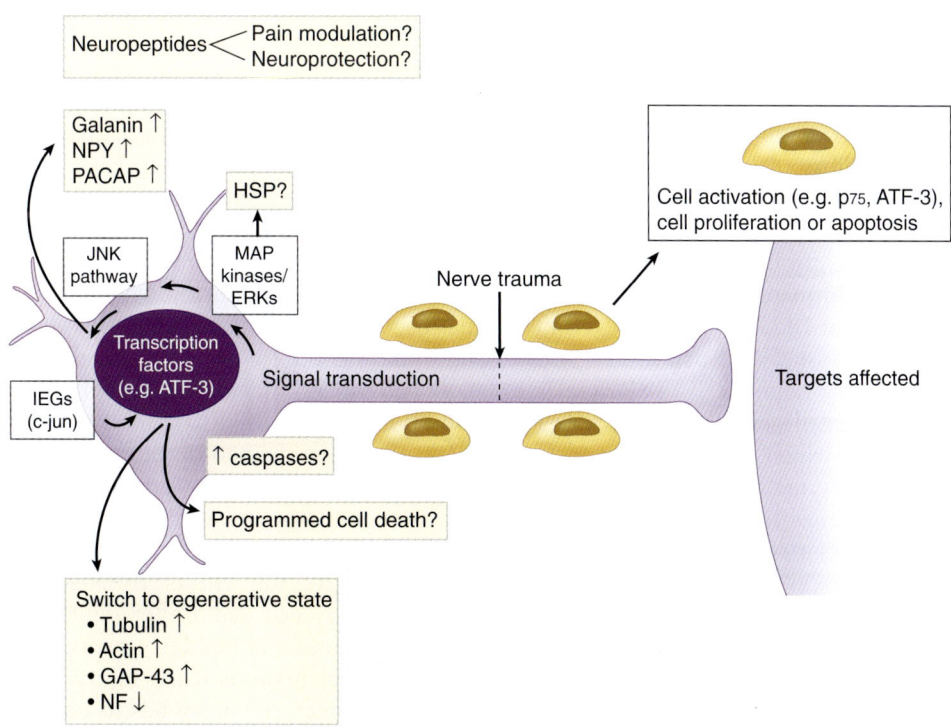

Figure 1–4   Schematic drawing of some alterations in signal transduction and their effects in neurons and non-neuronal cells after nerve trauma. (Modified from Dahlin LB. The biology of nerve injury and repair. J Am Soc Surg Hand 2004;4:143–55,[180] with permission.)

regulated in DRG after injury. Interestingly, GDNF promotes survival of peripheral neurons, but only if TGF-β is present.[87]

Injury-initiated changes in the neurotrophins and their receptors for BDNF and other substances (e.g., LIF, CNTF) in adult sensory and motor neurons should also be mentioned,[88–91] where gene expression in sensory neurons for BDNF, but not for NGF and NT-3, is increased at 24 hours post-injury in mice.[76] The response after nerve injury regarding PACAP also differs depending on the size of the sensory neurons, and can be modulated by exogenous supply of NT-3 and NGF, and has also been observed for ATF-3 and NPY.[73,92,93] NGF and NT-3 can also modulate the BDNF expression in sensory neurons differentially.[94] Exogenous supply of BDNF and particularly GDNF are beneficial for motor neuron survival and axonal regeneration with a less pronounced effect after an avulsion injury.[95,96]

Up-regulation of the neuropeptide galanin is dependent on interleukin-6 (IL-6) and LIF.[97] A signal for induction of IL-6[98] is believed to be retrogradely transported from the site of injury,[99] and interestingly LIF, in contrast to IL-6, is not up-regulated in sensory neurons, but transported from the site of injury preferentially by neurons expressing trkA and galanin.[100] IL-6 is fascinating in view of the release from macrophages, which are migrating into the distal nerve segment and to the site of injury after nerve transection and other injuries. In this context, the suppressor of cytokine signaling-3 (SOCS-3) is appealing since it binds to one unit of the IL-6 receptor. Surprisingly, there are also potential inhibitors of proliferation that are up-regulated in the DRG (Gadd-45-alpha, Gadd-45-gamma, IGFBP-3, interferon-beta), which may be related to the proliferation of the satellite cells surrounding the neurons.[76,103]

There are also other "assorted" genes that are up-regulated in DRG after injury. Amphiregulin may be an endogenously produced trophic factor in DRG. Amphiregulin is found also in Schwann cells and has been reported to stimulate proliferation of Schwann cells and to induce neurite formation.[104] There are transcripts present after injury in DRG that are involved in the reorganization of the cytoskeleton such as RB3 and TC10 in motor and sensory neurons.[105,106] SPRR1a is another regeneration-associated gene that is expressed after injury in DRG, and which seems to stimulate regeneration of adult sensory neurons.[107] There is also another large number of genes that are up-regulated, and one function of these "assorted" group of genes may be reorganization of the extracellular matrix, cytoskeleton, transcriptional machinery, and control of signal transduction. As pointed out previously, they all contribute to the alterations in the neuron transferring it from a transmitting mode to a growth mode.[79] Understanding of the signal transduction pathways in cells, particularly in neurons and non-neuronal cells, after injury is a very exciting research area. Recently, it was reported that electrical stimulation of the proximal nerve segment could modify regeneration-associated gene expression in motor neurons after injury.[108] In the future, we may be able to further manipulate injured peripheral neurons and non-neuronal cells, making it possible to interact with the signal transduction systems and gene expression. However, the complexity of these pathways and the details have to be further clarified.

Morphology and Cell Death

The morphologic signs of injury observed in a nerve cell body are unspecific, and include dissolution of Nissl bodies (chromatolysis), nuclear displacement, nuclear enlargement, and alterations in the volume of the cell body and the nucleus.[109] The extent of these changes has, however, been related to the survival of the neuron (see review by Fu and Gordon[79]). There may be an inappropriate activation of the gene program after injury to initiate regeneration, but a cascade mechanism that leads to programmed cell death (apoptosis) via activation of caspases, particularly caspases 3 and 9, may be activated.[110] Mitochondria likely play a pivotal role by releasing pre-apoptotic molecules that can trigger the cascade of caspases.[111] Morphologically, apoptosis includes fragmentation of DNA, cell shrinkage, condensation of chromatin, fragmentation of the nucleus and the cell, and formation of apoptotic bodies. The extent of cell death in DRG varies, and is species dependent, but up to as much as 50% of the sensory neurons may disappear after nerve transection,[112–114] which may also be related to the level of injury.[115] It should be emphasized that the response of motor and sensory neurons depends on the type of injury, such as root avulsion compared to distal transection. A more proximal injury compared to a distal injury as well as an avulsion injury compared to transection of a nerve has a more profound and extensive impact on the neurons. The sensory neuronal death probably begins within 24 hours after injury which indicates that any pharmacologic treatment should be initiated within that time period.[72,116,117] As pointed out previously, many substances, including GDNF, BDNF, HSP27, and HSP70, have been used to inhibit sensory and motor cell death, where the neuroprotective effect of HSP27 is related to processes downstream of cytochrome c release from mitochondria and upstream of caspase-3 activation.[118,119] Interesting results with potential clinical implications are the effects of N-acetyl-cysteine to prevent sensory cell death after injury.[72] Cell death is more pronounced and rapid in sensory neurons as compared to motor neurons if the injury is located in the periphery. In fact, an injury has to be located close to spinal cord (e.g., avulsion injury) to severely affect motor neurons.[95,120–126]

INJURY-INDUCED CHANGES IN DISTAL NERVE SEGMENT AND TARGETS

Wallerian Degeneration

It has long been known that when the peripheral nerve trunk is transected, the distal part of the axons disintegrate and undergoes Wallerian degeneration due to the loss of contact with its cell body.[127] Proteases, which are calcium dependent, are activated in the axon distal to the injury leading to a proteolytic process that disintegrates the axoplasm.[128] Thus, there are remnants of the distal part of disintegrating axons, including myelin debris, which are digested not only by the invading macrophages, but also to some extent of proliferating Schwann cells.[129,130] The relative importance of macrophages and Schwann cells for myelin removal is considered to vary with time after injury.[130] The Schwann cells react rapidly to transection of the axons and drop their myelin sheath, a process that may be regulated by a positive signal from the injured axons or by the absence of a signal normally provided by the intact axon.

Reaction of Schwann Cells

The Schwann cells seem to react very quickly to an injury with regard to intracellular processes. It has been reported that already within 30 minutes, an injury-activated MAP kinase cascade is initiated with a subsequent induction of mRNA for NGF, IL-6, and LIF.[131] There are a number of genes that are up- and down-regulated during activation of Schwann cells, which are partly shared by the response seen in DRG.[132] For example, in a transected sciatic nerve 370 and 157 genes were up- and down-regulated, respectively, of almost 10,000 spotted genes,[133] and these genes had a broad spectrum of function. There seems also to be a spatial differential response in the peripheral nerve trunk since it has been observed that ERK-activation (MAPK pathway) may be of importance in the more distal part of a transected nerve, while the JAK/STAT cascade activation pathway may be important to control the cellular response close to the site of injury.[134] JAK ("just another kinase") tyrosine kinases are associated with cytokine receptors and, along with the STAT transcription factors, are central components of pathways that result in the activation of gene expression upon cytokine stimulation. STATs are both signal transducers in the cytoplasm and activators of transcription in the nucleus.

Following the peripheral nerve injury, the Schwann cells proliferate and de-differentiate,[135] and the former process occurs very early following nerve transection.

Interestingly, it has been observed that the response may be faster in nonmyelinated Schwann cells.[136,137] Within the basal lamina, the Schwann cells proliferate, thereby forming bands of Büngner. There are indications that macrophages may play a role for the induction of Schwann cell proliferation, since such response is temporarily correlated to the migration of macrophages in the distal nerve segment. The up-regulation of interleukin-1 (IL-1) in macrophages may also trigger the increase in NGF transcription and NGF receptor density in Schwann cells.[138,139] Macrophages seem to have a pivotal role for the regulation of the Schwann cell response, since myelin digesting macrophages can secret mitogenes for Schwann cells, including PDGF and FGF.[140]

It is not only in the neurons that the transcription factor ATF-3 is up-regulated; non-neuronal cells (mainly Schwann cells) in the distal stump of a transected nerve express ATF3 already within a day.[141] The response increases for 1 to 2 weeks, and thereafter the response is decreased if the distal nerve segment is not attached to a proximal nerve end.[141a] In contrast, the ATF-3 induction subsides differently when proximal versus a distal nerve segment is attached, and regeneration is allowed into the distal nerve segment.[141] Interestingly, only around 65% of all endoneurial cells (and no perineurial cells) express ATF-3 after injury. The pattern of expression of ATF-3 positive cells in damaged nerves resembles that of other transcription factors and immediate early genes, like c-jun.[18,142,143] In contrast, CREB, Jun B, and D are not up-regulated in Schwann cells after injury.[18] Interestingly, forskolin, which improves Schwann cell proliferation and myelination and down-regulates c-jun, indicates that c-jun is not necessary for such processes.[18] The activation of the transcription factor ATF-3 and its "upstream" steps precede the observed changes in gene expression in Schwann cells. GAP-43 up-regulation in non-myelin–forming Schwann cells also are mediated by ATF-3.[69,144]

Schwann Cells, Neurotrophic Factors, and Surface and Extracellular Matrix Molecules

The Schwann cells and cells of other origin in the distal nerve segment up-regulate the synthesis of neurotrophic factors, which regulate survival and growth of axons. The expression of, for example, surface molecules (e.g., NCAM and L-1), extracellular matrix molecules (e.g., collagens, laminin, and tenascin), and neurotrophic factors and their receptors (e.g., NGF, NT-4, and BDNF) are increased (NT-3 decreased) in the endoneurial space.[145,146] The factors that regulate survival and growth of axons can be classified into various groups, such as neurotrophins (NGF, BDNF, NT-3, NT-4), neuropoetic cytokines (CNTF, IL-6, LIF), fibroblast growth factors (e.g., β FGF), and other groups (e.g., IGFs (including GDNF) and interleukins).[48,146–151] The neurotrophins bind to the family of tyrosine kinase receptors with its extracellular ligand-binding part and the intracellular part that regulates the steps of the signal transduction cascades as mentioned above. The binding occurs with high affinity (e.g., NGF receptor, trk A/p140; BDNF/NT-4 receptor, trk B/p145; NT-3 receptor, trk C/p145).[146] There is also the low-affinity NGF receptor (p75), which binds all known neurotrophins, and can act independently or as a co-receptor. The p75 receptor seems to have a dual mission after a nerve injury. Denervated Schwann cells up-regulate the low-affinity receptor p75, whose signaling via NGF has been reported to mediate Schwann cell apoptosis.[152–154] In contrast, this up-regulation also conducts the advancement of the axon, the growth cone/filopodia, and Schwann cell migration during development (see below).[155] TGF-β is involved in regeneration by influencing the synthesis of neurotrophins, matrix molecules, and LIF in Schwann cells.[156] Furthermore, TGF-β can in concert with TNF-α affect the viability of Schwann cells.[157]

The time pattern for up-regulation of all these molecules in Schwann cells may vary,[151] and, together with the time course of, for example, induction of ATF-3, may be of importance for the decision of timing of nerve repair and nerve reconstruction.[141a] An example of the variation between factors are the up-regulation of NGF and BDNF, which has a different time course and spatial pattern after injury.[158] A clinical finding is that nerve regeneration is impaired if the repair or reconstruction procedure is performed 6 months after the injury. This can be explained by the fact that Schwann cells atrophy and die (by apoptosis) or may not respond to stimulation[159,160] when the denervation is prolonged, which may be mediated by an unresponsiveness to glial growth factor (GGF) and down-regulation of c-erbB tyrosine kinase receptors.[161–164] As in the neurons, HSP27 is also of interest for the Schwann cells due to its presence in Schwann cell columns. HSP27 could possibly contribute to cytoskeletal dynamics in the Schwann cells.[165]

Injury-Induced Changes in Targets

After an injury, there is a degeneration of the distal part of the axon and secondary changes in skin receptors and muscles occur due to deprivation of anterograde transport to the disturbed part of the transected axon.[146,166–169] However, the details of such changes are beyond the scope of this review.

THE OUTGROWTH OF AXONS AFTER NERVE REPAIR

After the surgeon has adapted the transected proximal and distal nerve segment, initially there is an early inflammatory process in the gap, which includes accumulation of different cells and injury and growth factors.[170,171] The fibrin matrix that bridges the nerve segments contains the important macrophages with their wide range of potentially useful substances that are important for stimulation of the migrating Schwann cells and outgrowing axons.[172] The matrix, whose size depends on the length of the gap and the thickness of the adapted nerve segments, is later invaded by migrating Schwann cells, regenerating axons, and blood vessels. A new perineurium is created and axons are formed in minifascicles.

The regeneration of axons is a very delicate phenomenon (Fig. 1–5), with a great amount of navigation orchestrated by signal transduction. Numerous sprouts are formed by each parent axon, and in the terminal part of each sprout a growth cone, which expresses receptors for molecular guidance cues that, via their activated cytoplasmic signaling, regulate the cytoskeleton to control the advance of the growth cone. The growth cone initiation after injury that is created within hours after injury is dependent on local protein synthesis and degradation controlled by several signal transduction pathways.[173] The growth cone extends their finger-like extensions, filopodia, from the lamellipodial region (lamellipodia are veil-like structures) that palpates the environment. The filopodia can be considered as "long-distance" sensors for the growth cone.[174] These structures are rich in and dependent on polymerization and organization of actin filaments (F-actin, polymerized from monomeric G-actin subunits) taking place predominantly at the tip of the filopodia, and at the edge of the lamellipodia.[174–176] There is local recycling via retrograde flow of the actin subunits in the growth cone. The rate of F-actin polymerization and recycling decides the rate of advancement of the filopodial tip. The local regulation of the directional guidance of the growth cones at the site of injury is directed by local signal transduction mechanisms. A variety of proteins are involved, including Rho-family GTPases (see review by Guan and Row[177]). Microtubules also extend in the growth cone and are polymerized there with an interaction with the F-actin. The outgrowing axons from the proximal segment advance in concert with the migrating Schwann cells, just as in acellular nerve grafts,[22,178,179] in the distal nerve segment where extensive changes, as delineated above, have prepared the growth milieu for the axons.

Delicate mechanisms steer the axons with involvement of both attractive and repulsive mechanisms

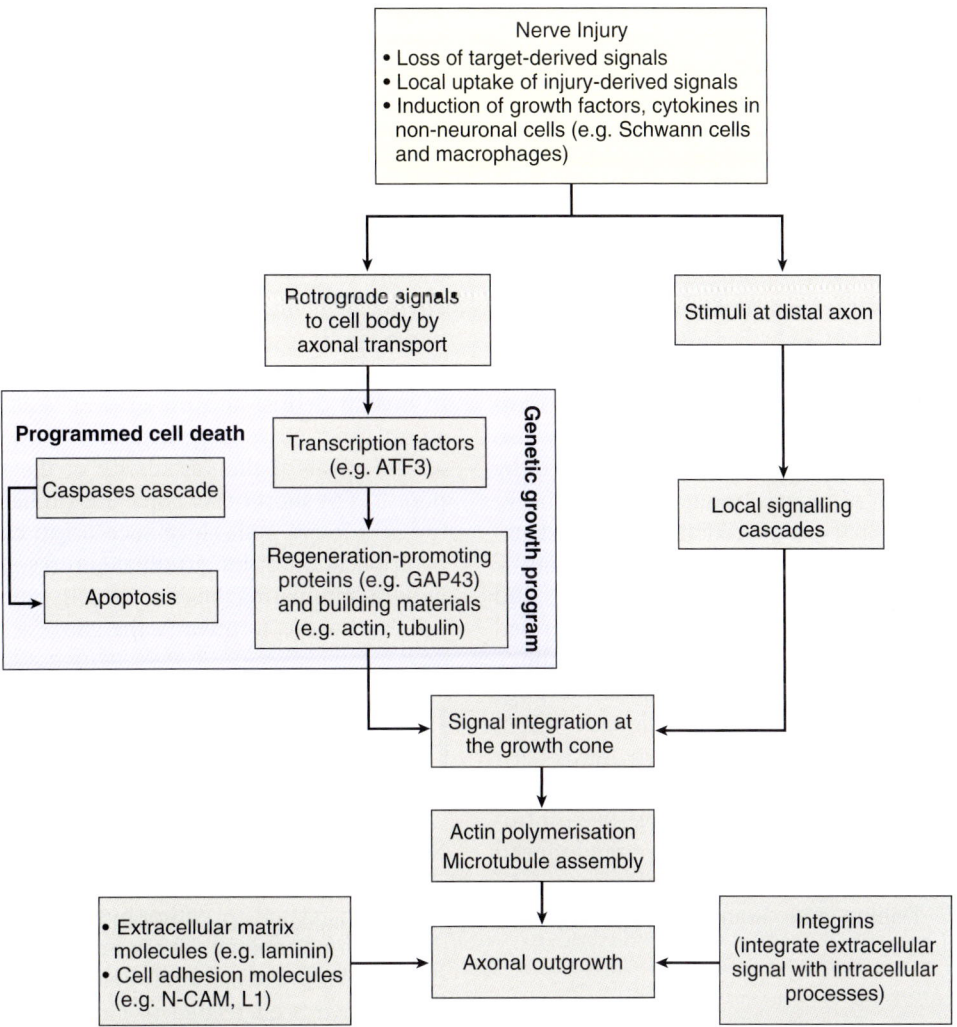

Figure 1–5 Simple figure showing different steps that put the neuron into a regenerative state. A nerve injury induce local changes and initiate signals up to the nerve cell body where the genetic growth program is activated by transcription factors inducing regeneration-related proteins. In some cells a cascade of caspases are initiated inducing programmed cell death. At the distal tip of the axon—for instance, the growth cone—there is integration of the signal from the growth program of the neuron with local signals that helps to direct the growth of the axon, which occurs via actin polymerization and microtubuli assembly influenced by attraction and repulsion cues. (Modified from Snider WD, Zhou FQ, Zhong J, et al. Signaling the pathway to regeneration. Neuron 2002;35:13–6,[256] with permission.)

which can be chemical and contact mediated (see reviews by Dahlin[180] and Dahlin and Brandt[181]). Cell–cell and cell–matrix adhesion is important since "neurite-promoting factors" (cell adhesion factors and extracellular matrix molecules), such as laminin, fibronectin, tenascin, and collagens, promote outgrowth.[21,182] A modifier of cell adhesion (MOCA) has been described that is associated with F-actin, and can modulate the organization of the actin cytoskeleton, at least during neuronal differentiation.[183] Cell surface glycoproteins integrins are receptors for the extracellular matrix molecules.[15,184] Members of the laminin family, particularly laminin-2 expressed by Schwann cells and laminin-8, exert their stimulatory effect via integrins to the intracellular actin in the growth cone and filopodia, thereby influencing the navigation of the axon.[185] The

growth factors, which are diffusible and soluble molecules, work at a distance.[186] The complexity of the local signal transduction mechanisms steering the axons is indicated by the fact that a specific molecule, acting via the same receptor on the growth cone/filopodia, can repulse or attract depending on cAMP status. Findings indicate that the response of growth cones to axon guidance molecules is dynamic, and can be rapidly and differentially modulated by neurotrophins.[187] Specifically, attachment of neurotrophins to trk and p75 receptors on growth cones can trigger changes in dynamics of actin filaments that regulate the behavior of the growth cone. Activation of the trk receptors mediates a local accumulation of actin filaments, while neurotrophin binding to the low-affinity receptor p75 triggers a local decrease in RhoA signaling that promotes lengthening of the filopodia.[174] Negative guidance cues, such as semaphorin IIIA (collapsin) and ephrin-A2, trigger repulsion via collapse of the growth cones/filopodia, probably through changes in the activity of Rho GTPases. For review of the local events of axonal outgrowth, see Gallo and Letourneau,[174–177] Goodman,[188] Kater and Rehder,[189] Kolodkin,[190] Kuffler,[191] Mueller,[192] and Tessier-Lavigne and Goodman.[193]

The outgrowth of axons is more complex after a transection injury with subsequent repair as compared to a simple crush injury, not only because axons can use existing precise pathways after a crush, but also that the response at the cell body level may be different. Outgrowth-stimulating substances such as FK506 may also have a type of injury-specific effect, as indicated by results where FK506 stimulates outgrowth after a nerve crush, but not after nerve transection and reconstruction.[194] The growth direction after nerve repair can be influenced by the mechanism reviewed above, and different types of specific growth have been described and shown (for review of specificity, see Dahlin[180] and Brushart[195]). Furthermore, experimentally a large number of substances, such as the mentioned FK506, and methods, such as hyperbaric oxygen, have been used to stimulate the outgrowth of axons after injury, but, unfortunately, no such treatment have been introduced and tested clinically in a prospective randomized study (for review of experimentally described methods, see Dahlin,[180] Dahlin and Brandt,[181] and Gordon, Sulaiman, and Boyd[196]).

The Nerve Graft

When there is a gap that cannot be overcome by adaptation of nerve segments without tension, the gap has to be bridged by a nerve graft, which serves both as a mechanical and a biological conduit. A variety of biological and artificial graft types have been reported,[197,198] but the optimal clinical graft is still an autologous nerve graft. The pioneering work by Millesi et al. describes the interfascicular nerve grafting procedure.[199] Autologous nerve grafts that are placed between severed nerve segments survive initially by diffusion and revascularization starts by the third postoperative day.[200,201] Wallerian degeneration occurs independently of the circulation, but is markedly delayed if macrophage invasion is inhibited.[202] Nerve regeneration is dependent on the presence of Schwann cells, as well as macrophages,[22,202,203] which make different acellular graft alternatives less suitable in clinical practice. However, attempts have been made to add cultured Schwann cells to such alternatives but the time for producing and culturing is still far beyond acceptable for clinical use. A method in which Schwann cells can be dissociated within a couple of hours and added to a sil-

icone tube or a tendon autograft used to bridge a nerve gap was recently shown to stimulate regeneration.[204,205] Axonal outgrowth is far better in pre-degenerated (number of days or weeks) nerve grafts, due to the proliferation of Schwann cells, than in freshly harvested nerve grafts.[203] Interestingly, axonal outgrowth is better in a nerve graft that has been pre-degenerated and frozen than in a fresh frozen nerve graft, indicating that the pre-degeneration process also can modify the local environment in the graft.[22] Theoretically, vascularized nerve grafts can be an option to secure circulation, improve macrophage invasion, stimulate cleaning up of myelin debris, and preserve Schwann cells, thereby stimulating nerve regeneration,[206] but may only be advantageous if the vascularity of the recipient site is poor.[207] For short nerve gaps, it is probably unnecessary to use a nerve graft since such a gap can be overcome by application of longitudinal sutures, with or without growth-stimulating factors, which can help Schwann cells and axons to traverse the gap.[208,209]

PATHOPHYSIOLOGY OF NERVE COMPRESSION

Nerve compression lesions are far more common than nerve transection injuries, thus deserving specific consideration related to pathophysiology, such as data on the pathophysiology of peripheral nerve compression.[210] Various pathophysiologic mechanisms and events have been related to clinical stages, symptoms, findings, and pressure levels in such conditions, especially in CTS. Various experimental setups have been used including acute (perspex chamber giving graded pressure to nerve[30,211]) and chronic (silicone tube of different internal diameters[212–214]) compression. Pressures have been measured clinically around different nerves in the upper extremity in normal subjects and in patients with nerve compression disorders. For example, the pressure in the carpal tunnel in patients is normally around 2 to 3 mm Hg, and it increases to 30 mm Hg in patients with CTS and with the wrist in neutral position.[215] The pressure increases up to 100 mm Hg when the wrist is flexed (Phalen's test) or extended. The pressure varies along the carpal tunnel and during the day and night.[216,217] Such pressure levels can be correlated to findings in peripheral nerve trunks compressed in experimental studies.

The magnitude of the pressure applied to a peripheral nerve trunk and the duration of compression are important for the injury.[210] Initially, experimental nerve compression affects the microcirculation in epineurial venules at a pressure of 20 to 30 mm Hg.[218] The intrafascicular blood flow observed in capillaries is impaired at 40 to 50 mm Hg, and at 80 to 120 mm Hg a complete stop in circulation is found experimentally,[218,219] with a subsequent decrease of nerve function.[220] Such pressures have also been correlated to development of symptoms and changes in diagnostic and neurophysiologic methods in patients with an experimentally induced CTS.[221] The disturbances in microcirculation induce an increase in permeability of epineurial and endoneurial vessels, leading to an epineurial and intrafascicular edema, which increase the intrafascicular pressure.[30,222] Such an increase of pressure in the endoneurial space may further impair microcirculation due to a valve mechanism since the blood vessels from the epineurium to the endoneurium pierce the perineurial barrier obliquely.[223] Already at the low compression levels (30 mm Hg), demyelination, based on Schwann cell necrosis and apoptosis, and involvement of macrophages,[224–226] is seen. The Schwann cells react very quickly with up-regulation of the immediate early gene c-jun[143] and a nuclear translocation of the transcription factor ATF-3, important for a proliferative response[227] (Fig. 1–6). A higher pressure of 80 mm Hg induces axonal pathology.[228] The axonal pathology is not uniformly distributed in the fascicle, since mainly subperineurial axons are affected, sparing axons in the core of the fascicle.[228]

The susceptibility of axons to a compression trauma varies, depending not only on the location in the fascicle, but also on the size of the fiber. Large-diameter myelinated nerve fibers (A1) are most susceptible to compression, and thinner myelinated fibers (A2) are less vulnerable, while nonmyelinated axons (C-fibers) are very resistant to nerve compression.[229] Sympathetic activity can normally influence the conduction properties (decrease of amplitude) in such C-fibers. Surprisingly, the response of C-fibers to sympathetic stimulation after severe nerve compression changes leading to an increase of the C-fiber amplitude,[230] which is interesting in view of pain aggravation in different types of nerve injuries during increased sympathetic activity.

Axonal transport is of crucial importance for the signaling after a nerve injury irrespective of magnitude and therefore the neuron use the same system to signal an injury during and after nerve compression (Fig. 1–7). Application of low pressures (20 to 30 mm Hg) inhibits fast and slow anterograde and retrograde axonal transport, depending on the duration of the pressure.[211,231,232] Thereby, the distal part of the axons is deprived of axonal transported material, not only necessary for synapse function, but also cytoskeletal components are affected. Later, an increased axonal transport of tubulin relative to actin is observed.[233] The inhibition of retrograde transport has a severe impact on the cell bodies in DRGs and in the spinal cord. It has been suggested that local injury-induced mechanisms are involved, elicited by, for example, presence of macrophages at the site of compression. Therefore, nerve compression can educe alterations in the cell body similar to those observed after nerve transection although the extent may be less pronounced (Fig. 1–7). Morphologic changes, similar to what is observed after nerve transection, are induced in the cell bodies.[234] Such alterations are unspecific, but more importantly, up-regulation of the neuropeptides galanin, NPY, and PACAP, preceded by induction of ATF-3 in the nucleus, is observed within days in sensory and motor neurons[81,227,235,236] (Fig. 1–8). The response of galanin and PACAP after nerve compression is different from, for example, partial and complete transection and a peripheral inflammation with respect to the size of the affected neurons and the number of neurons involved. This may reflect a different ability or capacity of the

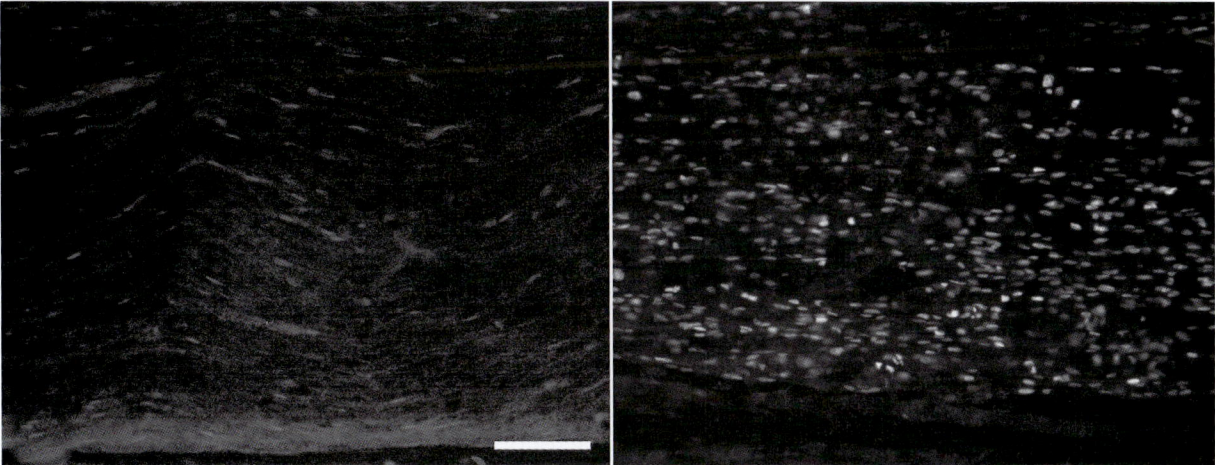

Figure 1–6 Immunocytochemical staining of the transcription factor ATF-3 in Schwann cells in an uninjured **(left)** and a compressed rat sciatic nerve **(right).** Compression induces a pronounced induction of ATF-3 in mainly Schwann cells. (Modified from Isacsson A, Kanje M, Dahlin LB. Induction of activating transcription factor 3 (ATF3) by peripheral nerve compression. Scand J Plast Reconstr Surg Hand Surg 2005;39:65-72,[227] with permission.)

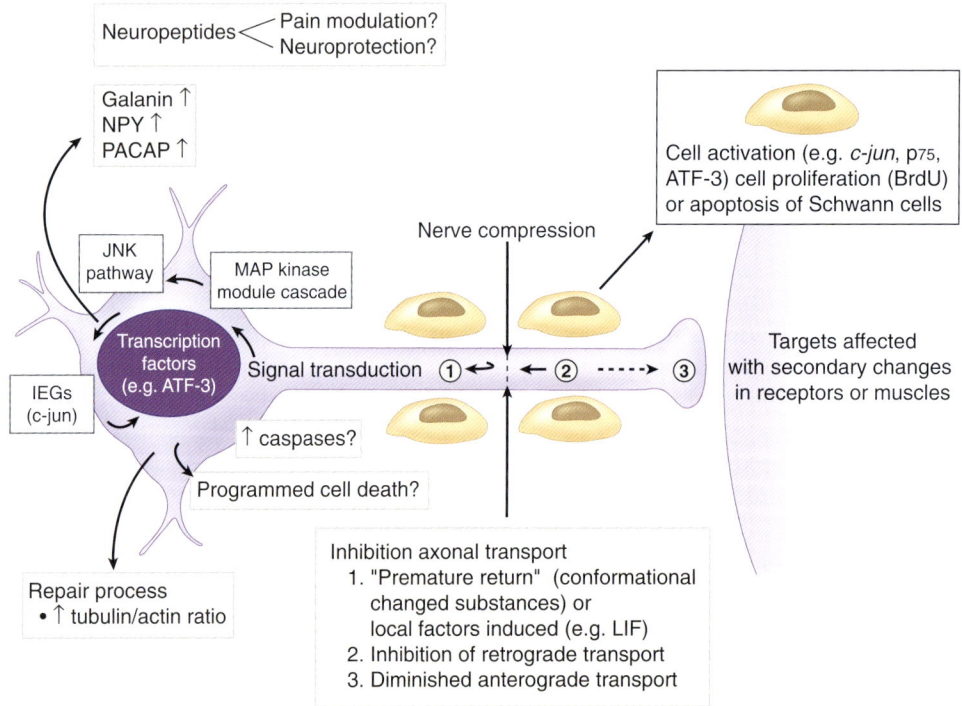

Figure 1–7 Schematic drawing of a neuron and Schwann cells and the targets with the initiating signals at the site of compression as well as examples of signal transduction steps and possible effects of the neuron and the Schwann cells induced by a peripheral nerve compression. (Modified from Dahlin LB. The biology of nerve injury and repair. J Am Soc Surg Hand 2004;4:143–55,[180] with permission.)

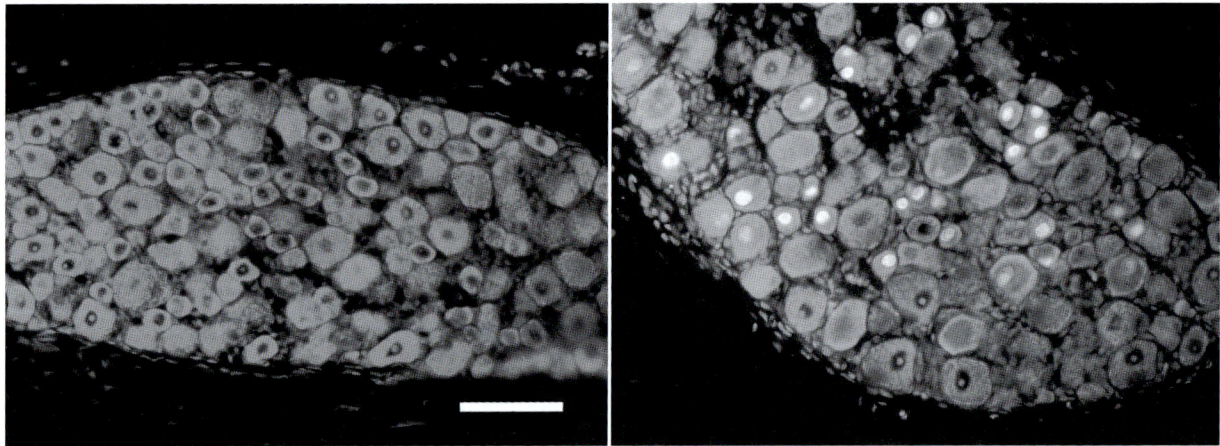

Figure 1–8 Immunocytochemical staining of the transcription factor ATF-3 in a dorsal root ganglion where the sciatic nerve was not injured **(left)**, and from dorsal root ganglion where the sciatic nerve was compressed **(right)**. Note the induction of ATF-3 in sensory neurons after compression. (Modified from Isacsson A, Kanje M, Dahlin LB. Induction of activating transcription factor 3 (ATF3) by peripheral nerve compression. Scand J Plast Reconstr Surg Hand Surg 2005;39:65-72,[227] with permission.)

sensory neurons to modulate any pain or disturbing allodynia and hyperesthesia during and after various nerve injuries.

Interestingly, CTS is more common in diabetic subjects compared to healthy individuals, and the question arises whether such subjects are more susceptible to compression trauma. Rats with streptozotocin-induced diabetes exhibit a pronounced inhibition of fast axonal transport at low pressures (30 mm Hg[237]), which can be

partly prevented by treatment with an aldose reductase inhibitor.[238] The prominent inhibition of axonal transport in rats with spontaneously developing diabetes leads to an induction of ATF-3 in a higher number of sensory neurons in DRG than in healthy rats,[239] reflecting an increased vulnerability of nerves to compression in diabetes. The "sick neuron" in diabetes may therefore be more sensitive to trauma (Fig. 1–9). However, the cause(s) has to be clarified in order to improve the diag-

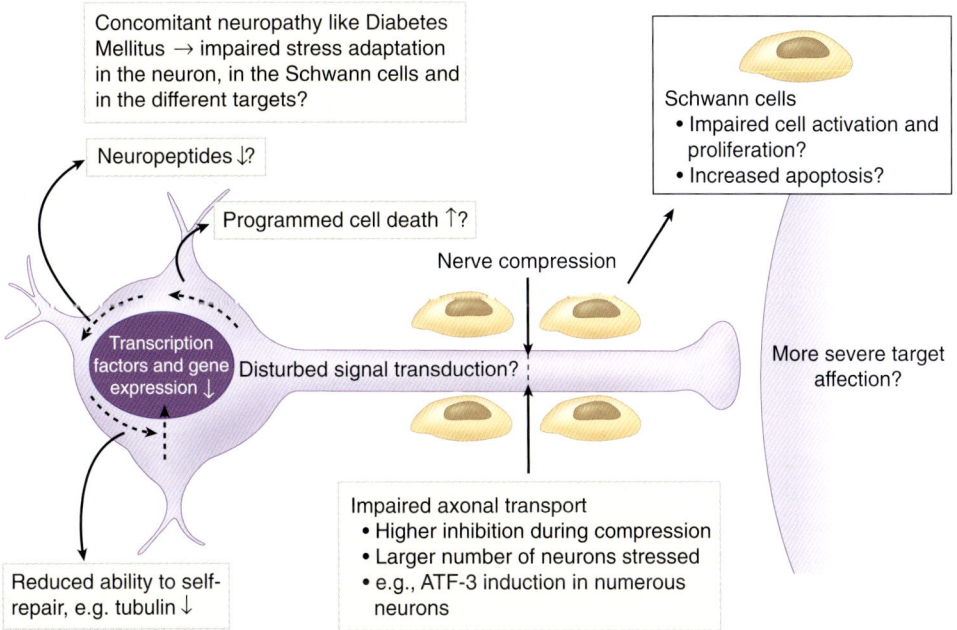

Figure 1–9 Schematic drawing of a neuron and Schwann cells in a "sick nervous system," such as in diabetes mellitus, and the possible changes that may occur in such subjects due to a peripheral nerve compression. Compression can induce a more pronounced inhibition of axonal transport and induction of ATF-3.[237,239] (Modified from Dahlin LB. The biology of nerve injury and repair. J Am Soc Surg Hand 2004;4:143–55,[180] with permission.)

nostic and therapeutic strategies in diabetic patients with or without neuropathy.

In accordance with findings in subjects with diabetes, where the peripheral nervous system is not healthy and basic disturbances in axonal transport is observed, a distal or a proximal nerve compression may confer an increased susceptibility to compression along the same nerve trunk. This hypothesis—double crush syndrome—was introduced by Upton and McComas already 1973,[240] initially suggesting that a proximal compression (e.g., spinal root level) can make a distal part of the same neuron (e.g., CTS) more susceptible due to an impaired anterograde axonal transport. On the other hand, distal nerve compression (e.g., CTS) can, via inhibition of retrograde axonal transport, make proximal parts of the same neuron (e.g., pronator syndrome) more sensitive to trauma (known as reversed double crush syndrome).[241]

THE DYNAMIC BRAIN AFTER NERVE INJURY

The outcome of nerve repair depends not only on all local events with slow and misdirected outgrowth as well as nerve cell death, but also to large extent to factors in the central nervous system,[9] including functional reorganization of cortical processes, which is caused by the de-afferentiation and the misdirected

outgrowth.[242,243] Misdirected outgrowth at the repair site was already demonstrated by Ramon y Cajal,[10] and means that reinnervation occurs of incorrect peripheral targets with subsequent reorganization at the somatosensory and motor cortex, as well as at several subcortical levels such as in the dorsal horn, cuneate and gracile nuclei, and thalamus.[244] These changes seem to be induced within minutes after the injury, but are apparent also for a considerable time after the injury.[244] Recently, it was observed that the contralateral hand function could be acutely improved during an acute deafferentiation induced by a tourniquet.[245]

Concerning sensation, tactile stimuli from the hand are considered to be processed in area 3b in the somatosensory cortex where its projection relative to other parts of the body is extensive. The information about stimuli is processed mainly to the contralateral hemisphere, but also to some extent to ipsilateral hemisphere, which is also shown for motor function.[246–248] In the motor and somato-sensory areas, different parts of the hand (and the rest of the body) are projected to areas constituted as well-defined individual bands. This cortical hand map, with its synaptic organization, can rapidly be changed and modified,[244] which indicates that the brain has a considerable plasticity. The rapid changes that occur after de-afferentiation, such as after a nerve injury, occur already after minutes, and are based on an unmasking of previously present, but functionally inactive synaptic connections that can lead to expansion of adjacent territories. The mechanisms behind the unmasking of latent synapses can be caused by, for example, reduction of GABAergic inhibition, contribution of excitatory glutaminergic synapses, and involvement of NMDA receptors and alterations in synapses.[249,250] Another phenomenon that occurs during cortical reorganization and which may occur over a long time period is the tiny protrusions from dendritic extensions of the neuron–neuronal spines. There is a certain turnover of spines, but the density and activity of these spines may vary because of environmental influence (see, for example, Johansson[251]).

A nerve injury with subsequent repair results in an immediate but also a progressively developing change in the cortical maps at several levels.[244,252–254] It is of crucial importance during the rehabilitation period after nerve injury and repair to start sensory retraining to improve the perceptual function. Experimental data indicate that an enriched sensory experience after the repair can modulate the size of the receptive field in cortical areas with refinement of the sensory resolution in a particular finger.[254] There are reasons to believe that a bilateral training method may be important during this phase of the rehabilitation and that the training should be started very early with most probably contribution of the multimodal approach (see review by Lundborg[9]).

The cortical motor representation can also go through changes after, for example, a nerve transfer. When intercostal nerves are used as nerve transfers to the musculocutaneous nerve to restore biceps function after brachial plexus injuries there are indications that the biceps representation move laterally from the intercostal area to the arm area.[255] In conclusion, the brain has a remarkable capacity for reorganization after injury and repair. Such capacity should be used in rehabilitation after injury and repair, where we could use a large number of molecular events peripherally and centrally to improve function in humans—from molecule to man.

NERVE INJURIES: CONCLUDING REMARKS AND A LOOK TO THE FUTURE

In modern hand surgery, the peripheral nerve injuries, irrespective of type or origin, still represent a major problem since the individual patient with an injury may suffer severely impaired hand function. Such an injury may have a considerable impact on the quality of life of the patient and his/her ability to work, thereby causing substantial costs for society. Nerve transection and avulsion injuries, especially at the brachial plexus level, produce high costs in each case, but even minor conditions such as nerve compression lesions can, due to the large number of patients, result in considerable costs for society. Surgical techniques may have reached a limit,

and new therapeutic approaches and strategies must be introduced. Therefore, we must improve our knowledge about all types of peripheral nerve injuries from the basic molecular level, and learn more about the delicate cellular mechanisms in peripheral and central neurons and non-neuronal cells in response to a trauma, and along a number of steps up to enhanced rehabilitation methods after the surgical or nonsurgical treatment—from molecule to man—to relieve as much pain and restore as much function as possible for our patients who suffer from diverse nerve injuries.

Acknowledgments

Research of the Peripheral Nerve Group in Malmö–Lund is supported by grants from the Medical Research Council (5188), Region Skåne (ALF), Craafords Foundation, Zoegas Fund for Medical Research, and Segerfalk's Fund, as well as funding from University Hospital Malmö and a number of regional funds. For space reasons, all references relevant in this research field have not been included, and I apologize to authors who have not been properly referenced. I am grateful to Professor Martin Kanje, Department of Cell and Organism Biology, Lund University, Lund, and my secretary Tina Folker for a substantial amount of help and advice during the preparation of this manuscript.

Dedication

To Anne, Erik, and Emma.

REFERENCES

1. Rosén B. The Sensational Hand. Clinical Assessment After Nerve Repair. PhD thesis, Lund University, 2000.
2. Rosberg HE, Dahlin LB. Epidemiology of hand injuries in a middle-sized city in southern Sweden: a retrospective comparison of 1989 and 1997. Scand J Plast Reconstr Surg Hand Surg 2004;38:347–55.
3. Rosberg HE, Steen-Carlsson K, Höjgård S, et al. Injury to the human median and ulnar nerves in the forearm—analysis of costs for treatment and rehabilitation of 69 patients in southern Sweden. J Hand Surg Br 2005;30:35–9.
4. Rosberg HE, Carlsson KS, Hojgard S, et al. What determines the costs of repair and rehabilitation of flexor tendon injuries in zone II? A multiple regression analysis of data from southern Sweden. J Hand Surg Br 2003;28:106–12.
5. Atroshi I, Gummesson C, Johnsson R, et al. Prevalence of carpal tunnel syndrome in a general population. JAMA 1999;282:153–8 [see comments].
6. Bekkelund SI, Pierre-Jerome C, Torbergsen T, et al. Impact of occupational variables in carpal tunnel syndrome. Acta Neurol Scand 2001;103:193–7.
7. Rayan GM, Asal NR, Bohr PC. Epidemiology and economic impact of compression neuropathy. In: Omer GE, Spinner M, Van Beak A, eds., Management of Peripheral Nerve Problems. Philadelphia: W.B. Saunders, 1998:484–93.
8. Slattery TJ. Back, carpal tunnel claims mounting. Paper presented at Risk & Insurance Management Society Annual Meeting, Anaheim, California, 1992.
9. Lundborg G. Richard P. Bunge memorial lecture. Nerve injury and repair—a challenge to the plastic brain. J Peripher Nerv Syst 2003;8:209–26.

10. Ramon y Cajal SR. Degeneration and Regeneration of the Nervous System. London: Oxford University Press, 1928.

11. Reimer M, Kanje M. Peripheral but not central axotomy promotes axonal outgrowth and induces alterations in neuropeptide synthesis in the nodose ganglion of the rat. Eur J Neurosci 1999;11:3415–23.

12. Takenaka T, Kawakami T, Hori H, et al. Axoplasmic transport and its signal transduction mechanism. Jpn J Physiol 1998; 48:413–20.

13. Miller CC, Ackerley S, Brownlees J, et al. Axonal transport of neurofilaments in normal and disease states. Cell Mol Life Sci 2002;59:323–30.

14. Gallant PE. Axonal protein synthesis and transport. J Neurocytol 2000;29:779–82.

15. van der Flier A, Sonnenberg A. Function and interactions of integrins. Cell Tissue Res 2001;305:285–98.

16. Jessen KR, Mirsky R. Signals that determine Schwann cell identity. J Anat 2002;200:367–76.

17. Esper RM, Loeb JA. Rapid axoglial signaling mediated by neuregulin and neurotrophic factors. J Neurosci 2004;24: 6218–27.

18. Stewart HJ. Expression of c-Jun, Jun B, Jun D and cAMP response element binding protein by Schwann cells and their precursors in vivo and in vitro. Eur J Neurosci 1995;7: 1366–75.

19. Miner JH, Patton BL, Lentz SI, et al. The laminin alpha chains: expression, developmental transitions, and chromosomal locations of alpha1-5, identification of heterotrimeric laminins 8-11, and cloning of a novel alpha3 isoform. J Cell Biol 1997; 137:685–701.

20. Patton BL, Miner JH, Chiu AY, et al. Distribution and function of laminins in the neuromuscular system of developing, adult, and mutant mice. J Cell Biol 1997;139:1507–21.

21. Wallquist W, Patarroyo M, Thams S, et al. Laminin chains in rat and human peripheral nerve: distribution and regulation during development and after axonal injury. J Comp Neurol 2002;454:284–93.

22. Danielsen N, Kerns JM, Holmquist B, et al. Predegeneration enhances regeneration into acellular nerve grafts. Brain Res 1995;681:105–8.

23. Davies AM. The neurotrophic hypothesis: where does it stand? Philos Trans R Soc Lond B Biol Sci 1996;351:389–94.

24. Davies AM. Paracrine and autocrine actions of neurotrophic factors. Neurochem Res 1996;21:749–53.

25. Jessen KR, Mirsky R. Schwann cells and their precursors emerge as major regulators of nerve development. Trends Neurosci 1999;22:402–10.

26. Shy ME, Shi Y, Wrabetz L, et al. Axon-Schwann cell interactions regulate the expression of c-jun in Schwann cells. J Neurosci Res 1996;43:511–25.

27. Mirsky R, Parmantier E, McMahon AP, et al. Schwann cell-derived desert hedgehog signals nerve sheath formation. Ann NY Acad Sci 1999;883:196–202.

28. Scherman P, Lundborg G, Kanje M, et al. Neural regeneration along longitudinal polyglactin sutures across short and extended defects in the rat sciatic nerve. J Neurosurg 2001; 95:316–23.

29. Lundborg G. Ischemic nerve injury. Experimental studies on intraneural microvascular pathophysiology and nerve function in a limb subjected to temporary circulatory arrest. Scand J Plast Reconstr Surg Hand Surg Suppl 1970;6:3–113.

30. Rydevik B, Lundborg G. Permeability of intraneural microvessels and perineurium following acute, graded experimental nerve compression. Scand J Plast Reconstr Surg Hand Surg 1977;11:179–87.

31. Richardson PM, Lu X. Inflammation and axonal regeneration. J Neurol 1994;241:57–60.

32. Zhou XF, Deng YS, Chie E, et al. Satellite-cell-derived nerve growth factor and neurotrophin-3 are involved in noradrenergic sprouting in the dorsal root ganglia following peripheral nerve injury in the rat. Eur J Neurosci 1999;11:1711–22.

33. Ramer MS, Thompson SW, McMahon SB. Causes and consequences of sympathetic basket formation in dorsal root ganglia. Pain 1999;(Suppl 6):S111–20.

34. Giuffrida R, Rustioni A. Dorsal root ganglion neurons projecting to the dorsal column nuclei of rats. J Comp Neurol 1992; 316:206–20.

35. Muragaki Y, Timothy N, Leight S, et al. Expression of trk receptors in the developing and adult human central and peripheral nervous system. J Comp Neurol 1995;356:387–97.

36. McMahon SB, Armanini MP, Ling LH, et al. Expression and coexpression of Trk receptors in subpopulations of adult primary sensory neurons projecting to identified peripheral targets. Neuron 1994;12:1161–71.

37. Ernfors P, Lee KF, Kucera J, et al. Lack of neurotrophin-3 leads to deficiencies in the peripheral nervous system and loss of limb proprioceptive afferents. Cell 1994;77:503–12.

38. Wright DE, Snider WD. Neurotrophin receptor mRNA expression defines distinct populations of neurons in rat dorsal root ganglia. J Comp Neurol 1995;351:329–38.

39. Paratore C, Hagedorn L, Floris J, et al. Cell-intrinsic and cell-extrinsic cues regulating lineage decisions in multipotent neural crest-derived progenitor cells. Int J Dev Biol 2002;46:193–200.

40. Acosta CG, Fabrega AR, Masco DH, et al. A sensory neuron subpopulation with unique sequential survival dependence on nerve growth factor and basic fibroblast growth factor during development. J Neurosci 2001;21:8873–85.

41. Mou K, Adamson CL, Davis RL. Time-dependence and cell-type specificity of synergistic neurotrophin actions on spiral ganglion neurons. J Comp Neurol 1998;402:129–39.

42. Farinas I, Cano-Jaimez M, Bellmunt E, et al. Regulation of neurogenesis by neurotrophins in developing spinal sensory ganglia. Brain Res Bull 2002;57:809–16.

43. Kirstein M, Farinas I. Sensing life: regulation of sensory neuron survival by neurotrophins. Cell Mol Life Sci 2002;59: 1787–802.

44. Farinas I, Wilkinson GA, Backus C, et al. Characterization of neurotrophin and Trk receptor functions in developing sensory ganglia: direct NT-3 activation of TrkB neurons in vivo. Neuron 1998;21:325–34.

45. Yawo H, Kuno M. Calcium dependence of membrane sealing at the cut end of the cockroach giant axon. J Neurosci 1985;5: 1626–32.

46. Fukunaga K, Miyamoto E. Role of MAP kinase in neurons. Mol Neurobiol 1998;16:79–95.

47. Ambron RT, Walters ET. Priming events and retrograde injury signals. A new perspective on the cellular and molecular biology of nerve regeneration. Mol Neurobiol 1996;13:61–79.

48. Lee P, Zhuo H, Helke CJ. Axotomy alters neurotrophin and neurotrophin receptor mRNAs in the vagus nerve and nodose ganglion of the rat. Brain Res Mol Brain Res 2001;87:31–41.

49. Zigmond RE, Sun Y. Regulation of neuropeptide expression in sympathetic neurons. Paracrine and retrograde influences. Ann NY Acad Sci 1997;814:181–97.

50. Curtis R, Scherer SS, Somogyi R, et al. Retrograde axonal transport of LIF is increased by peripheral nerve injury: correlation with increased LIF expression in distal nerve. Neuron 1994; 12:191–204.

51. Curtis R, Tonra JR, Stark JL, et al. Neuronal injury increases retrograde axonal transport of the neurotrophins to spinal sensory neurons and motor neurons via multiple receptor mechanisms. Mol Cell Neurosci 1998;12:105–18.

52. Sun Y, Zigmond RE. Leukaemia inhibitory factor induced in the sciatic nerve after axotomy is involved in the induction

of galanin in sensory neurons. Eur J Neurosci 1996;8:2213–20.

53. Tonra JR. Classical and novel directions in neurotrophin transport and research: anterograde transport of brain-derived neurotrophic factor by sensory neurons. Microsc Res Tech 1999;45:225–32.

54. Campana WM, Myers RR, Rearden A. Identification of PINCH in Schwann cells and DRG neurons: shuttling and signaling after nerve injury. Glia 2003;41:213–23.

55. Hanz S, Perlson E, Willis D, et al. Axoplasmic importins enable retrograde injury signaling in lesioned nerve. Neuron 2003; 40:1095–104.

56. Neves SR, Ram PT, Iyengar R. G protein pathways. Science 2002;296:1636–9.

57. Rajagopal R, Chen ZY, Lee FS, et al. Transactivation of Trk neurotrophin receptors by g-protein-coupled receptor ligands occurs on intracellular membranes. J Neurosci 2004;24: 6650–8.

58. Denhardt DT. Signal-transducing protein phosphorylation cascades mediated by Ras/Rho proteins in the mammalian cell: the potential for multiplex signalling. Biochem J 1996;318: 729–47.

59. Cobb MH, Schaefer EM. MAP kinase signaling pathways. Promega Notes Mag 1996;59:37.

60. Rubinfeld H, Seger R. The ERK cascade as a prototype of MAPK signaling pathways. Methods Mol Biol 2004;250:1–28.

61. Ham J, Eilers A, Whitfield J, et al. c-Jun and the transcriptional control of neuronal apoptosis. Biochem Pharmacol 2000;60: 1015–21.

62. Herdegen T, Leah JD. Inducible and constitutive transcription factors in the mammalian nervous system: control of gene expression by Jun, Fos and Krox, and CREB/ATF proteins. Brain Res Brain Res Rev 1998;28:370–490.

63. Kenney AM, Kocsis JD. Peripheral axotomy induces long-term c-Jun amino-terminal kinase-1 activation and activator protein-1 binding activity by c-Jun and junD in adult rat dorsal root ganglia in vivo. J Neurosci 1998;18:1318–28.

64. Lindwall C, Dahlin L, Lundborg G, et al. Inhibition of c-Jun phosphorylation reduces axonal outgrowth of adult rat nodose ganglia and dorsal root ganglia sensory neurons. Mol Cell Neurosci 2004;27:267–79.

65. Nakagomi S, Suzuki Y, Namikawa K, et al. Expression of the activating transcription factor 3 prevents c-Jun N-terminal kinase-induced neuronal death by promoting heat shock protein 27 expression and Akt activation. J Neurosci 2003; 23:5187–96.

66. Lonze BE, Ginty DD. Function and regulation of CREB family transcription factors in the nervous system. Neuron 2002; 35:605–23.

67. Liang G, Wolfgang CD, Chen BP, et al. ATF3 gene. Genomic organization, promoter, and regulation. J Biol Chem 1996;271: 1695–701.

68. Hai T, Hartman MG. The molecular biology and nomenclature of the activating transcription factor/cAMP responsive element binding family of transcription factors: activating transcription factor proteins and homeostasis. Gene 2001;273:1–11.

69. Weber JR, Skene JH. The activity of a highly promiscuous AP-1 element can be confined to neurons by a tissue-selective repressive element. J Neurosci 1998;18:5264–74.

70. Tsujino H, Kondo E, Fukuoka T, et al. Activating transcription factor 3 (ATF3) induction by axotomy in sensory and motoneurons: a novel neuronal marker of nerve injury. Mol Cell Neurosci 2000;15:170–82.

71. Allen-Jennings AE, Hartman MG, Kociba GJ, et al. The roles of ATF3 in glucose homeostasis. A transgenic mouse model with liver dysfunction and defects in endocrine pancreas. J Biol Chem 2001;276:29507–14.

72. Hart AM, Terenghi G, Kellerth JO, et al. Sensory neuroprotection, mitochondrial preservation, and therapeutic potential of n-acetyl-cysteine after nerve injury. Neuroscience 2004; 125:91–101.

73. Averill S, Michael GJ, Shortland PJ, et al. NGF and GDNF ameliorate the increase in ATF3 expression which occurs in dorsal root ganglion cells in response to peripheral nerve injury. Eur J Neurosci 2004;19:1437–45.

74. Herdegen T, Fiallos-Estrada CE, Schmid W, et al. The transcription factors c-JUN, JUN D and CREB, but not FOS and KROX-24, are differentially regulated in axotomized neurons following transection of rat sciatic nerve. Brain Res Mol Brain Res 1992;14:155–65.

75. Jenkins R, Hunt SP. Long-term increase in the levels of c-jun mRNA and jun protein-like immunoreactivity in motor and sensory neurons following axon damage. Neurosci Lett 1991; 129:107–10.

76. Nilsson A. Gene Expression in the Dorsal Root Ganglion and the Role of PAI-1 and Amphiregulin during Regeneration. PhD thesis, Lund University, 2004.

77. Tanabe K, Bonilla I, Winkles JA, et al. Fibroblast growth factor-inducible-14 is induced in axotomized neurons and promotes neurite outgrowth. J Neurosci 2003;23:9675–86.

78. Cowell IG. E4BP4/NFIL3, a PAR-related bZIP factor with many roles. Bioessays 2002;24:1023–9.

79. Fu SY, Gordon T. The cellular and molecular basis of peripheral nerve regeneration. Mol Neurobiol 1997;14:67–116.

80. Widerberg A, Kanje M, Dahlin LB. C-terminal flanking peptide of neuropeptide Y in DRG following nerve compression. Neuroreport 2001;12:3193–6.

81. Dahlin LB, Stenberg L, Kanje M. Galanin expression in sensory neurons after nerve compression or transection. Neuroreport 2003;14:359–62.

82. Landry M, Aman K, Dostrovsky J, et al. Galanin expression in adult human dorsal root ganglion neurons: initial observations. Neuroscience 2003;117:795–809.

83. Jongsma H, Danielsen N, Sundler F, et al. Alteration of PACAP distribution and PACAP receptor binding in the rat sensory nervous system following sciatic nerve transection. Brain Res 2000;853:186–96.

84. Noguchi K, Senba E, Morita Y, et al. Alpha-CGRP and beta-CGRP mRNAs are differentially regulated in the rat spinal cord and dorsal root ganglion. Brain Res Mol Brain Res 1990;7: 299–304.

85. Lewis SE, Mannion RJ, White FA, et al. A role for HSP27 in sensory neuron survival. J Neurosci 1999;19:8945–53.

86. Costigan M, Mannion RJ, Kendall G, et al. Heat shock protein 27: developmental regulation and expression after peripheral nerve injury. J Neurosci 1998;18:5891–900.

87. Krieglstein K, Henheik P, Farkas L, et al. Glial cell line-derived neurotrophic factor requires transforming growth factor-beta for exerting its full neurotrophic potential on peripheral and CNS neurons. J Neurosci 1998;18:9822–34.

88. Hammarberg H, Piehl F, Risling M, et al. Differential regulation of trophic factor receptor mRNAs in spinal motoneurons after sciatic nerve transection and ventral root avulsion in the rat. J Comp Neurol 2000;426:587–601.

89. Hammarberg H, Wallquist W, Piehl F, et al. Regulation of laminin-associated integrin subunit mRNAs in rat spinal motoneurons during postnatal development and after axonal injury. J Comp Neurol 2000;428:294–304.

90. Kashiba H, Senba E. Up- and down-regulation of BDNF mRNA in distinct subgroups of rat sensory neurons after axotomy. Neuroreport 1999;10:3561–5.

91. Tonra JR, Curtis R, Wong V, et al. Axotomy upregulates the anterograde transport and expression of brain-derived neu-

rotrophic factor by sensory neurons. J Neurosci 1998;18: 4374–83.

92. Jongsma Wallin H, Danielsen N, Johnston JM, et al. Exogenous NT-3 and NGF differentially modulate PACAP expression in adult sensory neurons, suggesting distinct roles in injury and inflammation. Eur J Neurosci 2001;14:267–82.

93. Kerekes N, Landry M, Lundmark K, et al. Effect of NGF, BDNF, bFGF, aFGF and cell density on NPY expression in cultured rat dorsal root ganglion neurones. J Auton Nerv Sys 2000;81: 128–38.

94. Karchewski LA, Gratto KA, Wetmore C, et al. Dynamic patterns of BDNF expression in injured sensory neurons: differential modulation by NGF and NT-3. Eur J Neurosci 2002; 16:1449–62.

95. Yuan Q, Wu W, So KF, et al. Effects of neurotrophic factors on motoneuron survival following axonal injury in newborn rats. Neuroreport 2000;11:2237–41.

96. Boyd JG, Gordon T. Glial cell line-derived neurotrophic factor and brain-derived neurotrophic factor sustain the axonal regeneration of chronically axotomized motoneurons in vivo. Exp Neurol 2003;183:610–9.

97. Thompson SW, Priestley JV, Southall A. gp130 cytokines, leukemia inhibitory factor and interleukin-6, induce neuropeptide expression in intact adult rat sensory neurons in vivo: time-course, specificity and comparison with sciatic nerve axotomy. Neuroscience 1998;84:1247–55.

98. Ito Y, Yamamoto M, et al. Differential temporal expression of mRNAs for ciliary neurotrophic factor (CNTF), leukaemia inhibitory factor (LIF), interleukin-6 (IL-6), and their receptors (CNTFR alpha, LIFR beta, IL-6R alpha and gp130) in injured peripheral nerves. Brain Res 1998;793:321–7.

99. Murphy PG, Borthwick LS, Johnston RS, et al. Nature of the retrograde signal from injured nerves that induces interleukin-6 mRNA in neurons. J Neurosci 1999;19:3791–800.

100. Thompson SW, Vernallis AB, Heath JK, et al. Leukaemia inhibitory factor is retrogradely transported by a distinct population of adult rat sensory neurons: co-localization with trkA and other neurochemical markers. Eur J Neurosci 1997;9:1244–51.

101. Murphy PG, Grondin J, Altares M, et al. Induction of interleukin-6 in axotomized sensory neurons. J Neurosci 1995; 15:5130–8.

102. Bruck W. The role of macrophages in Wallerian degeneration. Brain Pathol 1997;7:741–52.

103. Lu X, Richardson PM. Inflammation near the nerve cell body enhances axonal regeneration. J Neurosci 1991;11:972–8.

104. Kimura H, Schubert D. Schwannoma-derived growth factor promotes the neuronal differentiation and survival of PC12 cells. J Cell Biol 1992;116:777–83.

105. Iwata T, Namikawa K, Honma M, et al. Increased expression of mRNAs for microtubule disassembly molecules during nerve regeneration. Brain Res Mol Brain Res 2002;102:105–9.

106. Tanabe K, Tachibana T, Yamashita T, et al. The small GTP-binding protein TC10 promotes nerve elongation in neuronal cells, and its expression is induced during nerve regeneration in rats. J Neurosci 2000;20:4138–44.

107. Bonilla IE, Tanabe K, Strittmatter SM. Small proline-rich repeat protein 1A is expressed by axotomized neurons and promotes axonal outgrowth. J Neurosci 2002;22:1303–15.

108. Al-Majed AA, Tam SL, Gordon T. Electrical stimulation accelerates and enhances expression of regeneration-associated genes in regenerating rat femoral motoneurons. Cell Mol Neurobiol 2004;24:379–402.

109. Lieberman A. The axon reaction: a review of the principal features of perikaryal response to axonal injury. Int Rev Neurobiol 1971;14:99–124.

110. Nicholson DW, Thornberry NA. Caspases: killer proteases. Trends Biochem Sci 1997;22:299–306.

111. Budd SL, Nicholls DG. Mitochondria in the life and death of neurons. Essays Biochem 1998;33:43–52.

112. Vestergaard S, Tandrup T, Jakobsen J. Effect of permanent axotomy on number and volume of dorsal root ganglion cell bodies. J Comp Neurol 1997;388:307–12.

113. Shi TJ, Tandrup T, Bergman E, et al. Effect of peripheral nerve injury on dorsal root ganglion neurons in the C57 BL/6J mouse: marked changes both in cell numbers and neuropeptide expression. Neuroscience 2001;105:249–63.

114. Tandrup T, Woolf CJ, Coggeshall RE. Delayed loss of small dorsal root ganglion cells after transection of the rat sciatic nerve. J Comp Neurol 2000;422:172–80.

115. Ygge J. Neuronal loss in lumbar dorsal root ganglia after proximal compared to distal sciatic nerve resection: a quantitative study in the rat. Brain Res 1989;478:193–5.

116. McKay Hart A, Brannstrom T, Wiberg M, et al. Primary sensory neurons and satellite cells after peripheral axotomy in the adult rat: timecourse of cell death and elimination. Exp Brain Res 2002;142:308–18.

117. Wilson AD, Hart A, Brannstrom T, et al. Primary sensory neuronal rescue with systemic acetyl-L-carnitine following peripheral axotomy. A dose–response analysis. Br J Plast Surg 2003;56:732–9.

118. Benn SC, Perrelet D, Kato AC, et al. Hsp27 upregulation and phosphorylation is required for injured sensory and motor neuron survival. Neuron 2002;36:45–56.

119. Tidwell JL, Houenou LJ, Tytell M. Administration of Hsp70 in vivo inhibits motor and sensory neuron degeneration. Cell Stress Chaperones 2004;9:88–98.

120. Livesey FJ, Fraher JP. Experimental traction injuries of cervical spinal nerve roots: a scanning EM study of rupture patterns in fresh tissue. Neuropathol Appl Neurobiol 1992;18: 376–86.

121. Novikov L, Novikova L, Kellerth JO. Brain-derived neurotrophic factor promotes survival and blocks nitric oxide synthase expression in adult rat spinal motoneurons after ventral root avulsion. Neurosci Lett 1995;200:45–8.

122. Wu W. Expression of nitric-oxide synthase (NOS) in injured CNS neurons as shown by NADPH diaphorase histochemistry. Exp Neurol 1993;120:153–9.

123. Li L, Houenou LJ, Wu W, et al. Characterization of spinal motoneuron degeneration following different types of peripheral nerve injury in neonatal and adult mice. J Comp Neurol 1998;396:158–68.

124. Koliatsos VE, Price WL, Pardo CA, et al. Ventral root avulsion: an experimental model of death of adult motor neurons. J Comp Neurol 1994;342:35–44.

125. Ma J, Novikov LN, Kellerth JO, et al. Early nerve repair after injury to the postganglionic plexus: an experimental study of sensory and motor neuronal survival in adult rats. Scand J Plast Reconstr Surg Hand Surg 2003;37:1–9.

126. Hart AM, Wiberg M, Youle M, et al. Systemic acetyl-L-carnitine eliminates sensory neuronal loss after peripheral axotomy: a new clinical approach in the management of peripheral nerve trauma. Exp Brain Res 2002;145:182–9.

127. Koeppen AH. Wallerian degeneration: history and clinical significance. J Neurolog Sci 2004;220:115–7.

128. George EB, Glass JD, Griffin JW. Axotomy-induced axonal degeneration is mediated by calcium influx through ion-specific channels. J Neurosci 1995;15:6445–52.

129. Perry VH, Brown MC. Macrophages and nerve regeneration. Curr Opin Neurobiol 1992;2:679–82.

130. Hirata K, Kawabuchi M. Myelin phagocytosis by macrophages and nonmacrophages during Wallerian degeneration. Microsc Res Tech 2002;57:541–7.

131. Zrouri H, Le Goascogne C, Li WW, et al. The role of MAP kinases in rapid gene induction after lesioning of the rat sciatic nerve. Eur J Neurosci 2004;20:1811–8.

132. Cameron AA, Vansant G, Wu W, et al. Identification of reciprocally regulated gene modules in regenerating dorsal root ganglion neurons and activated peripheral or central nervous system glia. J Cell Biochem 2003;88:970–85.

133. Kubo T, Yamashita T, Yamaguchi A, et al. Analysis of genes induced in peripheral nerve after axotomy using cDNA microarrays. J Neurochem 2002;82:1129–36.

134. Sheu JY, Kulhanek DJ, Eckenstein FP. Differential patterns of ERK and STAT3 phosphorylation after sciatic nerve transection in the rat. Exp Neurol 2000;166:392–402.

135. Hall S. Nerve repair: a neurobiologist's view. J Hand Surg Br 2001;26:129–36.

136. Salonen V, Aho H, Röyttä M, et al. Quantitation of Schwann cells and endoneurial fibroblasts-like cells after experimental nerve trauma. Acta Neuropathol (Berl) 1988;75:331–6.

137. Clemence A, Mirsky R, Jessen KR. Non-myelin-forming Schwann cells proliferate rapidly during Wallerian degeneration in the rat sciatic nerve. J Neurocytol 1989;18:185–92.

138. Lindholm D, Heumann R, Meyer M, et al. Interleukin-1 regulates synthesis of nerve growth factor in non-neuronal cells of rat sciatic nerve. Nature 1987;330:658–9.

139. Taniuchi M, Clark HB, Johnson JEM. Induction of nerve growth factor receptor in Schwann cells after axotomy. Proc Natl Acad Sci USA 1986;83:4094–8.

140. Davis JB, Stroobant P. Platelet-derived growth factors and fibroblast growth factors are mitogens for rat Schwann cells. J Cell Biol 1990;110:1353–60.

141. Hunt D, Hossain-Ibrahim K, Mason MR, et al. ATF3 upregulation in glia during Wallerian degeneration: differential expression in peripheral nerves and CNS white matter. BMC Neurosci 2004;5:9 (http://www.biomedcentral.com/1471-2202/5/9).

141a. Kataoka K, Kanje M, Dahlin LB. Time- and injury-dependent expression of activating transcription factor 3 (ATF3) in neurons and non-neuronal cells of the rat sciatic nerve system. Program no. 29.8.2005 abstract viewer/itinerary planner. Washington, DC, Society for Neuroscience, 2005. Online.

142. Soares HD, Chen SC, Morgan JI. Differential and prolonged expression of Fos-lacZ and Jun-lacZ in neurons, glia, and muscle following sciatic nerve damage. Exp Neurol 2001;167:1–14.

143. Kanje M, Stenberg L, Ahlin A, et al. Activation of non-neuronal cells in the rat sciatic nerve in response to inflammation caused by implanted silicone tubes. Restor Neurol Neurosci 1995;8:181–7.

144. Curtis R, Stewart HJ, Hall SM, et al. GAP-43 is expressed by nonmyelin-forming Schwann cells of the peripheral nervous system. J Cell Biol 1992;116:1455–64.

145. Martini R. Expression and functional roles of neural cell surface molecules and extracellular matrix components during development and regeneration of peripheral nerves. J Neurocytol 1994;23:1–28.

146. Funakoshi H, Frisen J, Barbany G, et al. Differential expression of mRNAs for neurotrophins and their receptors after axotomy of the sciatic nerve. J Cell Biol 1993;123:455–65.

147. Hammarberg H, Piehl F, Cullheim S, et al. GDNF mRNA in Schwann cells and DRG satellite cells after chronic sciatic nerve injury. Neuroreport 1996;7:857–60.

148. Lewin GR, Barde YA. Physiology of the neurotrophins. Annu Rev Neurosci 1996;19:289–317.

149. Sendtner M, Stockli KA, Thoenen H. Synthesis and localization of ciliary neurotrophic factor in the sciatic nerve of the adult rat after lesion and during regeneration. J Cell Biol 1992;118:139–48.

150. Trupp M, Ryden M, Jornvall H, et al. Peripheral expression and biological activities of GDNF, a new neurotrophic factor for avian and mammalian peripheral neurons. J Cell Biol 1995;130:137–48.

151. Boyd JG, Gordon T. Neurotrophic factors and their receptors in axonal regeneration and functional recovery after peripheral nerve injury. Mol Neurobiol 2003;27:277–324.

152. Petratos S, Butzkueven H, Shipham K, et al. Schwann cell apoptosis in the postnatal axotomized sciatic nerve is mediated via NGF through the low-affinity neurotrophin receptor. J Neuropathol Exp Neurol 2003;62:398–411.

153. Syroid DE, Maycox PJ, Soilu-Hanninen M, et al. Induction of postnatal schwann cell death by the low-affinity neurotrophin receptor in vitro and after axotomy. J Neurosci 2000;20:5741–7.

154. Ferri CC, Bisby MA. Improved survival of injured sciatic nerve Schwann cells in mice lacking the p75 receptor. Neurosci Lett 1999;272:191–4.

155. Bentley CA, Lee KF. p75 is important for axon growth and schwann cell migration during development. J Neurosci 2000;20:7706–15.

156. Matsuoka I, Nakane A, Kurihara K. Induction of LIF-mRNA by TGF-beta 1 in Schwann cells. Brain Res 1997;776:170–80.

157. Creange A, Barlovatz-Meimon G, Gherardi RK. Cytokines and peripheral nerve disorders. Eur Cytokine Netw 1997;8:145–51.

158. Meyer M, Matsuoka I, Wetrose C, et al. Enhanced synthesis of brain-derived neurotropic factor in the lesioned peripheral nerve: different mechanisms are responsible for the regulation of BDNF and NGFmRNA. J Cell Biol 1992;119:45–54.

159. Sulaiman OA, Gordon T. Effects of short- and long-term Schwann cell denervation on peripheral nerve regeneration, myelination, and size. Glia 2000;32:234–46.

160. Sulaiman OA, Voda J, Gold BG, et al. FK506 increases peripheral nerve regeneration after chronic axotomy but not after chronic schwann cell denervation. Exp Neurol 2002;175:127–37.

161. Ekström PA. Neurones and glial cells of the mouse sciatic nerve undergo apoptosis after injury in vivo and in vitro. Neuroreport 1995;6:1029–32.

162. Li H, Terenghi G, Hall SM. Effects of delayed re-innervation on the expression of c-erbB receptors by chronically denervated rat Schwann cells in vivo. Glia 1997;20:333–47.

163. Li H, Wigley C, Hall SM. Chronically denervated rat Schwann cells respond to GGF in vitro. Glia 1998;24:290–303.

164. Hall SM. The biology of chronically denervated Schwann cells. Ann NY Acad Sci 1999;883:215–33.

165. Hirata K, He J, Hirakawa Y, et al. HSP27 is markedly induced in Schwann cell columns and associated regenerating axons. Glia 2003;42:1–11.

166. Grinnell AD. Trophic interaction between nerve and muscle. In: Engel AG, Franzini-Armstrong C, eds., Myology Basic and Clinical. New York: McGraw-Hill, 1994:303–32.

167. Hall ZW, Sanes JR. Synaptic structure and development: the neuromuscular junction. Cell 1993;72(Suppl):99–121.

168. Stark B, Carlstedt T, Risling M. Distribution of TGF-beta, the TGF-beta type I receptor and the R-II receptor in peripheral nerves and mechanoreceptors; observations on changes after traumatic injury. Brain Res 2001;913:47–56.

169. Magnusson C. Effects of Denervation on Gene Expression in Skeletal Muscle. Kalmar, Sweden: Department of Chemistry and Biomedical Sciences. PhD thesis, University of Kalmar, 2003.

170. Danielsen N, Dahlin LB, Thomsen P. Inflammatory cells and mediators in the silicone chamber model for nerve regeneration. Biomaterials 1993;14:1180–5.

171. Danielsen N, Varon S. Characterization of neurotrophic activity in the silicone chamber model for nerve regeneration. J Reconstr Microsurg 1995;11:231–5.

172. Dahlin LB, Zhao Q, Bjursten LM. Nerve regeneration in silicone tubes: distribution of macrophages and interleukin-1β in the formed fibrin matrix. Restor Neurol Neurosci 1995;8:199–203.

173. Verma P, Chierzi S, Codd AM, et al. Axonal protein synthesis and degradation are necessary for efficient growth cone regeneration. J Neurosci 2005;25:331–42.

174. Gallo G, Letourneau PC. Regulation of growth cone actin filaments by guidance cues. J Neurobiol 2004;58:92–102.

175. Gallo G, Letourneau P. Axon guidance: proteins turnover in turning growth cones. Curr Biol 2002;12:R560–2.

176. Gallo G, Letourneau PC. Neurotrophins and the dynamic regulation of the neuronal cytoskeleton. J Neurobiol 2000;44:159–73.

177. Guan KL, Rao Y. Signalling mechanisms mediating neuronal responses to guidance cues. Nat Rev Neurosci 2003;4:941–56.

178. Kerns JM, Danielsen N, Zhao Q, et al. A comparison of peripheral nerve regeneration in acellular muscle and nerve autografts. Scand J Plast Reconstr Surg Hand Surg 2003;37:193–200.

179. Brandt J, Dahlin LB, Kanje M, et al. Spatiotemporal progress of nerve regeneration in a tendon autograft used for bridging a peripheral nerve defect. Exp Neurol 1999;160:386–93.

180. Dahlin LB. The biology of nerve injury and repair. J Am Soc Surg Hand 2004;4:143–55.

181. Dahlin LB, Brandt J. Basic science of peripheral nerve repair—Wallerian degeneration/growth cone. Oper Tech Orthop 2004;14:138–45.

182. Jerregård H. Factors influencing nerve growth in situ and in vitro. PhD thesis, Linköping University, 2001.

183. Chen Q, Chen TJ, Letourneau PC, et al. Modifier of cell adhesion regulates N-cadherin-mediated cell-cell adhesion and neurite outgrowth. J Neurosci 2005;25:281–90.

184. Sonnenberg A. Integrins and their ligands. Curr Top Microbiol Immunol 1993;184:7–35.

185. Agius E, Cochard P. Comparison of neurite outgrowth induced by intact and injured sciatic nerves: a confocal and functional analysis. J Neurosci 1998;18:328–38.

186. Zheng M, Kuffler DP. Guidance of regenerating motor axons in vivo by gradients of diffusible peripheral nerve-derived factors. J Neurobiol 2000;42:212–9.

187. Tuttle R, O'Leary DD. Neurotrophins rapidly modulate growth cone response to the axon guidance molecule, collapsin-1. Mol Cell Neurosci 1998;11:1–8.

188. Goodman CS. Mechanisms and molecules that control growth cone guidance. Annu Rev Neurosci 1996;19:341–77.

189. Kater SB, Rehder V. The sensory-motor role of growth cone filopodia. Curr Opin Neurobiol 1995;5:68–74.

190. Kolodkin AL. Growth cones and the cues that repel them. Trends Neurosci 1996;19:507–13.

191. Kuffler D. Promoting and directing axon outgrowth. Mol Neurobiol 1994;9:233–43.

192. Mueller BK. Growth cone guidance: first steps towards a deeper understanding. Annu Rev Neurosci 1999;22:351–88.

193. Tessier-Lavigne M, Goodman CS. The molecular biology of axon guidance. Science 1996;274:1123–33.

194. Kvist M, Danielsen N, Dahlin LB. Effects of FK506 on regeneration and macrophages in injured rat sciatic nerve. J Peripher Nerv Syst 2003;8:251–9.

195. Brushart TME. Trophic and tropic influences on peripheral nerve regeneration. In: Omer G, Spinner M, Van Beak A, eds., Management of Peripheral Nerve Problem. Philadelphia: W.B. Saunders, 1998:235–42.

196. Gordon T, Sulaiman O, Boyd JG. Experimental strategies to promote functional recovery after peripheral nerve injuries. J Peripher Nerv Syst 2003;8:236–50.

197. Dahlin LB, Lundborg G. Experimental nerve grafting—towards future solutions of a clinical problem. J Hand Surg 1998;3:165–73.

198. Doolabh V, Hertl MC, Mackinnon SE. The role of conduits in nerve repair: a review. Rev Neurosci 1996;7:47–84.

199. Millesi H, Meissl G, Berger A. The interfascicular nerve grafting of the median and ulnar nerve. J Bone Joint Surg Am 1972;54:727–50.

200. Almgren KG. Revascularization of free pheripheral nerve grafts. An experimental study in the rabbit. Acta Orthop Scand Suppl 1975;154:1–104.

201. Best TJ, Mackinnon SE, Midha R, et al. Revascularization of peripheral nerve autografts and allografts. Plast Reconstr Surg 1999;104:152–60.

202. Dahlin LB. Prevention of macrophage invasion impairs regeneration in nerve grafts. Brain Res 1995;679:274–80.

203. Kerns JM, Danielsen N, Holmquist B, et al. The influence of predegeneration on regeneration through peripheral nerve grafts in the rat. Exp Neurol 1993;122:28–36.

204. Nilsson A, Dahlin LB, Lundborg G, et al. Graft repair of a peripheral nerve without the sacrifice of a healthy donor nerve by the use of acutely dissociated autologous Schwann cells. Scand J Plast Rec Surg Hand Surg 2005;31:1–6.

205. Brandt J. Tendon Autografts for Bridging Nerve Defects. Malmö, Sweden: Department of Hand Surgery, PhD thesis, Lund University, 2002.

206. Koshima I, Harii K. Experimental studies on vascularized nerve grafts in rats. J Microsurg 1981;2:225–6.

207. Breidenbach W, Terzis JK. The anatomy of free vascularized nerve grafts. Clin Plast Surg 1984;11:65–71.

208. Scherman P, Kanje M, Dahlin LB. Local effects on triiodothyronine-treated polyglactin sutures on regeneration across peripheral nerve defects. Tissue Eng 2004;10:455–64.

209. Scherman P, Kanje M, Dahlin LB. Bridging short nerve defects by direct repair under tension, nerve grafts or longitudinal sutures. Restor Neurol Neurosci 2004;22:65–72.

210. Rempel D, Dahlin L, Lundborg G. Pathophysiology of nerve compression syndromes: response of peripheral nerves to loading. J Bone Joint Surg 1999;81:1600–10.

211. Dahlin LB, Rydevik B, McLean WG, et al. Changes in fast axonal transport during experimental nerve compression at low pressures. Exp Neurol 1984;84:29–36.

212. Weisl H, Osborne GV. The pathological changes in rats' nerves subject to moderate compression. J Bone Joint Surg 1964;46B:297–306.

213. MacKinnon SE, Dellon AL, Hudson AR, et al. Chronic nerve compression. An experimental model in the rat. Ann Plast Surg 1984;13:112–20.

214. Dahlin LB, Kanje M. Conditioning effect induced by chronic nerve compression. Scand J Plast Reconstr Surg Hand Surg 1992;26:37–41.

215. Gelberman RH, Hergenroeder PT, Hargens AR, et al. The carpal tunnel syndrome—a study of carpal canal pressure. J Bone Joint Surg Am 1981;63:380–3.

216. Luchetti R, Schoenhuber R, Nathan P. Correlation of segmental carpal tunnel pressures with changes in hand and wrist positions in patients with carpal tunnel syndrome and controls. J Hand Surg Br 1998;23:598–602.

217. Luchetti R, Schoenhuber R, Alfarano M, et al. Serial overnight recordings of intracarpal canal pressure in carpal tunnel syndrome patients with and without wrist splinting. J Hand Surg 1994;19B:35–7.

218. Rydevik B, Lundborg G, Bagge U. Effects of graded compression on intraneural blood flow. An in vitro study on rabbit tibial nerve. J Hand Surg Am 1981;6:3–12.

219. Matsumoto N. [Experimental study on compression neuropathy—determination of blood flow by a hydrogen washout technic]. Nippon Seikeigeka Gakkai Zasshi. J Jpn Orthop Assoc 1983;57:805–16.

220. Dahlin LB, Danielsen N, Ehira T, et al. Mechanical effects of compression of peripheral nerves. J Biochem Eng 1986;108:120–2.

221. Lundborg G, Gelberman RH, Minteer-Convery M, et al. Median nerve compression in the carpal tunnel—functional response to experimentally induced controlled pressure. J Hand Surg 1982;7:252–9.

222. Lundborg G, Myers R, Powell H. Nerve compression injury and increase in endoneurial fluid pressure: a miniature compartment syndrome. J Neurol Neurosurg Psychiatry 1983;46:1119–24.

223. Myers RR. Anatomy and microanatomy of peripheral nerve. Neurosurg Clin N Am 1991;2:1–20.

224. Gupta R, Rowshan K, Chao T, et al. Chronic nerve compression induces local demyelination and remyelination in a rat model of carpal tunnel syndrome. Exp Neurol 2004;187:500–8.

225. Gupta R, Steward O. Chronic nerve compression induces concurrent apoptosis and proliferation of Schwann cells. J Comp Neurol 2003;461:174–86.

226. Gupta R, Lin YM, Bui P, et al. Macrophage recruitment follows the pattern of inducible nitric oxide synthase expression in a model for carpal tunnel syndrome. J Neurotrauma 2003;20:671–80.

227. Isacsson A, Kanje M, Dahlin LB. Induction of activating transcription factor 3 (ATF3) by peripheral nerve compression. Scand J Plast Reconstr Surg Hand Surg 2005;39:65–72.

228. Powell HC, Myers RR. Pathology of experimental nerve compression. Lab Invest 1986;55:91–100.

229. Dahlin LB, Shyu BC, Danielsen N, et al. Effects of nerve compression or ischemia on conduction properties of myelinated and non-myelinated nerve fibres. An experimental study in the rabbit common peroneal nerve. Acta Physiol Scand 1989;136:97–105.

230. Shyu BC, Danielsen N, Andersson SA, et al. Effects of sympathetic stimulation on C-fibre response after peripheral nerve compression. An experimental study in the rabbit common peroneal nerve. Acta Physiol Scand 1990;140:237–43.

231. Dahlin LB, Sjostrand J, McLean WG. Graded inhibition of retrograde axonal transport by compression of rabbit vagus nerve. J Neurolog Sci 1986;76:221–30.

232. Dahlin LB, McLean WG. Effects of graded experimental compression on slow and fast axonal transport in rabbit vagus nerve. J Neurolog Sci 1986;72:19–30.

233. Dahlin LB, Archer DR, McLean WG. Axonal transport and morphological changes following nerve compression. An experimental study in the rabbit vagus nerve. J Hand Surg Br 1993;18:106–10.

234. Dahlin LB, Nordborg C, Lundborg G. Morphological changes in nerve cell bodies induced by experimental graded nerve compression. Exp Neurol 1987;95:611–21.

235. Pettersson LM, Dahlin LB, Danielsen N. Changes in expression of PACAP in rat sensory neurons in response to sciatic nerve compression. Eur J Neurosci 2004;20:1838–48.

236. Bergmark M, Kanje M, Widerberg A, et al. Experimental nerve compression and upregulation of CPON in DRG. Neuroreport 2001;12:3783–6.

237. Dahlin LB, Meiri KF, McLean WG, et al. Effects of nerve compression on fast axonal transport in streptozotocin-induced diabetes mellitus. Diabetologia 1986;29:181–5.

238. Dahlin LB, Archer DR, McLean WG. Treatment with an aldose reductase inhibitor can reduce the susceptibility of fast axonal transport following nerve compression in the streptozotocin-diabetic rat. Diabetologia 1987;30:414–8.

239. Dahlin LB, Stenberg L, Isacsson A, et al. Nerve compression induces nuclear translocation of the transcription factor ATF3 in sensory neurons and non-neuronal cells in healthy and diabetic rats. Society for Neuroscience, annual meetings, New Orleans, LA, Nov. 8–12, 2003.

240. Upton ARM, McComas AJ. The double crush in nerve entrapment syndromes. Lancet 1973;ii:359–62.

241. Dahlin LB, Lundborg G. The neurone and its response to peripheral nerve compression. J Hand Surg 1990;15B:5–10.

242. Wall JT, Kaas JH, Sur M, et al. Functional reorganization in somatosensory cortical areas 3b and 1 of adult monkeys after median nerve repair: possible relationships to sensory recovery in humans. The J Neuroscience 1986;6:218–33.

243. Merzenich MM, Jenkins WM. Reorganization of cortical representations of the hand following alterations of skin inputs induced by nerve injury, skin island transfers, and experience. J Hand Ther 1993;6:89–104.

244. Wall JT, Xu J, Wang X. Human brain plasticity: an emerging view of the multiple substrates and mechanisms that cause cortical changes and related sensory dysfunctions after injuries of sensory inputs from the body. Brain Res Brain Res Rev 2002;39:181–215.

245. Bjorkman A, Rosen B, Westen DV, et al. Acute improvement of contralateral hand function after deafferentation. Neuroreport 2004;15:1861–5.

246. Hansson T, Brismar T. Tactile stimulation of the hand causes bilateral cortical activation: a functional magnetic resonance study in humans. Neurosci Lett 1999;271:29–32.

247. Bodegård A, Geyer S, Naito E, et al. Somatosensory areas in man activated by moving stimuli. Neuroreport 2000;11:187–91.

248. Ehrsson HH, Fagergren A, Jonsson T, et al. Cortical activity in precision- versus power-grip tasks: an fMRI study. J Neurophysiol 2000;83:528–36.

249. Chen R, Cohen LG, Hallett M. Nervous system reorganization following injury. Neuroscience 2002;111:761–73.

250. Kaas J. Plasticity of sensory and motor maps in adult mammals. Ann Rev Neurosci 1991;14:137–68.

251. Johansson BB. Brain plasticity and stroke rehabilitation. The Willis Lecture. Stroke 2000;31:223–30.

252. Florence SL, Garraghty PE, Wall JT, et al. Sensory afferent projections and area 3b somatotopy following median nerve cut and repair in macaque monkeys. Cerebral Cortex 1994;4:391–407.

253. Florence S, Jain N, Pospichal M, et al. Central reorganization of sensory pathways following peripheral nerve regeneration in fetal monkeys. Nature 1996;381:69.

254. Florence SL, Boydston LA, Hackett TA, et al. Sensory enrichment after peripheral nerve injury restores cortical, not thalamic, receptive field organization. Eur J Neurosci 2001;13:1755–66.

255. Mano Y, Nakamuro T, Tamura R, et al. Central motor reorganization after anastomosis of the musculocutaneous and intercostal nerves following cervical root avulsion. Ann Neurol 1995;38:15–20.

256. Snider WD, Zhou FQ, Zhong J, et al. Signaling the pathway to regeneration. Neuron 2002;35:13–6.

2

Primary Nerve Repair

Michael E. Jabaley

INTRODUCTION

Over the past 50 to 75 years, the techniques of primary nerve suture have changed.[1] A better understanding of nerve healing and repair techniques, combined with technologic improvements in optics, instruments, and suture material, have combined to alter surgical approaches and methods of repairing the transected peripheral nerve. As a result, the definition of the ideal nerve repair and the aims of nerve suture today are far different from the objectives and definitions of the early 20th century. At the beginning of the 21st century, one might even observe that technology and modern suture techniques have progressed as far as they can and that, except for minor modifications, further progress in nerve repair will require entirely new approaches. These future advances may rely heavily on pharmaceuticals, electronics, robotics, and other currently untried techniques to identify and join nerve ends, and stimulate abundant axon regrowth to accurately selected distal targets. For the present, however, nerve repair remains largely a technical exercise, and surgeons must work diligently to maximize the effects of those factors within their control so as to offset the limitations in those areas that they cannot influence.

In the early 20th century and after World War I, the principal objective of nerve suture was physical union of the ends at almost any cost. As a result, such maneuvers as lengthy mobilizations, extreme joint flexion, "bulb suture," bone shortening, and the use of relatively large-diameter suture material were employed to bridge gaps and hold the ends together. There was little regard for tension at the repair site, and the outcome of nerve suture under these conditions was frequently disappointing.

World War II focused attention on timing of repair, techniques, and most importantly, on results. In-depth study of outcomes in thousands of war-wounded patients by the British and American governments offered new insights into those factors that affected outcome, and set the stage for the major advances of the next 4 to 5 decades that have brought us to our current state of understanding.

The goals of this chapter are to define primary nerve repair, discuss the timing of repair, and describe the anatomic terms that will be used in discussing repair techniques. For completeness, several types of repair will be described, but the emphasis will be on fascicular identification, alignment, and methods of maintaining coaptation with little or no tension. For completeness, current practices that introduce newer variations and methods will be noted.

Primary nerve repair is defined as nerve suture performed immediately after or within the first several days following injury. The concept of a several day window of time for repair is important, for it affords the surgeon the option of selecting the time of repair, a luxury in keeping with the importance of the procedure. Because nerve suture is one of the most sophisticated and demanding reconstructive procedures that surgeons perform, it should be carried out under ideal conditions whenever possible.

Timing. From a practical standpoint, primary repair can be performed either on an emergency basis immediately after the injury is diagnosed or as a semi-elective procedure within the first several days. This latter is referred to as a delayed primary repair. In either case, repair is carried out during the first phase of wound healing (inflammatory phase). The common factor is that it is performed in the absence of scarring, and in a wound that heals primarily and does not suppurate.

A typical scenario is when a patient is seen in an emergency room or primary care setting, the diagnosis is made, the wound is cleansed (and possibly sutured), and the patient is referred for treatment. If the surgeon concurs in the diagnosis, elective repair can be scheduled. It matters little whether the wound has been sutured or not. So long as the edges can still be separated easily with a hemostat, the repair can be classified as primary. The significance of all this is that there is no visible collagen (scar) in the wound and the nerve has neither retracted nor fibrosed. It can still be drawn out to its original length and direct suture is possible. If the injury results from a sharp transection, the nerve ends need not be re-cut to perform a repair. If they are ragged or crushed, they should be trimmed appropriately. The space created by the nerve's natural recoil plus the length of nerve that has been damaged or may be excised constitutes the *nerve gap*. The tension required to overcome this gap determines whether the transected ends can be approximated.

It is helpful to distinguish between immediate and delayed primary repair. The latter offers several advantages. The patient can be counseled and advised about the nature of the injury and the proposed treatment. The procedure can be performed when it is logistically advantageous and the anesthetic of choice can be selected. Bleeding has usually stopped, and nonviable muscle can be better detected and excised. The threat of infection should be less. Finally, the nerve cell has begun to mobilize those factors and undergo those changes that result in axon regeneration.

PERTINENT ANATOMY

The microanatomy of peripheral nerves has been clearly described and is well understood.[2,3] A nerve is always under slight tension and this causes the ends to retract when it has been transected. This elasticity may not be easily overcome when one tries to rejoin nerve ends with microsuture and may sometimes frustrate the microsurgeon.

For surgical purposes, a nerve can be divided into two easily visible components: the fascicles and the epineurium (Fig. 2–1). The fascicles contain the axons and their Schwann cell sheaths. Axons may or may not be myelinated, and they are surrounded by the endoneurium. Each fascicle is bounded by the perineurium, which is a tough lamellar structure that serves several functions. It is a diffusion barrier that maintains the internal environment of the fascicle. Pressure within the perineurium is 1 to 2 mm Hg greater than the outside tissue, and accounts for the phenomenon of "mushrooming" when a fascicle is transected.

The location of fascicles varies somewhat within a nerve, and there are cross-connections between them as fibers migrate from one fascicle to another.[4] These connections can easily be seen with the aid of magnification. This migration of fibers occurs because fibers destined for a specific branch or function may arise at more than one level of the spinal cord. As fibers proceed distally, an inevitable sorting and rearranging is required to ultimately form a branch. This effect is more pronounced in the proximal limb than in those portions nearer the final target areas. Damage to the perineurium (as in passing a suture through it) renders axons nonfunctional, and should be avoided when possible.

Outside the fascicles is the epineurium, both internal or external. It is looser in nature, contains collagen and larger blood vessels, and provides structural integrity to the nerve. Sunderland showed that the amount of epineurium varies throughout a nerve, and is generally greater around joints. Epineurium, both internal and external, is the surgical plane of dissection within a nerve. Its surgical significance is that it can be can be incised, excised, or otherwise dissected, and it can be sutured without harm to fascicles so long as

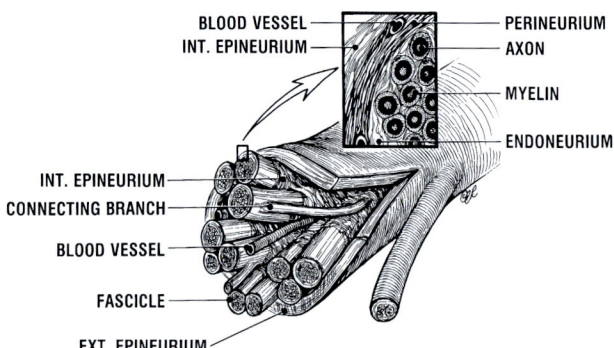

Figure 2–1 Anatomy of a peripheral nerve. The epineurium is divided into internal and external epineurium, and is the plane of dissection. It contains blood vessels and serves a nutritional as well as a structural role in the nerve. Individual fascicles are bounded by the perineurium and contain the conducting portion of the nerve (axons). There may be connecting branches between the fascicles. These and the perineurium should not be injured during the dissection. (From Jabaley ME. Modified techniques of nerve repair: epineurial splint. In: Gelberman RH, ed., Operative Nerve Repair and Reconstruction. Philadelphia: J.B. Lippincott, 1991:315–26,[14] with permission.)

interfascicular connections are recognized and protected. If the perineurium is not violated during dissection, axons contained therein can be expected to regrow and eventually to recover function. A number of studies have shown dissection distances for specific branches of nerves, and these can be helpful to the surgeon in trying to decipher the functional makeup of a nerve.[4–6]

These techniques of dissection permit one to separate and identify fascicles for later repair. Interestingly, epineurium is both the source of strength between the united ends and the source of fibroblasts and eventual scarring at the site of juncture. If nerve ends are joined with sutures, epineurium, whether external or internal, is the structure in which they should be placed. Since it is also the source of fibroblasts and collagen that form the scar bridge across which regenerating axons must cross, repair techniques must take its disposition into account.

PERTINENT PHYSIOLOGY

Nerve cells, their response to injury, and subsequent repair are unique in many respects.[7] The cell body resides in the spinal cord or dorsal root ganglia, while axons and accompanying Schwann cell apparatus stretch out to the periphery. The axon may comprise over 90% of the entire nerve cell volume, since it stretches from the cell all the way to the periphery. When transected, the process of Wallerian degeneration begins immediately, affecting both the cell body and peripheral axons. Although studies in recent years have described agents that may retard the process of degeneration, to date the only thing available clinically that directly influences this process is regenerating axons. There is a direct correlation between the degree of degeneration and the time interval between injury and repair. As distal microtubules collapse and myelin is absorbed, regenerating axons are impeded. The surgical implication of this phenomenon is obvious: *repair should be carried out as soon as it is safely possible.*

The pressure within a fascicle has been measured and is 1 to 2 mm Hg. When a nerve is cut, an immediate bulging or "mushrooming" at the cut end occurs. For this reason, it may sometimes be necessary to trim away this mushroom cap to perform a satisfactory nerve suture. Individual fascicles can be easily trimmed with microscissors to improve coaptation.

Histologic examination of the proximal ends of nerves within a few hours after transection shows axon sprouting and growth cones. Many of these growth cones enter the endoneurial tubes and ultimately reach the peripheral targets while others are pruned away. Successful nerve repair requires that as many axons as possible complete the process of regrowth. Since the surgeon has no hope of correctly aligning individual

TABLE 2–1
The Ideal Nerve Repair
1. Performed primarily, either immediate or delayed.
2. Well-vascularized bed with little or no scarring.
3. Viable nerve ends.
4. No hematoma.
5. Accurate fascicular alignment.
6. Fewest number of stitches, placed in epineurium.
7. Minimal tension.
8. Minimal or moderate joint flexion.

nerve fibers, the best that he or she can hope for is that fascicles can be accurately joined, and that all efforts should be directed toward forming this juncture.

One can envision the *milieu* that would provide the best opportunity for successful nerve regeneration (Table 2–1). It would be a bed of viable well-vascularized tissue, free of debris or foreign bodies. The nerve ends themselves would be viable, unscarred, and well vascularized. They should meet without undue tension, and the fascicular pattern of each nerve end should match. The ends should coapt, and this coaptation should be held with the fewest number of sutures, correctly placed in either the external or internal epineurium. Lastly, this should be accomplished without undue flexion of joints.

INDICATIONS

Candidates for nerve repair are identified by the circumstances of the injury. A patient with a previously normal nervous system who develops a motor or sensory nerve deficit after an injury should be presumed to have a nerve injury. Age and poor health are rarely contraindications to nerve repair, since the anesthetic and postoperative care are relatively uncomplicated, but the results of surgery are better in childhood and adolescence than in later life.

The principal indication for surgery is a wound with a nerve deficit that does not recover within 1 to 2 days (in low-velocity gunshot wounds, temporary nerve deficits are not uncommon, but these frequently recover quickly). Furthermore, if a wound is surgically explored and the patient has a nerve deficit, the status of the nerve should be clarified before wound closure and then addressed at a later date (Fig. 2–2).

Nerves can only be cut, crushed, or stretched, although injuries frequently combine these factors. Whichever mechanism produces the nerve wound plus whatever other trauma has occurred directly to the nerve determines whether the nerve can be sutured immediately or after a delay.

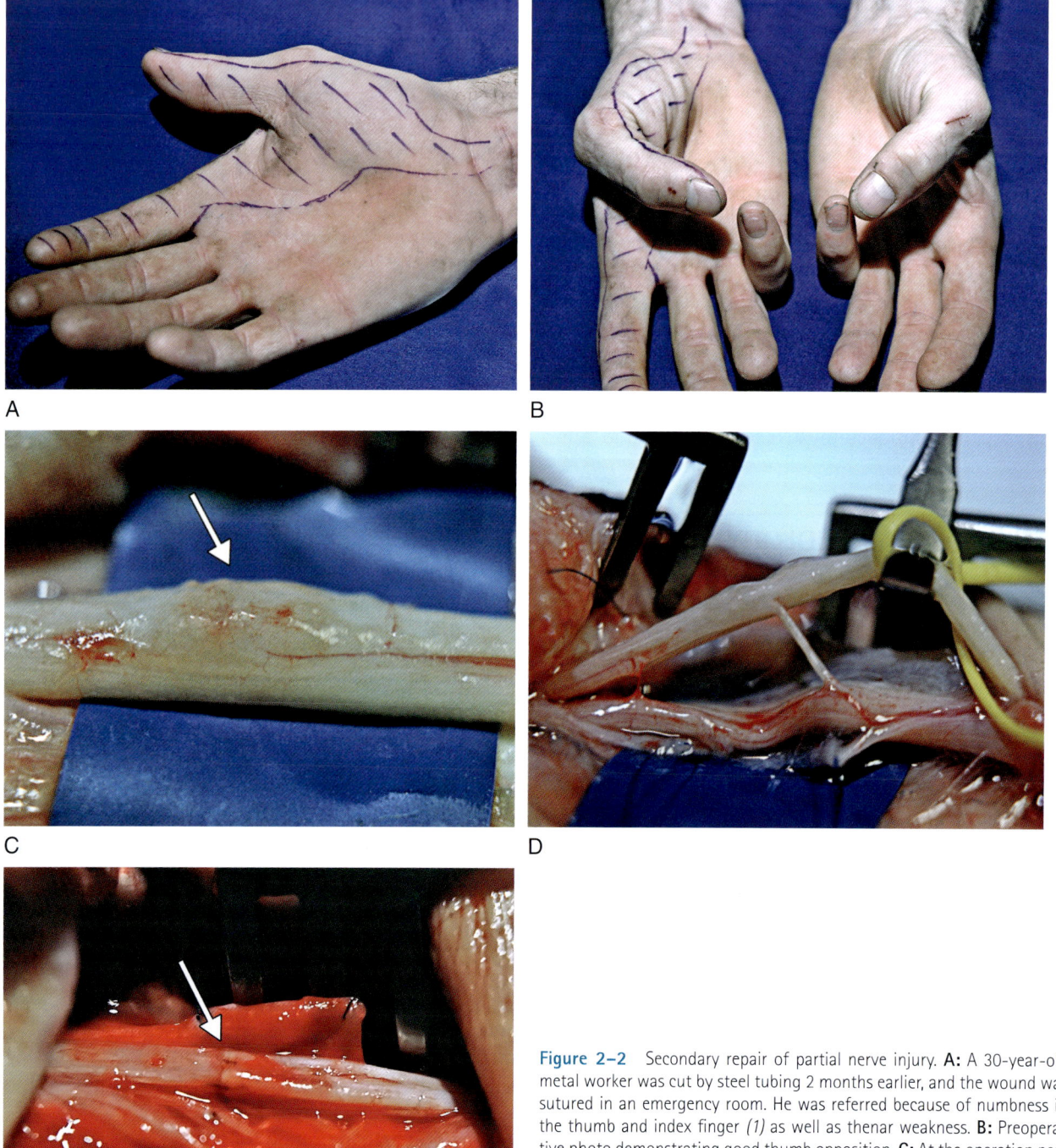

Figure 2–2   Secondary repair of partial nerve injury. **A:** A 30-year-old metal worker was cut by steel tubing 2 months earlier, and the wound was sutured in an emergency room. He was referred because of numbness in the thumb and index finger *(1)* as well as thenar weakness. **B:** Preoperative photo demonstrating good thumb opposition. **C:** At the operation performed with intravenous Lidocaine, scar and neuroma formation within the intact nerve could be seen and an incomplete lesion diagnosed. **D:** An awake stimulation verified function in the intact ulnar portion, and confirmed identification of proximal sensory and motor fascicles. **E:** General anesthesia was then administered to permit interfascicular repair of transected fascicles with 10-0 nylon.

If the wound is tidy and the nerve sharply transected (e.g., sharp objects like glass, knife, or razor), one may proceed to immediate suture (Fig. 2–3 A to H). Similarly, if untidy nerve ends can be trimmed and converted to a more satisfactory condition, direct suture can and should still be performed (Fig. 2–4 A to C). It is only when there is a major area of crushed (e.g., a punch press) or stretched (major joint dislocation or high-velocity missile) nerve over an unknown distance that one should consider wound debridement, cleansing, and waiting a few days to reassess the nerve before carrying out repair. This approach of staged repair has

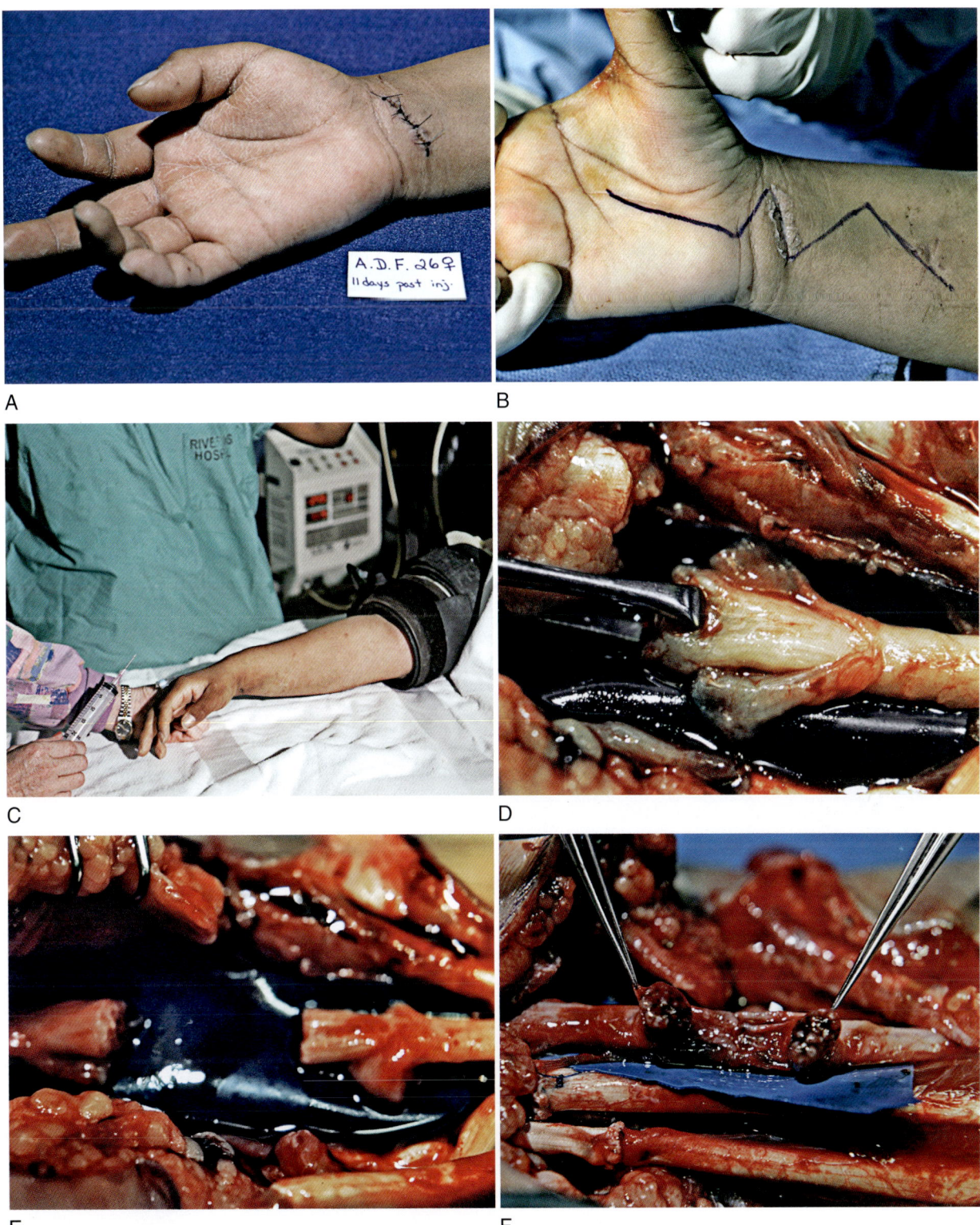

Figure 2–3 Secondary repair median nerve, seven flexor tendons. **A:** A 26-year-old woman was referred 11 days after a wrist laceration because of numbness and loss of flexion in the thumb, index, and long fingers. **B:** Surgical approach for median nerve exposure. **C:** At the operation 17 days after injury, an intravenous Lidocaine block was performed. **D:** The epineurium was trimmed back and the developing neuroma excised. **E:** Freshened nerve ends are visible. **F:** Epineurial splint has been constructed.

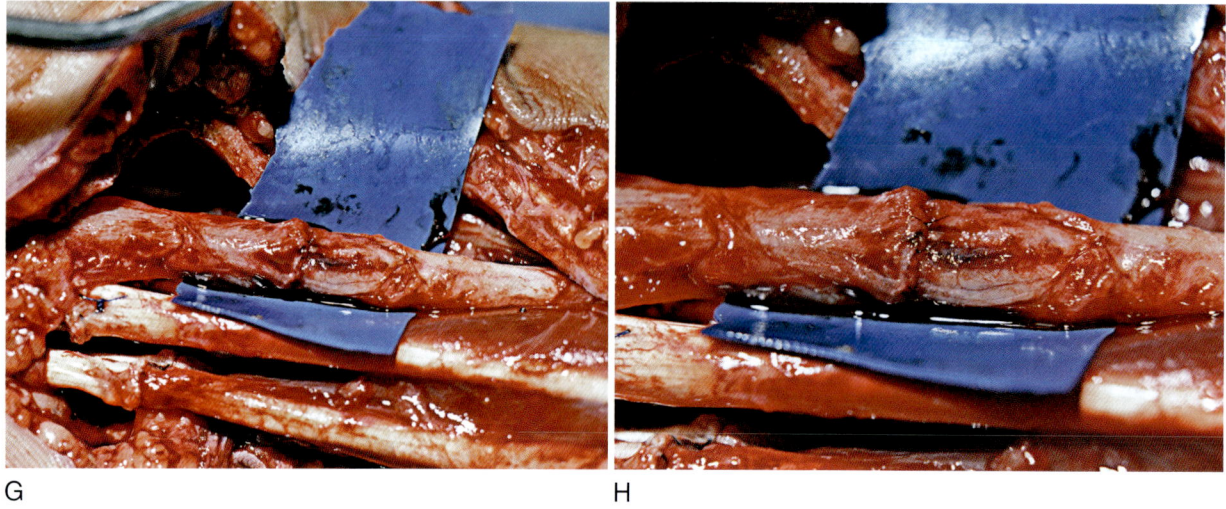

G   H

Figure 2–3—Cont'd **G:** Nerve fascicles are allowed to fall together. **H:** Fascicles will then be sutured using interfascicular technique.

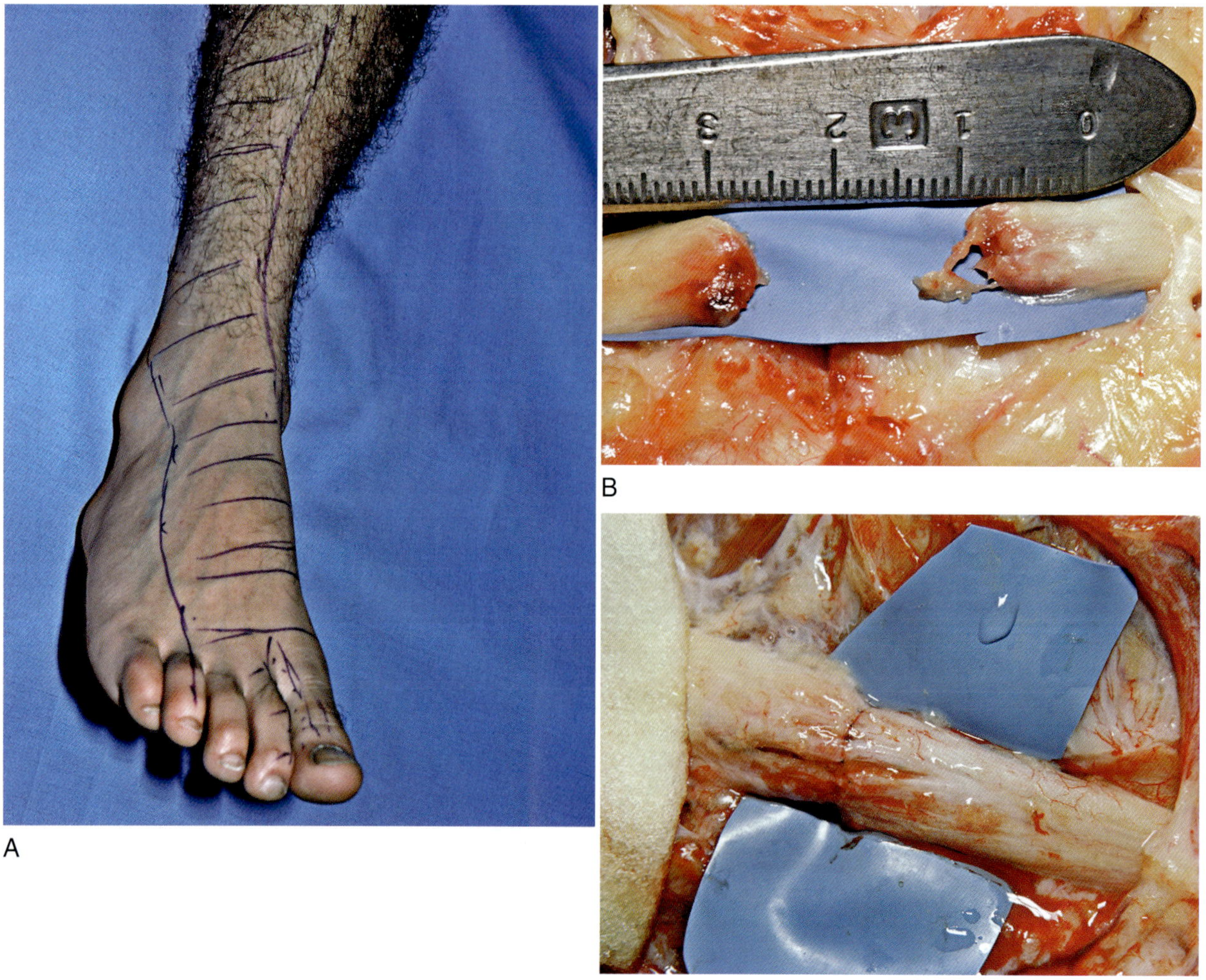

A

B

C

Figure 2–4   Delayed primary repair. **A:** A 20-year-old college student transected the superficial peroneal nerve while running through a dorm. Numbness in the lower leg and foot was evident at examination. **B:** Nerve gap of approximately 2.0 cm results from elastic contracture. Gap increased to 3.0 cm with trimming. **C:** This was easily overcome with epineurial splint technique (Fig. 2–7). (From Jabaley ME. Modified techniques of nerve repair: epineurial splint. In: Gelberman RH, ed., Operative Nerve Repair and Reconstruction. Philadelphia: J.B. Lippincott, 1991:315–26,[14] with permission.)

proven successful in past wars, and is equally applicable in civilian injuries.

Wound contamination also affects the timing of repair. Blast injuries that are heavily impregnated with debris or bacteria are better treated by staged reconstruction. This approach may include one or more debridements in the operating room. Nerves should not be repaired until the wound can be sutured with a reasonable expectation that it will heal without suppuration. Nerve repair in an infected wound is doomed to failure.

Not surprisingly, there are few absolute contraindications to primary nerve repair, but some of the relative contraindications mentioned above should be emphasized. The nature of a wound—particularly as affected by contamination and muscle of questionable viability—may stay the surgeon's hand and lead him to a delayed primary repair. Similarly, if the degree of the longitudinal injury cannot be determined, it may be best to delay. If the history suggests a long area of stretch, or if the crush extends for several centimeters away from a transection, definitive nerve suture is best deferred. It is an exercise in futility to sew nerve ends of questionable viability and have the repair fail. Unfortunately, there is no reliable test at this time to determine whether crushed or stretched nerve has the capacity to regenerate.

SURGICAL TECHNIQUE

At its heart, nerve repair is nothing more than the exercise of sound surgical principles, but certain aspects are relatively unique and bear emphasis.

Microsurgical Technique

Accurate analysis of a nerve end requires appropriate magnification. Fortunately, high-quality operating microscopes are available in most operating suites and they should be used. Highest magnifications work best for nerve inspection and fascicular alignment, whereas minimum magnifications of 4 to 5× are sufficient for accurate suture placement and tying. Zoom capability allows the surgeon to move up and down in magnification with more precision.

Microsurgical instruments are very much the surgeon's choice. I find straight and curved needle holders, relatively short (about 10 cm in length) and without a lock to be most comfortable for hand and extremity work. A variety of jeweler's forceps complete the list of most frequently used instruments. Microsuture of high quality is readily available in most operating rooms. Nylon remains the standard and is swaged onto tapered or tapercut needles. Suture diameters range from 9-0 to 11-0. The latter is relatively difficult

to manipulate and is reserved for special situations. Spatula-tipped needles may be useful in secondary procedures where there is epineurial thickening or scarring, but they are relatively traumatic in the freshly-cut nerve. For this reason, I prefer a tapercut needle.

Anesthesia

For major nerve repair or repair in conjunction with injuries to other structures, general anesthesia is preferred. Modern anesthetic agents and monitoring equipment have reduced the likelihood of error to such a low degree that many surgeons rarely, if ever, use axillary or supraclavicular blocks.

If electrical stimulation is planned, paralyzing agents must be avoided. If one does not wish to use a general anesthetic, intravenous lidocaine is an excellent technique and may be employed instead. The nerve ends can be quickly identified and the wound infiltrated with local anesthetic and the tourniquet deflated. One may then proceed directly to fascicular identification and repair. Lastly, local infiltration can be used for repair of digital nerves or other procedures of this magnitude.

What one should avoid is the situation where fractures have been fixed or tendons repaired using a block that then wears off or the patient becomes restless just as the nerve repair is begun. Nerve suture in a writhing and awake patient will quickly make one a disciple of general anesthesia.

Tourniquet

A cuff, whether inflated or not, should be in place for all nerve repairs. If the injury is in the upper arm, a sterile cuff can be placed higher and toward the axilla, thereby adding several centimeters of possible proximal exposure.

If the cuff is to be inflated, it should only be to the lowest pressure that stops blood flow, usually in the range of systolic pressure plus 100 to 125 mm Hg. There is a tendency among surgeons to set tourniquet pressure at a level that is higher than necessary. Tourniquet pressure is as important as tourniquet time in avoiding nerve injury but, unfortunately, is less emphasized in most operating rooms. If nerve repair is performed in conjunction with other procedures, such as tendon and bone work, the tourniquet can usually be deflated during some portions, thereby limiting the duration of tourniquet inflation.

Wound Cleansing

Once satisfactory anesthesia is achieved, local cleansing begins. The tourniquet may or may not be inflated for this portion. All the skin surrounding the wound should be manually scrubbed with a surgical brush to remove the inevitable dirt and debris often associated with accidental wounds. Once skin cleansing is complete, the wound itself can be scrubbed with gauze sponges or irrigated with pressure but using only sterile saline to which weak topical antibiotic has been added. These techniques will rid the raw surfaces of foreign body and debris, but they do not remove contaminated material impregnated deep in soft tissue. For this, there is no substitute for surgical excision, and it should be performed next.

Incisions

The surgeon should be prepared to extend wounds proximally and distally where necessary to identify vital structures in uninjured tissue. This means that extremities should be widely prepped and draped. This is quicker and usually easier than searching for nerve ends in a bloodstained wound. Such extensions of incisions should follow physiologic lines to protect the viability of skin and subcutaneous tissue and to avoid later contractures or troublesome scars. Where possible, incisions should be designed so that they cross the paths of nerves and arteries diagonally. In this way, repairs are overlain by viable flaps of skin and fat rather than directly connected to skin scars.

Wound Toileting and Debridement

The purpose of wound extension and subsequent cleansing is to convert a contaminated wound to a surgically clean one. Once mechanical scrubbing and/or pressure irrigation are completed, the surgeon must assess the wound for dead tissue or other contaminated material. If these are present, one must resort to surgical excision (debridement) for their removal. Techniques vary, but scissors are my choice for excising soft tissue of questionable viability. This procedure still requires surgical boldness, and one should not hesitate to perform an adequate excision.

Fascicular Identification

Many types of sophisticated equipment are available for intraoperative nerve stimulation and assessment in the acute case, and these can be useful in identifying specific motor and sensory branches. At the simplest, one can use disposable stimulators. Most operating suites have stimulators which permit the operator to vary the intensity and pulse duration of a stimulus, a must for awake stimulation. In recent years, more elaborate models with computer-assisted stimulators and recording devices have appeared, and these greatly enhance the surgeon's capabilities to measure and record responses. In principle, however, all these techniques for studying the transected nerve in the acute situation rely on the patient's ability either to perceive a stimulus applied to the cut proximal end of the nerve or to generate a motor response when stimulating the distal end.

Fascicular identification can be carried out at various times by different techniques, depending on the timing and circumstances. In the first few days after injury, direct electrical stimulation of distal motor fascicles will elicit a response and can be helpful in identifying motor bundles. After 3 to 5 days, this response disappears and the technique is no longer applicable. Awake stimulation, however, a technique whereby proximal fascicles are excited by low-voltage stimulation can still be employed[8–10] (Figs. 2–2 and 2–4). Using this technique, the cooperative patient can identify proximal sensory fascicles with considerable accuracy. In immediate repairs, either or both of these two techniques can be applied.

Once the distal response has been lost, the surgeon must rely on other techniques to identify motor fascicles. At appropriate levels, such as the terminal portions of the ulnar and median nerves, distal motor branches can be dissected directly from the main trunk and positively identified. This requires a knowledge of dissection distances for each such branch in order not to transect fibers crossing from one fascicle to another. Alternatively, the cross-sectional maps of Sunderland can be used because specific fascicles can be localized to an individual quadrant of a nerve and will retain that general location over a considerable distance. The Sunderland maps trace the fibers of each branch of major nerves through the entire extremity. The appearance of fascicles may change at a specific level, but their functional location remains more consistent, allowing the surgeon to make an educated guess about alignment.

Over the years, many attempts have been made to use histologic techniques to identify fascicles. All of these involve harvesting sections for analysis and time delay. They have not been widely accepted, and I have no experience with them.

If the wound conditions permit primary repair and positive fascicular identification can be made, the surgeon can proceed with the actual nerve suture. This consists in principle of the four steps outlined by Millesi and Terzis[11]: (1) preparation of the nerve stumps, (2) approximation of the ends, (3) coaptation of the ends, and (4) maintenance of the coaptation.

SURGICAL TECHNIQUE

Preparation of the Stumps

This step involves inspection and trimming of the nerve stumps. For successful recovery of function, it is most important that nerve ends be viable and capable of regeneration. The history of the injury and visual examination are the guides to suitability of nerve ends for repair, but magnification is also important in making this assessment. Trimmed fascicles should be of the same length, but it is unnecessary to trim away the mushrooming that normally occurs from the cut end of a nerve. As noted earlier, this results from the positive pressure within the fascicle and it will recur despite trimming the fascicle ends.

Approximation of the Ends

The surgeon must estimate the gap created by the natural elastic retraction of the nerve plus whatever lengths of nerve have been destroyed by the injury or resected by the surgeon. This is the true distance that must be overcome by nerve suture. In the process of approximation, tension is created which must be overcome and will directly affect the scar interface which forms as the nerve ends heal. If tension is deemed marginal, modest joint flexion may be sufficient to overcome it, but if it is excessive, alternative methods of union must be considered.

By dissecting the nerve from its bed, grasping each end with forceps, and manipulating adjacent joints, one can make a determination of whether the nerve ends can be satisfactorily joined by suture. Unfortunately, no hard and fast rules can be offered as to how much tension is too much. Some surgeons feel that gaps of up to 2.5 cm in a major forearm nerve can be overcome. Others have stated that repairs that can be held with microsuture are under acceptable tension. The ultimate decision as to what is acceptable falls to the surgeon's judgment. In my opinion, if the repair site lies comfortably with only modest joint flexion, tension is not excessive.

In *coaptation,* the surgeon must also examine the cut ends and determine how they should be matched. This is a critically important step in repair, especially in mixed motor and sensory nerves. As noted earlier, electrical stimulation can be helpful when identifying fascicles and can be applied in both immediate or delayed primary repairs. Before beginning the actual nerve suture, it is helpful to make a drawing of each end and note those fascicles or groups to be joined. A temporary suture for orientation may also be placed in the epineurium of each nerve end.

Maintenance of the Coaptation

In most instances, coaptation is maintained by individual stitches. Although tube repairs either with autogenous vein or synthetic materials have been described and can be successful, they are relatively new and are not in general use today. If tube repairs prove to yield results that are comparable to nerve suture, they offer decided advantages since there is less tension and fewer technical errors.

For most repairs, the surgeon should be prepared to join the nerve ends with a nonreactive suture of appropriate caliber. My choices are 9-0 or 10-0 monofilament nylon, on a 75- to 100-micron tapercut needle. The principal objective of these sutures is to maintain the alignment, not to hold the nerve ends together. For this reason, the nerve juncture must be protected during healing to prevent disruption (see external epineurial splint). Traditionally, repairs have been protected for at least 3 weeks. I have found that a splint that limits extension (for a repair on the flexor surface) may permit a measure of further flexion, thereby making further rehabilitation simpler.

In the past, authors have described several techniques of nerve suture, each advocating one or another form and location of suture placement.[12] It should be obvious from these remarks that suture placement is less important than respect for underlying principles. With an understanding of these principles, the surgeon should have an armamentarium which includes all of the techniques of nerve suture. Several of these will be described with suggestions as to when they might be employed.

TECHNIQUES OF NERVE SUTURE

External Epineurial Suture

This technique is sufficient for nerves of one or two fascicles, such as digital nerves. Here, the fascicles make up a large percentage of the cross-sectional area and matching is not a problem. A few well-placed sutures in the external epineurium will maintain alignment of major fascicles one to another and such sutures can be easily placed in the external epineurium. Because one typically uses only a few sutures, modest joint flexion only is necessary to avoid undue tension and distraction of the repair during the healing phase.

Perineurial Suture

This technique is mentioned only to emphasize that it is rarely used. Sutures passed through the perineurium will likely injure nerve fibers in that area of the fascicle and are best avoided except in situations where no other alternative exists. Although perineurial suture repairs have been described, they have enjoyed little popularity and are rarely employed. This is largely due to the tedious nature of their placement and the time required. When epineurium has been trimmed away, however, there may be no other tissue in which to place sutures and perineurium becomes the only choice. If this is so, every effort should be made to grasp only the outer portion of perineurium and protect the endoneurium and axons.

Group Fascicular Suture

Transected nerves with a larger number of fascicles are candidates for group fascicular repair, and this technique is the most frequently used in major mixed nerves of the forearm and arm. In these nerves, the amount of internal epineurium is greater and fascicular grouping more complex. Here, it is especially important to identify the motor components for separate repair. For a group fascicular repair, one examines each cut end of the nerve and selects groups of fascicles to be sutured. In a major nerve such as the median or ulnar, four or five groups may be chosen for suture. These are then matched appropriately with the opposite end and the approximation is held by the placement of sutures in the internal epineurium, external epineurium, or some combination thereof. If group fascicular suturing is performed, it is unnecessary to buttress the repair with additional external epineurial sutures.

External Epineurial Splint

Because of the elastic recoil of cut nerve ends, it is sometimes frustrating and difficult to hold the approximation while individual small caliber sutures are placed. Nerve holding devices have been described for this task and can be helpful if they are available. Similar to vessel approximators, these devices transfix the nerve ends with small needles which pierce the external epineurium and slide along a bar, allowing the ends to move toward each other. They must be removed at the completion of the procedure, of course.

Another technique which can be employed uses the external epineurium as a splinting device.[13,14] This method takes advantage of the engineering principle described by Saint Vernant (Fig. 2–5). The principle basically states that sutures placed at least 1-1/2 nerve diameters away from the cut end will relieve tension on the ends, allowing the surgeon to place a number of small sutures in the internal epineurium to maintain the coaptation. The late Kenya Tsuge described a "suture at a distance" technique to accomplish this end[15] (Fig. 2–6). Rather than using sutures to accomplish this, however, the external epineurium can be left attached and its free ends joined by suture to form a "splint." In this way, tension is transferred away from the cut end and fascicles easily and precisely joined.

The *technique* follows. If necessary, the nerve ends are trimmed appropriately prior to suture. If it appears that a direct suture can be performed without excessive tension, the external epineurium is incised longitudinally on its superficial surface and dissected away (but not discarded) from the underlying fascicles, either with

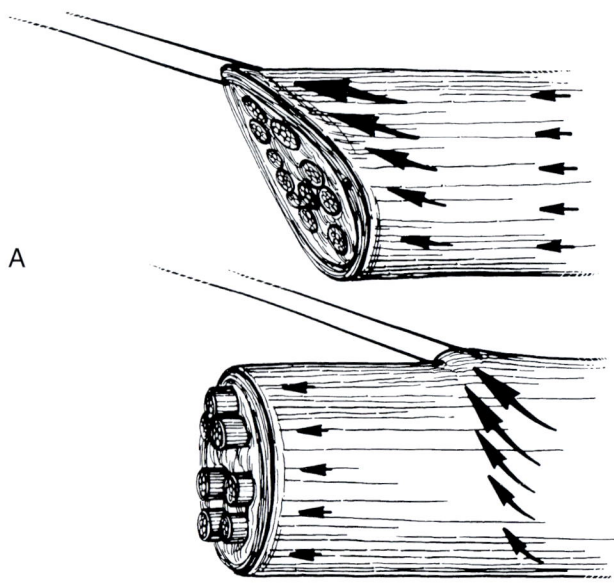

A

B

Figure 2–5 The principles of St. Vernant (modified). A suture placed at the end of a nerve **(A)** produces uneven tension, and is difficult to place and hold during repair. If placed at least 1-1/2 diameters from the cut end, the tension is evenly distributed, permitting a tension-free juncture of fascicles **(B)**. (From Jabaley ME. Modified techniques of nerve repair: epineurial splint. In: Gelberman RH, ed., Operative Nerve Repair and Reconstruction. Philadelphia: J.B. Lippincott, 1991:315–26,[14] with permission.)

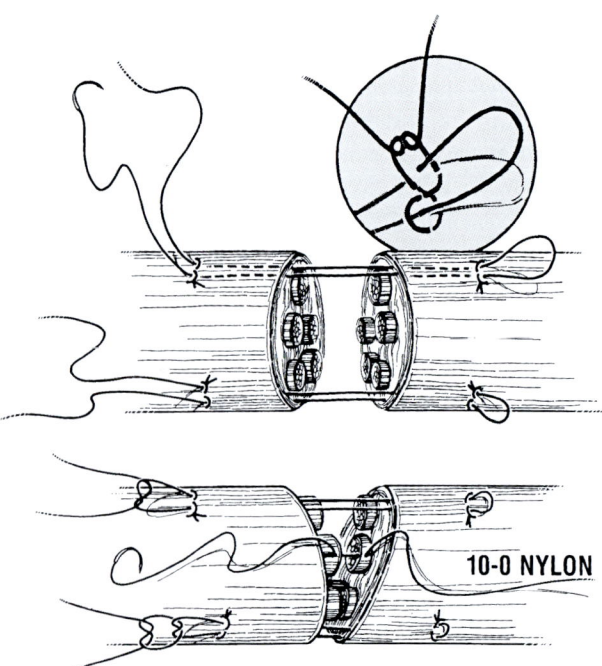

10-0 NYLON

Figure 2–6 The Tsuge "suture at a distance." This method employs the same technique as the Tsuge tendon repair. Tension is relieved by external epineurial sutures placed at a distance from the cut ends **(top)**. Pullout sutures of 10-0 nylon placed through fascicles may be difficult to remove and harmful to axons **(bottom)**. (From Jabaley ME. Modified techniques of nerve repair: epineurial splint. In: Gelberman RH, ed., Operative Nerve Repair and Reconstruction. Philadelphia: J.B. Lippincott, 1991:315–26,[14] with permission.)

knife or scissors. This maneuver is analogous to "peeling a banana" (Fig. 2–7 A to C).

The epineurium is left attached on the deep surface, several millimeters from each nerve end. By grasping the free ends of these strips of external epineurium, the surgeon can then quickly determine whether the ends will meet satisfactorily. If they do, a few interrupted sutures of 8-0 nylon can be placed to join the ends of the external epineurial strips *on the deep surface only, completing the construction of the "splint."* This maneuver relieves tension on the nerve ends, which now abut easily against each other. The surgeon can approximate individual fascicles or groups of fascicles which have been previously selected for repair with little or no tension.

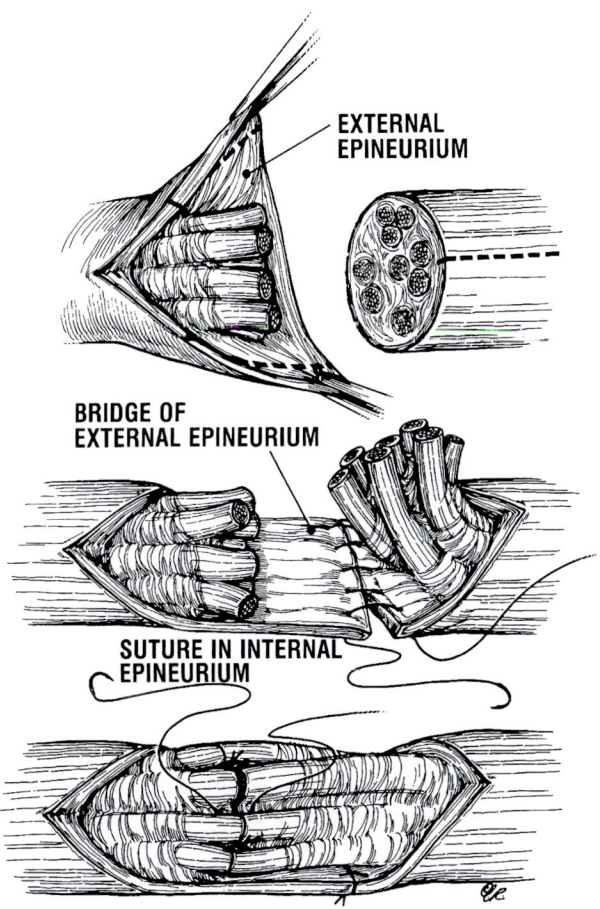

EXTERNAL EPINEURIUM

BRIDGE OF EXTERNAL EPINEURIUM

SUTURE IN INTERNAL EPINEURIUM

Figure 2–7 The epineurial splint technique **(top).** The external epineurium is incised longitudinally and peeled back but not removed **(top)** to expose the individual fascicles **(middle).** External epineurium is joined on the deep surface of the nerve with 8-0 nylon sutures to relieve tension and allow fascicle ends to fall together **(bottom).** Fascicles are then aligned and the coaptation maintained with 9-0 or 10-0 sutures placed in the internal epineurium. (From Jabaley ME. Modified techniques of nerve repair: epineurial splint. In: Gelberman RH, ed., Operative Nerve Repair and Reconstruction. Philadelphia: J.B. Lippincott, 1991:315–26,[14] with permission.)

It is important to note that no effort is made to close the epineurium around the entire circumference of the nerve. The superficial surface is specifically left open and devoid of external epineurium. In this way, the surgeon can inspect the final coaptation and make certain that is satisfactory.

Once the repair is complete and prior to wound closure, the surgeon should visually inspect the repair site as adjacent joints are placed in various degrees of flexion and extension. In this way, a position can be selected which allows the repair site to lie comfortably without excessive tension. The wound is then closed in whatever manner the surgeon chooses. If a subcutaneous layer is present, it is helpful to approximate it with a few sutures to interpose a layer of fat between the nerve repair and skin scar. Drains are rarely necessary.

In most instances, external splintage with plaster is sufficient to maintain the coaptation, but children may require casting. The position of joints is usually not changed for the first 3 weeks. At that time, joint mobilization can be begun with no precautions other than to avoid immediate hyperextension. In some respects, nerve repairs behave like tendon repairs relative to surrounding structures, that is, they glide freely in some areas but are more likely to adhere against bone or fascia in other areas. Repairs in synovial tissue or surrounded by muscle are less likely to adhere and can be mobilized more easily. The importance of nerve gliding following repair has been stressed by Wilgis[15a] and others and plays an important role in the ultimate result. Gliding exercises can be part of the postoperative routine.

CONTROVERSIES

With the availability of operating microscopes and microsuture, there came controversy about techniques of repair. Some authors recommended discarding external epineurial suture as inadequate, and advocated suturing fascicular groups and even individual fascicles instead. More recently, these arguments have largely dissipated and the principles have become clearer. The factors that influence the outcome of nerve repair are gentle handling of nerve ends, assurance of viability, and accurate placement of sutures that do not damage the perineurium or the structures within it. Specifically, sutures are not placed in the endoneurium or through the perineurium but in the epineurium, either internal, external, or in combination. It is also important that fascicle ends not overlap or gap excessively. If a particular fascicle appears too long, it should be shortened. Regardless of the technique selected, the repair must be performed without excessive tension.

When tension seems excessive, the surgeon is left with no alternative except to bridge the resultant defect with nerve grafts (see Chapter 3). Although nerve grafting introduces several variables (limited availability of donor nerve, two sutures lines instead of one, additional operating time, additional foreign body, and numbness at the donor site), its advantages far outweigh the disadvantages of a repair between nonviable ends or one with excessive tension. One should have no misgivings about turning to a nerve graft when direct suture violates the principles which have been outlined. The results of grafting are clearly better than those of a repair under improper circumstances.

The role of conduit (or tubes) is still being examined.[16] Autogenous veins and a variety of synthetic absorbable conduits have been described and are now available. The literature suggests that short gaps in small nerves of the hand and fingers may be treated as effectively with tubes as with direct suture or nerve graft. If this is so, conduits offer clear benefits from the standpoint of postoperative positioning and mobilization. If regeneration through a tube is equally good, this technique may be preferable to repair by more traditional techniques.

In larger nerves, such as the major forearm or upper arm nerve, the use of tubes is presently experimental and should only be used when patients have been informed and surgeons recognize their unproven nature. Still, there are carefully controlled studies under way which may clarify the role of conduits in major forearm nerves such as the median and ulnar and they hold promise for the future.

One of the more difficult challenges facing the surgeon is in follow-up of patients who have undergone nerve repair. In the repair of major extremity nerves, a follow-up period of 3 to 5 years is ideal, for improvement in muscle function and sensation may continue for at least this long. At present, an advancing Tinel's sign and careful muscle testing are as reliable as any method for following progress of regenerating nerve. These, combined with careful baseline studies and subsequent examinations gives the surgeon some insight into the pace of recovery (Fig. 2–8 A to K). Electrical studies have been used extensively to study intact nerves following decompression, notably in the median nerve after carpal tunnel surgery. No such studies of repaired nerves exist and the surgeon is left to his clinical judgment and serial testing to evaluate the results of nerve suture (Fig. 2–9 A to G).

THOUGHTS FOR THE FUTURE

For the past several decades, surgical efforts have centered on removing impediments to axon regrowth and allowing recovery to occur at a more normal rate. As a result of these efforts, surgeons typically use fewer sutures which are small in caliber and which are correctly placed. It is not likely that further improvement will result from future refinement of these techniques. Investigators are now looking at several other areas to enhance the outcome of nerve repair.[17]

The limiting factors in functional recovery now seem to be (1) the inability of the proximal nerve cell to speed up axon regrowth, and (2) the maintenance of motor and sensory receptors distally while regeneration is occurring. The final result of a nerve repair now depends on the outcome of the race between regenerating axons and atrophying distal receptors. Although intensive research in the area of the nerve cell has been ongoing for quite some time, the clinical spin-off has been meager at best. The absence of a pharmacologic stimulant to axon regeneration is clearly one of the limiting factors in functional recovery following nerve suture, especially in proximal lesions.

In a similar vein, the process of Wallerian degeneration and subsequent collapse of endoneurial tubes appears to be counterproductive and to retard axon regrowth. If this process can be successfully retarded, regeneration may occur more quickly. Finally, technology is now available that permits implantable stimulators to excite muscle intermittently and slow the process of atrophy.[18] Clinical studies that incorporate these devices offer hope for patients who undergo repair of proximal extremity injuries.

The problem of distal atrophy resulting from injury has dogged surgeons for as long as repairs have been done. Recovery following proximal repairs is often minimal, even though a satisfactory nerve suture has been performed. When this occurs, the only remaining option is one or more tendon transfers to rebalance the remaining muscles. Experience in a variety of circumstances over the past century has taught us that transferred tendons and their muscles can relearn tasks which are quite dissimilar to their original function.

In recent years, the concept of nerve transfers has been a clear refinement of this technique and has clearly shortened the time to recovery, thereby mitigating the problem of muscle atrophy.[19,20] Successful nerve transfer depends on the availability of an expendable branch of a functional nerve which can be transferred to a more distal location, thereby shortening the time to recovery and minimizing the effect of muscle atrophy. The importance of the technique is underscored by the devotion of two chapters in this book to its application. The overpowering advantage of a nerve transfer is the ability to convert a proximal nerve injury into a distal one with little or no cost in donor nerve selection. Resourceful surgeons will doubtlessly explore the possible combinations of donor and recipient nerves, but these remain the food for future editions of this book.

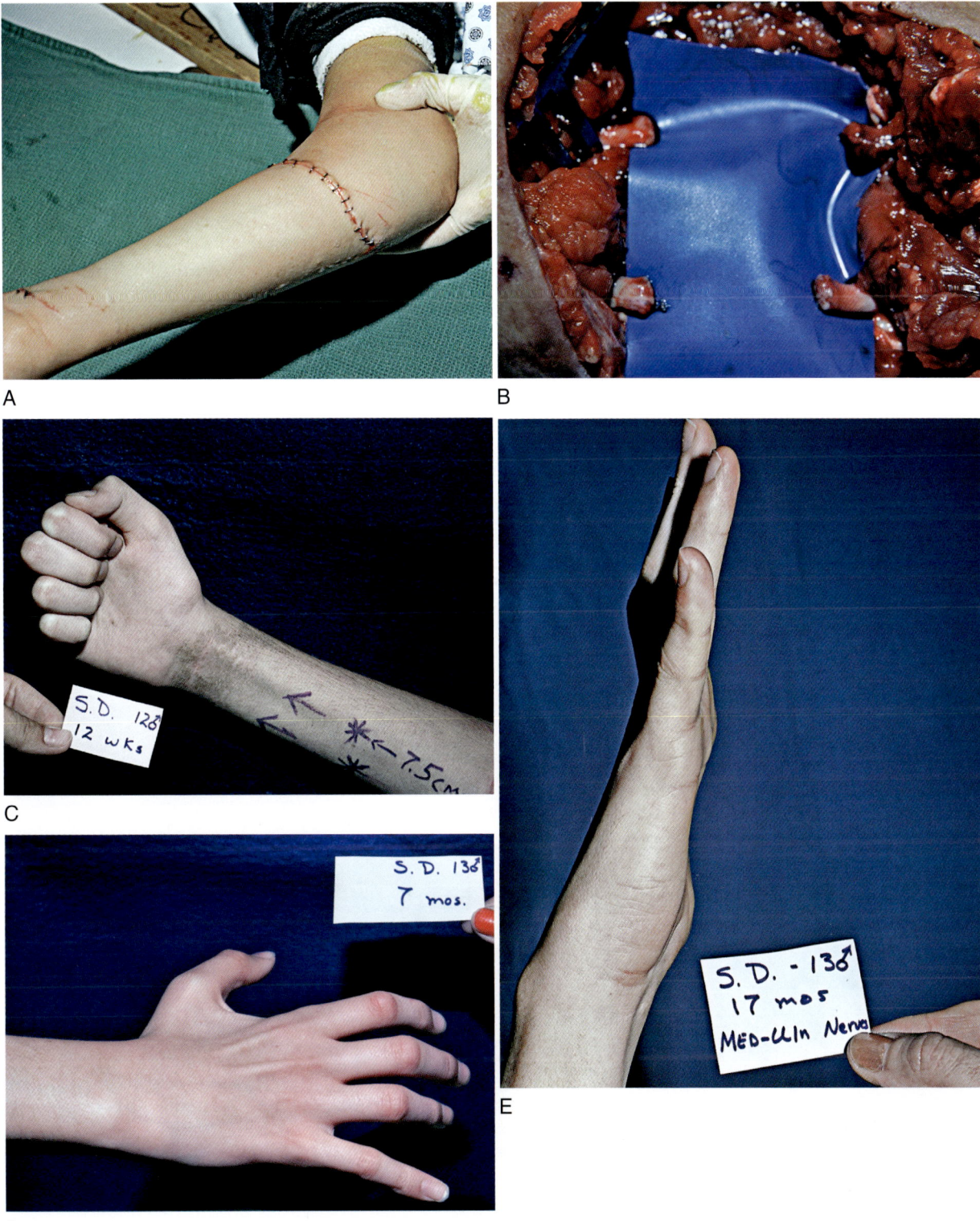

Figure 2–8 Proximal median nerve repair, long-term follow-up. **A:** A 12-year-old boy suffered a deep laceration of the proximal forearm while running with a glass jar that broke when he fell. He underwent surgery initially to stop bleeding, and then was referred for treatment. **B:** Surgery, performed 48 hours after injury, repaired both median and ulnar arteries and nerves as well as all forearm flexor muscle bellies except FDP to index and FPL. **C:** At 12 weeks, moving Tinel's sign (*) function in finger flexors, and intrinsic palsy of thumb. **D:** Intrinsic atrophy and clawing are visible at 7 months. **E:** By 17 months, clawing has disappeared.

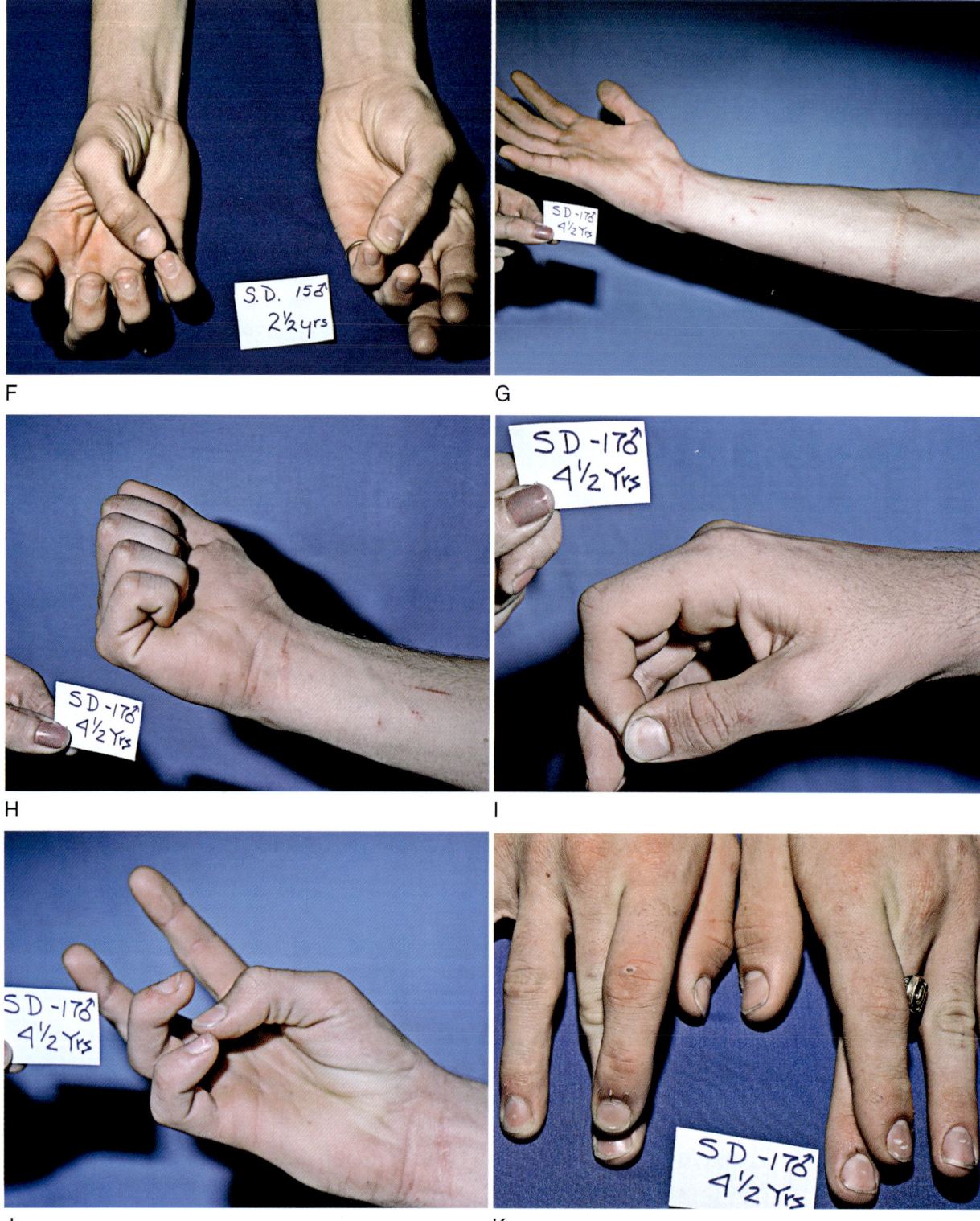

Figure 2–8–Cont'd **F:** Intrinsic function is recovering by 2.5 years. Note the visible abductor pollicus brevis during thumb oppostion. **G:** Further recovery is seen at 4.5 years. Note the increased bulk of the thenar and hypothenar muscles. **H:** Median innervated muscles and ulnar innervated intrinsics are fully functional, although not quite as strong as opposite hand. **I:** Note the absent Froment's sign with key pinch. **J:** Good thumb opposition. **K:** The patient is able to cross fingers. Two-point discrimination returned to 3 to 4 mm.

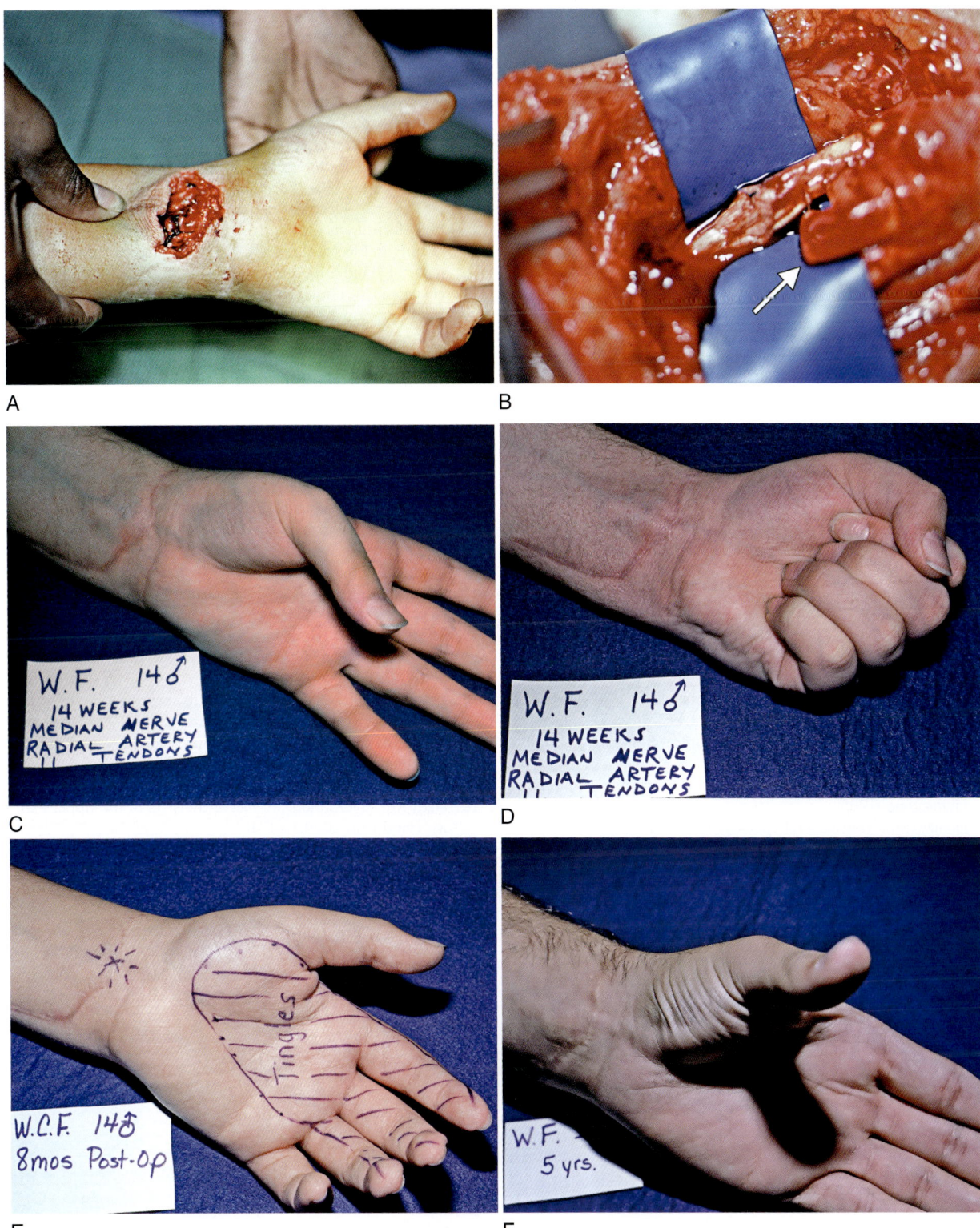

Figure 2–9 Low median nerve repair, long-term follow-up. **A:** A 14-year-old boy lacerated his wrist when his hand went through a windowpane as he attempted to open it. Surgery was performed on the day of injury. Preoperative view of the wound, just proximal to the wrist crease. **B:** An intraoperative view shows a partially completed median nerve repair. Tendon ends *(arrow)* have not yet been sutured. Primary repairs of the median nerve, radial artery, and 11 tendons were performed. **C:** At 14 weeks, there is full recovery of tendon function (except FDP). **D:** At 14 weeks, opposition is weak. **E:** At 8 months, paresthesias are present in the fingers and Tinel's sign (*) is at the repair site. At 9 months, a secondary procedure was performed to shorten the FDP tendon of the index, and to perform an external neurolysis of the repaired median nerve. **F:** A 5-year follow-up illustrates satisfactory recovery of thenar muscles.

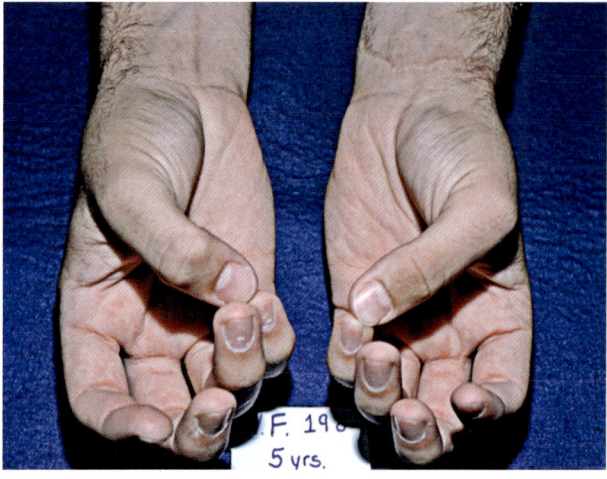

G

Figure 2–9—Cont'd **G:** Note the good bulk of the thenar muscles. Opposition was almost as strong as the uninjured side. Best subjective sensation was in the radial side of the ring finger and progressively less toward the index. On sensory testing, two-point discrimination was 4 to 5 mm, moving two-point discrimination was 2 mm, and von Frey monofilament was normal in all areas.

REFERENCES

1. Naff NJ, Ecklund JM. History of peripheral nerve surgery techniques. Neurosurg Clin N Am 2001;12:197–209.
2. Sunderland S. Nerves and Nerve Injuries, 2nd ed. Edinburgh: Churchill-Livingstone, 1971.
3. Lundborg G. Nerve Injury and Repair. Edinburgh: Churchill-Livingstone, 1988.
4. Jabaley, ME, Wallace WH, Heckler FR. Internal topography of major nerves of the forearm and hand: a current view. J Hand Surg 1980;5:1–18.
5. Chow JA, Van Beek AL, Bilos ZJ, et al. Anatomical basis for repair of ulnar and median nerves in the distal part of the forearm by group fascicular suture and nerve grafting. J Bone Joint Surg Am 1986;68:273–80.
6. Williams HB, Jabaley ME. The importance of internal anatomy of the peripheral nerves to nerve repair in the forearm and hand. Hand Clin 1986;2:689–707.
7. Dahlin LB. The biology of nerve injury and repair. J Am Soc Surg Hand 2004;4:143–55.
8. Jabaley, ME. Electrical nerve stimulation in the awake patient. Bull Hosp Jt Dis Orthop Inst 1984;44:248–59.
9. Gaul JS Jr. Electrical fascicle identification as an adjunct to nerve repair. J Hand Surg 1983;8:289–96.
10. Hakstian RW. Funicular orientation by direct stimulation. J Bone Joint Surg Am 1968;50:1178–86.
11. Millesi H, Terzis JK. Problems of terminology in peripheral nerve surgery. Microsurgery 1983;4:51–6.
12. Sunderland S. The pros and cons of funicular nerve repair. J Hand Surg 1979;4:201–11.
13. Jabaley ME. Technical aspects of peripheral nerve repair. J Hand Surg 1984;9:14–9.
14. Jabaley ME. Modified techniques of nerve repair: epineurial splint. In: Gelberman RH, ed., Operative Nerve Repair and Reconstruction. Philadelphia: J.B. Lippincott, 1991:315–26.
15. Tsuge K, Ikuta Y, Sakaue M. A new technique for nerve suture: the anchoring funicular suture. Plast Reconstr Surg 1975;56:496–500.
15a. Wilgis EF, Murphy R. The significance of longitudinal excursion in peripheral nerves. Hand Clin 1986;4:761–6.
16. Meek MF, Coert JH. Clinical use of nerve conduits in peripheral nerve repair: Review of the literature. J Reconst Microsurg 2002;18:97–109.
17. Frostick SP, Kemp GJ. Schwann cells, neurotrophic factors, and peripheral nerve regeneration. Microsurgery 1998;18:397–405.
18. Nicolaidis SC, Williams HB. Muscle preservation using an implantable electrical system after nerve injury and repair. Microsurgery 2001;21:241–7.
19. Nath RK, MacKinnon SE. Nerve transfers in the upper extremity. Hand Clin 2000;16:131–9.
20. Weber RV, Mackinnon SE. Nerve transfers in the upper extremity. J Am Soc Surg Hand 2004;4:200–13.

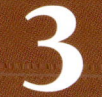

3 Nerve Grafting

Hanno Millesi

INTRODUCTION

The bed of a nerve (e.g., the median nerve) has a certain length from the formation of the nerve by its two roots from the medial and the lateral cord, to its final division at the exit of the carpal tunnel if the elbow joint is extended. Since the nerve and its bed are not located in the plane of the axis of the elbow joint, but to its palmar side the bed becomes shorter if the elbow joint is flexed. The nerve is loosely located in its bed. If the wrist joint and the fingers are extended, the median nerve is elongated; with flexion of the elbow joint the median nerve becomes shorter.

Measurement of the median nerve in cadavers (extended elbow)[1] revealed the following values for adults: wrist and fingers in middle position, 516.6 ± 10.4 mm; elongation by extension of the wrist and the fingers, +23.4 ± 7.1 mm = 540 mm (+4.5%); and shortening by flexion of the elbow joint, −77.1 ± 8.9 mm = 439.5 mm (−15%).

The nerve is able to accommodate to this changes in length because it (1) can move passively in the longitudinal direction against the surrounding tissue via its gliding apparatus (perineurium); (2) the fascicles are arranged loosely in the interfascicular epineurium and can move against each other; (3) the perineurium has a certain elastic extensibility; (4) the nerve fibers within the endoneurium are arranged in an undulated way and can elongate and shorten by changing the wavy course[2–4]; and (5) there is sufficient space for accommodation (the elongated nerve is thinner, the shortened nerve is thicker).

Sunderland and Bradley[5] performed stress strain tests with human cadaver nerves (median and ulnar nerve). Elongations of at least 6% to 8% were tolerated without any irreversible changes in the mechanical behavior.

WHAT HAPPENS AFTER SHARP TRANSECTION OF A NERVE?

A *clean transection* causes the loss of continuity of the nerve, and the two stumps spread apart due to the elasticity of the nerve tissue *(elastic retraction)*. Since the transection was caused by a sharp instrument, very little damage was inflicted to the nerve tissue in the close neighborhood of the transection. In order to restore and maintain continuity, the force causing the elastic retraction has to be overcome and there is no necessity of compensatory elongation.

The situation becomes more complicated if the attempt to restore continuity is performed at a later date. Any living tissue has the tendency to shrink if there is no constant stress of elongation. This shortening is more important if a fibrosis develops (*fibrotic retraction*).

In a late secondary repair of continuity, even if there is no defect at all, some *compensatory elongation* of normal nerve tissue is necessary in order to restore the full original length of the nerve. The *fibrotic retraction* is more severe if a segment of the nerve proximal and distal to the site of the transaction has developed edema and a fibrotic reaction.

Thus far, there is no actual nerve defect. This *distance* between the two stumps is caused by the elastic retraction as mentioned above, but it is strongly influenced by the position of the adjacent joints. For the median nerve, it becomes shorter with flexion and longer with extension of the elbow joint.

A *nerve defect* is created if a segment of nerve tissue is lost or was so badly damaged that it had to be resected. The same is true in cases of a rupture if the adjacent segments of the nerve have suffered a severe traction lesion before the rupture occurred. In this case, the original length of the nerve can be restored only by compensatory elongation of the remaining segments of the nerve or by adding new tissue.

NERVE DEFECT MANAGEMENT

There are five basic ways to manage a nerve defect:

1. Restoration of continuity by end-to-end coaptation.
2. Restoration of continuity by adding tissue.
3. Bypassing a defect by transfer of synergistic nerve fibers of equal destination as suggested by Schmidhammer et al.[6]: transfer of motor fibers for the deep head of the flexor pollicis brevis to the other thenar muscles by end-to-side coaptation via nerve graft.
4. Bypassing a defect by nerve fiber transfer from another nerve if the proximal stump is lacking.
5. Nerve–muscle neurotization if the distal stump is lacking.

For purposes of this chapter, points 1 and 2 are of interest.

Restoration of Continuity by End-to-End Coaptation

This is the simplest and most logical way to restore the continuity of a transected nerve. If there is no defect, the cross-sections correspond perfectly and an optimal coaptation can be obtained. The forces of the elastic retraction only have to be overcome and the nerve must not be elongated. The surgeons were so convinced that end-to-end repair was the treatment of choice that this technique was used for increasingly longer defects. The so-called "critical" resection length was defined as the segment of a nerve that can be overcome by end-to-end

coaptation after maximal approximation of the two stumps by flexing the adjacent joints with good chances of success. In the 1920s, the critical resection length was estimated with up to 25 cm.[7]

The high number of failures caused shrinkage of the critical resection length to 7 to 10 cm in the 1950s. With a closer look at the problem, it became evident that the figures of Sunderland's stress strain studies[5] are based on a cadaver nerve outside the body. If a nerve segment was studied in situ, the stress strain curve is much stiffer due to the friction within the body. If a long segment of the median or the ulnar nerve including branches were studied within the body, the necessary force to obtain elongation became very high (Fig. 3–1).[1]

My conclusion from our study was that tension at the site of repair has a negative influence on healing of repaired nerves and the regeneration across the repair site. The argument against this conclusion is based on limb elongation. A gradual elongation of the nerves is possible without any harm. This argument cannot be applied, however, for trauma cases. In limb elongation, we elongate normal nerves. The elongation can be distributed over a long distance, and each segment has to elongate a small amount only. There is an intact gliding apparatus, and there are no adhesions. In spite of these facts, one can observe once in a while a paralysis during such a lengthening procedure.

Gradual elongation after end-to-end nerve repair in flexed position of the adjacent joints had been tried already in the 18th century without much success. In a recent paper,[8] good results in experiments with the median nerve of rabbits were reported if the repair was performed tensionless in flexed position of the elbow joint with gradual elongation after 2 weeks of complete immobilization. The results were superior to the repair by nerve grafts. However, this experiment suffers from

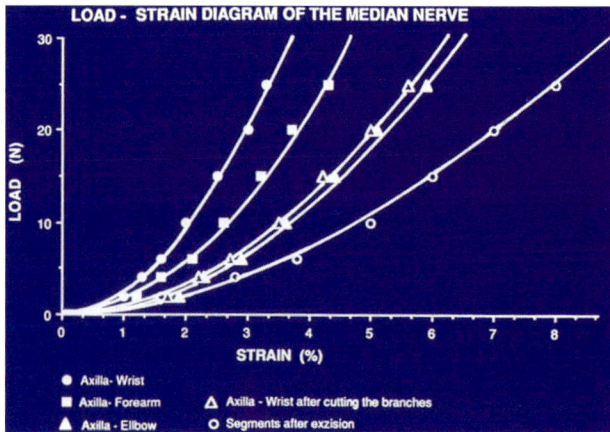

Figure 3–1 Load strain diagram of the median nerve. Human cadaver. The stress strain curve is much stiffer if measured with the end inside the body, and even stiffer yet if a segment with branches is examined.

a severe mistake. After nerve grafting, the involved limb of the experimental animals was not immobilized at all compared to two other series with immobilization. Consequently, this experiment violates a basic rule of experimental surgery, which is to provide equal conditions for techniques to be repaired.

Attempts to cover defects by elongating nerve segment before a repair using expander-like devices did not become popular.

The statement that a repair under tension is unfavorable for regeneration does not mean that a repair under tension excludes useful regeneration. One of the reasons that I questioned nerve repair under tension was the classic report of Nicholson and Seddon.[9] A large series of median nerve lesions was studied. In median nerve repairs at the wrist with defects of less than 2.5 cm, a result of M3 was achieved in 70% of cases. The M3 result was achieved in only 50% of cases with a defect of more than 2.5 cm. This shows that even with defects of more than 2.5 cm, an M3 result could be reached, albeit the percentage was lower. Everyone would agree that a failure rate of 50% in a technically rather simple surgery is too high.

In summary, end-to-end repair offers an optimal chance for successful regeneration if there is no or a very small defect. With rising defects, the chances of end-to-end repair decrease. A strict limit cannot be given because there are many variables, such as body constitution, site of lesion in relation to branches, extension of the trauma, and so on.

Adding New Tissue

The alternative technique to end-to-end repair is adding new tissue. Two basic techniques, nerve grafting and alternatives to same, are available. A nerve graft is living tissue that provides circumstances comparable to a distal stump. Regenerating axons should meet conditions similar to those in a distal stump. Alternatives are devices that provide favorable conditions for minifascicles from the proximal stump to proceed in the direction of the distal stump.

Alternatives

After transection of a nerve, a series of processes commences. Transected axons produce axon sprouts proceeding in a distal direction. Schwann cells proliferate, as well as fibroblasts from the perineurium and the epineurium. New capillaries are formed. Thus, a great number of minifascicles containing capillaries, axons, and connective tissue cells surrounded by some kind of perineurium are created. In a resected neuroma, these minifascicles proceed in an irregular way, which is regarded by many surgeons as the main characteristic of a neuroma. If there is a directional factor of any kind,

the minifascicles proceed in the desired direction. This phenomenon was described by Schröder und Seiffert,[10] and termed "neuromateous neurotization."

Alternatives are valid for short defects only. The following is a partial list of materials used:

Vein grafts
Silicon chamber
Millipore chamber
Polyglycol tubes
Freeze thawed muscle
Cialite preserved nerve
Lyophilized nerve

Nerve Grafting

The logical way to replace a missing segment of a nerve seems to be a nerve graft. The axons of the graft undergo Wallerian degeneration as in any distal nerve segment after it had been separated from the donor nerve. In contrast to a skin graft, the nerve graft must not only cover the defect between the two stumps but provide optimal conditions for the regenerating axons such as a distal stump after Wallerian degeneration (endoneurial structures, Schwann cells, etc.).

The axon sprouts grow along the endoneurial structures to reach the distal end of the graft and to cross to the distal stump. By the Schwann cells of the graft, new nerve fibers with all special properties are formed. A new nerve is the result, but there is no accumulation of mini-fascicles. *This is the neurotization of the graft.*

Therefore, the condition for a successful grafting procedure is how well it copes with the task to provide optimal conditions for regenerating axons. This means that a 100% survival of all structures of the nerve has to occur, including the delicate structures of the endoneurium and the Schwann cells.

Philipeaux and Vulpian,[11] who performed the first experimental nerve graft in 1870, demonstrated that the graft will be neurotized from the proximal stump regardless of whether it is interposed in an orthodromic or antidromic manner.

Albert,[12] who performed free nerve grafting in humans as early as 1876, used nerve trunks like the median or the ulnar nerves as donors and had no success. Bielschowsky and Unger[13] studied such nerve grafts histologically, and showed that a great part of the nerve tissue had undergone fibrosis, apparently because the spontaneous revascularization by connections between the vessels on the surface of the nerve, and the vessels of the recipient site did not provide revascularization in due time to prevent necrobiosis of the structures most sensitive to anoxia such as the Schwann cells and the endoneurium.

In this way, the nerve graft became transformed from living nerve tissue such as at the distal stump of a severed nerve to a connective tissue strand. Even so, neurotization may occur as neuromatous neurotization mentioned above when discussing the alternatives. There were some useful results; however they were much inferior to an end-to-end repair of the continuity when a defect was not too long. Such a fibrotic nerve graft behaves like an alternative. Before the 1970s, such a development was regarded as the normal outcome of a free nerve grafting.[14] In a textbook on peripheral nerve surgery, which appeared in 1995, the fibrosis and disorganization in a graft, especially in the distal segment, are mentioned.[15]

In those days, it was generally accepted that Schwann cells could not survive free grafting. Only the brilliant experiment of Aguayo et al.[16] with the trembler mouse demonstrated clearly that Schwann cells are able to survive the initial ischemic period of free grafting. Under optimal conditions in a well-supplied bed, connections between blood vessels of the surface of the graft and the recipient site are established in 24 to 48 hours.

Full survival is then a question of the tissue mass of the graft in relation to its surface. In 1915, Foerster[17] suggested the use of cutaneous nerves as grafts. Grafts of this size usually survive the grafting procedure very well. The different caliber of such cutaneous nerve grafts and the thick nerve trunks to be repaired created a new problem: the *calibre difference*.

On the other hand, the harvesting of a cutaneous nerve as a nerve graft does not cause an important loss of function. Cutaneous nerves are available in great numbers in contrast to trunk grafts. Of course, the development of a neuroma has to be avoided.

The intention to avoid any ischemic period stimulated the development of so-called pedicled nerve grafts in an analogy to a pedicled skin flap in contrast to a free skin graft. The first nerve graft without an ischemic period was performed by Barnes et al. in 1946.[18] Shelden et al.[19] and Strange[20,21] published case reports treated by such techniques. A long defect of a single nerve was managed by sacrificing another nerve parallel to it. The method was applied mainly in cases with long defects of the median and ulnar nerves. The median nerve was repaired at the expense of the ulnar nerve. In the first stage, the distal end of the ulnar nerve was sutured to the distal end of the median nerve, which formed a loop. After sufficient circulation had been established at the suture site, the ulnar nerve was transected very proximal to gain a segment long enough to cover the defect of the median nerve. The blood supply of the graft depended now on vessels entering the ulnar nerve across the repair site with the median nerve.

The ulnar nerve was turned down and the end of the nerve was connected to the distal stump of the median nerve. The transplant now covered the defect in an antidromic fashion. Shelden et al.[19] modified the technique so as to allow an orthodromic repair.

Some recovery, especially as far as sensibility is concerned, was reported, but the method never become popular.[22] The advantage to maintain the circulation during the grafting procedure is far less important than the disadvantages of sacrificing an important nerve, loss of time, and the fact that the course of the regenerating axons along the nerve trunk is not predictable and therefore an aimed connection is impossible.

The problem of the caliber difference when using cutaneous nerve segments was solved by Seddon[23] by forming a cable of the size of one thick nerve to be repaired by assembling several thin skin nerves using stitches or glue (*cable graft technique*).

Assembling several skin nerves to form a cable means that a part of the surface of these grafts is in contact with another free graft, and is not available for contact with the recipient site. Some segments of a graft may survive better, other segments may develop disorder and fibrosis as described by Hudson et al.[14]

The decisive disadvantage of the cable graft technique could be avoided by changing the approach by 180 degrees. Instead of combining the cutaneous nerve segment to form a cable, the two nerve stumps are dissected by interfascicular dissection into major fascicles and fascicle groups. Corresponding fascicles and groups of fascicles in the proximal and distal nerve stumps are connected by multiple cutaneous nerve grafts, which are individually placed. These grafts survive very well, and preserve their Schwann cells and the delicate structure of the endoneurium. The isolated and individual interposition of nerve grafts allows the surgeon to connect any given elected point on the proximal stump with any specific point on the distal stump ("aimed connection").[24–27]

It is interesting to note that this simple consideration is still not fully understood by surgeons dealing with nerve grafting. Otherwise, it cannot be explained why in a recent experimental study on nerve repair, the authors still considered the cable graft technique to be the "gold standard" that was used for comparing the results of other techniques.[28]

A free graft must form adhesions to survive. It is therefore extremely sensitive against longitudinal traction and tension at the suture site. This will be discussed later.

Taylor and Ham[29] introduced the technique of free vascularized nerve grafting. A pedicled nerve graft is analogous to a pedicled skin flap; similarly, a free vascularized nerve graft is analogous to a free microvascular skin flap. In both cases, nerve ischemia is avoided. Schwann cells and the structures of the endoneurium survive and are fully preserved. The vascularized nerve graft is a perfect size match for the the severed distal nerve stump. Another advantage over a free nerve graft is the fact that no spontaneous connections between the vessels of the surface of the graft and the recipient site have to be established, and consequently no adhesions have to be formed. The paraneurium, the gliding tissue around the nerve, remains intact. The vascularized graft is therefore much less sensitive to longitudinal traction and tension.

Great expectations were stimulated by this technique and many surgeons thought this technique would revolutionize nerve repair. In special investigations the anatomy of the vascular pedicles of different nerves was studied,[30] and particular techniques elaborated. Attempts were made to avoid sacrificing a major nerve trunk for use as a graft by using a cutaneous nerve such as the sural nerve[31] or the saphenous nerve.

Doi et al.[32] held the view that nerve defects longer than 10 cm can be managed only by vascularized nerve grafts. The big disadvantage of vascularized nerve grafts is the fact that there is no way to influence the course of an axon within the graft, and one cannot predict where an axon will exit the distal stump relative to its entry site.

In spite of remarkable successes, the revolution failed to appear and vascularized nerve grafting has become a technique with special indications under rather rare conditions.

PERSONAL EXPERIENCE: FREE NERVE GRAFTING

My first nerve grafting procedure was performed in 1958.[33] A young boy suffered a high-voltage electrical injury. He lost one leg and one hand at the forearm level. The contralateral forearm suffered necrosis of the soft tissue at the palmar side of the forearm, including the median and the ulnar nerve, all flexor tendons, and the little finger. The skin of the forearm was replaced by a pedicled skin flap, and the flexor tendons were reconstructed by tendon grafts. Useful gripping function was restored, but there was no sensibility. For this reason, the continuity of the median nerve was restored by a long trunk graft harvested from the ulnar nerve of the amputated forearm. Based on an experimental study,[34] the distal site of coaptation was resected, and the two stumps reconnected by a secondary end-to-end repair. Some protective sensibility returned.

In 1962, I reported my results on nerve repair[35] which included six cases of nerve grafting, all of which were cable grafts. In all cases with nerve grafts longer than 3 cm, a resection of the distal site of coaptation had to be performed in order to remove the scar tissue at the distal site of coaptation, which prevented the crossing of the axons into the distal stump. This reflects the main problem of nerve repair by nerve grafts. The axons have to cross two site of coaptation to reach the distal stump. For surgeons of the 1960s, it was evident that a

technique with two suture sites had to be inferior to one with a single coaptation. But this problem is mainly a question of time. The longer the nerve graft is, and the slower axon sprouts proceed distally, the stronger the development of the scar at the distal coaptation, and the more effective the block will be. This problem was regarded as so important that Bosse[36] suggested a nerve grafting procedure in two steps. The proximal coaptation is performed as the first step, leaving the distal end free. The distal coaptation is performed in a second step procedure at a time when it could be assumed that the axon sprouts have reached the distal end of the graft.

I was not pleased with the cable graft technique. From the experiments of Hudson et al.,[14] it can clearly be seen that there is no full survival of these grafts. The reason, assembling to a cable, was already mentioned. As a matter of fact, Seddon himself was not very pleased with the technique, as he stopped using it. In 1947, when Seddon published the cable graft technique, he reported 13 cases,[23] compared to 22 cases in 1963,[37] and another 22 cases in 1972.[38] In other words, in the 16 years between 1947 and 1963, he had operated on nine cases, and in the 9 years between 1963 and 1972, not even one case.

For me it became clear that forming of a cable should be avoided. Each cutaneous nerve graft should be placed individually, exposing the entire circumference of the graft so as to make it available for contact with the recipient site. Under this condition, we can expect a full structural survival of each graft.

The second reason for the poor result of this grafting concept was the fact that Seddon recommended shortening the gap by approximating the two nerve stumps as much as possible, and then grafting the "remaining" defect.[39] This was due to the erroneous but widespread opinion that the result of nerve grafting was dependent on the length of the graft. In fact, the result depends more on the length of the defect of nerve tissue. The longer the defect, the more intraneural topography changes; hence, it becomes increasingly difficult to connect corresponding locations of the cross-section. Of course, a longer defect needs longer grafts. In a given defect, however, the length of the graft that is needed to cover the "distance" between the stumps, which in turn is influenced by the position of the adjacent joints, is irrelevant to the final result.

The axon sprouts are able to cross the proximal and distal sites of coaptation much quicker and in greater numbers if the nerve stumps are coapted without interposed collagenous connective tissue. Such an optimal coaptation can be achieved only if there is no tension between the stumps. Tension produces some degree of separation between the stumps. This gap is filled with collagenous tissue, which makes regeneration more difficult. Experiments proved that axon sprouts are able to cross two optimal sites of coaptation much easier than a less than optimal site.[40,41] Tension focuses at the sites of coaptation. The two ends of the grafts are fixed secondary to the adhesions, which revascularize the grafts and are essential for their survival in contrast to the movable proximal and distal free segment of the damaged nerve.

Under optimal conditions, the grafts are neurotized much quicker. The block at the distal site of coaptation occurred in only 14% of grafts longer than 3 cm in the first 50 cases in whom the new approach was applied. With increasing experience, this problem has been eliminated. In spite of this fact, one should not forget that axonal frustration may occur in rare instances. This problem occurs when there is a failure of the advancement of the Tinel's sign at the distal site of coaptation.

INTERFASCICULAR NERVE GRAFTING TECHNIQUE

This technique was developed based on clinical and experimental experience as mentioned above. The term "interfascicular" was elected because it reflects at best the difference from the cable graft technique. The cutaneous segments of the graft are not sutured or glued together to form a cable the same size as the nerve to be repaired. The two stumps are dissected by interfascicular dissection into minor units (big fascicles or fascicle groups), which are then individually connected by a cutaneous nerve graft. However, according to my experience, there are many factors influencing the outcome, in addition to the quality of the coaptations. All these factors have to be considered, and I shall try to discuss these factors in the following pages.

To begin with, I have to state that "the nerve graft" as a technique per se does not exist. If a person compares a new technique with "nerve grafting" or "conventional nerve grafting" without explaining the details of the technique involved, this reveals that he or she has not really understood the problems connected with nerve grafting. The factors involved and the individual technical steps can best be explained by a case demonstration.

Case 1

Z.K., age 38 years, male railway worker suffered a severe accident to his left arm by being hit by a train. The accident caused:

1. Lesion of the brachial artery and vein with impairment of circulation. Restoration of continuity of the brachial artery by a vein graft reestablished the circulation. A forearm fasciotomy was performed.

2. Fracture of the humerus, which was treated by osteosynthesis with a plate.
3. Lesion of musculocutaneous nerve.
4. Lesion of radial nerve.
5. Lesion of median nerve.

The ulnar nerve remained intact and is still functional. The preoperative situation is demonstrated in Fig. 3–2. There is a complete loss of the radial-nerve innervated muscle, except the triceps. Continuity was restored by nerve grafts in an extra-anatomical bed. There was complete paralysis of the biceps and brachial muscle due to destruction of the musculocutaneous nerve distal to the coracobrachial muscle. Neurotization of the biceps was achieved by nerve grafts coapted end to side to the proximal musculocutaneous nerve and introduced into the biceps muscle as a nerve–muscle neurotization. There was complete loss of motor function and sensibility in the territory of the median nerve with a strongly positive Tinel-Hoffmann sign at midarm level.

Along with the surgery on the musculocutaneous and the radial nerve, the continuity of the median nerve was restored by nerve grafts. This procedure will be described here as an example of interfascicular nerve grafting.

Case 2

Patient P.F., male, age 13 years. The injury was located at the distal forearm with a subsequent transection of

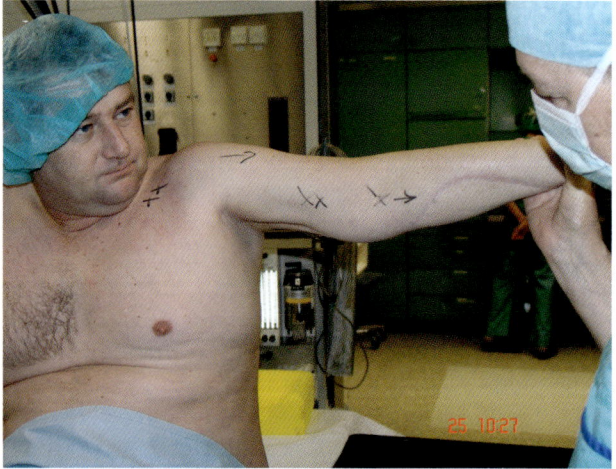

Figure 3–2   Case 1: Z.K., 38-year-old male railway worker suffered a severe injury to his left arm upon being hit by a train. The accident caused: (1) A lesion of the brachial artery and vein with impairment of the circulation. Restoration of the continuity of the brachial artery by a vein graft reestablished the circulation. A forearm fasciotomy was performed. (2) A fracture of the humerus, which was treated by osteosynthesis with a plate. (3) Lesion of the musculocutaneous nerve. (4) Lesion of the radial nerve. (5) Lesion of the median nerve. The ulnar nerve remained intact and was still functional.

the median and the ulnar nerve. A primary neurorrhaphy was performed but there were no signs of regeneration within the expected time frame. The Tinel-Hoffmann sign was positive at the site of primary repair (Fig. 3–3). This case will be shown as an example of interfascicular nerve repair after failed primary repair.

Case 3

Patient H.E., female, age 28 years. Injury by a motor boat propeller at the gluteal area during professional activities as a surfing teacher. The injury caused a destruction of the sciatic nerve over a long distance with severe skin loss. This case will be discussed as an example of skin repair before nerve surgery, and as an example of a long nerve defect (Figs. 3–4 and 3–5).

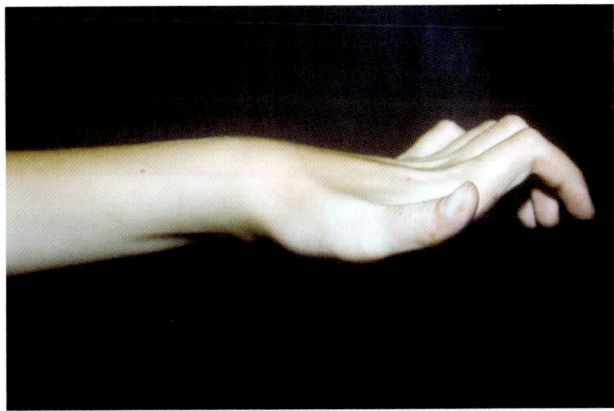

Figure 3–3   Patient P.F., 13-year-old male. Injury was located at the distal forearm. Transection of the median and the ulnar nerve, primary neurorrhaphy was performed without signs of regeneration in proper time. The Tinel-Hoffmann sign was positive at the site of primary repair.

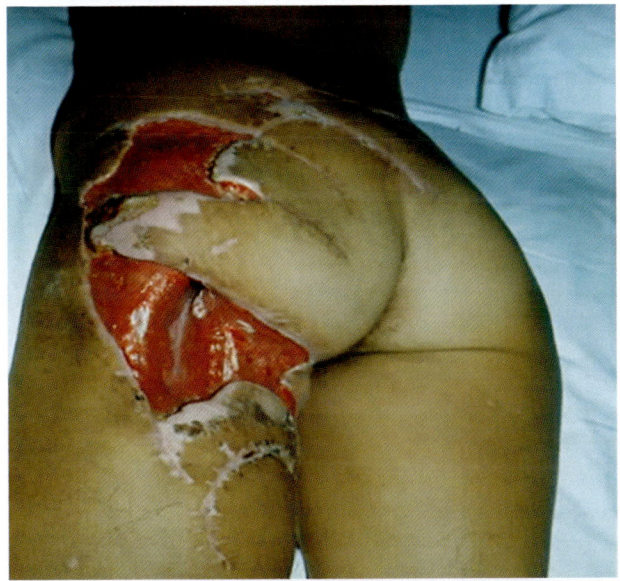

Figure 3–4   Patient H.E., 28-year-old female. Injury by a motor boat propeller at the gluteal area during professional activities as a surfing teacher. The injury caused destruction of the sciatic nerve over a long distance with severe skin loss.

In such a case, adequate grafting material does not exist. One possibility is to elect that part of the distal cross-section of the damaged nerve that has the best chances to provide recovery when neurotized.

Case 4

Patient M.Ch., male, age 35 years. After an injury, there was a defect of the radial nerve. Continuity was restored by interfascicular nerve grafting (Fig. 3–6). There were no signs of recovery after appropriate time period.

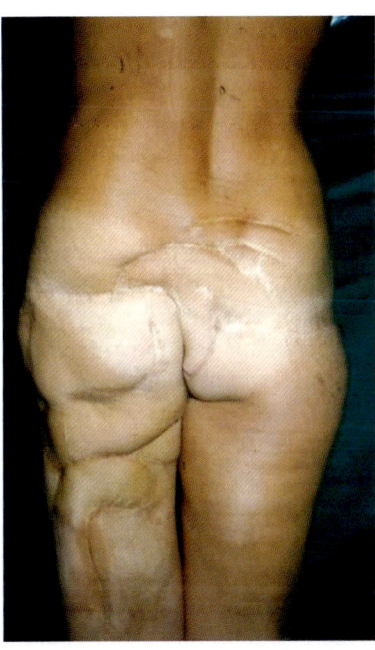

Figure 3–5   Reconstruction of soft tissues as a preparation for nerve repair.

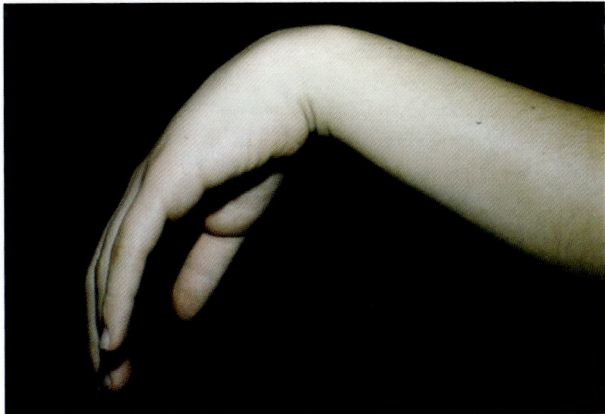

Figure 3–6   Patient M.Ch., 35-year-old male. After injury, there was a defect of the radial nerve. Restoration of continuity by interfascicular nerve grafting.

Approach

The election of a proper approach is extremely important. The approach should provide a sufficient view to perform an easy dissection, but it should not excessively expose the nerve.

The surgical scar should be distant to the nerve and the site of nerve repair to avoid a negative effect of the scar on the healing of the nerve. Under no circumstances should the final skin scar have a constricting effect on the nerve. At present, there is a trend to use minimal scars; in certain cases, this offers advantages. It is easy to explore a peroneal nerve using a longitudinal incision following the course of the nerve. According to my experience, such a scar is usually hypertrophic and has a negative influence on the underlying nerve. To explore the peroneal nerve using a sequence of transverse incisions with undermining the skin between the incisions provides a much better environment for the nerve. In contrast to this consideration, using a pre-existing transverse scar at the wrist may have a constricting effect. In such a case, a midlateral incision may be more advisable, even if it requires more effort on the part of the surgeon and becomes rather long. This type of approach, however, allows for good grafts, and the possibility of enlarging the forearm circumference if necessary by applying a skin graft.

In Case 1, we had to expect a defect of the median nerve at the medial aspect of the upper arm. At this level, there was also the vein graft repair of the brachial artery. There was already a longitudinal scar from the primary surgery that could have been used. However, I preferred to use two transverse incisions proximal and distal to the site of the lesion.

Through the proximal incision, I could identify the median nerve and the artery in a healthy tissue plane (Fig. 3–7). The distal incision led into massive fibrous tissue. In order to avoid violating the rule of always exposing the nerve initially in unscarred tissue, the dissection was stopped. A third transverse incision was done in the cubital fossa. Even here, fibrous tissue was present in consequence of the swelling, but this area was not directly involved in the traumatic process. Here the cubital vein, cubital artery, and median nerve could be easily identified (Fig. 3–8).

After lifting the skin, the neurovascular structures could be followed as far distally as the level of the distal arm incision. The artery could be isolated and the distal stump identified (Fig. 3–9). With careful lifting of the skin, the exploration was finished.

Preparation of Nerve Stumps

There were two ways to prepare the stumps: (1) serial resections from the end in the proximal and distal

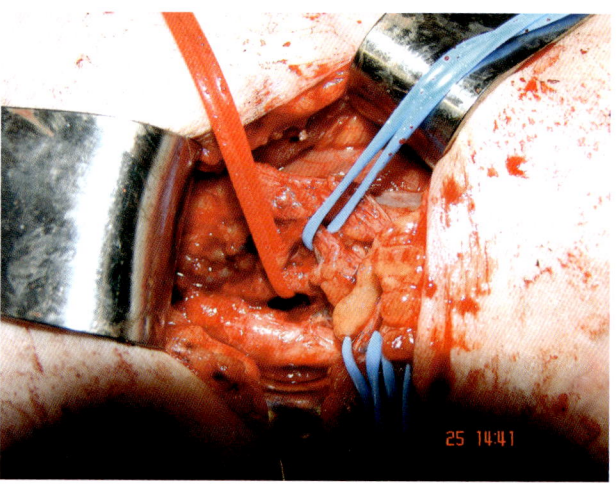

Figure 3–8 To define the anatomic structures in normal tissue, a third incision was performed in the cubital fossa and the vein, and the artery and the median nerve were defined.

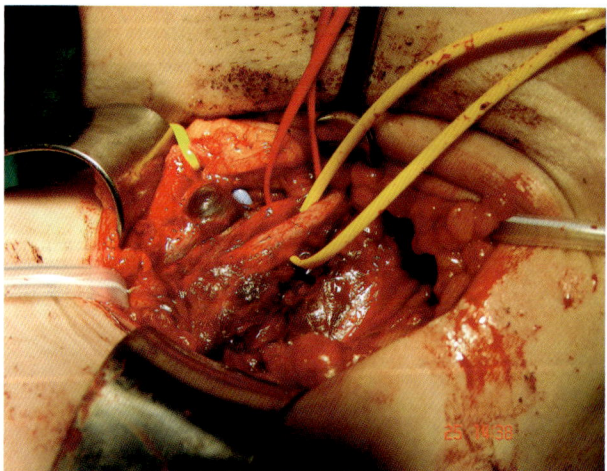

Figure 3–7 Case 1: Exploration of the site of the lesion by two transverse incisions. Definition of the artery and the proximal stump of the median nerve.

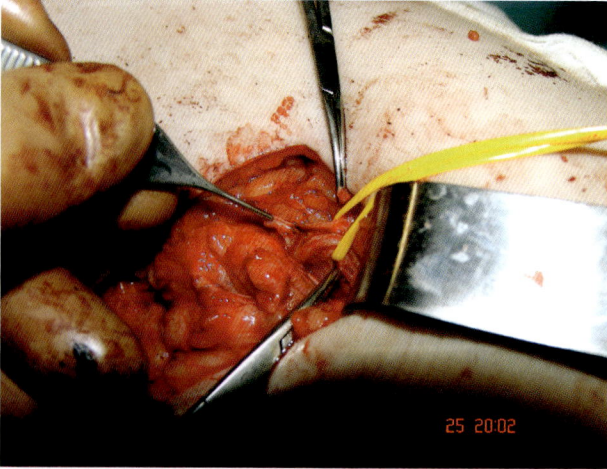

Figure 3–9 Dissecting from the cubital fossa to the medial aspect of the upper arm, the distal stump was defined at a level of the second incision at the upper arm.

directions, respectively, until normal-looking structures of the nerve are encountered, and (2) interfascicular dissection was then performed, starting in normal appearing nerve and proceeding distally towards the damaged stump. Any undamaged fascicles or fascicular groups were isolated and preserved. The epifascicular epineurium and perineurium were reflected and preserved deep to the stump in order to provide a supporting bed for the nerve grafts.

In Case 1, we could isolate at the proximal stump one large fascicle and two medium-sized ones (Fig. 3–10). At the distal stump, one large, a medium-sized, and two small fascicles were separated (Fig. 3–11).

A completely different situation occurred in Case 2. Here the trauma was much less extensive. Again, coming from healthy tissue, the two suture sites were

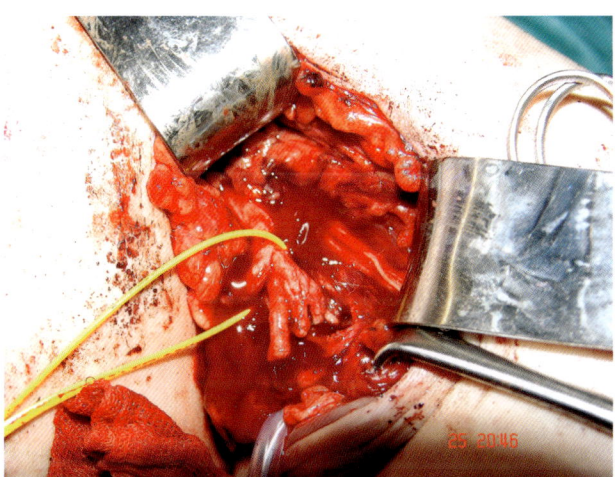

Figure 3–10 Preparation of the proximal stump by interfascicular resection. Isolation of one large- and two medium-sized fascicles. The two nerve grafts in the right aspect are grafts for the musculocutaneus nerve.

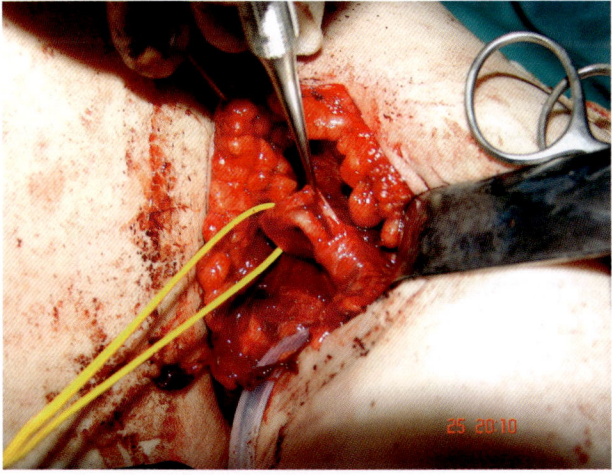

Figure 3–11 Interfascicular dissection of the distal stump. Finally, one large-, one medium-, and two small-sized fascicles could be isolated.

exposed. Interfascicular dissection started proximal and distal to the site of repair. Pre-existing fascicle groups were isolated, and the epifascicular epineurium and the paraneurium reflected. There was an acceptable fascicular alignment of the median nerve. An intraneural interfascicular neurolysis was performed. The fascicular alignment of the ulnar nerve, however, was poor and the site of repair was resected leaving two stumps with isolated groups of fascicles.

In Case 3, the wound had to be closed by plastic surgery before nerve repair could be considered. Again, the two stumps were approached from the healthy side prepared by interfascicular dissection.

Analysis of the Two Stumps

The next step was to analyze the two stumps in order to define which fascicle or which fascicle group of the proximal stump corresponded to which in the distal one. In Case 1, it seemed logical that the big fascicle of the proximal stump corresponded to the big fascicle of the distal stump. Most probably they contained the nerve fibers for the hand. The smaller fascicles were already separated in preparation to branch off in the proximal forearm. We needed therefore one or two cutaneous nerve segments for the big fascicle, and one for each medium fascicle of the proximal stump to be connected to the medium fascicle and the two small fascicles of the distal stump. We assumed that these fascicles contained mainly motor nerve fibers. If we wanted to know exactly to which part of the forearm muscles they went, we would have had to continue the dissection to the midforearm and follow the muscle branches by retrograde tracing to the distal stump. The big fascicle contained, according to our assumption, motor and sensory nerve fibers for the hand. At this level of nerve section, the motor and sensory fascicles are distributed diffusely over the cross-section of the nerve; hence, staining or any other technique of senso-motor differentiation would not be of practical value.

In Case 2, a fascicular pattern as depicted in Figs. 3–12 and 3–13 was encountered. In the proximal stump, two fascicle groups were located at the palmar side, and a major group with many small fascicles at the dorsal side. The situation is depicted from an intraoperative sketch. In the distal stump (Figs. 3–14 and 3–15), we encountered again the major group with the many small fascicles, and three groups at the palmar side apparently formed by divison of the two fascicular groups of the proximal stump.

The decisive question was which of these groups contained the motor nerve fibers and would form the deep branch of the ulnar nerve. In this situation, a staining technique may help. But it is easier to extend the dissection in the distal direction, define the division of the ulnar nerve in the superficial and deep branches, and

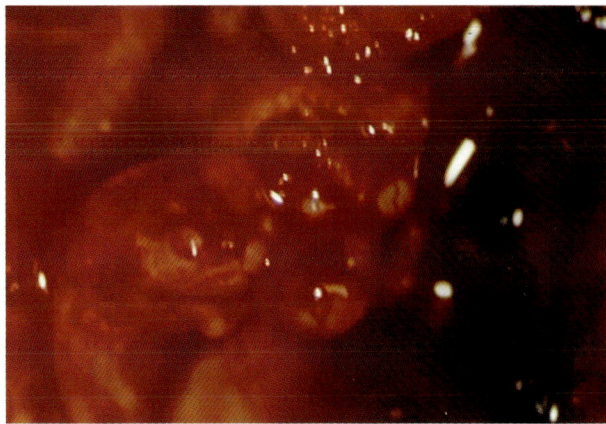

Figure 3-12 In the proximal stump, two fascicle groups are located at the palmar side, and a major group with many small fascicles at the dorsal side.

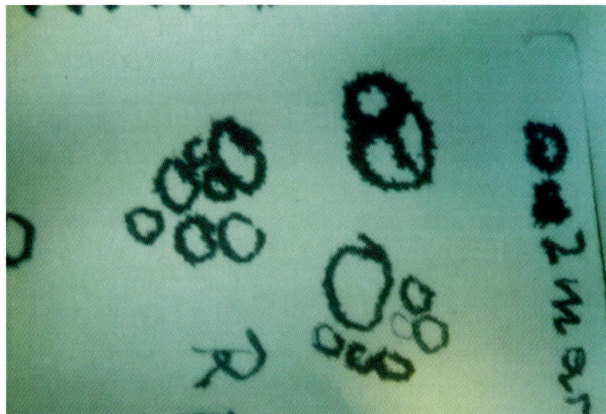

Figure 3-13 Intraoperative sketch of the proximal stump.

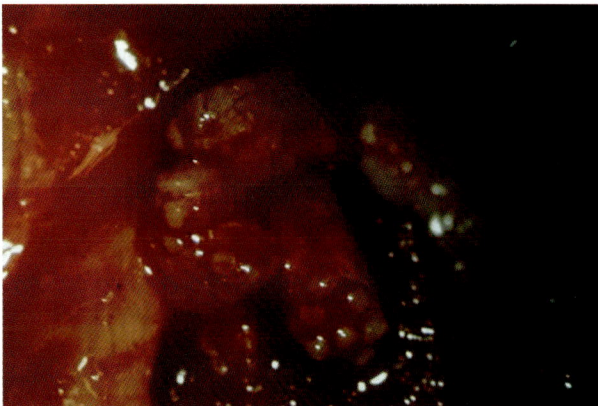

Figure 3-14 In the distal stump, we meet again the major group with the many small fascicles, and three groups at the palmar side apparently formed by divison of the two fascicular groups of the proximal stump.

follow the deep branch by retrograde tracing to the distal stump. In Case 2, the larger fascicle group with many fascicles formed the deep branch, and these groups were connected by two segments of the sural nerve.

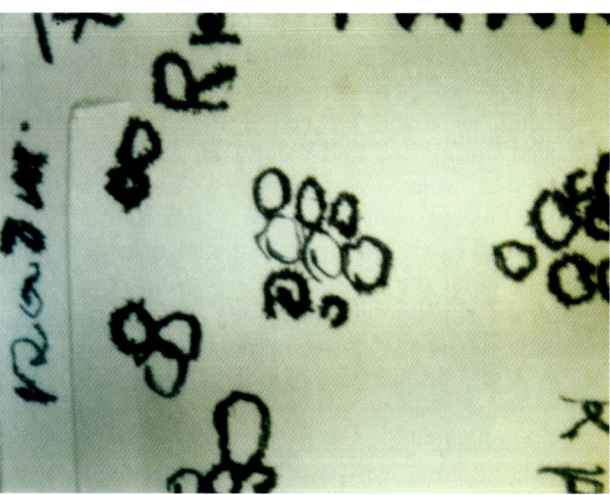

Figure 3-15 Intraoperative sketch of the distal stump.

In Case 3, we had to deal with a thick nerve that may have contained between 30 and 120 fascicles. It was impossible to cover the cross-section with autologous nerve grafts. This situation may justify the application of allografts or the combination of autografts and alternatives. The best solution, of course, would have been the application of artificially designed nerve grafts consisting of a proper stroma and Schwann cells from the host.

In our case, we decided to interpose our autografts between areas that we knew contained mainly nerve fibers for the tibial nerve. In the proximal segment close to the pelvis, these fibers are mainly concentrated in the caudal part of the cross-section, and in the medial segment at the level of the thigh.

Determination of Distance Between the Two Stumps

The defect was determined by the trauma and the damage of the tissue of the two stumps, which made a proper resection necessary. The distance between the two stumps to the nerve defect could be manipulated by changing the angle of the adjacent joints. By flexing these joints the distance can be minimized (Fig. 3-16). This means that the length of graft is minimized, but the two sites of coaptation are exposed to tension at the site where the mobile proximal and distal stumps meet the fixed grafts, which have developed adhesions in order to survive. By extending the joints in the close neighborhood, the distance is maximized. Longer grafts are needed but the sites of coaptation are rather relaxed when mobilization starts (Fig. 3-17). It is my strong recommendation to elect the maximal distance.

For Case 1, the estimated distance was 11.5 cm; Case 2, about 6 cm, and Case 3, 20 cm.

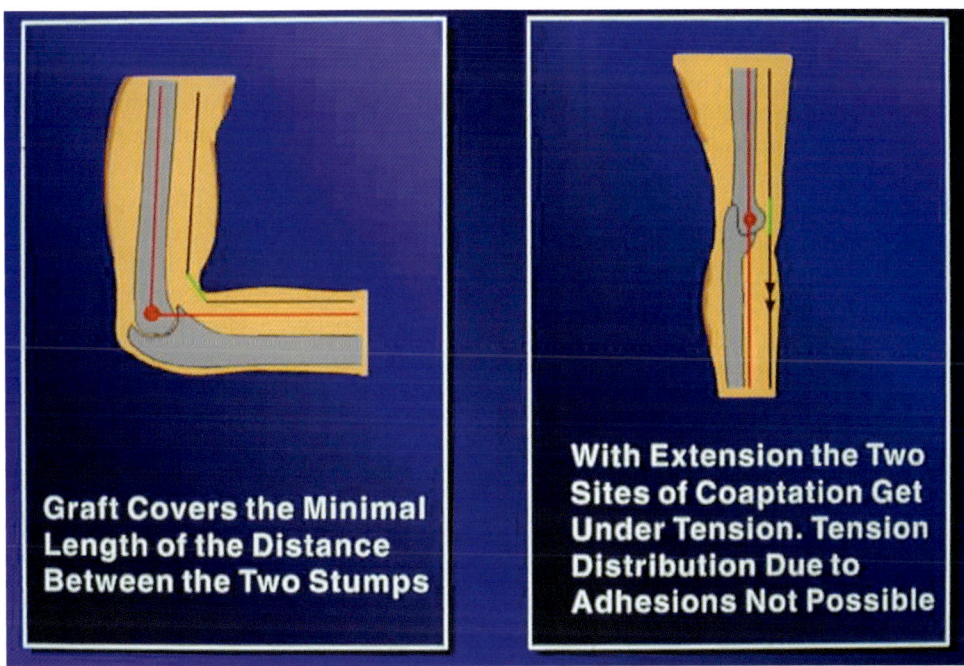

Figure 3-16 Minimal distance between the two stumps.

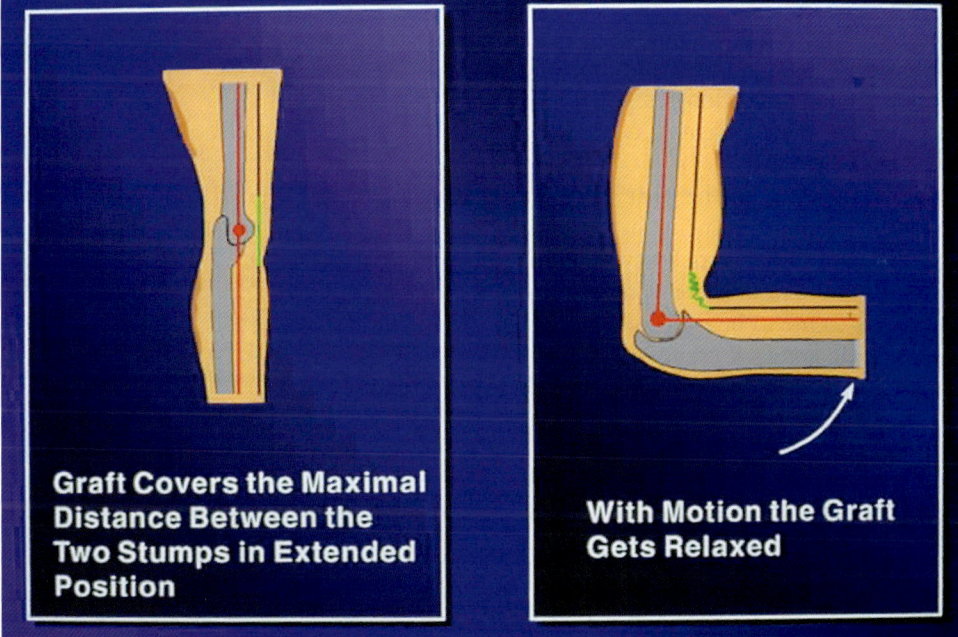

Figure 3-17 Maximal distance between the two stumps.

Harvesting Nerve Grafts

The first choice of a cutaneous nerve graft was the two sural nerves. According to the body length of the patient, a graft length of 36 to 45 cm can be gained. The sural nerve is formed by a source from the tibial nerve joined by nerve fibers from the peroneal nerve (Ramus communicans peroneus).

The two sources meet at different levels, and this creates some difficulties when harvesting the sural nerve. The nerve is easily found dorsal of the lateral malleolus, somewhat deeper to the V. saphena parva. We exposed the nerve by a small transverse incision at this level. Another incision was made 3 cm proximal to the distal incision. The nerve was defined here as well. By traction on the nerve at this level, one can easily see whether the already defined nerve at the distal incision is the only one or if there are already branches that have to be transacted independently. If all branches are transected, the nerve can easily extracted by the more proximal incision. By pulling at the distal end of the nerve and careful palpation, the nerve can be followed in proximal direction. If by gentle traction at the distal end of the nerve the sural nerve can be mobilized by 2 to 3 cm, we have the ideal situation of a sural nerve without important branches or contributions. In this case, the nerve can be palpated easily below the fossa poplitea isolated between the two gastrocnemius muscles after transection of the fascia transected and harvested. Easy harvesting of the nerve by a stripper would be possible as an alternative.

In case of a contribution or branches, the nerve cannot be mobilized. The level of branches or contributions is identified by palpation. An additional transverse incision has to be made to isolate the nerve there. This has to be continued until the full length of the nerve has been isolated. The two or even three proximal sources of the nerve are cut and the nerve extracted. In this case, the use of a nerve stripper would destroy these contributing branches.

If a longer nerve graft is desired, two more transverse incisions are used at and above the level of the popliteal fossa, and the sural nerve is followed within the tibial or even within the sciatic nerve as long as possible. In many cases, the sural nerve is present at a high level such as a distinct fascicle group.

Since Wallerian degeneration in the graft will occur anyway, we must not treat the sural nerve or any other potential donor nerve with the same delicacy as a functioning nerve. Harvesting the sural nerve using an endoscopic technique seems to me to be over-treatment.

A longitudinal incision along the entire calf produces an ugly scar, which seems counterproductive, especially in a female patient. At about midcalf level, the sural nerve perforates the fascia and is the situated in the subcutaneous tissue. If the nerve is transacted here, the danger of developing a painful neuroma is high. If the entire length of the sural nerve is excised and the proximal stump disappears in the depth of the subfascial space, this danger is nill.

Other donor nerves include the following:

Medial cutaneous antebrachial nerve.
Lateral cutaneous femoral nerve. (This nerve should be cut high up within the pelvis to avoid a painful neuroma.)
Superficial branch of the radial nerve. (This nerve has a high risk of neuroma formation and should be harvested only in brachial plexus cases with a high-level lesion.)
Saphenous nerve.
Posterior cutaneous antebrachial nerve.

Lateral cutaneous antebrachial nerve.
Posterior cutaneous femoral nerve.

If a nerve trunk without function is available—for example, in case of a limb amputation or as a residual segment of a vascularized nerve graft—a graft suitable for free grafting can be produced by splitting the trunk graft into minor units (Fig. 3–18). Sunderland's postulation of the continuing plexiform structure of a nerve trunk[5] is not true for fascicle groups. Segments of heavy exchange between fascicle groups alternate with long segments without any exchange[42] (Fig. 3–19).

Determining Length of Cutaneous Nerve Graft

The harvested donor nerve is transected into segments about 10% longer than the distance between the two stumps. Additionally one must decide which fascicular group in the cutaneous graft to use for the corresponding fascicular groups in the recipient nerve. The sural nerve has a changing fascicular pattern from proximal to distal. At the proximal end, the nerve frequently has

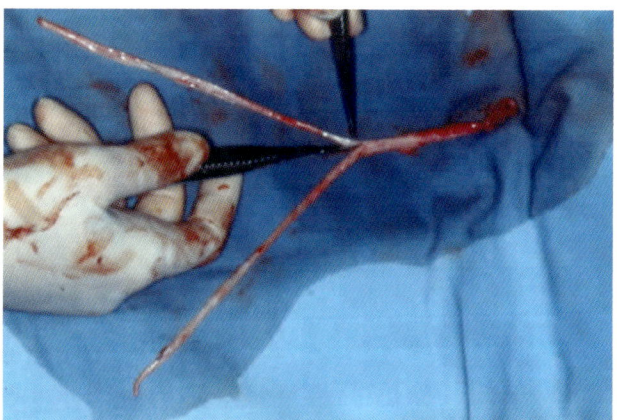

Figure 3–18 Splitting a trunk graft into minor units at the group level.

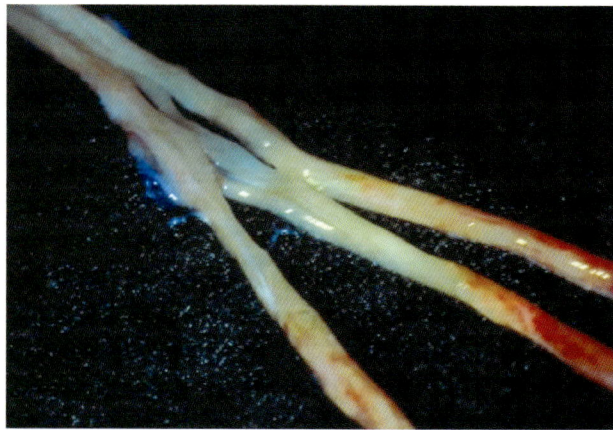

Figure 3–19 In a nerve trunk, the plexiform arrangement of the fascicles, as described by Sunderland,[5] are followed by long segments without interchanges between the fascicle groups.

a monofascicular pattern. During its course, the fascicles divide; at the distal end the nerve may have a polyfascicular pattern with six to eight small (nonmanageable) fascicles. The fascicular pattern with the best fit in the graft segment is matched to a corresponding fascicular group in the stump. The sural nerve as well as any other donor nerve is embedded in paraneurium.

The paraneurium is a layer of loose connective tissue that provides the gliding capacity of the nerve, and links the nerve to the surrounding tissue or to other structure like vessels within a neurovascular bundle. After harvesting the nerve, the paraneurium remains on the surface of the nerve.

When cutting the nerve graft to the proper length, some overlapping of the paraneurium may occur, even with the sharpest instruments. This redundant paraneurium forms an obstacle for the axons upon crossing the line of coaptation. Fibroblasts originating from the paraneurium disturb the healing process. It is therefore extremely important to shift the paraneurium and the epifascicular epineurium away from the cross-section when cutting the nerve.

In my experience, sharps scissors with serrated blades are the best instrument to accomplish this. Of course, the cutaneous nerve is not cut in one bite, but rather in several delicate bites. Each time, the tissue on the surface is shifted away and the fascicular tissue is exposed (Fig. 3–20 A and B). The proper segments are prepared for Case 1 (Fig. 3–21).

Interposition of Nerve Grafts Between the Two Stumps

The nerve grafts are now introduced in the gap between the two stumps. This can be done one by one or, connecting them as a half-tube for easier handling. The main point is that the grafts are kept separate from each other and the two ends of each graft are identified in order to allow a proper coaptation.

Coaptation

Each end of each graft is now coapted to the previously defined fascicle or fascicle group. One fine stitch is used to achieve this without touching the graft with forceps. The small cuff of perineurial tissue mentioned above helps to avoid displacement of the deeply placed fascicles in the graft.. If there are several fascicles or fascicle groups each of them is transected at a different level This provides a certain stability (Fig. 3–22). The single stitch is sufficient; sometimes no sutures are required, and coaption can occur through natural fibrin clotting. We do not apply tissue glues.

The situation with Case 1 is demonstrated in Figs. 3–23 and 3–24. For Case 2, Fig. 3–25 shows the coaptation of two of the four grafts to the proximal stump of

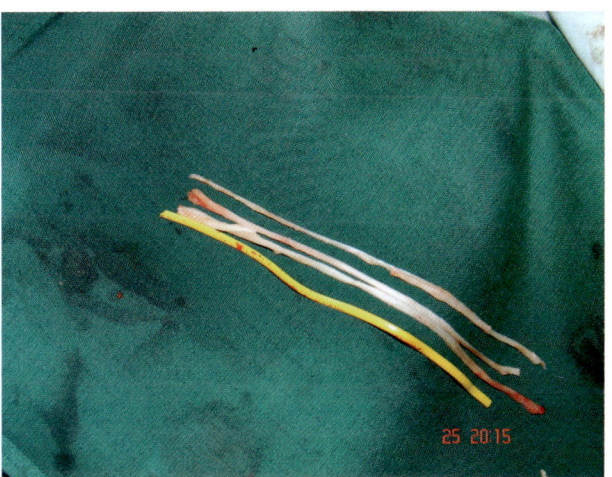

Figure 3–21   Three segments of the sural nerve are prepared to bridge the defect of the median nerve in Case 1.

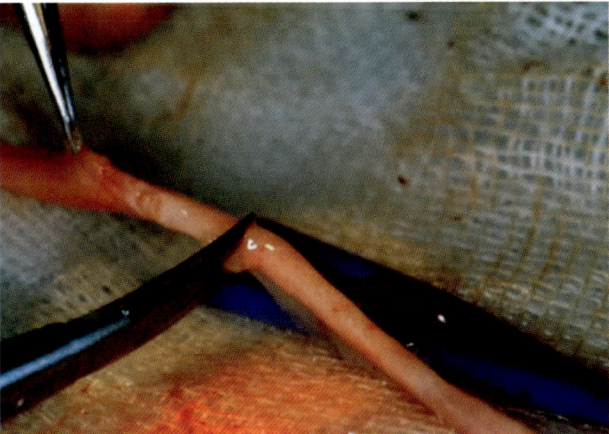
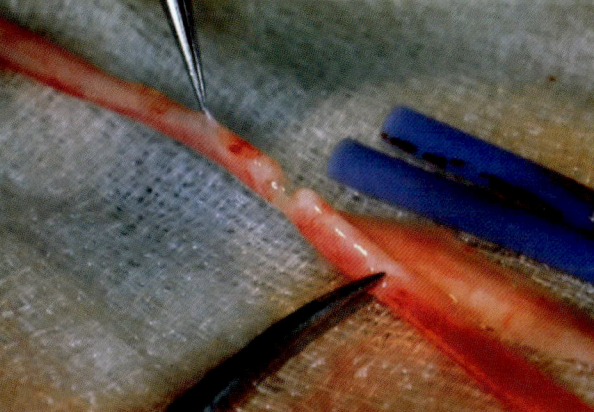

Figure 3–20   Transsection of a sural nerve graft into segments of proper length using a serrated scissors. The transsection is done in several bites **(left)**. With each bite, the paraneurium is shifted away from the site of cross-section **(right)** to avoid overlapping.

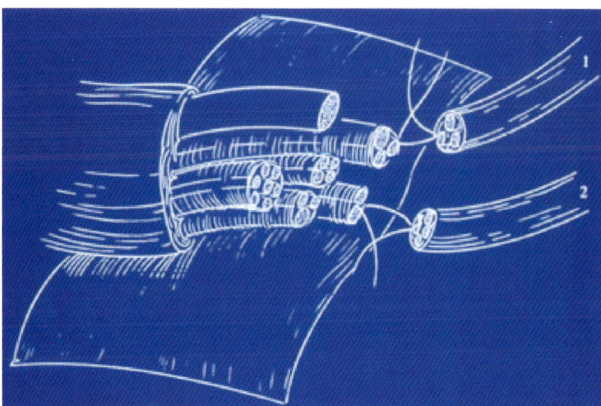

Figure 3–22   Two cutaneus nerve grafts segments are approximated to one fascicle group each. The stump is prepared by interfascicular dissection. The fascicle groups are transsected at different levels to provide stability by interdentation.

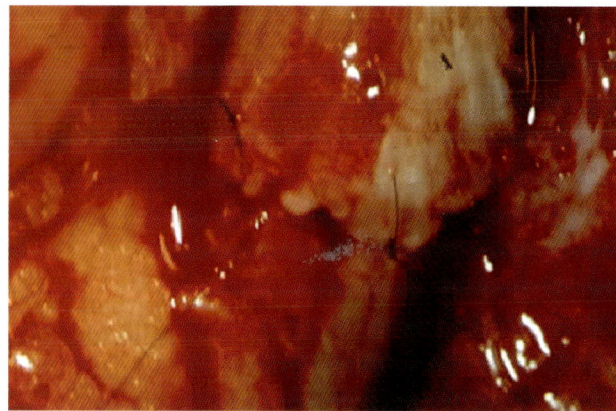

Figure 3–25   Proximal stump of the ulnar nerve in Case 2. Two sural nerve grafts have been already coapted to the stump. Note that an "exact" coaptation is not possible due to the different fascicular pattern. This rather rough coaptation does not preclude a very good result (Fig. 3–26).

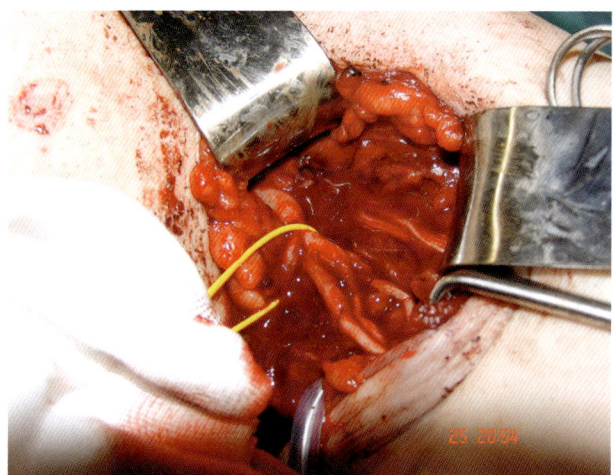

Figure 3–23   The proximal ends of the grafts are coapted to the isolated fascicle groups of the proximal stump (Case 1).

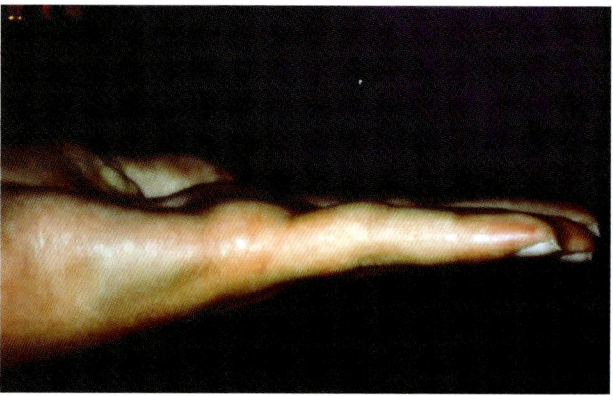

Figure 3–26   Result of the restoration of the continuity of the ulnar nerve by nerve grafts in Case 2.

the ulnar nerve. It can clearly be seen that the size and number of fascicles of the groups and of the grafts do not correspond very well, and only a loose coaptation can be achieved. Proper outgrowth of the axon sprouts occurs in this situation due to neurotropism and neurotrophism. The result speaks for itself (Fig. 3–26).

Wound Closure

After such a grafting procedure, all structures are extremely sensitive to traction and shearing forces. It is therefore important to avoid any shearing forces when the soft tissue wound and the skin wound are closed. This is an important part of the surgery that should be performed by an experienced surgeon who understands this problem.

Immobilization

After nerve grafting according to the interfascicular technique, absolute immobilization is mandatory. This

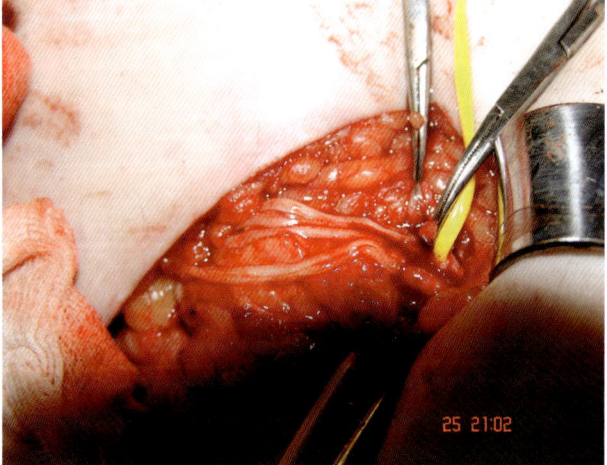

Figure 3–24   The distal ends of the grafts are coapted to the isolated fascicle groups of the distal stump. Note that the grafts are not in contact with each other.

relates to the wound closure as mentioned above and to the postoperative dressing. The involved limb has to remain in the exact position that it was in at the time the grafts were inserted. During limb elevation while applying the dressing, care must be taken to maintain the exact angle of the adjacent joints while a cast is applied.

For example, in a median nerve repair, the upper extremity is immobilized with shoulder abduction and elbow extension, with the wrist in a position of function. The position should be maintained for at least 3 or 4 days. The patient can be mobilized with arm elevation maintained with an IV pole.

The same is true for an ulnar nerve repair following anterior transposition or for radial nerve repair. If the ulnar nerve is left in the epicondylar, the arm is immobilized with elbow flexion. If the median or ulnar nerve repair is performed close to the wrist joint, the limb is immobilized with the elbow extended and the wrist in a position of function and the fingers extended.

From animal experiments, we know that after 2 days certain stability by natural fibrin clotting already exists. Therefore, the first 2 days are the most critical.

After 5 to 6 days, the danger of dehiscence is minimal and after 8 days no immobilization is necessary anymore. This is one of the big advantages of our grafting technique: after 8 days, active and passive range of motion exercises in physiotherapy can be started.

Postoperative Supervision

Every patient should remain under the postoperative supervision of the surgeon until wound healing is finished. The surgeon should also supervise the physiotherapy. The surgeon has to note the appearance and advancement of the Tinel-Hoffmann sign. If it stops at the proximal site of coaptation, something went wrong with the grafting procedure. Revision is indicated, and eventually the grafting has to be repeated.

If the Tinel-Hoffman sign stops at the distal site of coaptation, axonal advancement across the repair site might be blocked by the ingrowth of fibrous tissue. However, a good result can still be achieved if the distal site of coaptation is resected and a new coaptation performed.

Fortunately, this problem at present occurs in very rare instances, but the surgeon must be aware of it. A typical example is shown in Case 4.

The postoperative treatment includes active and passive exercises, measures to increase circulation, the administration of vitamin B1, and electrical stimulation.

Results

Case 1: The follow-up period is not long enough and no result can be presented.

Case 2: Excellent recovery of the ulnar nerve function (Fig. 3–26) after the nerve grafting. Excellent recovery of the median nerve after neurolysis of the primary suture site (Fig. 3–27).

Case 3: Satisfactory recovery of the tibialis innervated muscles. Restoration of extension of the ankle joint by tibialis posterior tendon transfer (Figs. 3–28 and 3–29). The patient could reassume her original profession as a surfing teacher (Fig. 3–30).

Case 4: Radial nerve lesion and restoration of continuity by nerve grafting. The Tinel sign did not advance beyond the distal site of coaptation. We had to assume that the further advancement of the axon sprouts was blocked. This is an indication to re-explore the distal site, which was fibrotic. The distal site of coaptation (Fig. 3–31) was resected, and a new coaptation performed, with very good results. (Figs. 3–32 and 3–33).

THE TECHNIQUE OF VASCULARIZED NERVE GRAFTING

My personal experience with vascularized nerve grafts is limited to application of this technique in brachial

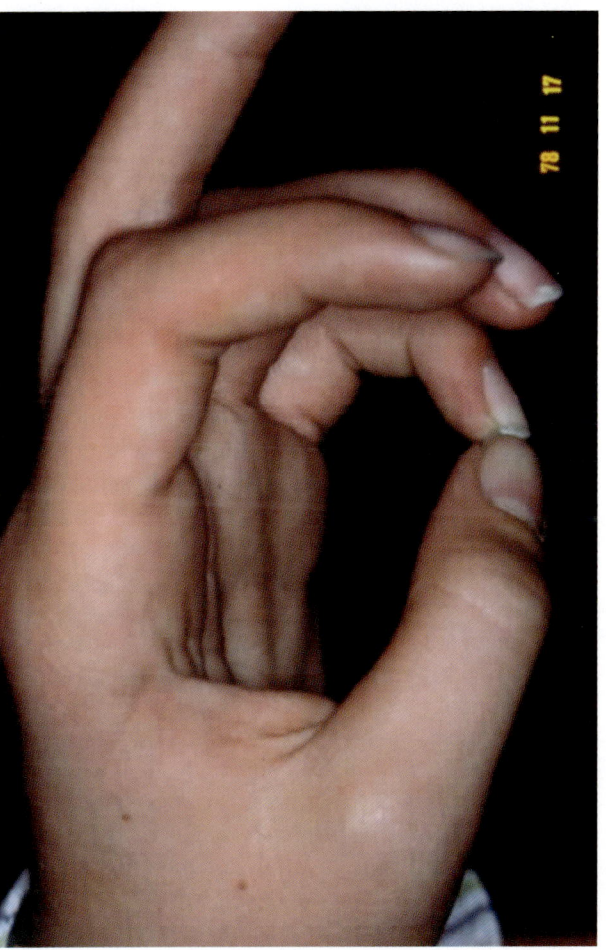

Figure 3–27 Result of the neurolysis, performed at the site of the primary repair of the median nerve in Case 2.

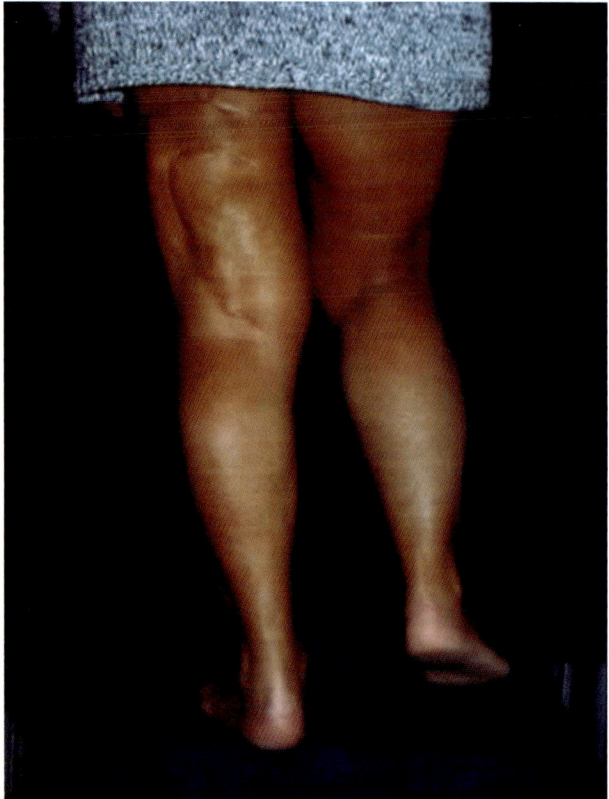

Figure 3–28 Case 3: Function result after restoring a defect of a sciatic nerve by 20-cm-long nerve grafts. Good recovery of the tibialis innervated muscles.

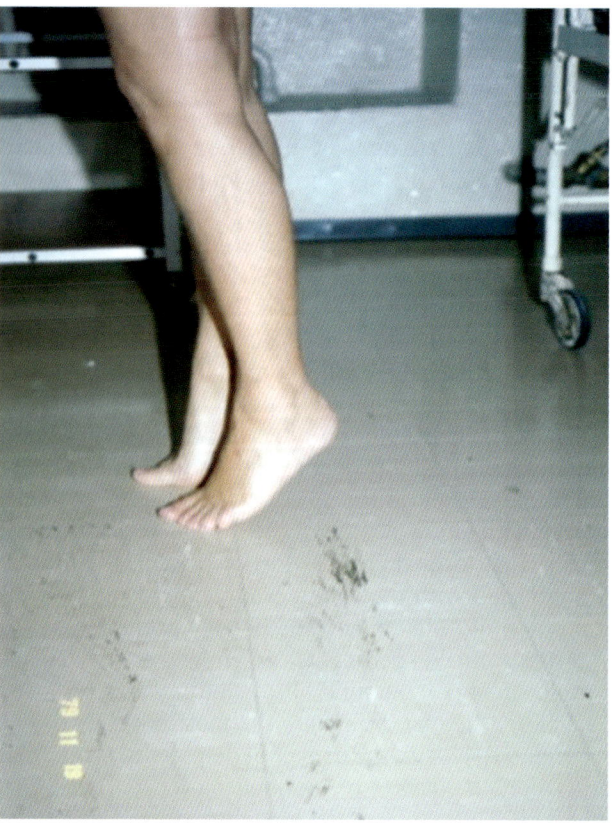

Figure 3–29 Restoration of extension of the ankle joint by tibialis posterior tendon transfer.

plexus surgery. In extensive brachial plexus lesions, the prognosis for functional recovery of ulnar nerve innervated muscles is poor; consequently, ulnar nerve reconstruction has the lowest priority. In a complete brachial plexus lesion with avulsion of C8 and T1, the ulnar nerve seems expendable and could be used as a donor graft. Of course, irreparable damage of C8 and T1 has to be proven by exploration. Indirect evidence of avulsion by MRI or CT-myelography is not sufficient to justify harvesting the ulnar nerve. There are well-documented cases of patients with signs suggesting an avulsion of C8 and/or T1 who recovered useful function in this area.

The main advantage of harvesting the ulnar nerve is that it provides an abundant source of grafts. I have always found it hard to understand why others have not used free ulnar nerve grafts as split grafts more frequently as we did many years ago. Following the suggestion of Julia Terzis, the superior collateral ulnar artery and vein can be used as vascular pedicle, which provides sufficient blood supply for the total length of the ulnar nerve.

The pedicle is long enough to provide sufficient freedom of movement to reach any point in the brachial plexus area. The vascularized graft is an island flap, and

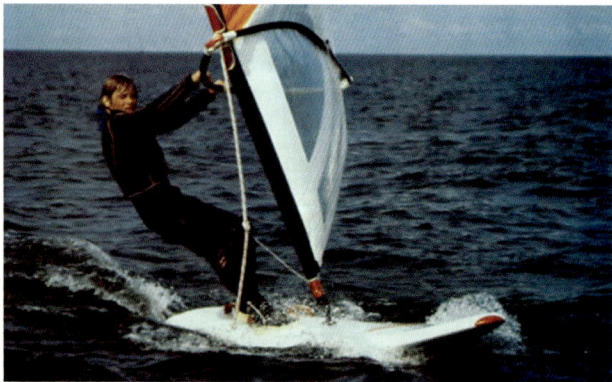

Figure 3–30 Case 3: The patient could reassume her profession as a surfing teacher.

the risk of performing a vascular anastomosis is avoided. There is only the risk of torsion or stretching the pedicle to eventually cause circulation breakdown. If everything goes well, there is no ischemic period.

The big disadvantage is fascicular mismatch, as mentioned above, due to the changing fascicular pattern of the ulnar nerve. Direct matching is only possible if grafting isolated motor or sensory fascicles in the proximal and distal stumps.

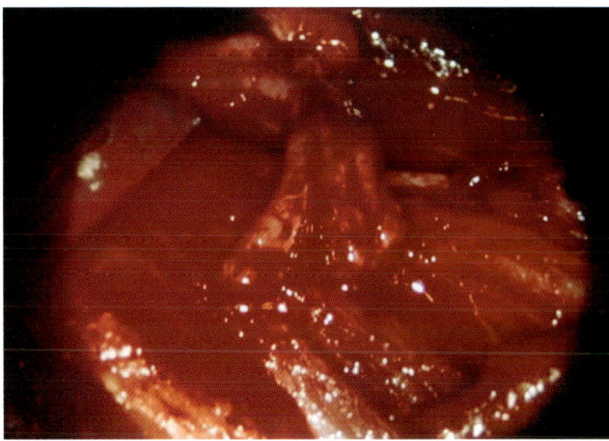

Figure 3–31 Case 4: After resection of the fibrotic distal suture site, the distal end of the nerve grafts, which survived the grafting very well, are clearly visible. A new coaptation is performed.

I applied this technique in two ways: (1) interpositional grafting of C6 to the musculocutaneous nerve, and (2) contralateral C7 transfer to the ipsilateral median nerve.

Interpositional Grafting C6 to Musculocutaneous Nerve

The ulnar nerve is isolated, and the vascular pedicle is identified. The ulnar nerve is transected as far distal as necessary to have a long enough segment. The nerve is transected at a proximal level. It is now an island flap connected to the body by the vascular pedicle only. The nerve is turned around by 180 degrees without impairing the circulation in the pedicle. The distal end is connected to the prepared stump of C6. The former proximal end—now the distal end—is connected to the distal stump of the transected musculocutaneous nerve. In some cases, I had a quick neurotization and an excellent recovery. Some cases were only partially successful, and some cases were failures.

In eight patients, we performed the following: interpositional grafting C6 to the musculocutaneous nerve as described above. Interpositional grafting from C7 to the radial nerve by free sural nerve grafts to preferentially neurotize the cross-sectional region from the origin of the fascicles to triceps muscle. As examples, two cases are described.

Case 5: Patient P.A., male, age 28 years. Vascularized ulnar nerve graft to the biceps (Fig. 3–34). Free sural nerve graft to the triceps. Excellent recovery of biceps function, alongside recovery of triceps muscle (Fig. 3–35).

Case 6: Patient Ch.A., male, age 24 years. Complete brachial plexus lesion on left side. Vascularized ulnar nerve graft for the biceps (Fig. 3–36). Free sural

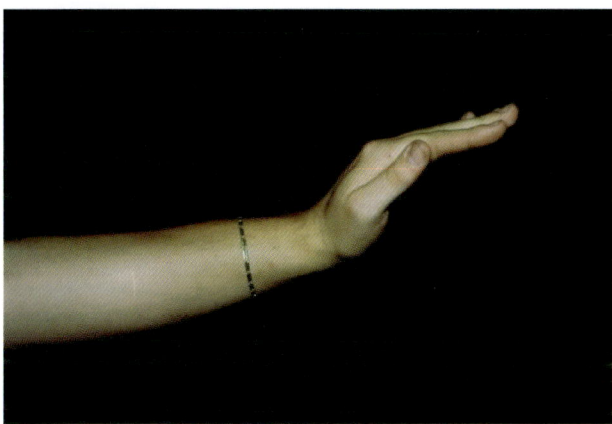

Figure 3–32 Case 4: Satisfactory result of a radial nerve repair after nerve grafting, blockage at the distal site of coaptation, resection of the coaptation site, and performing a new coaptation.

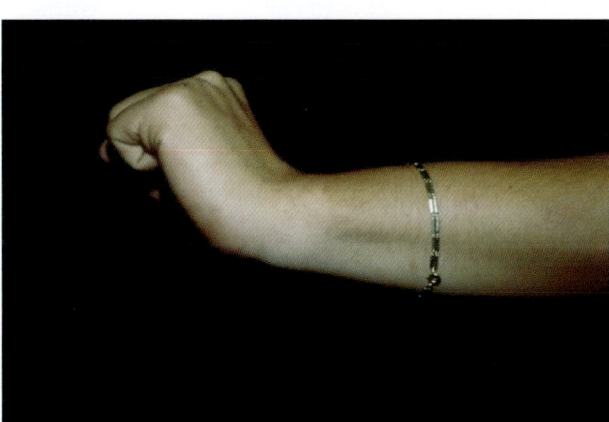

Figure 3–33 Case 4: Final result after radial nerve grafting.

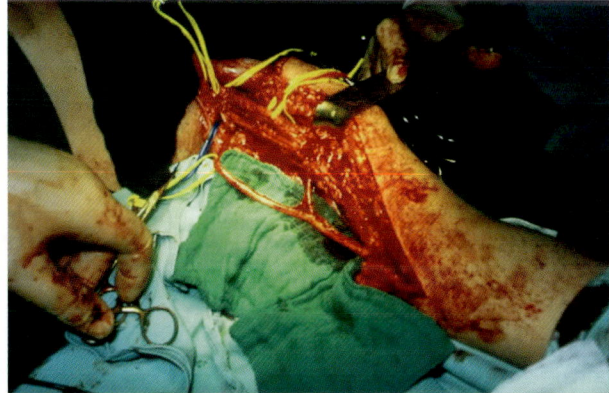

Figure 3–34 Case 5: Vascularized ulnar nerve graft prepared to neurotisize the musculocutaneus nerve. At the same time, the triceps was neurotisized by free nerve grafts.

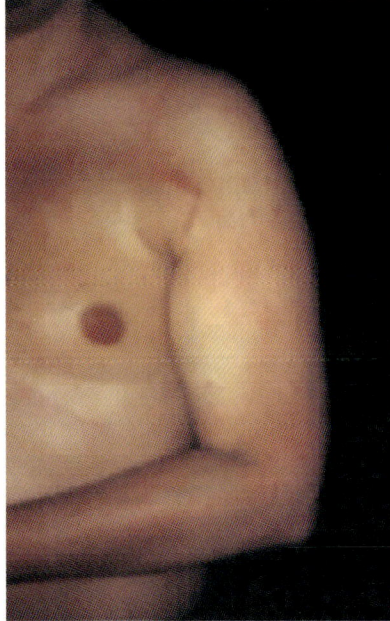

Figure 3–35 Case 5: Excellent recovery of the biceps muscle.

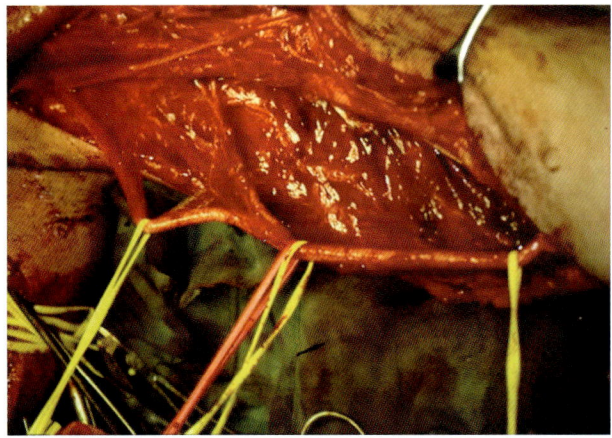

Figure 3–36 Case 6: Vascularized ulnar nerve graft to neurotisize the musculocutaneus nerve. At the same time, the triceps was neurotisized by free nerve grafts.

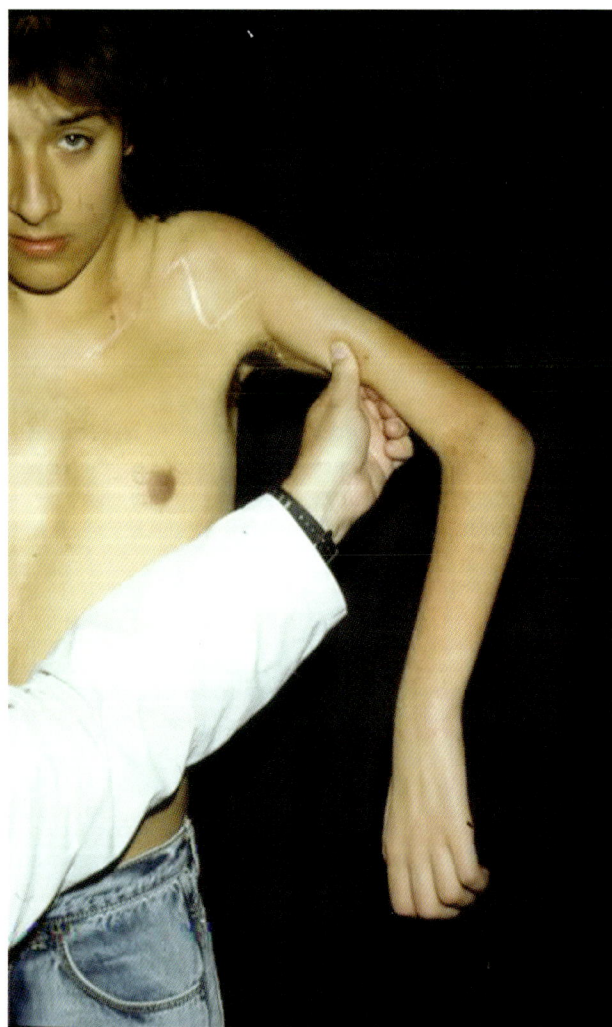

Figure 3–37 Case 6: No recovery of the biceps. Satisfactory recovery of the triceps.

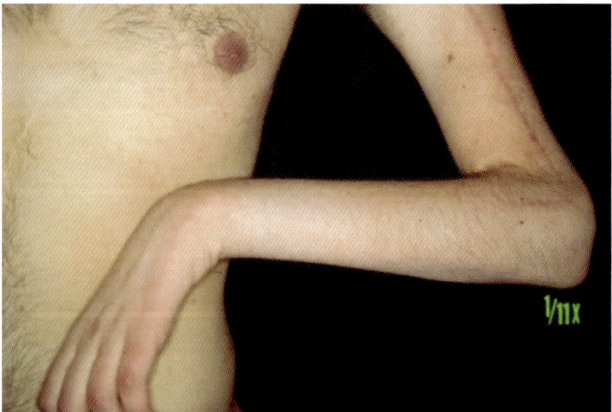

Figure 3–38 Case 6: Satisfactory elbow flexion after transfer of the triceps to the biceps tendon.

nerve graft for the triceps. No useful recovery at the biceps (Fig. 3–37), but useful recovery of the triceps. Restoration of elbow flexion by triceps transfer to the biceps tendon (Fig. 3–38).

Eight cases were in the study. The average outcome for biceps muscle strength (vascularized ulner nerve graft) was M2.5, and the average outcome for triceps muscle strength (free sural nerve graft) was M2.9. The conclusion of this study was that apart from theoretical considerations, there is no practical difference between free and vascularized nerve grafts. Avoidance of an ischemic period plays no role.

Contralateral C7 Transfer in Cases of Multiple Root Avulsions

Following the suggestions of Gu et al.,[43] I used the ulnar nerve—again as an island flap—to connect the former distal end of the nerve across the ventral side of the chest to the contralateral ventral branch of the spinal nerve C7. The former proximal end of the ulnar nerve—now the distal end—was coapted to the distal stump of the transected median nerve.

In a number of these cases, we found that there was useful motor recovery of the flexor digitorum superficialis muscle, the flexor pollicis longus, and the flexor carpi radialis. After arthrodesis of the wrist joint, and after surgery to bring the thumb to a better position, key grip function could be achieved after the flexor carpi radialis tendon had been transferred to extend the thumb and the fingers. There was also return of protective sensibility in the median nerve territory. In order to get sensibility in the ulnar nerve territory, the distal end of the ulnar nerve was coapted end to side to the median nerve.

Since that time, I have found that C7 transfer only works well in young patients within a short time from the injury. The best results can be achieved if the median and ulnar nerves are neurotized using the saphenous nerve as a free graft.

Case 7: Traction lesion of the left arm in an 8-year-old boy with avulsion of all five roots. In a first operation, important nerves were neurotized by local nerve transfers. Six months after the accident, nerve fibers from contralateral C7 were transferred to the median and ulnar nerves using saphenus nerve grafts with good success (Figs. 3–39, 3–40, 3–41, and 3–42).

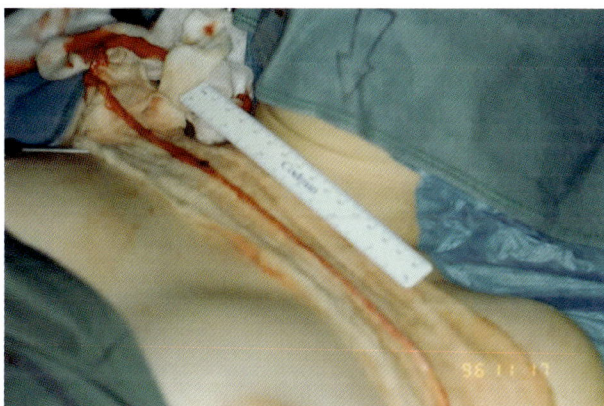

Figure 3–40 Case 7: C7 transfer using both saphenous nerves to connect C7 with the median and the ulnar nerve. (The image derives from a similar case.)

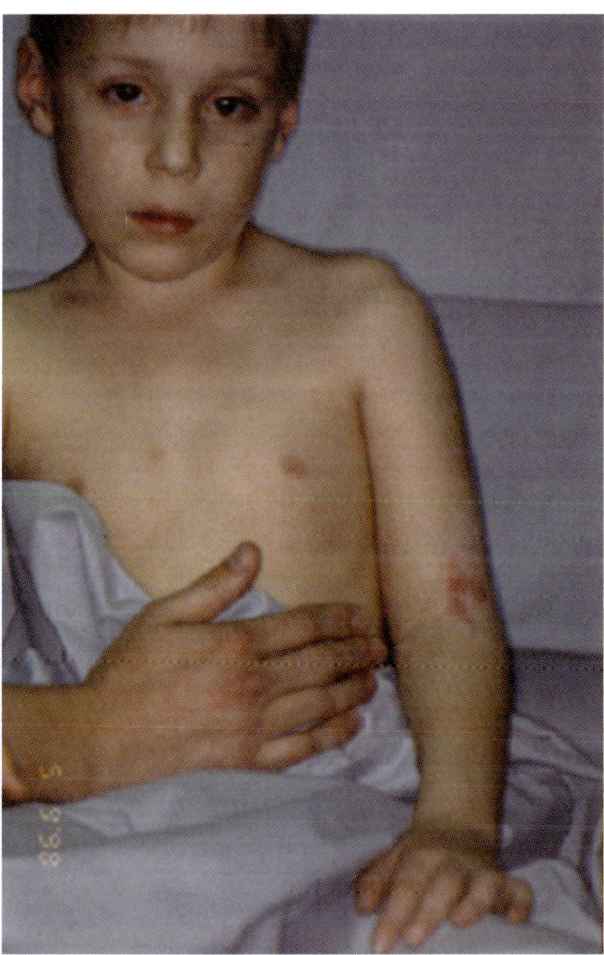

Figure 3–39 Case 7: Eight-year-old boy, traction lesion of the left arm, avulsion of all five roots. Neurotization of important muscles by nerve transfers.

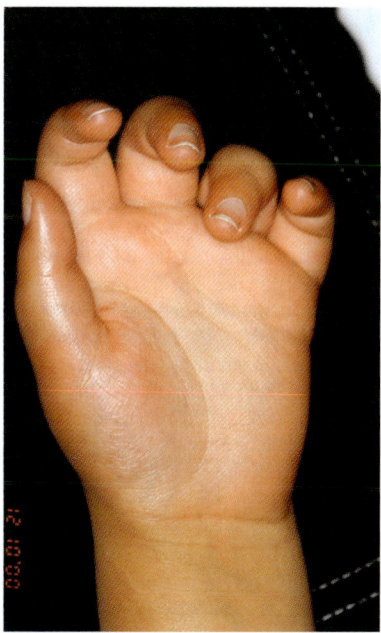

Figure 3–41 Case 7: Excellent recovery of finger flexors, flexor pollicis longus, and thenar muscles.

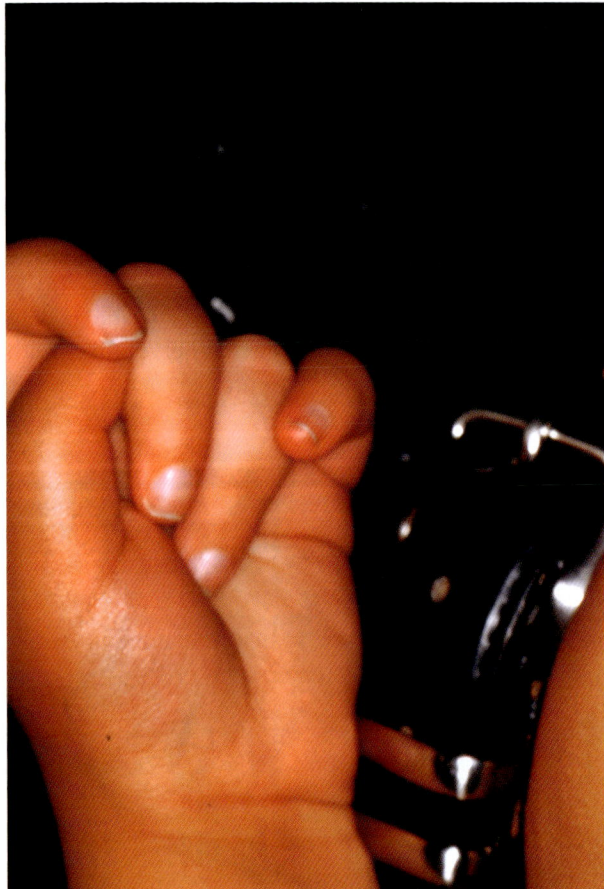

Figure 3–42 Note the active thumb and finger flexion.

REFERENCES

1. Zöch G, Reihsner R, Millesi H. Elastic behavior of the median nerve and the ulnar nerve in situ and in vitro. Handchir Mikrochir Plast Chir 1989;21:305–9.
2. Fontana F. Traité sur le Venin de la Vipère et sur les Poissons américains. Firenze: Nyon l'Ainé, 1781.
3. Clarke E, Bearn JG. The spiral nerve bands of Fontana. Brain 1972;95:1–20.
4. Sunderland S. The connective tissues of peripheral nerves. Brain 1965;88:841.
5. Sunderland S, KC Bradley. Stress-phenomena in human peripheral nerve trunks. Brain 1961;84:102.
6. Schmidhammer R, van der Nest D, Redl H, Millesi H. Synergistic terminal end to side nerve graft coaptation: investigation in a non human primate model. Eur Surg. In press.
7. Babcock W. A standard technique for operations on peripheral nerves with a special reference to the closure of large gaps. Surg Gynecol Obstet 1927;45:364.
8. Ruch DS, Deal DN, Ma J, et al. Management of peripheral nerve defects: external fixator-assisted primary neurorrhaphy. Bone Joint Surg Am 2004;86:1405–13.
9. Nicholson OR, Seddon HJ. Nerve repair in civil practice. Results of treatment of median and ulnar nerve lesions. BMJ 1957;2:1065.
10. Schröder JM, Seiffert KE. Die Feinstruktur der neuromatösen Neurotisation von Nerventransplantaten. Virchows Arch 1970; B5:219.
11. Philipeaux JM, Vulpian A. Note sur les essais de greffes d'un trocon de nerf lingual entre les deux bouts d'hypoglosse. Arch Physiol 1870;3:618.
12. Albert E. Einige Operationen am Nerven. Wien Med Press 1885;26:1285.
13. Bielschowsky M, Unger E. Die Überbrückung grosser Nervenlücken. Beiträge zur Kenntnis der Degeneration und Regeneration peripherer Nerven J Physiol Neurol 1916–1918; 22:267.
14. Hudson A, Hunter D, Kline D, et al. Histological studies of experimental interfascicular graft repairs. J Neurosurg 1979;31:333–40.
15. Hudson A, Kline D. Nerve injuries. Philadelphia: W.B. Saunders, 1995.
16. Aguayo AJ, Kasarjian J, Skamene E, et al. Myelination of mouse axons by Schwann cells transplanted from normal and abnormal human nerves. Nature 1977;268:753–5.
17. Foerster O. Vortrag Ausserordentliche Tagung der Deutschen Orthopädischen Gesellschaft. Münch Med Wschr 1916;63:283.
18. Barnes R, Bacsich P, Wyburn GM, et al. A study of the fate of nerve grafts in man. Br J Surg 1946;34:34–41.
19. Shelden CH, Pudenz RH, McCarty CS. Two stage autograft for repair of extensive median and ulnar nerve defects. J Neurosurg 1947;4:492–6.
20. Strange FGStC. An operation for nerve pedicle grafting. Preliminary communication. Br J Surg 1947;34:423.
21. Strange FGStC. Case report on pedicled nerve graft. Br J Surg 1950;37:331.
22. Brooks D. The place of nerve grafting in orthopaedic surgery. J Bone Joint Surg Am 1955;37:299.
23. Seddon HJ. The use of autogenous grafts for the repair of large gaps in peripheral nerves. Br J Surg 1947;35:151.
24. Millesi H. Zum Problem der Überbrückung von Defekten peripherer Nerven. Wien Med Wschr 1968;118:182.
25. Millesi H, Berger A, Meissl G. The interfascicular nerve grafting of the median and ulnar nerves. J Bone Joint Surg Am 1972;54:727–50.
26. Millesi H, Berger A, Meissl G. Experimentelle Untersuchung zur Heilung durchtrennter peripherer Nerven. Chir Plastica 1972;1:174–206.
27. Millesi H, Berger A, Meissl G. Further experiences with interfascicular grafting of the median, ulnar and radial nerves. J Bone Joint Surg Am 1976;58:227–30.
28. Ruch DS, Deal DN, Ma J, et al. Management of peripheral nerve defects: external fixator-assisted primary neurorrhaphy. J Bone Joint Surg Am 2004;86:1405–13.
29. Taylor GI, Ham FJ. The free vascularized nerve graft Plast Reconstr Surg 1976;57:413–26.
30. Breidenbach WB, Terzis JK. The anatomy of free vascularized nerve grafts. Clin Plast Surg 1984;11:65–71.
31. Townsend PLG, Taylor GI. Vascularised nerve grafts using composite arterialised neuro-venous systems. Br J Plast Surg 1984;37:1–17.
32. Doi K, Kuwata N, Kawakami F, et al. Free vascularized sural nerve graft. Microsurgery 1984;5:175–84.
33. Bsteh FX, Millesi H. Zur Kenntnis der zweizeitigen Nerventransplantation bei ausgedehnten peripheren Nervendefekten. Klin Med (Wien) 1960;12:571.
34. Bsteh FX. Experimentelles zur Frage der zweizeitigen Nerventransplantation. Zbl Neurochir 1953;13:23.
35. Millesi H. Nerve transplantation for reconstruction of peripheral nerves injured by the use of the microsurgical technic. Minerva Chir 1967;22:950–1.
36. Bosse JP. Diskussionsbeitrag. In: Gorio A, Millesi H, Mingrino S, eds., Posttraumatic Peripheral Nerve Regeneration: Experimental Basis and Clinical Implications. New York: Raven Press, 1981:347.
37. Seddon HJ. Nerve grafting. J Bone Joint Surg Br 1973;45:44.
38. Seddon HJ. Surgical Disorders of the Peripheral Nerves. Edinburgh: Churchill-Livingstone, 1972.

39. Seddon HJ. Surgical Disorders of the Peripheral Nerves, 2nd ed. Edinburgh: Churchill-Livingstone, 1975.

40. Millesi H, Berger A, Meissl G. Experimentelle Untersuchung zur Heilung durchtrennter peripherer Nerven. Chir Plast 1972;1:174–206.

41. Millesi H. Healing of nerves. Clin Plast Surg 1977;4:459–73.

42. Eberhard D, Millesi H. Split nerve grafting. J Reconstr Microsurg 1996;12:71–6.

43. Gu YD, Zhang GM, Chen DS, et al. Seventh cervical nerve root transfer from the contralateral healthy side for treatment of brachial plexus root avulsiones. J Hand Surg Br 1992;17:518–21.

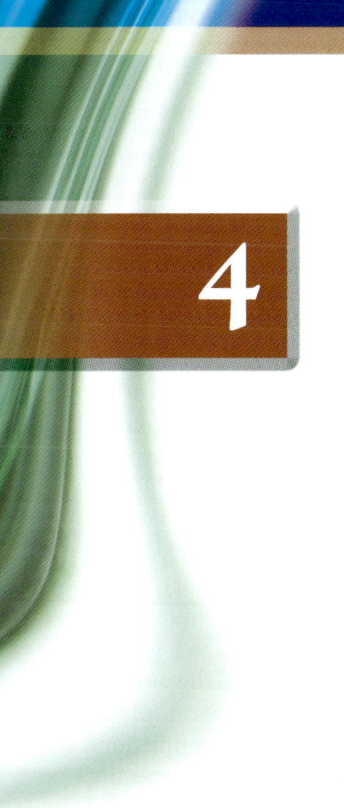

4

A Practical Approach to Nerve Grafting in the Upper Extremity

David J. Slutsky

What the heart has once owned and had, it shall never lose.

HENRY WARD BEECHER (1813–1887)

INTRODUCTION

In this era of tissue bioengineering, an autogenous nerve graft may be considered the ultimate biocompatible, resorbable nerve conduit, with a basil lamina, preformed guidance channels, a reserve of viable Schwann cells, and nerve growth factors. In addition, it is capable of developing an intrinsic circulation. The nerve graft provides a regenerating axon with a means for passage to the distal nerve stump, while protecting it from the surrounding environment. There is no foreign body reaction and no graft versus host response. The results of nerve grafting still remain the gold standard by which all new techniques are compared. The underlying cornerstone of nerve grafting hinges on an understanding of the nerve's response to injury as well as intimate knowledge of the specific nerve anatomy.

NERVE RESPONSE TO INJURY

Cell Body

The neuron consists of a central cell body, located within the central nervous system, and a peripheral axon. The axon represents a tremendously elongated process attached to the nerve cell body. Thousands of axons make up the substance of a peripheral nerve. The axon contains up to 90% of the axoplasmic volume. When a nerve is severed, one immediate consequence is loss of this vital fluid.[1] The normal retrograde transport of neurotrophic factors from the target organ ceases. The cell body undergoes chromatolysis, which includes mitochondrial swelling, migration of the nucleus to the periphery, and dispersal of Nissl substance. The more proximal the site of transection, the more intense the reaction, which peaks by 2 to 3 weeks. The cell body may die and is lost from the neuron pool. If it survives, however, the cell body then shifts its resources toward replacing the axoplasm and rebuilding the axon.

Distal Axon

The distal axon cannot survive without its connection to the cell body and disintegrates (i.e., Wallerian degeneration). Endoneurial edema occurs within a few hours.[2] The microtubules and neurofilaments of the distal axon that are responsible for axoplasmic transport undergo proteolysis by a calcium-activated neutral protease.[3] At 72 hours, the Schwann cells can be seen digesting the myelin sheath and axonal subcomponents.[4] Endoneurial collagen production from both Schwann cells and fibroblasts increases, causing progressive shrinkage of the distal tubules.[5] The Schwann cells rapidly proliferate, forming columns (the bands of Büngner) that appear to stimulate the direction and magnitude of axonal growth.

Proximal Axon

Following transection, there is demyelination of the distal stump. The axons degenerate to one or more proximal internodes. The distance varies with the severity of injury, ranging from a few millimeters with mild trauma to several centimeters with severe injury.[6] The endoneurial tube lies empty, consisting mostly of the Schwann cell basal lamina.

AXON REGENERATION

Nerve regeneration does not involve mitosis and multiplication of nerve cells. Instead, the cell body restores nerve continuity by growing a new axon. Axon sprouting has been demonstrated as early as 24 hours following nerve transection. One axon sends out multiple unmyelinated axon sprouts from the tip of the remaining axon, or collateral sprouts from a nearby proximal node of Ranvier. The distal sprout contains the growth cone. This sends out filopodia,[7] which adhere to sticky glycoprotein molecules in the basil lamina of Schwann cells, such as laminin and fibronectin (neurite-promoting factors).[8] The filopodia contain actin, which aid in pulling the growth cone distally.[9] The basil lamina of two abutting Schwann cells form a potential endoneurial tube into which the regenerating axon grows. These axons will deteriorate if a connection with a target organ is not reached. There are up to 50 advancing sprouts from a single axon. Initially there are many more nerve fibers crossing a nerve repair than in the parent nerve.[10] Although more than one axon may enter the same endoneurial tube, there is eventual resorption of the multiple sprouts, leaving one dominant axon.

Axons grow between 1 and 2 mm/day.[11] The normal 16-day turnover rate of acetylcholine receptors is shortened in denervated muscle to about 4 days.[12] For practical purposes, the maximum length that a nerve can grow to restore motor function is approximately 35 cm.

This in part accounts for the poor motor recovery when grafting nerve defects proximal to the elbow in adults. Sensory end organs remain viable since there is no end plate, and retain the potential for reinnervation.[13] Nerve grafting a digital nerve defect may provide protective sensation even after many years.

Role of Schwann Cells

The importance of maintaining Schwann cell viability in the nerve graft is evident. Following nerve transection, the Schwann cell removes the axonal and myelin debris in both the severed nerve ends and the nerve graft. Schwann cells produce an immediate source of nerve growth factor (NGF) that helps to support the proximal stump.[14] The Schwann cell expresses NGF receptors that aid in directing the advancing growth cone.[15] It also increases its production of other neurotrophic factors, including ciliary neurotrophic factor, brain-derived neurotrophic factor, and fibroblast growth factor, which promote axonal growth.[16] The laminin and fibronectin in the Schwann cell basil lamina act as a rail for the advanced axon sprouts to grow down. The Schwann cell produces a myelin sheath for the immature axon sprout. Cell biologists have attempted to mimic these functions by incorporating Schwann cells, laminin, fibronectin, and nerve growth factors into synthetically engineered nerve conduits.

Role of Nerve Graft

The nerve graft acts to provide a source of empty endoneurial tubes through which the regenerating axons can be directed. Any tissue that contains a basil lamina such as freeze-dried muscle or tendon, can be substituted,[17] but only the autogenous nerve graft also provides a source of viable Schwann cells. In order to do be effective, the graft must acquire a blood supply. If the nerve graft survives, the Schwann cells will also survive.[2]

Graft Incorporation

Once separated from its blood supply, the graft undergoes Wallerian degeneration. Schwann cells can survive for up to 7 days, depending purely on diffusion.[18,19] By 3 days after implantation, there is invasion of the nerve graft by endothelial buds from the surrounding tissue bed, with evidence of high nerve blood flows by 1 week.[20,21] This segmental vascular sprouting from extraneural vessels is not limited by the length of the graft.[22,23] The length of the graft is, within certain limits, of no significance to the end result, provided there is tension-free anastomosis.[24] The ingrowth of vessels from the ends of the graft (inosculation) does not appear to be of major importance, unless the recipient bed is poorly vascularized.[23] The late phase of nerve graft incorporation demonstrates migration of Schwann cells from the proximal nerve end into the graft as well as from the graft into both host nerve ends.[25]

Graft Diameter

Small diameter grafts spontaneously revascularize but large diameter grafts do so incompletely.[26] Thick grafts undergo central necrosis with subsequent endoneurial fibrosis. This ultimately impedes the advancement of any ingrowing axon sprouts. Cable nerve grafts are similar to thick grafts. They consist of a number of nerve grafts that are sutured or glued together to match the caliber of the recipient nerve. Since a large percentage of the surface is in contact with another graft and not in contact with the recipient bed, the central portions may not revascularize. Millesi has stressed that with large diameter recipient nerves it is hence preferable to use multiple smaller caliber grafts to bridge fascicular groups in the proximal and distal stumps in order to increase the surface area that is in contact with the recipient bed.

Nerve Biomechanics

A normal nerve has longitudinal excursion, which subjects it to a certain amount of stress and strain in situ. Peripheral nerve is initially easily extensible. It rapidly becomes stiff with further elongation due to the stretching of the connective tissue within the nerve.[27] Chronically injured nerves become even stiffer.[28] Elasticity decreases by as much as 50% in the delayed repair of nerves in which Wallerian degeneration has occurred.[29] Experimentally, blood flow is reduced by 50% when the nerve is stretched 8% beyond its in vivo length. Complete ischemia occurs at 15%.[30] Suture pullout does not occur until a 17% increase in length. This suggests that ischemia and not disruption of the anastomosis is the limiting factor in acute nerve repairs.[31] This observation is also applicable to nerve grafting.

Nerves are viscoelastic tissue in that when low loading in tension is applied over time the nerve elongates, without a deterioration in nerve conduction velocities. Stress relaxation results in recovery of blood flow within 30 minutes, at 8% elongation.[29] Intriguing experimental work has been done with gradual nerve elongation to overcome nerve gaps using tissue expansion[32] and external fixation,[33] but this cannot be considered an accepted standard of treatment as yet.

A normal nerve can compensate for the change in length with limb flexion and extension because it is surrounded by gliding tissue that permits longitudinal movement. The change in length is distributed over the entire nerve, so that the elongation of each nerve segment is small. A nerve graft becomes welded to its recipient bed by the adhesions through which it becomes vascularized. As a consequence, the nerve graft is exquisitely sensitive to tension because it has no longitudinal excursion. The harvested length of the graft must be long enough to span the nerve gap without tension while the adjacent joints are extended. This is also the position of temporary immobilization. If the limb or digit is immobilized with joint flexion, the graft will become fixed in this position. When the limb is then mobilized at 8 days, the proximal and distal stumps will be subject to tension even though the graft was initially long enough. Early attempts at lengthening the graft will lead to disruption of the anastomosis.

GRAFTING VERSUS PRIMARY REPAIR

A tension-free repair is the goal for any nerve anastomosis. When there is a clean transection of the nerve and the gap is caused by elastic retraction, an acute primary repair is indicated. When treatment of a nerve laceration is delayed, fibrosis of the nerve ends prevents approximation; hence, nerve grafting is indicated even though there is no loss of nerve tissue. As a general rule, primary nerve repair yields superior results to nerve grafting, provided that there is no tension across the anastomotic site.[34] Grafting can obtain similar results to primary repair under ideal conditions.[35] If a nerve is repaired under tension though, the results will actually be superior with an interpositional graft.[36] Axon sprouts are able to cross two tension-free anastomotic sites easier than crossing one anastomosis that is under tension.[37]

Nerve grafting is indicated to bridge a defect when more than 10% elongation of the nerve would be necessary to bridge the gap.[29] This is a better indication for grafting than the nerve gap per se, although 4 cm is often used as the critical defect for grafting in the limb.[38] Defects less than this may be overcome by nerve rerouting and transposition in some instances.

THE NERVE GAP

There is a difference between the nerve gap and a nerve defect. A nerve gap refers to the distance between the nerve ends, whereas a nerve defect refers to the actual amount of nerve tissue that is lost. With simple nerve retraction following division, the fascicular arrangement is similar. As the defect between the proximal and distal stumps increases, there is a greater fascicular mismatch between the stumps, which leads to poorer outcomes. Gaps exceeding 5 cm have been reported to adversely affect the result.[39]

CONSIDERATIONS FOR DONOR NERVE GRAFTS

A number of conditions must be met in order for a nerve to be considered as a potential graft. First, the relation between the surface area and the diameter of the graft must be optimal to allow rapid revascularization. The donor site defect from sacrifice of any given nerve must be acceptable for the patient. The harvested nerve must be long enough to ensure a tension-free anastomosis with the adjacent joints in full extension. Finally, the cross-sectional area and number of fascicles should match those of the recipient nerve at the level of injury as closely as possible. For these reasons, most of the available grafts are cutaneous nerves.

Most donor grafts will be an imperfect match of the recipient nerve. The fascicular arrangement of the nerve graft is dissimilar to the nerve being repaired, in size, number, and fascicular topography. The branching pattern of the grafts usually changes from an oligofascicular pattern proximally to a polyfascicular pattern distally, which does typically correspond to the branching pattern of the recipient nerve. There may be some loss of axon sprouts due to growth down peripheral branches that leave the nerve graft. Some authors have recommended inserting the grafts in a retrograde manner for this reason, but others feel this is not warranted.[24]

The choice of nerve graft will be dictated by the by the length of the nerve gap, the cross-sectional area of the recipient nerve, the available expendable donor nerves for that particular nerve injury, and the surgeon's preference.

DONOR NERVE GRAFTS

As a general rule, it is good practice to divide the donor nerve in an intermuscular plane rather than in the subcutaneous tissue to diminish the risk of a painful neuroma. Innovative surgeons continue to provide novel ways in which to bridge nerve gaps, such as using the fascicular group to the third web space as a source of nerve graft material for bridging median nerve gaps,[40] and the distal anterior interosseous nerve to reconstruct neuromas of the recurrent motor branch of the median nerve.[41] Some of the more commonly used donor nerves are summarized below.

UPPER EXTREMITY GRAFTS

Medial Antebrachial Cutaneous Nerve

The medial antebrachial cutaneous nerve (MABCN) arises from either the medial cord or lower trunk of the brachial plexus. It travels down the arm medial to the brachial artery, and then pierces the deep fascia with the basilic vein about the middle of the arm. More than 90% of the time, the MABCN will bifurcate into an anterior and posterior branch proximal to the medial

epicondyle,[42] which provide sensation to the medial forearm and posteromedial elbow, respectively. It is preferable to use the anterior branch to avoid a bothersome sensory loss over the elbow. The anterior branch crosses the elbow between the medial epicondyle and the biceps tendon, usually in front of the cubital vein, and then travels superficial to the flexor carpi ulnaris muscle, ending 10 cm from the wrist. It is approached through an anteromedial incision on the proximal forearm. This nerve provides a graft of up to 20 cm.

Lateral Antebrachial Cutaneous Nerve

The lateral antebrachial cutaneous nerve (LABCN) is the distal continuation of the musculocutaneous nerve. It exits from underneath the biceps tendon, and then divides into anterior and posterior branch at the elbow crease. The donor site defect corresponds to the anterolateral forearm, but it may also innervate the volar radial or dorsoradial thumb. For this reason, it is not harvested for grafting a sensory nerve deficit to the thumb.[43] There is a partial or complete overlap of the sensory territory of the superficial radial nerve up to 75% of the time.[44] The nerve is approached through an anterolateral incision on the proximal forearm, as it passes deep to the cephalic vein (Fig. 4–1). The LABCN provides a nerve graft of 5 to 8 cm.

Posterior Cutaneous Nerve of the Forearm

The posterior cutaneous nerve of the forearm (PCNF) is a sensory branch of the radial nerve that may rarely be used as a source of graft material. It arises from the radial nerve in the spiral groove and pierces the lateral head of the triceps. It descends the lateral side of the arm and then travels down the dorsal forearm to the wrist where it communicates with terminal branches of the LABCN.

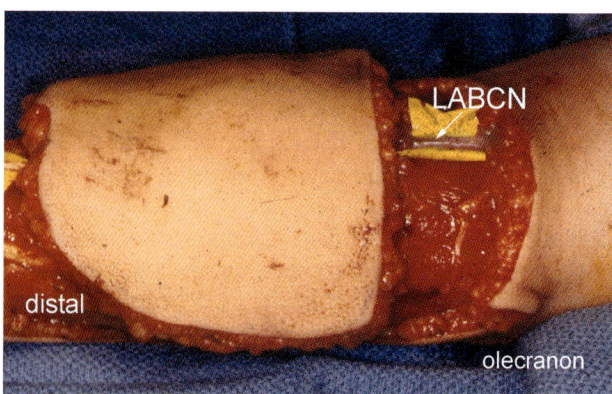

Figure 4–1 Isolation of the lateral antebrachial cutaneous nerve while harvesting a radial forearm flap. (From Slutsky DJ. A practical approach to nerve grafting in the upper extremity. Atlas of the Hand Clinics. Nerve Repair and Reconstruction: A Practical Guide, Vol. 10, No. 1. Philadelphia: W.B. Saunders, 2005:73–92, with permission.)

It supplies sensation to the posterolateral forearm. It is identified via a dorsolateral incision at the elbow between the junction of the brachioradialis (BR) and the extensor carpi radialis longus (ECRL). The PCNF provides 2 to 5 cm of graft material.[45]

Superficial Radial Nerve

The superficial radial nerve (SRN) is prone to painful neuroma formation after trauma; hence, it is not a first-line choice of graft. It may be used for proximal radial nerve injuries, where it is excluded from grafting unless it can be separated from the motor fibers. This is to prevent any regenerating motor nerve fibers from being misdirected to cutaneous reinnervation. The SRN separates from the radial nerve just distal to the elbow in the front of the lateral epicondyle, and then descends behind the brachioradialis along the lateral side of the upper forearm. It then branches into a major palmar and dorsal branch (Fig. 4–2). The SRN can be identified through a dorsolateral incision approximately 7 cm from the wrist, where it winds around the tendon of the BR to pierce the deep fascia. The area of hypoesthesia corresponds to the dorsum of the thumb and adjacent sides of the first and second web spaces. It can provide a nerve graft of up to 15 to 20 cm.

Dorsal Cutaneous Branch of the Ulnar Nerve

The dorsal cutaneous branch of the ulnar nerve (DCBUN) is an uncommon source of nerve graft that has been employed with clinical success. It is an appropriate size and length for use as a digital nerve graft. It can be identified at its takeoff from the main ulnar nerve, 5 cm proximal to the wrist. It passes distally under cover of the flexor carpi ulnaris (FCU), and then perforates the deep fascia. It runs along the dorsomedial aspect of the wrist and hand before dividing into two or three dorsal digital branches. The area of sensory loss corresponds to the dorsal ulnar aspect of the carpus and proximal parts of the ring and small fingers. Painful neuroma formation or loss of hand function related to the use of this nerve is not typical.[46] The nerve can be approached through a dorsomedial incision centered over the distal radioulnar joint. The DCBUN provides a graft of 4 to 6 cm (Fig. 4–3).

Posterior Interosseous Nerve

The terminal portion of the posterior interosseous nerve (PIN) provides proprioception to the joint capsule. Harvesting the nerve leaves no apparent motor nor sensory deficit. The PIN lies adjacent to the posterior interosseous artery on the dorsal surface of the interosseous membrane, deep to the fourth extensor compartment. It ranges from 1 to 5 mm and contains one to five fascicles. It is a good match for grafting digital nerve defects at the distal interphalangeal joint (DIP).[47] The nerve can be located through a dorsal wrist incision just proximal to Lister's tubercle, developing the plane between the 3rd and 4th extensor compartments. The mean length of the PIN from its terminal expansion at the wrist to its most distal muscular branch (to the extensor pollicus longus) is 6 cm.[48]

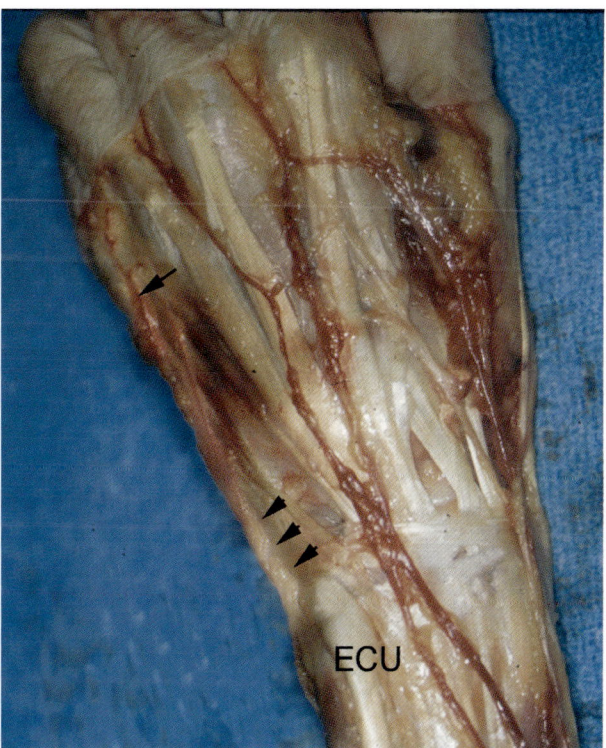

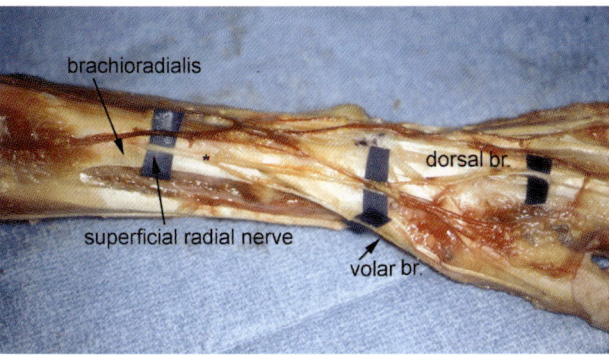

Figure 4–2 Superficial radial nerve arising from underneath the brachioradialis. Note the bifurcation (*) into a major dorsal and volar branch.

Figure 4–3 Dorsal cutaneous branch of the ulnar nerve *(arrows)* coursing dorsal and ulnar to the extensor carpi ulnaris *(ECU)* overlying the fourth intermetacarpal space.

Palmar Cutaneous Branch of the Median Nerve

The palmar cutaneous branch of the median nerve (PCBMN) is consistently present in anatomic studies.[49–51] It originates from the radial side of the median nerve an average 5.9 cm proximal to the distal wrist crease (range, 4.1 to 7.8 cm). Lying within its own tunnel, it courses distally in the interval between the flexor carpi radialis and the palmaris longus. It penetrates the antebrachial fascia at an average of 1.9 cm (range, 1.4 to 2.6 cm) proximal to the wrist crease. It then it travels superficial to the palmar aponeurosis, within 1.5 cm of the wrist crease. At the level of the distal wrist crease, the PCBMN is an average of 2 mm radial to the thenar crease (range 6 mm radial to 6 mm ulnar to the thenar crease). It often remains as one major cable, but it can have a variable branching pattern. The main trunk consists of an average of 1000 myelinated axons arranged in one to four fascicles.[52]

The palmar cutaneous branch of the median nerve, akin to the SRN, is also prone to painful neuroma formation after a laceration. It should be harvested from its point of origin off the median nerve to minimize this risk. The nerve can be located through a curved volar radial incision proximal to the wrist crease, developing the plane between the flexor carpi radialis and palmaris longus (if present). The median nerve is found lying underneath the sublimus tendons. The PCBMN is located on the radial side of the median nerve and followed distally (Fig. 4–4). It can provide a graft length

of 2 to 4 cm from its point of origin to where it pierces the deep fascia.

Anterior Interosseous Nerve

The terminal portion of the anterior interosseous nerve (AIN) also provides proprioception to the joint capsule. Harvesting the nerve similarly leaves no apparent motor nor sensory deficit. The nerve is located adjacent to the anterior interosseous artery on the anterior surface of the interosseous membrane, deep to the pronator quadratus (PQ). It can also be approached through a dorsal incision as for the PIN, after excising a window in the interosseous membrane (Fig. 4–5 A and B). The primarily motor fibers of the AIN provide an expendable donor of adequate size and fascicle number suitable for grafting the recurrent motor branch of the median nerve[41] or the deep motor branch of the ulnar nerve at the wrist.[53]

▌LOWER EXTREMITY GRAFTS

Sural Nerve

The sural nerve (SN) is a common source of nerve graft material. It is formed from the medial cutaneous sural nerve that originates from the tibial nerve. It descends between the two heads of the gastrocnemius piercing the deep fascia in the upper part of the leg, where it is joined by the lateral sural cutaneous branch off the peroneal nerve. It then passes downward near the lateral margin of the tendoachilles to the interval between the lateral malleolus and the calcaneus. After giving off a medial calcaneal branch, it runs forward, below the lateral malleolus, and is continued along the lateral side of the foot. It supplies the skin of the lateral and posterior part of the lower third of the leg. In order to harvest the nerve, the patient is positioned supine on the operating table, with a sandbag placed at midcalf level. The leg is then flexed with the foot on the sandbag to maintain the flexed knee position. The nerve is located via a longitudinal incision that is 1 cm posterior and superior to the lateral malleolus, where it is often accompanied by the lesser saphenous vein. Traction is placed on the nerve until it can be palpated 3 cm proximally, and then a second transverse incision is made. In this manner, the nerve is followed as high as the popliteal fossa by dividing all of the sural communicating branches. The SN provides graft lengths of 30 to 40 cm (Fig. 4–6 A, B).

Superficial Peroneal Nerve

The superficial peroneal nerve has been generally overlooked as a potential donor nerve graft. It is the major lateral branch of the common peroneal nerve that inner-

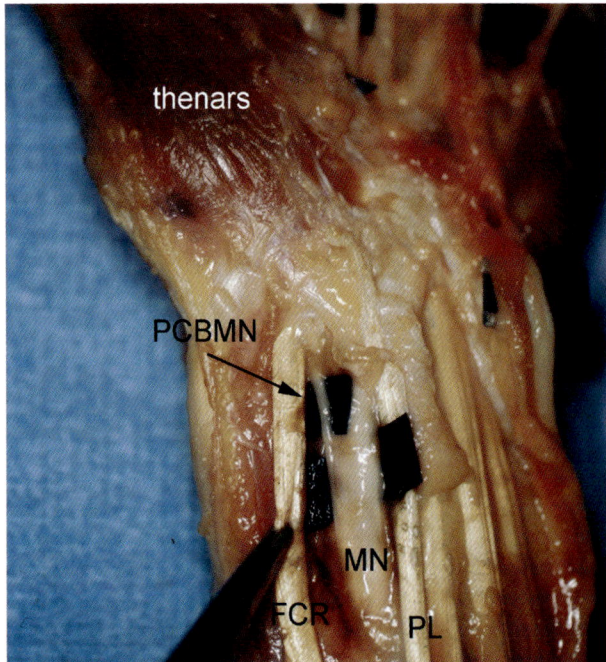

Figure 4–4 Palmar cutaneous branch of the median nerve *(PCBMN),* arising from the radial side of the median nerve *(MN),* in the interval between the flexor carpi radialis *(FCR)* and the palmaris longus *(PL).*

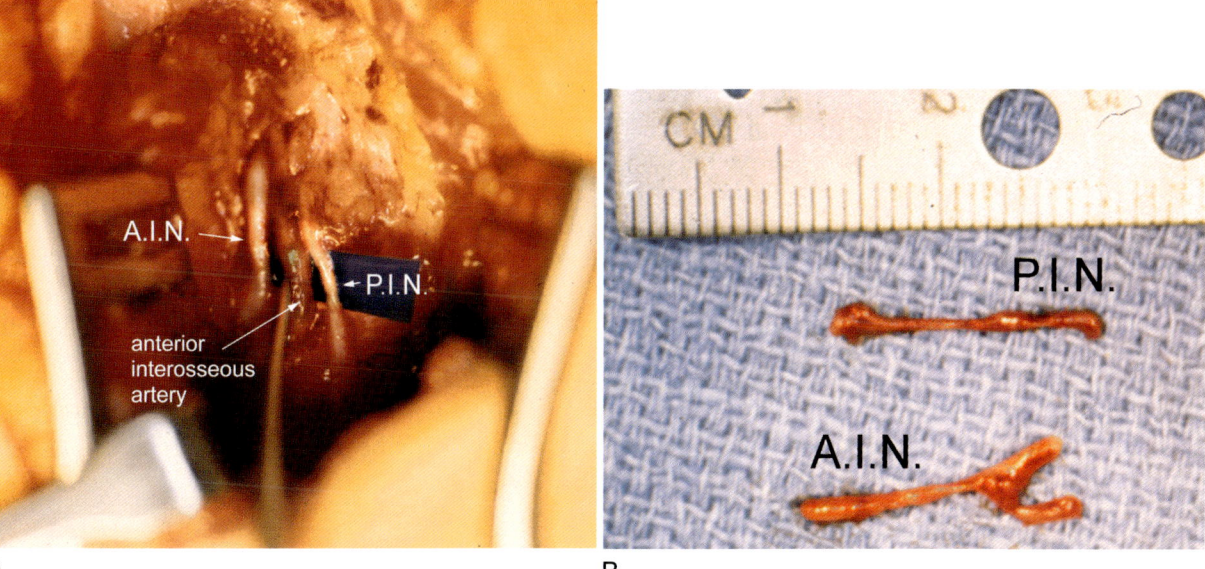

A   B

Figure 4–5   Anterior interosseous nerve *(AIN)* and posterior interosseous nerve *(PIN)* grafts. **A:** Intraoperative photo of PIN. A window in the interosseous membrane allowed isolation of the AIN. **B:** Typical size of harvested grafts. (From Slutsky DJ. A practical approach to nerve grafting in the upper extremity. Atlas of the Hand Clinics. Nerve Repair and Reconstruction: A Practical Guide, Vol. 10, No. 1. Philadelphia: W.B. Saunders, 2005:73–92, with permission.)

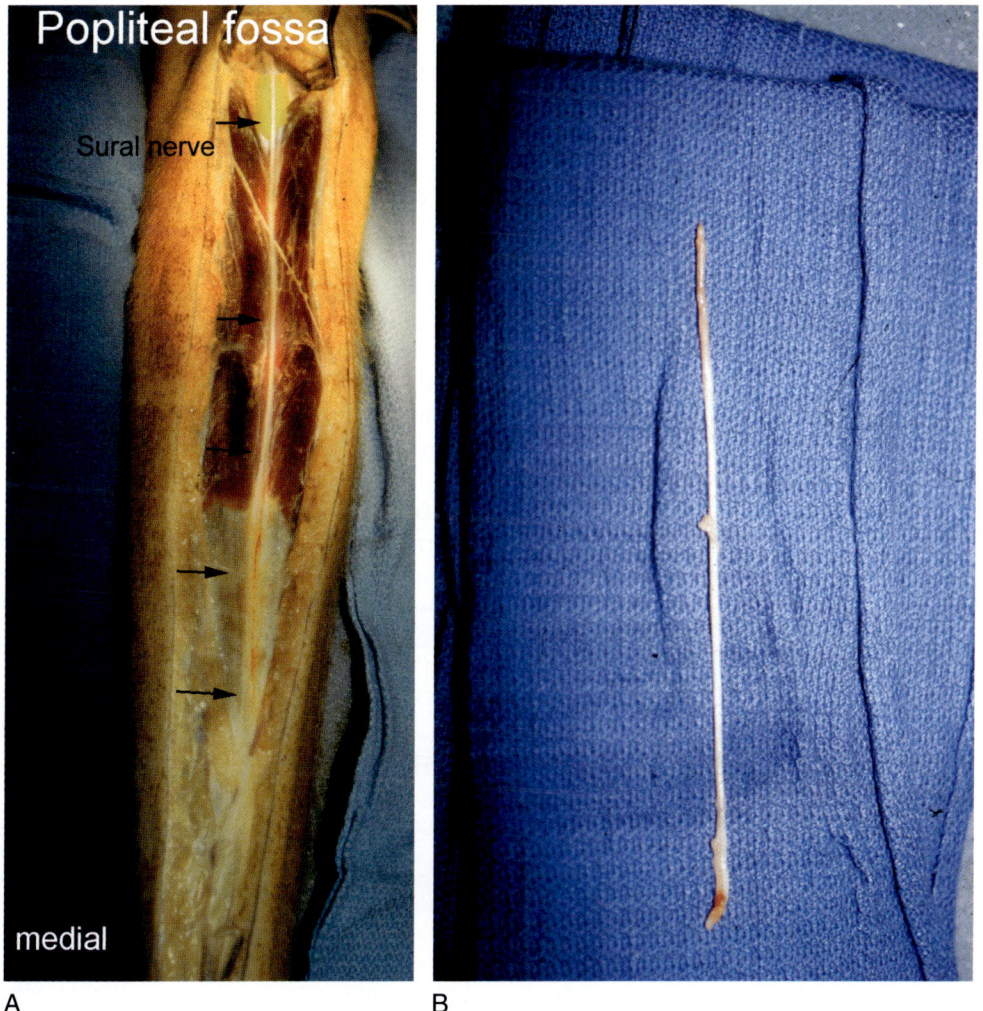

A   B

Figure 4–6   **A:** Demonstration of the sural nerve anatomy looking from the posterior aspect of a prone right leg *(arrows)*. **B:** Harvested sural nerve graft. (From Slutsky DJ. A practical approach to nerve grafting in the upper extremity. Atlas of the Hand Clinics. Nerve Repair and Reconstruction: A Practical Guide, Vol. 10, No. 1. Philadelphia: W.B. Saunders, 2005:73–92, with permission.)

vates the peroneus longus and brevis muscles, and provides sensation to the lateral aspect of the lower leg and dorsal foot. It begins at the bifurcation of the common peroneal nerve between the fibula and the proximal peroneus longus. It then descends on the interosseous membrane with the anterior tibial artery to the front of the ankle joint, where it divides into a lateral and medial terminal branch. It can be located through an anterolateral ankle incision and then followed proximally. It provides a consistently long graft comparable to the sural nerve. It has been used successfully for grafting of the median, radial, and ulnar nerves, including digital nerve defects. It is of particular use where multiple or very long nerve grafts are required.[54]

Lateral Femoral Cutaneous Nerve

This nerve is an independent branch off the lumbosacral plexus that provides sensation to the anterolateral aspect of the thigh. It pierces the fascia lata 2 cm below and medial to the anterior superior iliac spine. It is approached through an incision medial and inferior to the anterior superior spine. The nerve is identified where it becomes subcutaneous, just distal to the sartorius. It provides a graft 10 to 20 cm long.

Saphenous Nerve

This is the largest cutaneous branch of the femoral nerve. It descends on the lateral side of the femoral artery and enters the adductor canal. It descends along the medial side of the knee, and then becomes subcutaneous behind and between the tendons of the sartorius and gracilis. It passes down the medial side of the leg next to the saphenous vein. It divides into a medial and lateral branch in the lower third of the leg, continuing as far as the great toe. The nerve can be identified through a posteromedial incision adjacent to the long saphenous vein, midway between the medial malleolus and Achilles tendon. It provides a graft of up to 40 cm in length. It should not be harvested if the sural nerve is also being used due to large combined donor site defects.

NERVE GRAFT PREPARATION

Millesi has written extensively on this subject.[24,55] If the recipient nerve is the approximate diameter of the graft, the two stumps are transected until normal appearing tissue without fibrosis is seen. The graft is inserted by an epineurial repair. If the recipient nerve is larger than the graft the fascicular pattern determines the type of preparation. If the nerve contains one to four fascicles, the stump is resected until healthy tissue is encoun-

tered. Multiple nerve grafts are used to completely cover the cross-sectional area of each fascicle (that is 1:2 or 1:3 ratio).

When there are 5 to 12 fascicles that are the size of the nerve graft, then each fascicle is grafted individually. When there is a polyfascicular pattern with a group fascicular arrangement, interfascicular dissection is performed to isolate the fascicle groups, which are then grafted individually. He recommends sectioning each group of fascicles at different levels to prevent an overlap of the suture lines. If there is no group fascicular arrangement, interfascicular dissection is not performed. Graft insertion is then guided by the intraneural topography of the nerve for that specific level of injury.

MOTOR SENSORY DIFFERENTIATION

The use of intraoperative motor and sensory nerve differentiation can diminish the risk of fascicular mismatch when grafting a nerve. The anatomic method is based on separate identification of groups of fascicles,[56-59] the electrophysiologic method uses awake stimulation,[60] and histochemical methods rely on staining for enzymes specific to motor or sensory nerves.[61]

Electrical Fascicle Identification

Awake stimulation requires the cooperation of both the anesthesiologist and the patient. It is based on the observation that motor and sensory fascicles can be differentiated by direct stimulation.[62] The median and ulnar nerves in the distal forearm are most amenable to this technique.[60] It is especially useful when there is a nerve defect, due to the dissimilar fascicular pattern between the proximal and distal nerve ends. The initial nerve dissection is performed under a regional block with tourniquet control. The wound is infiltrated with local anesthetic prior to release of the tourniquet. After 20 minutes the patient is awakened. A low amperage stimulator is then applied to the major fascicles of the proximal nerve end in a systematic manner, starting at 0.2 to 0.5 milliampere. Sensory fascicles will elicit pain, and may be localized to a specific digit. Motor fascicles elicit no response at lower intensities and poorly localized pain at higher intensities. A cross-sectional sketch of the proximal stump is made (Fig. 4–7). The sensory fascicles are tagged with 10-0 nylon, and the patient is placed under general anesthesia. The distal stump is then stimulated in a similar fashion. The reverse picture will be seen, with motor fascicles eliciting a muscle twitch and sensory fascicles being silent. A cross-sectional map is again made, and used to match the proximal and distal motor and sensory fascicles.

Use of Nerve Action Potentials

Neuromuscular function in man as in other mammals disappears 3 to 5 days after nerve section.[63] The preservation of nerve action potentials (NAP) for up to 10 days following nerve transection can be used in place of the

Median Nerve: 20 cm proximal to styloid

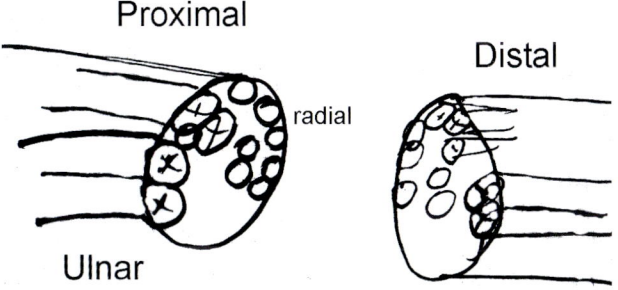

Figure 4–7 Intraoperative drawing of fascicular mapping. (From Slutsky DJ. A practical approach to nerve grafting in the upper extremity. Atlas of the Hand Clinics. Nerve Repair and Reconstruction: A Practical Guide, Vol. 10, No. 1. Philadelphia: W.B. Saunders, 2005:73–92, with permission.)

muscle twitch to map the distal stump.[64,65] This prevents the need to dissect the nerve to its distal motor branch. Nerve action potential recordings following acute nerve transection are characterized by diminishing amplitudes with preserved latencies until the action potential is no longer present. The compound motor action potential (CMAP) disappears at 7 to 9 days, and the sensory nerve action potential (SNAP) disappears at day 10 or 11.[66]

The initial dissection is performed under nitrous oxide, since fentanyl can abolish the response. The nerve stimulation is performed after the tourniquet has been deflated for 20 minutes using a pulse width duration of 0.05 millisecond and a repeat rate of 1 to 2 per second. Averaging is used for small amplitude NAPs. CMAPs are recorded from the thenar/hypothenar muscles, and SNAPs are recorded from either the index or small finger using ring electrodes (Fig. 4–8 A through D). A grouped fascicular repair is then performed as described above.

In chronic injuries, the awake stimulation of the proximal stump is unchanged. Since the NAPs are no longer present, it is necessary to dissect the distal motor

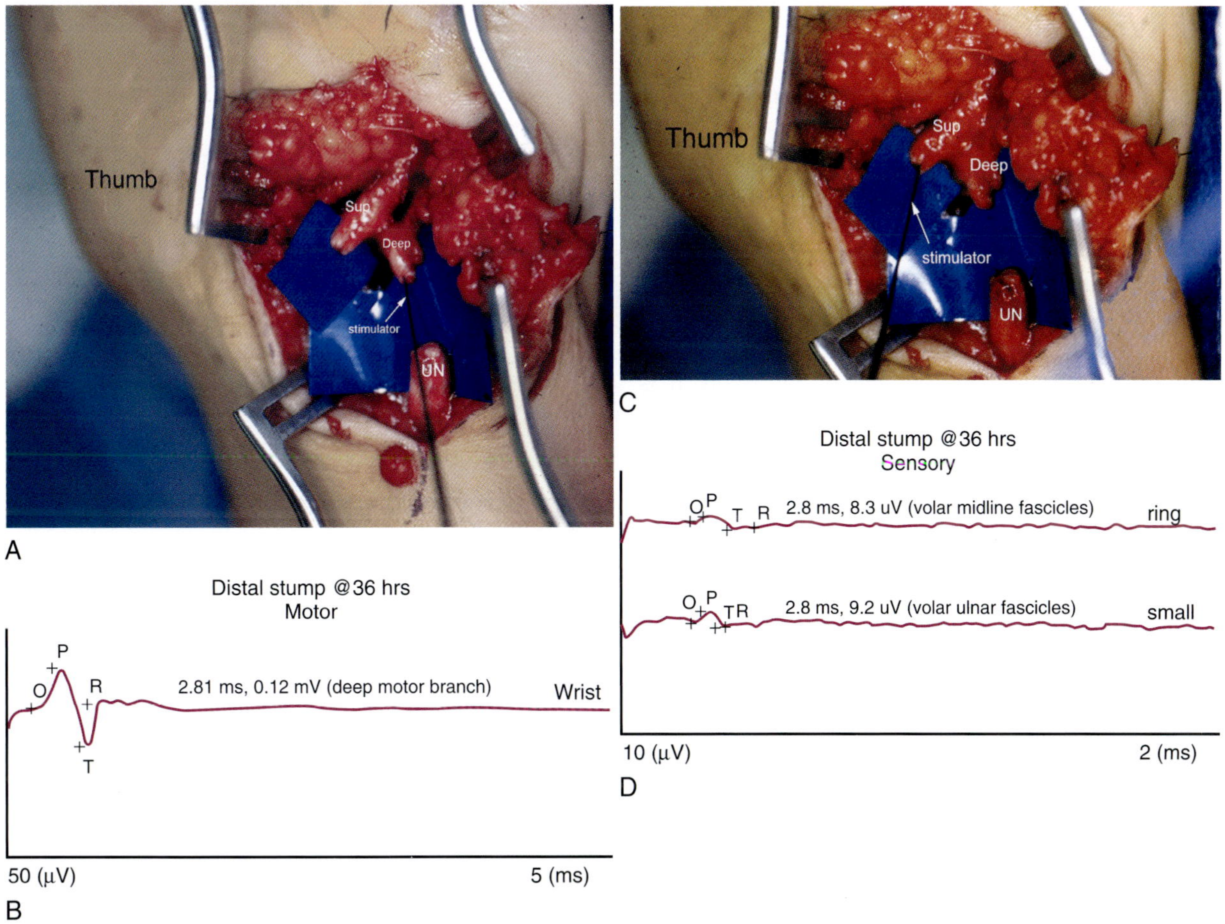

Figure 4–8 Intraoperative stimulation of ulnar nerve at wrist. **A:** Stimulation of deep motor branch. **B:** CMAP with normal latency but low amplitude (recorded from ADM). **C:** Stimulation of superficial *(Sup)* sensory fascicles. **D:** SNAPs with normal latencies but low amplitudes (recorded from small and ring fingers). (From Slutsky DJ. A practical approach to nerve grafting in the upper extremity. Atlas of the Hand Clinics. Nerve Repair and Reconstruction: A Practical Guide, Vol. 10, No. 1. Philadelphia: W.B. Saunders, 2005:73–92, with permission.)

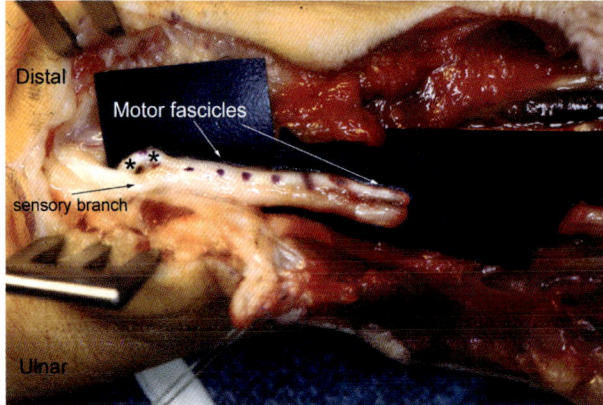

Figure 4–9 Ulnar nerve motor fascicles traced from the distal stump to the deep motor branch in the palm (*). (From Slutsky DJ. A practical approach to nerve grafting in the upper extremity. Atlas of the Hand Clinics. Nerve Repair and Reconstruction: A Practical Guide, Vol. 10, No. 1. Philadelphia: W.B. Saunders, 2005:73–92, with permission.)

branch, and then follow the motor fascicles proximally to the nerve stump (Fig. 4–9).

NERVE LESIONS IN CONTINUITY

Electrical stimulation is useful to determine if there are any intact fascicles in a neuroma in continuity.[67] Bipolar hook electrodes are used with the stimulating and recording electrodes separated by at least 4 cm. The stimulus frequency is two or three times/second with a pulse duration of less than 0.1 millisecond. The intensity is slowly increased to the range where a response is expected (3 to 15 V). The recorder sensitivity is increased to a maximum of 20 V/cm. The nerve is stimulated proximal to, across, and below the lesion. It is estimated that there must be at least 4000 myelinated axons for a recordable NAP to conduct through a neuroma[68] (Fig. 4–10 A and B). A neurolysis is performed to single out any normal-appearing fascicles. This is then confirmed electrically. Nonconducting fascicle are excised and grafted.

GRAFTING SPECIFIC NERVES

Median Nerve

Anatomy

The median nerve arises from the medial and lateral cords of the brachial plexus. It contains the nerve root fibers from C6–T1. It provides the motor supply to the pronator teres (PT), the flexor digitorum sublimus (FDS), the palmaris longus (PL), the flexor carpi radialis (FCR), the thenar muscles, and the two radial lumbricals. Its anterior interosseous branch supplies the

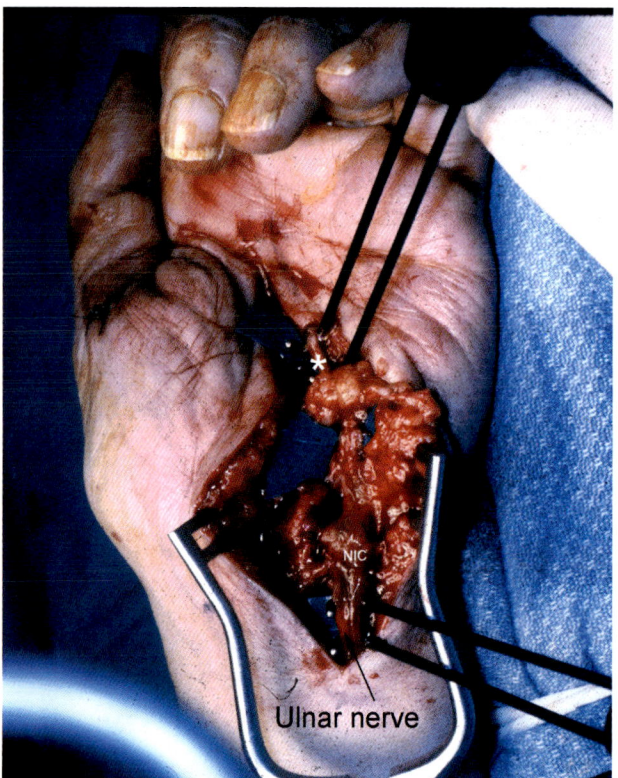

A

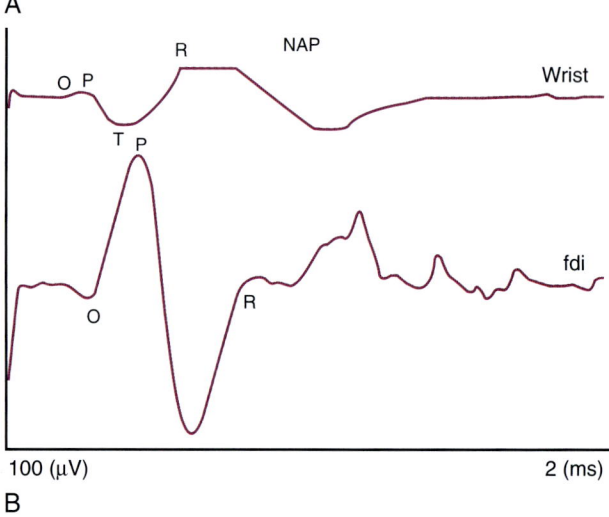

100 (μV)   2 (ms)

B

Figure 4–10 Neuroma in continuity of ulnar nerve. **A:** Nerve stimulation with bipolar electrodes proximal to a neuroma-in-continuity (NIC), with recording over a common digital nerve (*). **B:** Nerve action potential (NAP) recorded from the common digital nerve (top tracing). Nerve stimulation also elicited a compound motor action potential from the first dorsal interosseous (FDI). (From Slutsky DJ. A practical approach to nerve grafting in the upper extremity. Atlas of the Hand Clinics. Nerve Repair and Reconstruction: A Practical Guide, Vol. 10, No. 1. Philadelphia: W.B. Saunders, 2005:73–92, with permission.)

flexor pollicus longus, PQ, and flexor digitorum profundus (FDP) to the index and middle fingers. Its sensory distribution includes the palmar surface of the thumb, index, middle, and radial half of the ring finger. It lies lateral to the axillary artery, but then crosses medial to it at the level of the coracobrachialis. At the elbow it travels behind the bicipital aponeurosis but in front of the brachialis. It enters the forearm between the two heads of the pronator teres and is adherent to the undersurface of the FDS muscle until it becomes superficial, 5 cm proximal to the wrist. It then passes underneath the carpal transverse ligament, giving off the recurrent motor branch and sensory branches to the thumb and fingers.

Injury at the Elbow

The median nerve is located through an S-shaped anteromedial incision at the cubital fossa. The lacertus fibrosis is divided, taking care to preserve the LABCN. The median nerve and brachial vein lie medial to the artery. At this level, the motor branches of the median nerve consistently collect into three fascicular groups. There is an anterior group (to the PT and FCR), middle group (to the FDS and hand intrinsics), and a posterior group (to the AIN branch).[69] These branch groups can be traced proximally without harm, within the main trunk of the median nerve for 2.5 to 10 cm.[70]

Injury in the Forearm

The median nerve is approached through a S-shaped incision over the volar forearm. The nerve is identified on the undersurface of the sublimus muscle. In the upper third of the forearm, the motor branches usually lie peripherally, typically on the radial and ulnar sides. The motor fascicles from the recurrent motor branch are in a slightly radial position at 100 mm proximal to the radial styloid. The central core of the proximal stump should be connected distally with the motor and sensory components of the hand. Any large identifiable forearm motor branches should be attached about the periphery (Fig. 4–11 A to C).

Injury at the Wrist

The median nerve at the wrist has approximately 30 fascicles. The motor recurrent branch often consists of two fascicles that are situated in a volar position, with the various sensory groups in the radial, ulnar, and dorsal positions. The motor branch can be separated from the main trunk without harm for up to 100 mm proximal

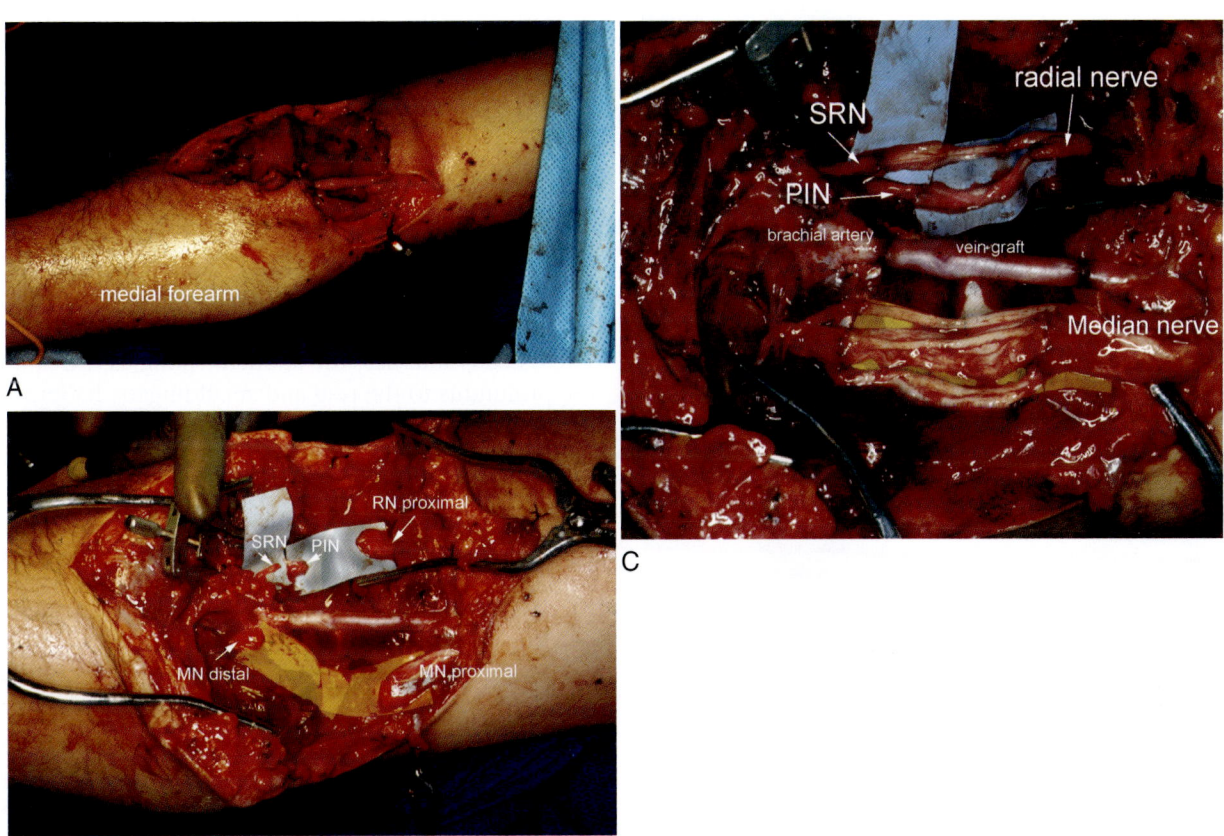

Figure 4–11 Proximal median and radial nerve grafts. **A:** Laceration through antecubital fossa. **B:** Note median nerve laceration *(MN)*, radial nerve *(RN)* laceration at bifurcation of superficial radial nerve branch *(SRN)*, and posterior interosseous nerve *(PIN)*. **C:** Multiple fascicular grafts to median nerve, superficial radial nerve, and PIN nerve. (From Slutsky DJ. A practical approach to nerve grafting in the upper extremity. Atlas of the Hand Clinics. Nerve Repair and Reconstruction: A Practical Guide, Vol. 10, No. 1. Philadelphia: W.B. Saunders, 2005:73–92, with permission.)

to the thenar muscles.[59] The motor fascicles in the recurrent motor branch are identified where they leave the median nerve trunk and then followed proximally to the distal nerve end. In order to maintain motor continuity when there is a median nerve gap at the wrist level, a sural nerve graft should be sutured to the large bifascicular group of fascicles along the volar aspect of the distal stump, and connected to a matching radial group of fascicles in the proximal stump (Fig. 4–12 A and B).

Injury in the Hand

The median nerve is approached through an extensile carpal tunnel approach, with division of the transverse carpal ligament (TCL). The recurrent motor branch is most commonly found distal to the TCL as it enters the thenar muscles (Fig. 4–13 A, B).[71] Topographically, the motor branch is located on the radial-volar aspect 60% of the time, the central-volar aspect 22%, and between those two locations in 18%. The motor branch passes through a separate distinct fascial tunnel before enter-

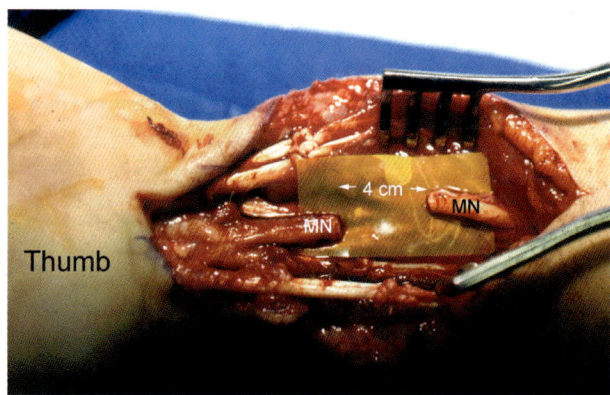

A

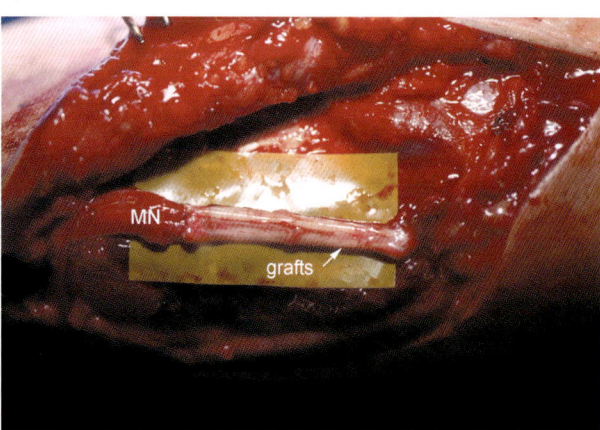

B

Figure 4–12 Median nerve laceration near wrist. **A:** Four-cm defect between median nerve *(MN)* ends. **B:** sural nerve grafts with matching of volar radial fascicle groups. (From Slutsky DJ. A practical approach to nerve grafting in the upper extremity. Atlas of the Hand Clinics. Nerve Repair and Reconstruction: A Practical Guide, Vol. 10, No. 1. Philadelphia: W.B. Saunders, 2005:73–92, with permission.)

ing the thenar muscles 56% of the time. The terminal portion of the AIN provides a good caliber match at this level.

The sensory fibers travel within the common digital nerves to the thumb and index and middle fingers, as well as the communicating branch to the third web space. The LACBN or MACBN is a suitable graft for nerve gaps at this level (Fig. 4–14 A to C). When the median nerve defect is greater than 5 cm and extends from the wrist to the common digital nerve bifurcation, sural grafts are more appropriate (Fig. 4–15 A to C).

Digits

Many authors recommend nerve grafting when the gap exceeds 1 cm, with the wrist and all three finger joints extended.[43] The digital nerves are approached though a midlateral or volar Brunner incision. The LACBN is a good caliber match at this level. The dorsal sensory branch, which arises from the proper digital nerve, can also be used as graft material. This branch most commonly arises proximal to the PIP flexion crease, and then crosses superficial or deep to the digital artery to lie just above the extensor mechanism, innervating the dorsum of the middle phalanx.[72] This branch can be provide a 1- to 2-cm nerve graft (Fig. 4–16). Distal to the DIP joint, the nerve trifurcates. The terminal PIN is a suitable graft at this level.

Ulnar Nerve

Anatomy

The ulnar nerve arises from the medial cord of the brachial plexus. It contains the nerve root fibers from C8 to T1. It provides the motor supply to the hypothenar muscles, the ulnar two lumbricals, the interosseous muscles, the adductor pollicus, FCU, and the profundus to the ring and small fingers. Its sensory distribution includes the palmar surface of the small and the ulnar half of the ring finger as well as the dorsoulnar carpus. It lies medial to the axillary artery and continues distally to the midarm, where it pierces the medial intermuscular septum. The nerve is often accompanied by the superior ulnar collateral artery. At the elbow, it lies between the medial epicondyle and the olecranon where it is covered by Osborne's ligament. It enters the forearm between the two heads of the FCU covered by a fibrous aponeurosis (the cubital tunnel). It runs deep to the FCU up to the distal forearm. At the wrist, it passes over the TCL, medial to the ulnar artery through Guyon's canal. The deep motor branch is given off at the pisiform and passes underneath a fibrous arch to lie on the palmar surface of the interossei. It crosses the palm deep to the flexor tendons, to terminate in the adductor pollicus and ulnar head of the flexor pollicis brevis.

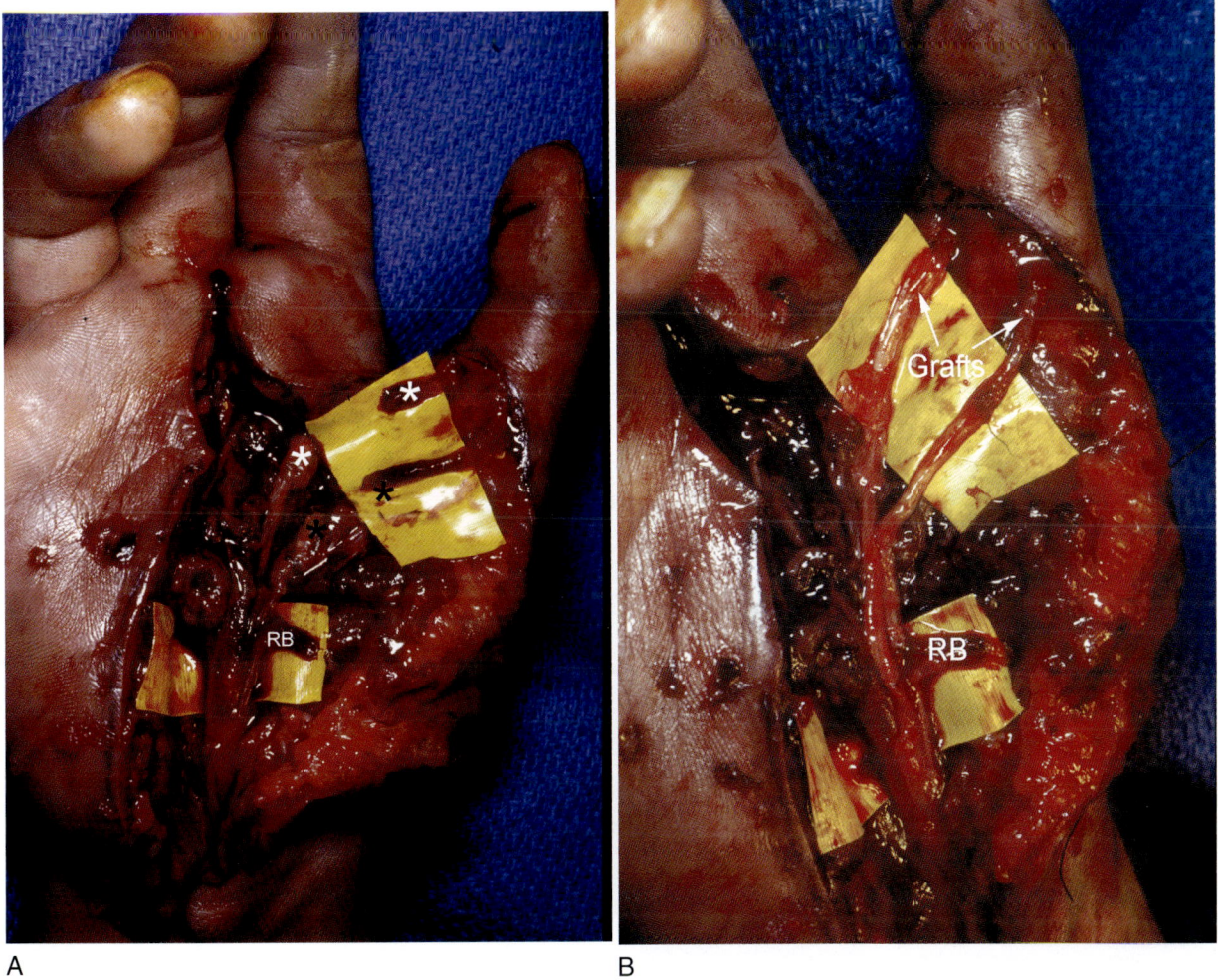

A   B

Figure 4–13   Median nerve laceration. **A:** Laceration of median nerve at junction of motor recurrent branch *(RB)* and digital sensory nerves to the thumb (*). **B:** Repair of recurrent branch, LABCN grafts to digital nerves. (From Slutsky DJ. A practical approach to nerve grafting in the upper extremity. Atlas of the Hand Clinics. Nerve Repair and Reconstruction: A Practical Guide, Vol. 10, No. 1. Philadelphia: W.B. Saunders, 2005:73–92, with permission.)

Injury at the Elbow

The ulnar nerve is located through a curved postero-medial incision behind the medial epicondyle. At the elbow, the ulnar nerve contains about 20 fascicles including the motor branches to the forearm muscles. The motor fascicles to the FCU and the intrinsics are centrally located, whereas the sensory fibers are superficially located. The proximal motor branches to the FCU and FDP can often be traced for up to 6 cm before interfascicular connections.[58] It is possible to distinguish between sensory and motor fascicles in the distal nerve end using low-intensity electrical stimulation, if performed within a few days of the injury. Occasionally, fascicles innervating the flexor muscles can be separated from those supplying the intrinsic muscles in the hand.[73] The sural nerve is commonly used as graft material at this level (Fig. 4–17 A to C).

Injury in the Forearm

The motor fascicles lie dorsal and slightly ulnarly to the sensory fascicles at the wrist level, and usually maintain a dorsal relationship as one moves proximally. The motor component remains as a distinct entity up to 90 mm proximal to the styloid.[56] At 50 to 85 mm proximal to the radial styloid, the dorsal sensory branch joins the other groups. At the level of the midforearm, 50 mm from the ulnar styloid the motor fascicles lie dorsal to the sensory fascicles.[59] A sural nerve graft should thus be placed in the dorsal quadrant of the proximal nerve end and the dorsoulnar quadrant of the distal nerve end to restore motor continuity.

Injury at the Wrist

The ulnar nerve has 15 to 25 fascicles at the wrist. It can be clearly divided into a volar sensory component

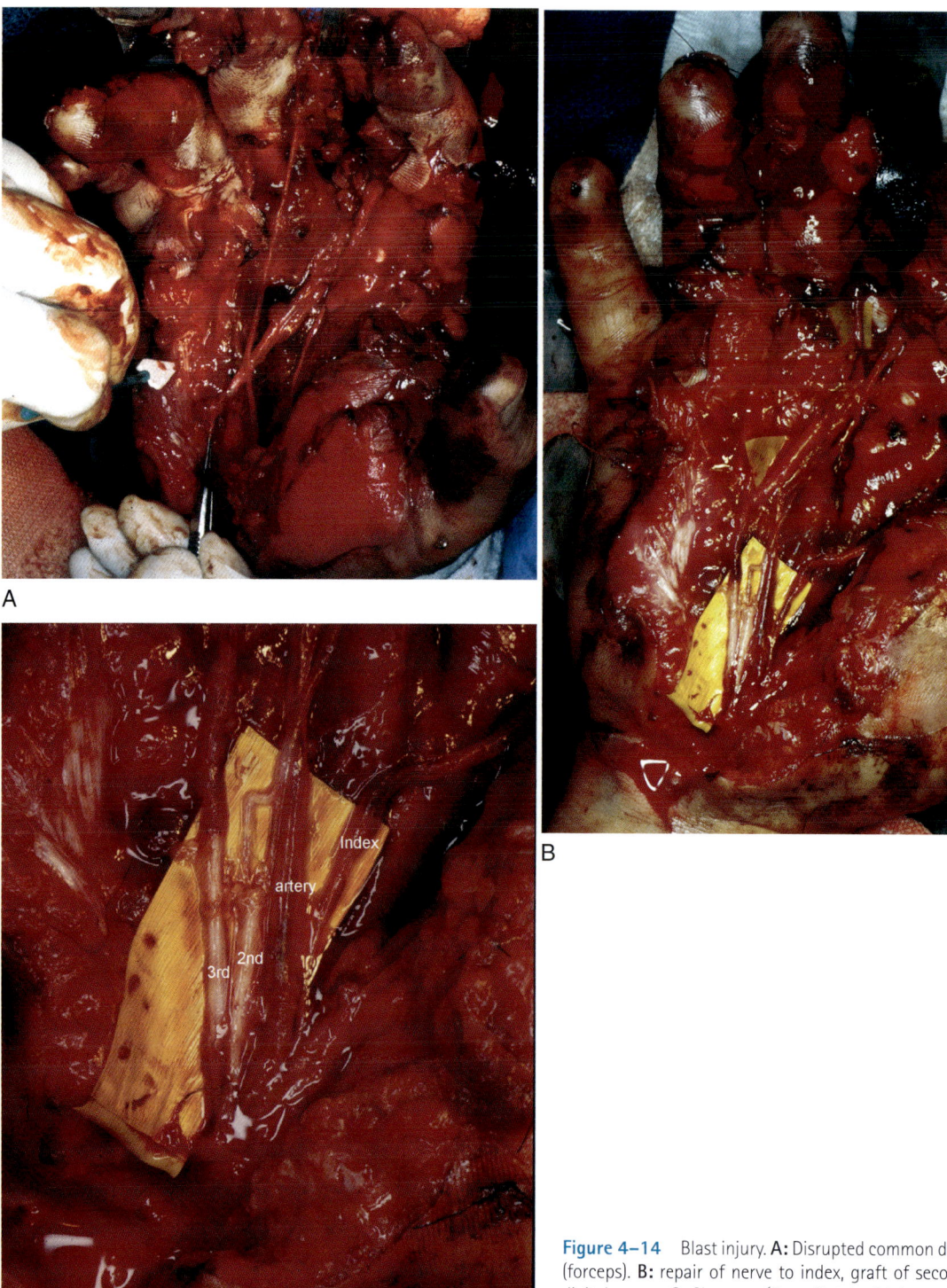

A

B

C

index

artery

2nd

3rd

Figure 4–14 Blast injury. **A:** Disrupted common digital nerves and artery (forceps). **B:** repair of nerve to index, graft of second and third common digital nerves. **C:** Close-up. (From Slutsky DJ. A practical approach to nerve grafting in the upper extremity. Atlas of the Hand Clinics. Nerve Repair and Reconstruction: A Practical Guide, Vol. 10, No. 1. Philadelphia: W.B. Saunders, 2005:73–92, with permission.)

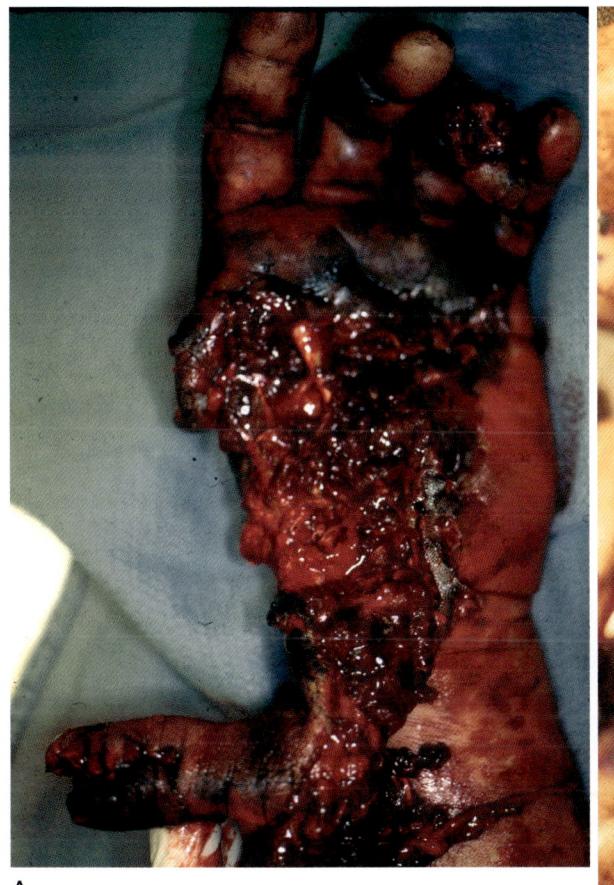

A

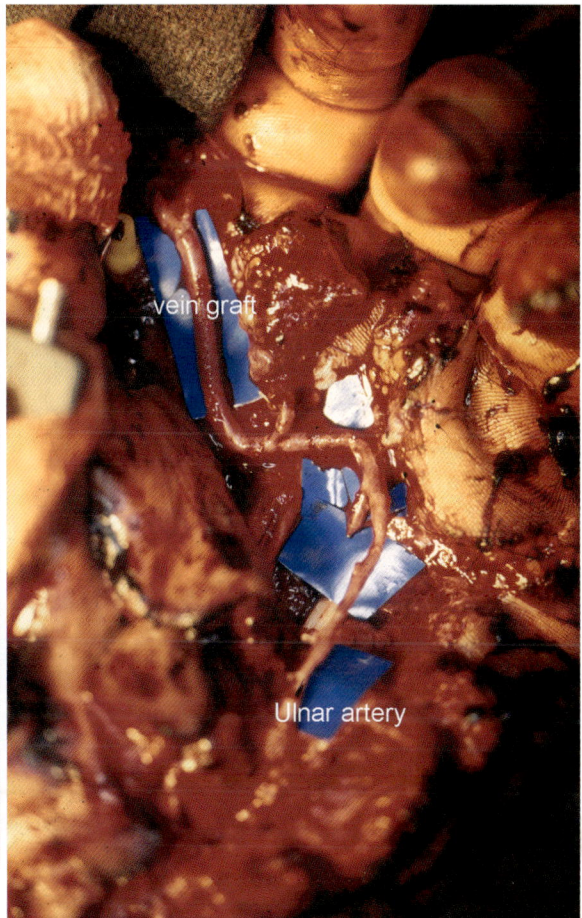

B

C

Figure 4–15 Avulsion injury. **A:** Thumb amputation associated with avulsion of the palmar arch and median nerve branches in the palm. **B:** Thumb replant plus reconstruction of palmar arch with vein graft. **C:** Twelve-cm sural nerve grafts from proximal median nerve *(MN)* to digital nerves *(DN)*. (From Slutsky DJ. A practical approach to nerve grafting in the upper extremity. Atlas of the Hand Clinics. Nerve Repair and Reconstruction: A Practical Guide, Vol. 10, No. 1. Philadelphia: W.B. Saunders, 2005:73–92, with permission.)

NERVE REPAIR AND RECONSTRUCTION

and a dorsal motor component. The ulnar nerve is approached through an S-shaped incision over the volar ulnar forearm. The nerve is identified medial to the ulnar artery underneath the FCU muscle. If a muscle twitch is no longer present, the motor branch can be

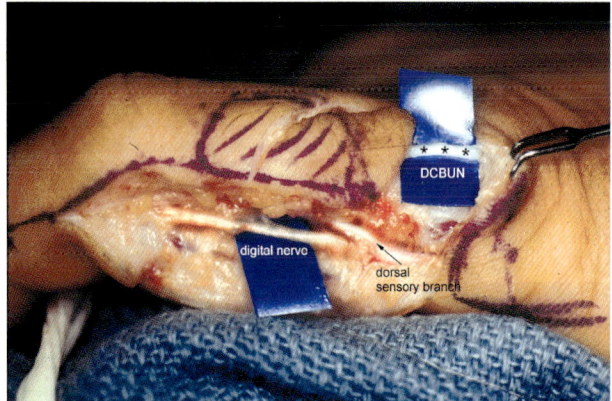

Figure 4–16 Dorsal sensory branch arising from the proper digital nerve of the small finger. DCBUN (*), dorsal cutaneous branch of the ulnar nerve. (From Slutsky DJ. A practical approach to nerve grafting in the upper extremity. Atlas of the Hand Clinics. Nerve Repair and Reconstruction: A Practical Guide, Vol. 10, No. 1. Philadelphia: W.B. Saunders, 2005:73–92, with permission.)

traced from the takeoff of the deep motor branch to the distal nerve end (Fig. 4–8 A).

Hand

The nerve is approached through a volar ulnar incision in line with the ring finger. The deep motor and more superficial sensory fascicles are easily separated at this level and allow separate grafting (Fig. 4–8 A and C). The sural nerve, LABCN, or MABCN provide suitably sized grafts. The DCBUN is not usually grafted since neuromas of this nerve are uncommon.

Digits

Grafting in the digits is similar to the median nerve.

Guidelines for Digital Nerve Graft Selection

Higgins et al.[74] investigated the fascicular cross-sectional area and number of fascicles of five nerve graft sites to specific digital nerve segments. In the fingertip distal to the distal interphalangeal joint (DIP), the AIN, PIN, and MABCN were all appropriate choices for caliber-matched grafts (Fig. 4–18 A to C). The LABCN, however, was the only similar donor nerve when the

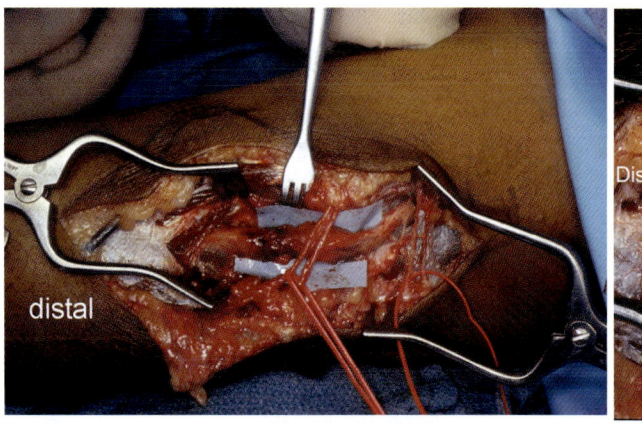

A

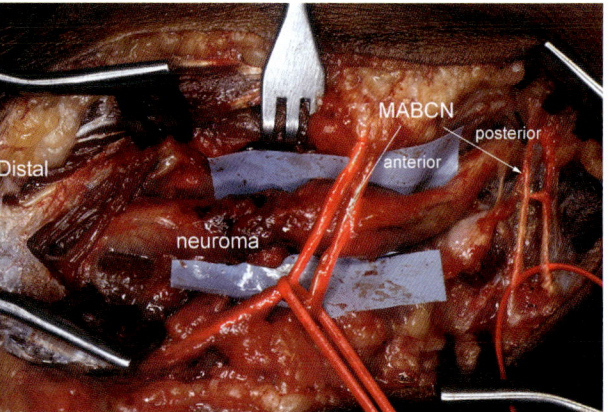

B

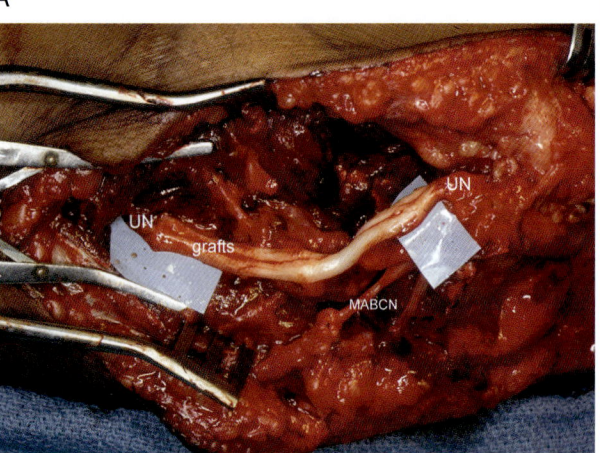

C

Figure 4–17 Neuroma of ulnar nerve at elbow. **A:** Medial aspect of the right elbow demonstrating an ulnar nerve neuroma. **B:** Close-up of neuroma. Note the anterior and posterior branches of the medial antebrachial cutaneous nerve *(MABCN)*. **C:** Sural nerve grafts to ulnar nerve *(UN)*. (From Slutsky DJ. A practical approach to nerve grafting in the upper extremity. Atlas of the Hand Clinics. Nerve Repair and Reconstruction: A Practical Guide, Vol. 10, No. 1. Philadelphia: W.B. Saunders, 2005:73–92, with permission.)

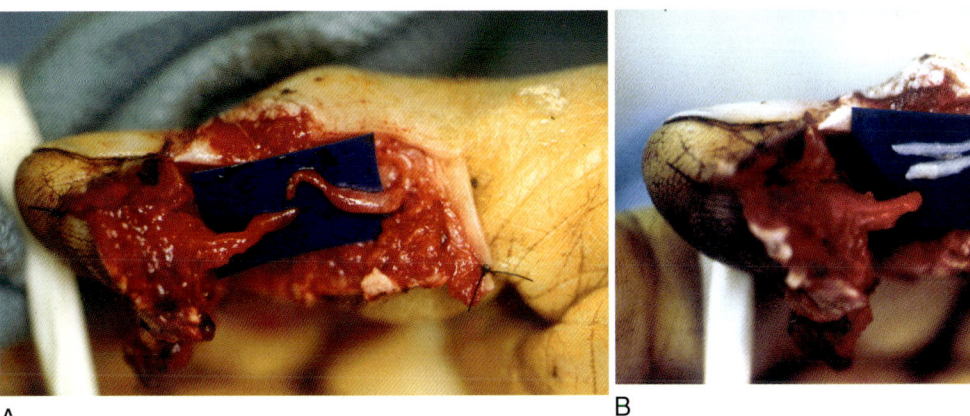

A

B

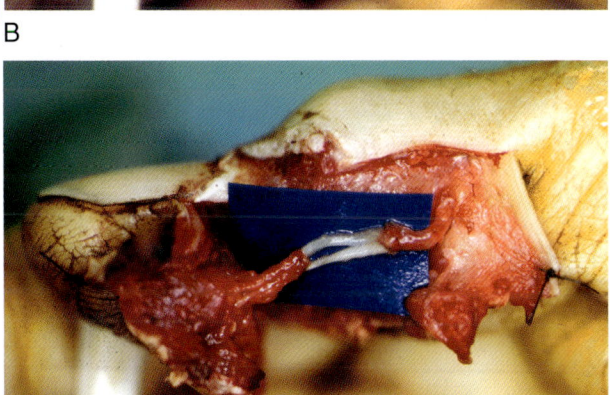

C

Figure 4–18   Digital nerve injury. **A:** Saw injury to the radial digital nerve of the thumb. **B:** One-cm nerve defect after debridement. The PIN graft is approximately one-half the diameter of the terminal portion of the radial digital nerve. **C:** PIN nerve graft interposed between the two fascicles of the terminal digital nerve.

number of fascicles was assessed. The LABCN is also the best match in caliber and fascicle number for digital nerve deficits between the metacarpophalangeal joint (MP) to the DIP joint, and from the common digital nerve bifurcation to the MP joint. The sural nerve was the most appropriate choice when grafting defects between the wrist and the common digital nerve bifurcation, even though there were considerably fewer fascicles and a smaller cross-sectional area than the common digital nerve.

Radial Nerve

Anatomy

The radial nerve arises from the posterior cord of the brachial plexus. It receives contributions from C5 through C8 spinal roots. The nerve contains approximately 16,000 myelinated fibers.[75] It runs medial to the axillary artery. At the level of the coracobrachialis, it courses posteriorly to lie in the spiral groove of the humerus. In the lower arm, it pierces the lateral intermuscular septum to run between the brachialis and brachioradialis. It divides 2 cm distal to the elbow into a superficial radial sensory branch (SRN) and a deep motor branch, the posterior interosseous nerve (PIN) (Fig. 4–19). It gives off branches to the extensor carpi radialis longus and brevis, and brachioradialis and anconeus before giving off the PIN branch. The PIN continues on between the superficial and deep head of the supinator muscle, to exit on the dorsal forearm. After it emerges from the distal border of the supinator, the PIN sends branches to the extensor digitorum communis, extensor carpi ulnaris, extensor digiti quinti, extensor pollicus longus and brevis, and the extensor indicis proprius in descending order, although there may be considerable variation.[76]

Injury at the Elbow

The volar approach to the radial nerve is through an anterolateral incision, developing the intermuscular interval between the brachialis and brachioradialis. Recurrent branches from the radial artery must be divided to gain access to both nerve branches. Separate grafting of the SRN and the PIN branch are relatively straightforward (Fig. 4–18).

Injury in the Forearm and Wrist

The PIN is approached dorsolaterally, developing the plane between the extensor carpi radialis brevis and the extensor digitorum communis. At this level, the PIN contains motor fibers only; hence, separate fascicle identification is unnecessary (Fig. 4–20 A to C). The PIN also has a short distance to travel to reinnervate the motor end plates, which accounts for generally

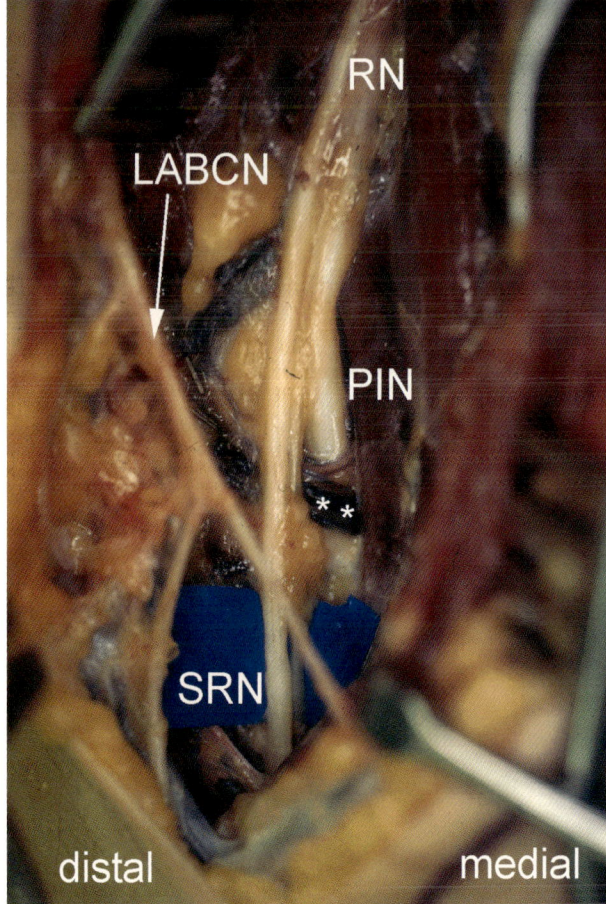

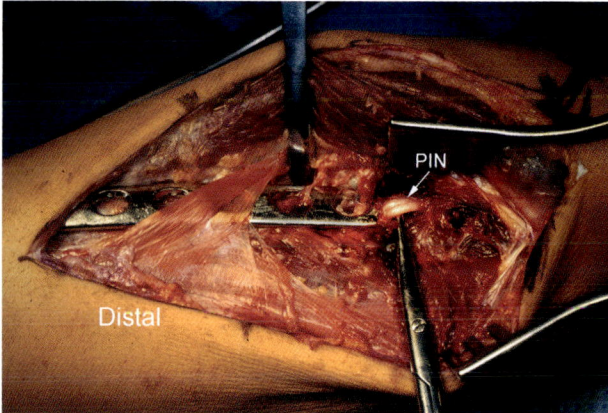

A

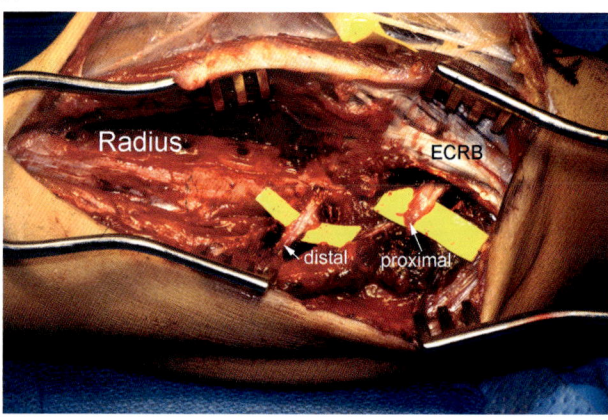

B

Figure 4–19   Anterior approach to the radial nerve at the elbow. Note the radial nerve *(RN)* dividing into the posterior interosseous nerve *(PIN)* and the superficial radial nerve *(SRN)*. LACBN, lateral antebrachial cutaneous nerve, radial recurrent vessels (*). (From Slutsky DJ. A practical approach to nerve grafting in the upper extremity. Atlas of the Hand Clinics. Nerve Repair and Reconstruction: A Practical Guide, Vol. 10, No. 1. Philadelphia: W.B. Saunders, 2005:73–92, with permission.)

favorable results.[77] Lacerations of the superficial branch in the forearm are not usually grafted, which allows harvest of the SRN for grafting adjacent nerve injuries. Some authors do advocate grafting the SRN at the wrist, mostly to prevent symptomatic neuroma formation.[78]

SUMMARY

Nerve grafting is a century-old art[79] that is honed by experience and limited only by the imagination. Clearly, myriad factors may influence the type of graft and the manner in which it is used. A sound knowledge of the intrafascicular topography combined with intraoperative aids for motor and sensory differentiation can lead to superior clinical results, especially with large nerve deficits.

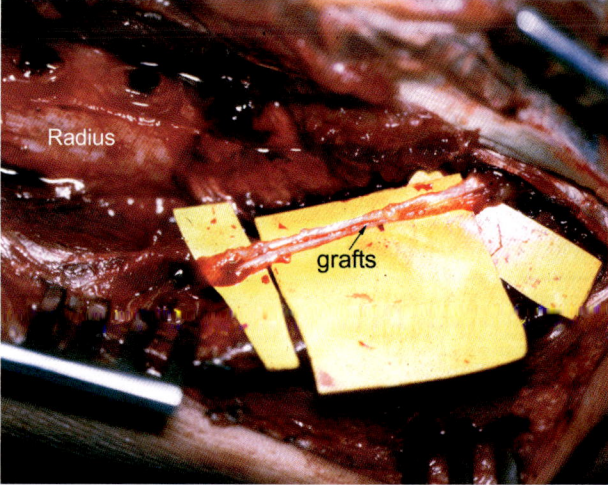

C

Figure 4–20   Posterior interosseous nerve injury. **A:** Dorsal approach to left forearm demonstrating a PIN injury after plating of a proximal radius fracture. **B:** Proximal and distal nerve ends isolated. **C:** Interposed nerve grafts. (From Slutsky DJ. A practical approach to nerve grafting in the upper extremity. Atlas of the Hand Clinics. Nerve Repair and Reconstruction: A Practical Guide, Vol. 10, No. 1. Philadelphia: W.B. Saunders, 2005:73–92, with permission.)

REFERENCES

1. Lundborg G. Ischemic nerve injury. Experimental studies on intraneural microvascular pathophysiology and nerve function in a limb subjected to temporary circulatory arrest. Scand J Plast Reconstr Surg Suppl 1970;6:3–113.

2. Mellick RS, Cavanagh JB. Changes in blood vessel permeability during degeneration and regeneration in peripheral nerves. Brain 1968;91:141–60.

3. Badalamente MA, Hurst LC, Stracher A. Calcium-induced degeneration of the cytoskeleton in monkey and human peripheral nerves. J Hand Surg Br 1986;11:337–40.

4. Haftek J, Thomas PK. Electron-microscope observations on the effects of localized crush injuries on the connective tissues of peripheral nerve. J Anat 1968;103:233–43.

5. Thomas PK. Changes in the endoneurial sheaths of peripheral myelinated nerve fibres during Wallerian degeneration. J Anat 1964;98:175–82.

6. Lubinska L. Demyelination and remyelination in the proximal parts of regenerating nerve fibers. J Comp Neurol 1961;117:275–89.

7. Yamada KM, Spooner BS, Wessells NK. Ultrastructure and function of growth cones and axons of cultured nerve cells. J Cell Biol 1971;49:614–35.

8. Timpl R, Rohde H, Robey PG, et al. Laminin—a glycoprotein from basement membranes. J Biol Chem 1979;254:9933–7.

9. Letourneau PC. Cell-to-substratum adhesion and guidance of axonal elongation. Dev Biol 1975;44:92–101.

10. Mackinnon SE, Dellon AL, O'Brien JP. Changes in nerve fiber numbers distal to a nerve repair in the rat sciatic nerve model. Muscle Nerve 1991;14:1116–22.

11. Buchthal F, Kuhl V. Nerve conduction, tactile sensibility, and the electromyogram after suture or compression of peripheral nerve;a longitudinal study in man. J Neurol Neurosurg Psychiatry 1979;42;436–51.

12. Bevan S, Steinbach JH. Denervation increases the degradation rate of acetylcholine receptors at end-plates in vivo and in vitro. J Physiol 1983;336:159–77.

13. Terzis JK, Michelow MB. Sensory receptors. In: Gelberman R, ed., Operative Nerve Repair and Reconstruction. Philadelphia: J.B. Lippincott & Company, 1991:85–105.

14. Levi-Montalcini R, Angeletti PU. Nerve growth factor. Physiol Rev 1968;48:534–69.

15. Taniuchi M, Clark HB, Schweitzer JB, et al. Expression of nerve growth factor receptors by Schwann cells of axotomized peripheral nerves: ultrastructural location, suppression by axonal contact, and binding properties. J Neurosci 1988;8: 664–81.

16. Thanos PK, Okajima S, Terzis JK. Ultrastructure and cellular biology of nerve regeneration. J Reconstr Microsurg 1998;14: 423–36.

17. Nishiura Y, Brandt J, Nilsson A, et al. Addition of cultured schwann cells to tendon autografts and freeze-thawed muscle grafts improves peripheral nerve regeneration. Tissue Eng 2004;10:157–64.

18. Fansa H, Schneider W, Keilhoff G. Revascularization of tissue-engineered nerve grafts and invasion of macrophages. Tissue Eng 2001;7:519–24.

19. Aguayo AJ, Kasarjian J, Skamene E, et al. Myelination of mouse axons by Schwann cells transplanted from normal and abnormal human nerves. Nature 1977;268:753–5.

20. Lind R, Wood MB. Comparison of the pattern of early revascularization of conventional versus vascularized nerve grafts in the canine. J Reconstr Microsurg 1986;2:229–34.

21. Daly PJ, Wood MB. Endoneural and epineural blood flow evaluation with free vascularized and conventional nerve grafts in the canine. J Reconstr Microsurg 1985;2:45–9.

22. Penkert G, Bini W, Samii M. Revascularization of nerve grafts: an experimental study. J Reconstr Microsurg 1988;4:319–25.

23. Prpa B, Huddleston PM, An KN, Wood MB. Revascularization of nerve grafts: a qualitative and quantitative study of the soft-tissue bed contributions to blood flow in canine nerve grafts. J Hand Surg Am 2002;27:1041–7.

24. Millesi H. Techniques for nerve grafting. Hand Clin 2000;16:73–91, viii.

25. Trumble TE, Parvin D. Physiology of peripheral nerve graft incorporation. J Hand Surg Am 1994;19:420–7.

26. Best TJ, Mackinnon SE, Evans PJ, et al. Peripheral nerve revascularization: histomorphometric study of small- and large-caliber grafts. J Reconstr Microsurg 1999;15:183–90.

27. Kwan MK, Woo SL-Y. Biomechanical properties of peripheral nerve. In: Gelberman R, ed., Operative Nerve Repair and Reconstruction. Philadelphia: J.B. Lippincott & Company, 1991:47–55.

28. Beel JA, Groswald DE, Luttges MW. Alterations in the mechanical properties of peripheral nerve following crush injury. J Biomech 1984;17:185–93.

29. Trumble TE, McCallister WV. Repair of peripheral nerve defects in the upper extremity. Hand Clin 2000;16:37–52.

30. Lundborg G, Rydevik B. Effects of stretching the tibial nerve of the rabbit. A preliminary study of the intraneural circulation and the barrier function of the perineurium. J Bone Joint Surg Br 1973;55:390–401.

31. Clark WL, Trumble TE, Swiontkowski MF, et al. Nerve tension and blood flow in a rat model of immediate and delayed repairs. J Hand Surg Am 1992;17:677–87.

32. Matsuzaki H, Shibata M, Jiang B, et al. Distal nerve elongation vs nerve grafting in repairing segmental nerve defects in rabbits. Microsurgery 2004;24:207–12.

33. Ruch DS, Deal DN, Ma J, et al. Management of peripheral nerve defects: external fixator-assisted primary neurorrhaphy. J Bone Joint Surg Am 2004;86:1405–13.

34. Terzis J, Faibisoff B, Williams B. The nerve gap: suture under tension vs. graft. Plast Reconstr Surg 1975;56:166–70.

35. Millesi H. The current state of peripheral nerve surgery in the upper limb. Ann Chir Main 1984;3:18–34.

36. Kalomiri DE, Soucacos PN, Beris AE. Nerve grafting in peripheral nerve microsurgery of the upper extremity. Microsurgery 1994;15:506–11.

37. Millesi H. Healing of nerves. Clin Plast Surg 1977;4:459–73.

38. Stevens WG, Hall JD, Young VL, et al. When should nerve gaps be grafted? An experimental study in rats. Plast Reconstr Surg 1985;75:707–13.

39. Frykman GK, Gramyk K. Results of nerve grafting. In: Gelberman R, ed., Operative Nerve Repair and Reconstruction. Philadelphia: J.B. Lippincott & Company, 1991:553–67.

40. Ross D, Mackinnon SE, Chang YL. Intraneural anatomy of the median nerve provides "third web space" donor nerve graft. J Reconstr Microsurg 1992;8:225–32.

41. Vernadakis AJ, Humphreys DB, Mackinnon SE. Distal anterior interosseous nerve in the recurrent motor branch graft for reconstruction of a median nerve neuroma-in-continuity. J Reconstr Microsurg 2004;20:7–11.

42. Masear VR, Meyer RD, Pichora DR. Surgical anatomy of the medial antebrachial cutaneous nerve. J Hand Surg Am 1989;14:267–71.

43. Nunley J. Donor nerves for grafting. In: Gelberman R, ed., Operative Nerve Repair and Reconstruction. Philadelphia: J.B. Lippincott & Company, 1991:545–67.

44. Mackinnon SE, Dellon AL. The overlap pattern of the lateral antebrachial cutaneous nerve and the superficial branch of the radial nerve. J Hand Surg Am 1985;10:522–6.

45. Hall HC, MacKinnon SE, Gilbert RW. An approach to the posterior interosseous nerve. Plast Reconstr Surg 1984;74:435–7.

46. Greene TL, Steichen JB. Digital nerve grafting using the dorsal sensory branch of the ulnar nerve. J Hand Surg Br 1985;10:37–40.

47. Waters PM, Schwartz JT. Posterior interosseous nerve: an anatomic study of potential nerve grafts. J Hand Surg Am 1993; 18:743–5.

48. Elgafy H, Ebraheim NA, Yeasting RA. The anatomy of the posterior interosseous nerve as a graft. J Hand Surg Am 2000;25:930–5.

49. Watchmaker GP, Weber D, Mackinnon SE. Avoidance of transection of the palmar cutaneous branch of the median nerve in carpal tunnel release. J Hand Surg Am 1996;21:644–50.

50. Martin CH, Seiler JG 3rd, Lesesne JS. The cutaneous innervation of the palm: an anatomic study of the ulnar and median nerves. J Hand Surg Am 1996;21:634–8.

51. DaSilva MF, Moore DC, Weiss AP, et al. Anatomy of the palmar cutaneous branch of the median nerve: clinical significance. J Hand Surg Am 1996;21:639–43.

52. Ahcan U, Arnez ZM, Bajrovic FF, et al. Nerve fibre composition of the palmar cutaneous branch of the median nerve and clinical implications. Br J Plast Surg 2003;56:791–6.

53. Ustun ME, Ogun TC, Buyukmumcu M, et al. Selective restoration of motor function in the ulnar nerve by transfer of the anterior interosseous nerve. An anatomical feasibility study. J Bone Joint Surg Am 2001;83:549–52.

54. Buntic RF, Buncke HJ, Kind GM, et al. The harvest and clinical application of the superficial peroneal sensory nerve for grafting motor and sensory nerve defects. Plast Reconstr Surg 2002;109:145–51.

55. Millesi H. Indications and techniques of nerve grafting. In: Gelberman R, ed., Operative Nerve Repair and Reconstruction. Philadelphia: J.B. Lippincott & Company, 1991:525–43.

56. Chow JA, Van Beek AL, Meyer DL, et al. Surgical significance of the motor fascicular group of the ulnar nerve in the forearm. J Hand Surg Am 1985;10:867–72.

57. Jabaley ME, Wallace WH, Heckler FR. Internal topography of major nerves of the forearm and hand: a current view. J Hand Surg Am 1980;5:1–18.

58. Watchmaker GP, Lee G, Mackinnon SE. Intraneural topography of the ulnar nerve in the cubital tunnel facilitates anterior transposition. J Hand Surg Am 1994;19:915–22.

59. Williams HB, Jabaley ME. The importance of internal anatomy of the peripheral nerves to nerve repair in the forearm and hand. Hand Clin 1986;2:689–707.

60. Gaul JS Jr. Electrical fascicle identification as an adjunct to nerve repair. Hand Clin 1986;2:709–22.

61. Deutinger M, Girsch W, Burggasser G, et al. Peripheral nerve repair in the hand with and without motor sensory differentiation. J Hand Surg Am 1993;18:426–32.

62. Hakstian RW. Funicular orientation by direct stimulation. An aid to peripheral nerve repair. J Bone Joint Surg Am 1968;50:1178–86.

63. Landau WM. The duration of neuromuscular function after nerve section in man. J Neurosurg 1953;10:64–8.

64. Slutsky D. Nerve conduction studies in hand surgery. J Am Soc Surg Hand 2002;3:1–18.

65. Slutsky DJ. A practical approach to nerve grafting in the upper extremity. Atlas of the Hand Clinics. Nerve Repair and Reconstruction: A Practical Guide, Vol. 10, No. 1. Philadelphia: W.B. Saunders, 2005:73–92.

66. Chaudhry V, Cornblath DR. Wallerian degeneration in human nerves: serial electrophysiological studies. Muscle Nerve 1992;15:687–93.

67. Happel LT, Kline KD. Nerve lesions in continuity. In: Gelberman R, ed., Operative Nerve Repair and Reconstruction. Philadelphia: J.B. Lippincott & Company, 1991:601–16.

68. Tiel RL, Happel LT Jr, Kline DG. Nerve action potential recording method and equipment. Neurosurgery 1996;39:103–9.

69. Zhao X, Lao J, Hung LK, et al. Selective neurotization of the median nerve in the arm to treat brachial plexus palsy. An anatomic study and case report. J Bone Joint Surg Am 2004;86:736–42.

70. Gunther SF, DiPasquale D, Martin R. The internal anatomy of the median nerve in the region of the elbow. J Hand Surg Am 1992;17:648–56.

71. Lanz U. Anatomical variations of the median nerve in the carpal tunnel. J Hand Surg Am 1977;2:44–53.

72. Tellioglu AT, Sensoz O. The dorsal branch of the digital nerve: an anatomic study and clinical applications. Ann Plast Surg 1998;40:145–8.

73. Teboul F, Kakkar R, Ameur N, et al. Transfer of fascicles from the ulnar nerve to the nerve to the biceps in the treatment of upper brachial plexus palsy. J Bone Joint Surg Am 2004;86:1485–90.

74. Higgins JP, Fisher S, Serletti JM, et al. Assessment of nerve graft donor sites used for reconstruction of traumatic digital nerve defects. J Hand Surg Am 2002;27:286–92.

75. Bonnel F. Microscopic anatomy of the adult human brachial plexus: an anatomical and histological basis for microsurgery. Microsurgery 1984;5:107–18.

76. Abrams RA, Ziets RJ, Lieber RL, et al. Anatomy of the radial nerve motor branches in the forearm. J Hand Surg Am 1997;22:232–7.

77. Young C, Hudson A, Richards R. Operative treatment of palsy of the posterior interosseous nerve of the forearm. J Bone Joint Surg Am 1990;72:1215–9.

78. Wray RC Jr. Repair of sensory nerves distal to the wrist. Hand Clin 1986;2:767–72.

79. Albert E. Einige Operationen am Nerven. Wien Med Press 1885;26:1285.

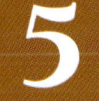

5

End-to-Side Neurorrhaphy: A Review of the Current Literature and Its Potential Applications in Neuroma Prevention, Functional Recovery, and Clinical Application

James R. Urbaniak, Erika G. Lumsden, and Tedman L. Vance

INTRODUCTION

End-to-side nerve repair, or termino-lateral neurorrhaphy, has the potential to solve numerous clinical scenarios. First noted in the literature 100 years ago, current literature abounds with the basic science and clinical research that supports the use of this technique when primary nerve repair, nerve transfers, or nerve grafting are not possible.[1]

Traumatic injuries with massive peripheral nerve defects, or brachial plexus nerve avulsions have traditionally been treated with free nerve grafts or nerve transfer, which require the donor nerve to sacrifice its original target. What distinguishes end-to-side neurorrhaphy is the use of a donor nerve to innervate the injured nerve without abandoning its own anatomic region. The advantages include the expanded source of donor nerves, and the reduced regeneration time when repairs are performed closer to end organs.

The clinical application extends to the treatment of symptomatic neuromas. Although several techniques have been described for the treatment of neuromas, including ligation, epineurial barriers, silicone capping, steroid injection, and implantation into bone or muscle, there is still little consensus regarding the best method of treatment.[2–5] Often the goal involves pain control, with function as a secondary issue. This chapter will review the basic science behind end-to-side neurorrhaphy and its use in treating symptomatic neuromas, and other peripheral nerve injuries in the upper extremity.

RATIONALE AND BASIC SCIENCE

The potential source of regenerating axons following end-to-side neurorrhaphy remains somewhat in question, although numerous laboratory studies have investigated this activity.[6-12] In vitro application of growth factors to noninjured intact axons has been shown to stimulate axonal sprouting.[13,14] The proximity of growth factors emanating from Schwann cells or the degenerating nerve stump may be adequate to stimulate intact axons to sprout collateral branches, and these sprouts may advance distally to reinnervate target end organs.[15,16]

The axons of the donor nerve should remain uninjured at the time of end-to-side nerve repair if care is taken in preparing the epineurial window. These concepts form the basis for end-to-side neurorrhaphy.

The standard end-to-side nerve repair involves making an epineurial window on the donor nerve (Fig. 5–1 A to D). The connection is made by epineurial-to-epineurial coaptation of the injured severed nerve to the windowed defect. Ideally, the axons of the donor nerve are not violated.

Initial investigations debated the source of the regenerating axons.[6-8,17] Many studies have shown that axonal sprouting can be induced in intact noninjured axons.[18,19] The release of neurotrophic factors from the injured nerve, Schwann cells, and surrounding tissue induce a quorum of axon sprouts that arise from nearby intact axons to reinnervate the injured nerve and its target area. Yamauchi et al.[20] demonstrated that the expression of growth-associated protein 43 (GAP-43), a marker of growth cone formation, as well as neurotrophin-3 (NT-3) and brain-derived neurotrophic factor (BDNF) is implicated in the mechanism of col-

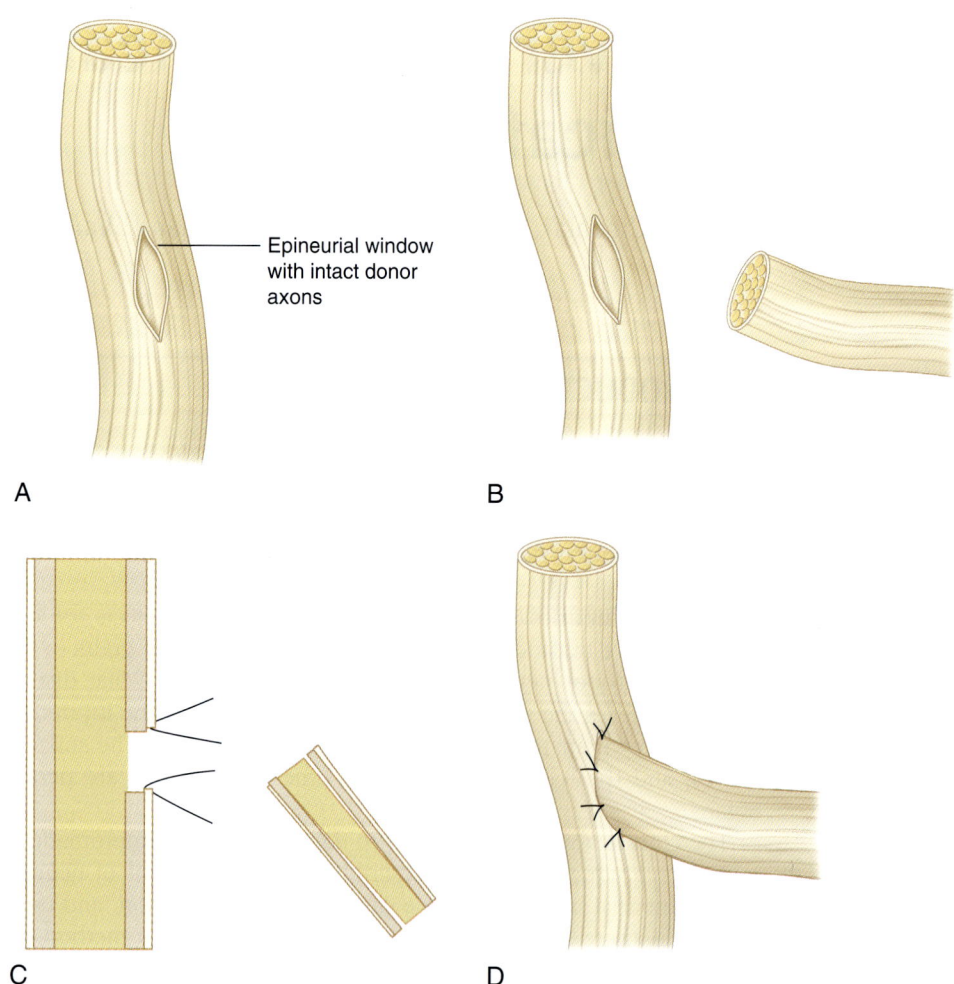

Epineurial window
with intact donor
axons

A

B

C

D

Figure 5–1 **A:** End-to-side nerve repair. **B:** Recipient nerve (peroneal nerve) is sharply cut and approximated to donor nerve (tibial nerve) window. **C:** Sutures are placed through epineurium of donor and recipient nerves. **D:** Final repair.

lateral sprouting of motor nerves in the end-to-side model. Verification of collateral sprouting as the source of regeneration has been confirmed visually with fluorescent dye tracer.[17]

In another rat model, Sananpanich et al.[21] reported the results of end-to-side and end-to-end neurorrhaphy of musculocutaneous and ulnar nerves. Retrograde labeling confirmed that the musculocutaneous and ulnar nerves received neurons from independent regions within the spinal cord, and that there was no overlap. In this study, 24 Sprague-Dawley rats were divided into two groups. In Group 1, 12 animals underwent an end-to-side neurorrhaphy with the distal musculocutaneous nerve stump sutured to the ulnar nerve through a 0.7-mm epineural window. In Group 2, 12 animals underwent an end-to-end neurorrhaphy with the distal end of the musculocutaneous sutured to the proximal end of the transected ulnar nerve. The reinnervating neurons were found to originate exclusively from the ulnar nerve pool.

Liu et al. recently evaluated the functional recovery after various techniques of end-to-side neurorrhaphy in 80 female rats.[10] They transected the peroneal nerve, which was then sutured to the tibia nerve in an end-to-side fashion after preparing an epineurial window. Their findings suggested that an end-to-side neurorrhaphy allows effective motor recovery. This was demonstrated by early improvement of the peroneal functional index, stronger muscle contractile function, greater muscle weight, and a higher density of regenerated axons as compared to an unrepaired nerve. The results also demonstrated that removal of the epineurium of the donor nerve at the nerve repair site increased the effectiveness of an end-to-side nerve repair. The removal of the epineurium did not affect the function of the donor nerves.

Pickering et al. investigated the application and functional recovery of animals following an end-to-side neurorrhaphy across segmental defects to determine whether collateral axonal sprouting can occur across gaps.[11] The functional recovery of gap-repaired lesions was compared to those repaired by direct suture.

In 96 female rats, the right peroneal nerve was sharply transected 3 mm distal to the bifurcation of the sciatic nerve. A perineural window sized to match the distal peroneal stump was made in the tibial nerve of each rat. In these groups, a 2-, 4-, or 6-mm ultra thin plastic tube (internal diameter 0.03 in) was sutured to the surrounding epineurium of the tibial nerve using 12-0 nylon (Fig. 5–2 A to C) The distal peroneal stump was then telescoped into the distal end of the tube using two 12-0 sutures. Results were assessed by an objective weekly gait analysis, specifically the peroneal functional index (PFI). This study demonstrated successful nerve regeneration across gaps of up to 6 mm that occurred following end-to-side nerve repair with functional rein-

nervation of a distal nerve (secondary to collateral axons sprouting). The study indicates a potential clinical use for end-to-side technique when using a plastic tube to bridge the gap. It is important to emphasize that in all of three of these studies in our laboratory, there was no significant histologic or functional deficit in the donor nerve.

Use of a large epineurial window helicoid technique was first explored by Yan et al.[22] as an improvement over the conventional end-to-side technique by providing a larger surface area from which axons can sprout into the recipient nerve. Peripheral nerve repairs are often unsatisfactory due to a paucity of sprouting fibers in the repaired nerve, which leads to muscle atrophy and motor end-plate degeneration before any significant reinnervation can occur. It was theorized that a larger surface area of repair would provide more available axons for regeneration, and thus improve motor end-plate reinnervation.

The helicoid method involves a 4-mm oblique-cut epineurial window, as opposed to the conventional 1-mm epineurial window, at the site of the donor nerve. This increases the axonal contact area by as much as five times the conventional surface area. The increased surface area associated with the helicoid neurorrhaphy resulted in an increased volume of axons sprouting into the recipient nerve, as demonstrated by greater fascicular number, diameter, and regularity.[22] The improved axon sprouting resulted in a statistically significant increased titanic force on moist muscle weight at the respected target fibers as compared with the traditional end-to-side technique. In the helicoid group, the number of regenerative nerve fibers approached 100% of the proximal stump or "normal" peroneal nerve. The comparison group of traditional end-to-side technique showed a 79% ratio of regenerated fibers.

INDICATIONS

The indications for end-to-side neurorrhaphy are generally infrequent based on our experience as well as that of others. This technique has limited clinical applications. Distinct applications for this method are yet to be fully defined because of the paucity of clinical reports. There are, however, specific situations when this method is of clinical value when no other reliable methods are available. We emphasize that first considerations for neurorrhaphy should be end-to-end repair, nerve grafting, or nerve transfers before selecting end-to-side repair. The four scenarios in which we have experienced good clinical results with end-to-side nerve repair follow:

1. Symptomatic distal neuromas in the hand
2. Avulsed digital nerves in the palm
3. Absent medial or ulnar nerve sensation in the hand

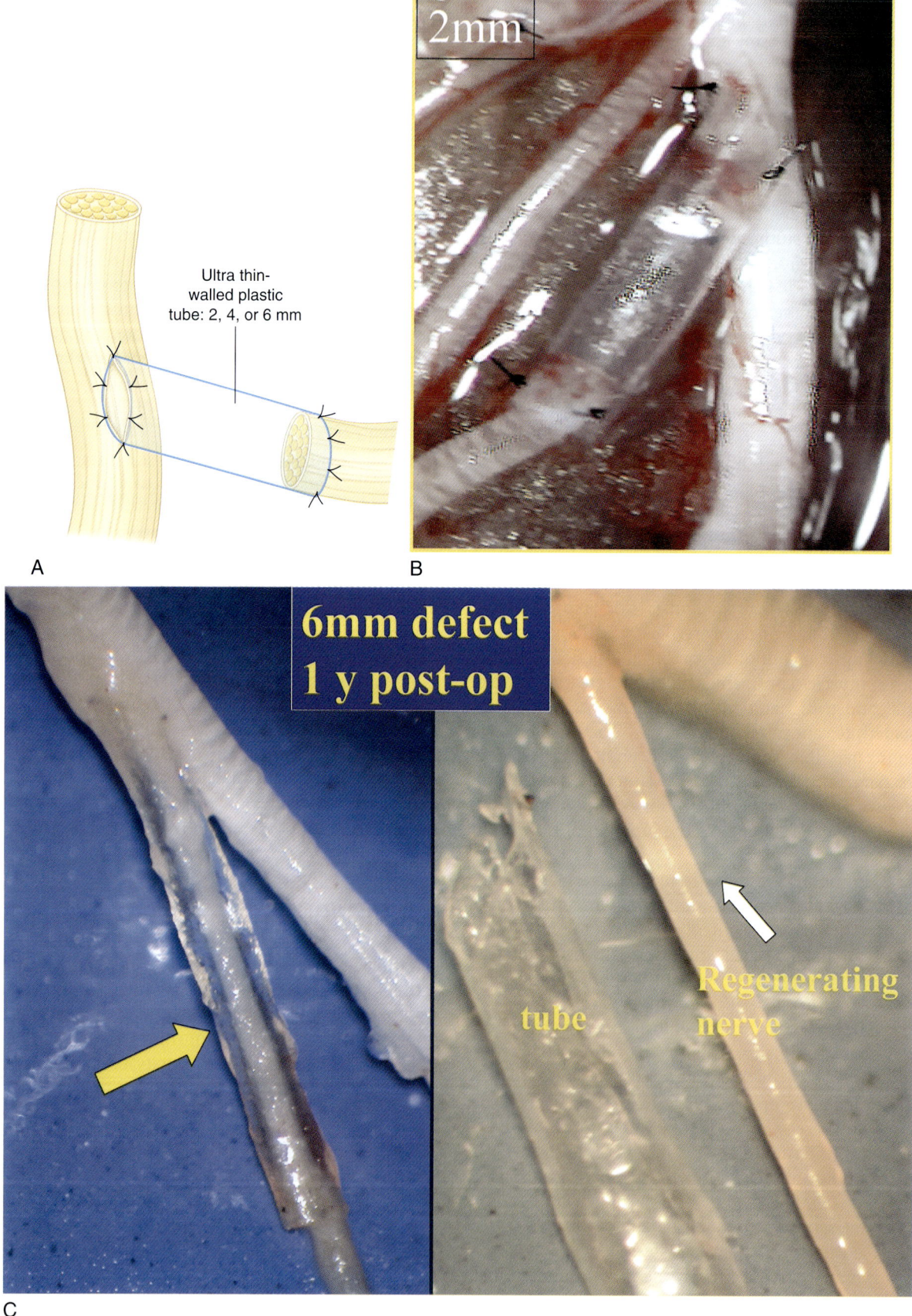

Figure 5–2 **A:** End-to-side nerve repair across a 6-mm gap. **B:** Thin plastic tube bridges 6-mm gap of rat peroneal nerve to tibial nerve. **C:** Examination 1 year after end-to-side nerve repair across the 6-mm gap. Plastic tube is then placed on the left and removed on the right to demonstrate regenerating peroneal nerve across the gap.

4. Motor branch of the musculocutaneous nerve to the median nerve

SYMPTOMATIC NEUROMAS

In our hands, the most useful application of end-to-side nerve repair has been in the management of symptomatic neuromas of the hand. We have been most successful using this technique originally described by Al-Qattan[23,24] to treat painful neuromas of the superficial radial nerve. Previous methods of treating painful neuroma or neuromas in continuity of the superficial radial nerve (the "nuisance nerve") have been unreliable. These methods include coverage with soft tissue transfers, proximal resections, mobilization, and implantation of the distal neuroma into deep tissue such as proximal muscle.

If a painful neuroma of a distal branch of the superficial radial nerve is present, the distal neuroma is excised, and the proximal nerve segment is sutured end to side into the intact superficial radial nerve (Fig. 5–3). The distal segment, if it can be located, may likewise be sutured into the intact superficial radial nerve more distally. We have had relief of symptoms and tenderness in seven patients who have been treated in this manner.

In theory, if a neuroma of the entire superficial radial nerve was present, the proximal segment of the superficial radial nerve could be inserted end to side into an intact nearby nerve such as the lateral antebrachial cutaneous nerve or median nerve, but we have had no clinical experience with this approach.

This method can also be successfully employed to satisfy the severed digital nerve in an index ray deletion by performing an end-to-side neurorrhaphy of the proximal segment of the digital nerve on the severed index finger into the intact digital nerve of the thumb or long finger.

We have also experienced success in treating a painful neuroma in the small remnant of a previously deleted supernumerary digit by performing an end-to-side nerve repair to the intact digital nerve.

DIGITAL NERVES IN PALM

With the avulsed digit or digits, the common digital nerves are often avulsed directly from the median or ulnar nerve proximally. With the replantation or revascularization procedure, the distal avulsed nerves, after debridement to normal appearing neural tissue may be too short for direct repair. In addition it is frequently difficult to find an ideal locus on the proximal median or ulnar nerve to reconnect the avulsed digital nerve, even with an interposition nerve graft. In this situation,

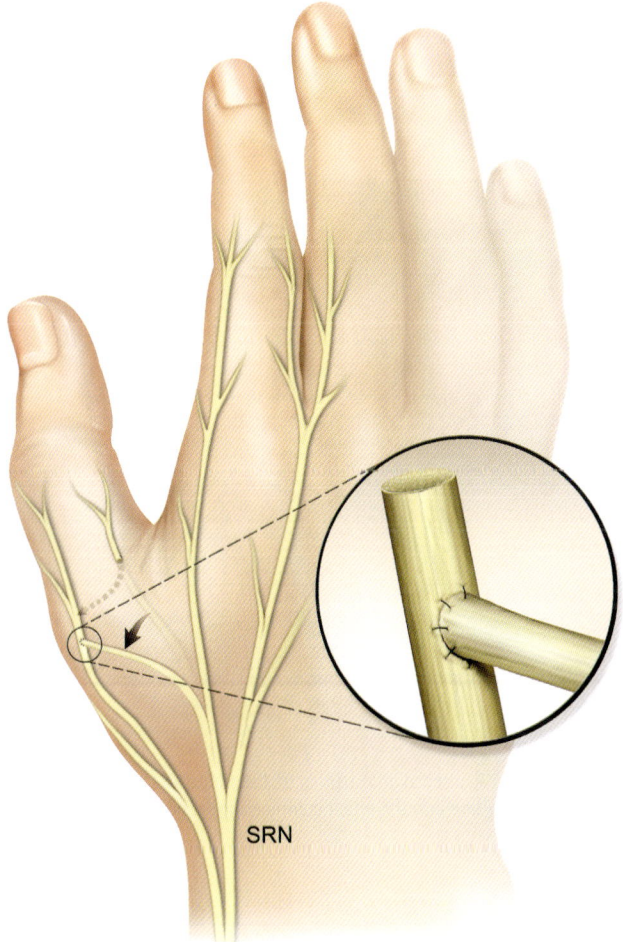

Figure 5–3 Painful neuroma in the branch of the superficial radial nerve (SRN) has been resected, and the branch sutured end to side into an intact branch of the superficial radial nerve. If the distal end can be located, it also can be sutured end to side into an intact branch of the superficial radial nerve (double dotted lines).

end-to-side nerve repair of the avulsed digital nerve to the adjacent intact common or proper digital nerves offers a salvage method (Fig. 5–4).

We have used this technique several times over the years in replantation of avulsed digits. The expected recovery is usually protective sensation, and to our knowledge the patients have had no painful neuromas.

Another application for this technique is when there is irreparable damage to the median or ulnar nerve proximal to the hand with loss of sensation. The common digital nerves of the median nerve can be sutured end to side into the functional ulnar nerve, or vice versa when there is irreparable damage to the ulnar nerve and the median nerve is intact.

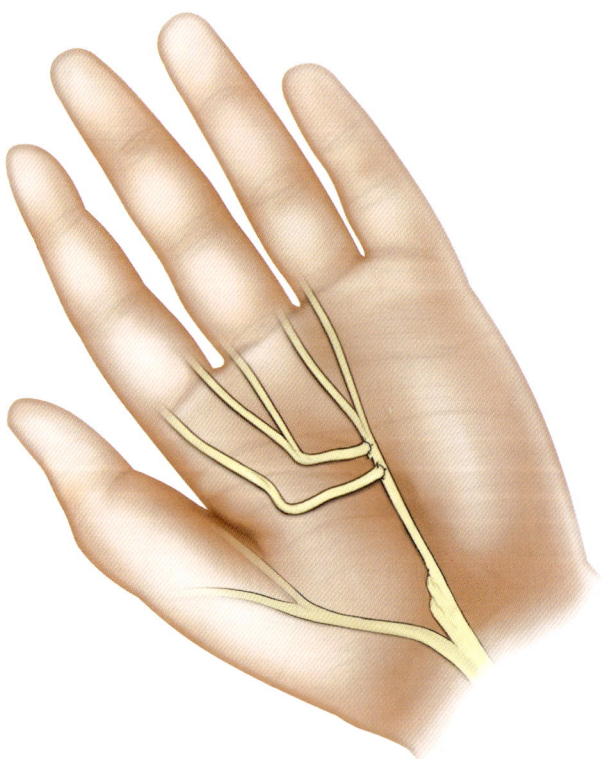

Figure 5–4 Avulsed digital nerves of the index and long fingers are sutured end to side into the intact common digital nerve to the long and ring finger.

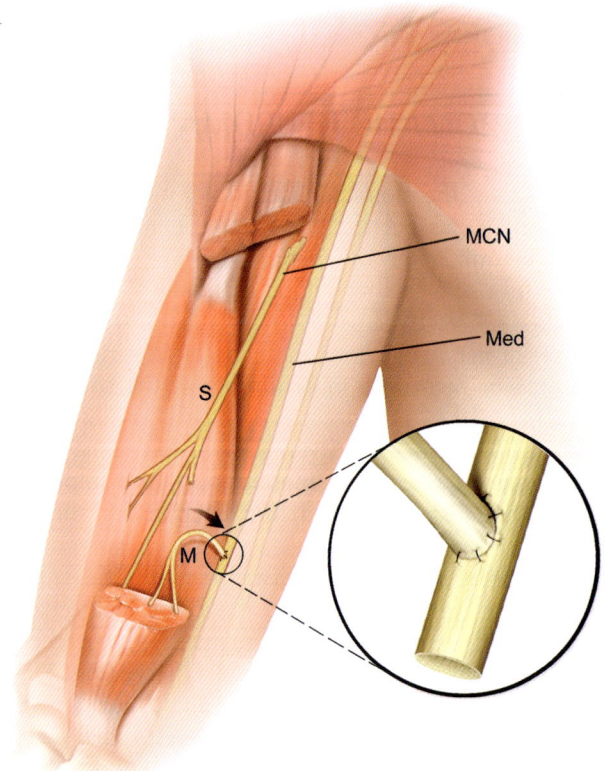

Figure 5–5 Motor branch *(M)* of the biceps muscle was dissected free from the sensory branch *(S)* of the musculocutaneous nerve *(MCN)* and sutured end-to-side into the intact median nerve *(Med)*.

MUSCULOCUTANEOUS NERVE TO MEDIAN NERVE

There are several methods to reinnervate the biceps muscle when it has been lost secondary to a brachial plexus injury. Various methods such as donors from fascicles of the ulnar nerve (Oberlin transfer), spinal accessory nerve, and intercostal muscle nerve are discussed in other chapters of this book.[25] Another viable option is an end-to-side repair with the musculocutaneous nerve into the median nerve. We have witnessed good functional recovery with the procedure and have seen excellent results in a patient of Minoru Shibato (Minoru Shibato, Professor, Niigata University School of Medicine, Niigata, Japan, personal communication, 2004).

When performing this procedure, it is important to dissect the motor branch of the musculocutaneous nerve from the sensory branch (lateral antebrachial cutaneous nerve). The clearly identified motor branch to the biceps is easily sutured end to side into the nearby median nerve in the upper arm (Fig. 5–5).

In this technique, the sprouting axons from the median nerve have only a short distance to travel through the motor branch to the target motor end plates of the biceps muscle. This setup may explain the good functional results that we have seen with this technique.

SURGICAL TECHNIQUE

The surgery is usually performed under tourniquet ischemia. Using loupe magnification, the donor nerve is exposed, and the recipient nerve is freely mobilized for ease of repair. As in all nerve repairs, the nerves should never be connected under tension. A blue soft rubber background mat is placed beneath the nerves to be repaired. This aids not only in better visibility, but also promotes easier handling of the delicate nerves. An operating microscope is recommended for the actual repair.

An epineurial helicoid window is made in the donor area to match the size of the recipient nerve end. As we demonstrated in the laboratory, this technique provides greater surface area for axonal regeneration.[22] Care is taken not to injure the intact fascicles, and we do not incise the perineurium as some investigators have suggested.[6–8] If there is a neuroma on the end of the recipient nerve, it is cleanly excised so that pouting fascicles are apparent on the severed nerve. Two 9-0 or 10-0 microsutures are placed 180 degrees apart in the epineurium of the recipient and donor nerves so that the cut end is perpendicular to the donor nerve. The repair is facilitated by passing the suture first through the recipient nerve and then into the donor nerve. It is less traumatic to the recipient nerve to pass the microneedle from outside in rather than inside out. Depending on the size of the nerve, one to four additional sutures may be placed.

The tourniquet is released and hemostasis obtained. Since the repair has been done under no tension, early motion is usually recommended.

Potential Pitfalls

1. Inadequate exposure of the donor nerve and inadequate mobilization of the recipient nerve.
2. Repairing the nerve under tension.
3. Making the window in the donor nerve too small rather than elliptical or helicoid.
4. Damage to the donor fascicles by penetrating the perineurium.

RESULTS

Since no large clinical series have been reported on end-to-side neurorrhaphy and our personal experience is limited, the expected clinical outcomes are yet to be accurately determined. However, in the few but specific examples described in this chapter we have definitely witnessed favorable results.

REFERENCES

1. Battal MN, Hata Y. A review on the history of end-to-side neurorrhaphy. Plast Reconstr Surg 1997;99:2110–1.
2. Battista A, Cravioto H. Neuroma formation and prevention by fascicle ligation in the rat. Neurosurgery 1981;8:191–204.
3. Durak N, Yuksel F, Kislaoglu E. Effectiveness of epineural barriers as a flap and free graft in reducing neuroma formation in the rat following sciatic nerve severance. Eur J Plast Surg 1995;18:272–5.
4. Goldstein SA, Sturim HS. Intraosseous nerve transposition for treatment of painful neuromas. J Hand Surg Am 1985;10:270–4.
5. Swanson AB, Boere NR, Lumsden RM. The prevention and treatment of amputation neuromata by silicone capping. J Hand Surg Am 1977;2:70–8.
6. Noah EM, Williams A, Fortes W, et al. A new animal model to investigate axonal sprouting after end-to-side neurorrhaphy. J Reconstr Microsurg 1997;13:317–25.
7. Noah EM, Williams A, Jorgenson C, et al. End-to-side neurorrhaphy: A histologic and morphometric study of axonal sprouting into an end-to-side nerve graft. J Reconstr Microsurg 1997;13.99–106.
8. Yan JG, Matloub HS, Sanger J, et al. Nerve Sprouting Behavior after Terminolateral Neurorrhaphy: Experimental Study in Rats. Annual meeting of American Association of Hand Surgery, Hawaii, January, 1999.
9. Chen LE, Pickering T, Qi WN, et al. One-year results following end-to-side neurorraphy. Trans Orthop Res Soc 2003;28:95.
10. Liu K, Chen LE, Seaber AV, et al. Motor functional and morphological findings following end-to-side neurorraphy in the rat model. J Orthop Res 1999;17:293–300.
11. Pickering T, Chen L, Seaber AV, et al. Motor functional recovery using nerve conduit in end-to-side neurorrhaphy. Trans Orthop Res Soc 2002;27:643.
12. Zhang F, et al. One donor nerve with two sites of end-to-side neurorrhaphy: an experimental study in rats. Trans Orthop Res Soc 2002;27:642.
13. Gurney ME, Yamamoto H, Kwon Y. Induction of motor neuron sprouting in vivo by ciliary neurotrophic factor and basic fibroblast growth factor. J Neurosci 1992;12:3241–7.
14. Isaacson LG, Saffran BN, Crutcher KA. Nerve growth factor-induced sprouting of mature, uninjured sympathetic axons. J Comp Neurol 1992;326:327–36.
15. Chen YG, Brushart TM. The effect of denervated muscle and schwann cells on axon collateral sprouting. J Hand Surg Am 1998;23:1025–33.
16. Lundborg G, Zhao Q, Kanje M, et al. Can sensory and motor collateral sprouting be induced from intact peripheral nerve by end-to-side anastomosis? J Hand Surg Br 1994;19:277–82.
17. Hayashi A, Yanai A, Komuro Y, et al. Collateral sprouting occurs following end-to-side neurorrhaphy. Plast and Reconstr Surg 2004;114:129–37.
18. Zhang Z, Soucacos PN, Bo J, et al. Evaluation of collateral sprouting after end-to-side nerve coaptation using a fluorescent double-labeling technique. Microsurgery 1999;19:281–6.
19. Rowan P, Chen LE, Urbaniak JR. End-to-side nerve repair: a review. Hand Clin 2000;16:151–9.
20. Yamauchi T, Maeda M, Tamai S, et al. Collateral sprouting mechanism after end-to-side nerve repair in the rat. Med Electron Microsc 2000;33:151–6.
21. Sanapanich K, Morrison WA, Messina A. Physiologic and morphologic aspects of nerve regeneration after end-to-end or end-to-side coaptation in a rat model of brachial plexus injury. J Hand Surg Am 2002;27:133–42.
22. Yan J, Matloub HS, Sanger JR, et al. A modified end-to-side method for peripheral nerve repair: large epineural window helicoid technique versus small epineural window standard end-to-side technique. J Hand Surg Am 2002;27:484–92.
23. Al-Qattan M. Terminolateral neurorraphy: review of experimental and clinical studies. J Reconstr Microsurg 2001;17:99–108.
24. Al-Qattan M. Prevention and treatment of painful neuromas of the superficial radial nerve by the end-to-side repair concept: an experimental study and preliminary clinical experience. Microsurgery 2000;20:99–104.
25. Oberlin C, Beal D, Leechavengvongs S, et al. Nerve transfer to biceps muscle using a part of ulnar nerve for C5–C6 avulsion of the brachial plexus: anatomical study and report of four cases. J Hand Surg Am 1994;19:232–7.

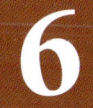

6

Upper Extremity Nerve Transfers

Renata V. Weber and Susan E. Mackinnon

INTRODUCTION

A nerve-to-nerve transfer is increasingly being used as the primary and often definitive treatment for nerve injuries, especially when direct repair or nerve grafting is not an option, or likely to result in a poor outcome because of proximal injuries or long nerve gaps. Whereas tendon transfers still have a role in the management of functional repair after long-term denervation, the advantages of a nerve transfer render it a better option in certain acute clinical setting. Improvement in microsurgical tools, advances in nerve repair, and a better understanding of the internal nerve topography have contributed to the creation and usage of nerve transfers. Nerve-to-nerve transfers offer a superior alternative for functional restoration in isolated or multiple nerve injuries when early reinnervation of the target end organ is necessary, such as in proximal injuries or delayed treatment. Expendable sensory or motor axons close to the end organ allow for earlier regeneration and preclude the need for nerve grafts. Given the number of nerve transfers created in the last decade, it may be surprising to realize that the first nerve transfers were performed at the turn of the 19th century.

BACKGROUND

Upper extremity motor nerve injuries have devastating consequences for the affected patient. The first nerve transfers were originally intended for otherwise irreparable brachial plexus root avulsion injuries.[1] These salvage procedures often had poor results and were largely abandoned. In 1948, Lurje[2] recommended using a neighboring nerve for nerve transfers in cases of brachial plexus injuries when direct nerve repair was not possible. He used the long thoracic nerve, thoracodorsal nerve, and triceps branch of the radial nerve for transfer to the suprascapular, musculocutaneous, and axillary nerves. During the same period, advances made in nerve grafting techniques, especially the modifications popularized by Hanno Millesi[3] in the late 1960s to early 1970s, led to abandoning nerve transfers in favor of nerve grafts. Millesi's introduction of interfascicular nerve grafts from the rudimentary "cable grafts" elevated nerve grafting to the standards now routinely employed.[4,5] Brachial plexus injuries were being treated with complete excision and primary grafting of the entire scarred area. The surgery is lengthy, requires significant harvest of expendable donor nerves, and is associated with significant morbidity. Recovery of function was greatly improved over previous attempts at repair, especially in the pediatric population; however, incomplete recovery continued to be a problem in adults. In obstetric brachial plexus injuries, grafting remains the gold standard, most likely because of the smaller distance that the nerve needs to regenerate to the target organ.

Interest in creating nerve transfers initially stemmed from SEM's experience with four specific areas: (1) the suboptimal recovery of function witnessed after brachial plexus surgery in the previous decades, (2) the stimulus provided by this patient population for creating alternatives methods for reconstruction, (3) an understanding of the internal topography of the of peripheral nerves, and (4) experience with tendon transfers. The latter, coupled with an understanding of the potential for motor re-education, set the stage for transfer of the nerves innervating the donor muscles rather than the tendons themselves.

In the early 1990s, we used several nerve transfers. The medial pectoral branches were routinely transferred to the musculocutaneous nerve to provide a nearby source of pure motor axons in upper plexus injuries.[6] The terminal branch of the anterior interosseous nerve was transferred to the deep motor branch of the ulnar nerve for reconstruction of high ulnar nerve injuries.[7] Satisfactory results from these transfers provided the stimulus for other transfers, including reconstruction of the radial nerve from expendable branches of the median nerve as well as reconstruction of pronation from redundant ulnar or median nerve transfers.[8,9] As we acquire a greater understanding of the internal topography of the peripheral nerve and evaluate the results of the current nerve transfers, we modify current practices and techniques. It is very likely that nerve transfers will become the surgical technique of choice for reconstruction of the majority of proximal and severe injuries.

The optimal correction is a direct repair whenever possible. Large nerve gaps, proximal injuries, and avulsion type injuries complicate the surgical management. Time constraints due to muscle atrophy after denervation negatively influence recovery. Nerve transfers offer a surgical alternative for restoration of function following severe proximal nerve injuries by delivering expendable sensory or motor axons close to the end organ. Until the last century, the results of nerve repair in the upper extremity and especially of the brachial plexus

were viewed with pessimism. In the latter half of the 20th century, advances in peripheral nerve surgery, improvements in nerve grafting techniques, and knowledge of internal topography, injury pattern and regenerative ability of the peripheral nerve have contributed to the advancement of peripheral nerve surgery, allowing for the development of nerve transfers.

Presurgical Evaluation

Epidemiology and Patient Selection

Devastating injuries to the brachial plexus that result in loss of motor function and sensation of the involved upper extremity involve young males in as many as 90% of cases.[10,11] Most of these cases are due to motor vehicle accidents, and motorcycle accidents have been implicated in up to 84% of cases.[12] Between 0.67% to 1.3% of motor vehicle accidents and up to 4.2% of motorcycle accidents result in some permanent brachial plexus injury.[10] In motorcycle accidents, the patient is less protected than in a motor vehicle accident, and brachial plexus is under greater traction forces; thus root avulsions injuries are more common. Crush injuries are seen more commonly after motor vehicle accidents. Other common causes of brachial plexus injuries include pedestrian/motor vehicle accidents, gunshot wounds, and sudden blows to the head or shoulder from sport or from occupational accidents such as from falling objects. Brachial plexus palsies may also occur from lower-velocity injuries including bicycling, skiing, falling from a height, or tripping down stairs.

Most patients will be referred from another consultant or from their primary physician 2 to 4 months after sustaining an injury to the upper arm with neurologic deficit that should have resolved spontaneously. Ideally, we prefer to evaluate these patients as close to the time of injury as possible, in order to follow the recovery process. Occasionally, the patients will be sent for a first evaluation 6 to 9 months after injury, at which point the urgency for repair becomes more immediate.

Nerve injuries are classified as six degrees of injury and can be found in Table 6–1.[13] They can be grouped

TABLE 6–1			
Classification of Nerve Injury			
Sunderland	**Seddon**	**Mackinnon**	**Injury**
Degree I	Neurapraxia	Degree I	Conduction block resolves spontaneously
Degree II	Axonotmesis	Degree II	Axonal rupture without interruption of the basal lamina tubes
Degree III		Degree III	Rupture of both axons and basal lamina tubes, some scarring
Degree IV		Degree IV	Complete scar block
Degree V	Neurotmesis	Degree V	Complete transection
		Degree VI	Combination of I through V and normal fascicles

into three categories. (1) injuries that will recover spontaneously (first and second degrees); (2) injuries that must be repaired (fifth degree or neurotmesis); and (3) injuries with partial recovery that will likely need surgery (third, fourth, and sixth degrees).

Preoperative Studies

Patients who sustain a transection of the nerve will benefit from early exploration (within 3 weeks) and primary repair or repair with a graft. If the nerve injury is very proximal, these patients may be candidates for a nerve transfer procedure. The determination is based on the entire clinical picture, location of the injury, time for reinnervation, and possible permanent loss of function because of delay for reinnervation. Patients with traction injuries are treated conservatively with observation for the first 3 months. During this time, physical therapy to maintain joint movement is critical for optimal recovery. If no sign of recovery is noted by 3 months, electrodiagnostic testing can be used to determine if spontaneous recovery is likely. Electromyographic (EMG) studies performed less than 4 to 6 weeks after injury may not be useful. A first- and second-degree nerve injury will recover spontaneously, and the interest of the EMG is to evaluate the extent of recovery in order to target management of potential surgery if there is evidence of lack of spontaneous regeneration. Initially, fibrillation potentials will be seen on serial EMGs. As muscle recovery progresses, the number of fibrillation potentials will decrease, and voluntary motor unit potentials (MUPs) will appear and increase.[14,15] The demonstration of MUPs indicates a favorable prognosis for functional recovery.

In addition to EMGs, plain films assist in determining the severity of the impact and extent of the injury. A transverse process fracture may lead us to suspect an avulsion of the corresponding root because the deep cervical fascia travels between the transverse processes of cervical vertebrae and the cervical roots.[16] A clavicular fracture may be associated with a laceration of the brachial plexus, and the presence of broken ribs may preclude the use of certain intercostal nerves as suitable donor nerves. Computerized tomography (CT) scanning and more importantly magnetic resonance imaging (MRI) are helpful in assessing the injury. MRI can visualize all portions of the brachial plexus, whereas CT/myelography will only evaluate possible root avulsion. The MRI is especially advantageous for imaging the distal brachial plexus because of its multiplanar capability.[17] Muscle, nerve, and vascular structures can be readily distinguished from each other, and pathologic lesions may be accurately localized in relation to surrounding structures. Post-traumatic neuromas can often be identified and in conjunction with EMG studies, a surgical plan is created.

Indications for Nerve Transfers

The surgical indications for nerve transfers are evolving as new donor sources for motor and sensory restoration are proposed and reproduced. While there is no absolute guideline for when a nerve transfer should be used, we prefer to reserve nerve transfers for the following situations: (1) a brachial plexus injury in which there is no graftable proximal nerve or nerve root; (2) a high proximal injury that requires a long distance for regeneration; (3) in order to avoid scarred areas in critical locations with potential for injury to vital surrounding structures; (4) in the case of major limb trauma with segmental loss of nerve tissue that would require several grafts; (5) as an alternative to nerve grafting when time from injury to reconstruction is prolonged; (6) in partial nerve injuries with a defined functional loss; (7) in spinal cord root avulsion injuries; and (8) in nerve injuries where the level of injury is uncertain, such as with idiopathic neuritides or radiation trauma and nerve injuries with multiple levels of injury.

The most devastating injury to the upper limb is a brachial plexus injury that encompasses the entire plexus, leaving the patient with an insensate functionless limb. The injuries most often seen are a result of a traction injury to the brachial plexus or avulsion injuries of the spinal cord roots. In traction injuries, the nerves are stretched and may regenerate spontaneously; however, in many cases, the nerves become scarred, effectively blocking the regenerative process. When there is more than one component of the brachial plexus injured resulting in partial residual loss of function, or no function at all, our reconstructive priority is first to restore elbow flexion. Shoulder abduction and external rotation is the next priority. The "best" donor nerves should be reserved to restore these critical functions. Often for extensive injuries, a combination of nerve transfers, tendon transfers, and free muscle transfers may be necessary to optimize the recovery of upper extremity function. Tendon transfers may be needed in case of a failed nerve reconstruction, or to augment a reconstruction that leaves the patient with some residual weakness.[18,19] Free muscle transfers are usually planned as an adjunct after primary nerve reconstruction in complex brachial plexus injuries. Sensory transfers are used to restore sensation, in particular to the ulnar side of the thumb and radial side of the index finger. As in any complex reconstruction, the transfer—nerve or musculotendinous—is customized to the deficits and the individual needs of the patient, especially given the limitations of donor nerves and innervated muscles.

Principles of Nerve Transfer

The more commonly used motor nerve transfers are modeled after their analogous tendon transfers; thus

TABLE 6–2
Criteria for Motor Nerve Transfer
Donor nerve near motor end plates of target muscle (shortest distance = shortest time for re-innervation)
Expendable or redundant donor motor nerve
Donor nerve with pure motor nerve fibers
Donor motor nerve with a large number of motor axons
Donor nerve innervates a muscle that is synergistic to the target muscle (preferred but not required to facilitate re-education)
Motor re-education improves functional recovery

TABLE 6–3
Criteria for Sensory Nerve Transfer
Donor sensory nerve near the target sensory nerve
Expendable donor sensory nerve (noncritical sensory distribution)
Donor sensory nerve with a large number of pure sensory axons
Denervated distal end of donor nerve repaired end to side to adjacent normal sensory nerve
Sensory re-education improves functional recovery

similar principles hold true for the two transfers. Only an expendable nerve fascicle or nerve branch is used. Nerves with expendable fascicles or branches make excellent donor nerves. Unlike a tendon transfer, a nerve transfer does not rely on amplitude and excursion of the tendon muscle unit, nor is it limited to the one tendon/one function and the straight line of pull principles. The type of muscle fiber unit and the insertion of the tendon will influence the ultimate effectiveness of that muscle's contraction in its new position.[20,21]

The major advantages of a nerve transfer over that of a tendon transfer are that (1) nerve transfers can restore sensibility in addition to motor function, (2) a nerve that innervates multiple muscle groups can be restored with a single nerve transfer, and (3) the insertion and attachments of the muscle(s) in question are not disrupted, and thus the original muscle function and tension are maintained. While a synergistic nerve transfer is ideal, antagonistic nerve transfers can be successfully used in some cases such as branches of median nerve used to restore radial nerve function.[22]

A significant advantage of nerve transfers over long nerve grafts is the ability to convert a proximal high-level nerve injury to a low-level nerve injury. This is especially important in high median nerve and ulnar nerve injuries. The donor nerves close to the injured nerve as well as to the motor end-plate are selected, and nerve grafts are rarely needed in addition to a nerve transfer. An internal neurolysis allows for separation of donor and recipient fascicles from the main nerve so that an end-to-end repair is performed. Nerve transfers for both motor and sensory nerves have similar criteria, and are listed in Table 6–2 and Table 6–3.[23,24]

When choosing the ideal donor nerves for transfer, a nerve that innervates a synergistic muscle group is preferable, as it facilitates postoperative motor re-education. While a nerve supplying a nonsynergistic, or even antagonistic muscle group may be used, more retraining may be necessary to learn to contract the newly reinnervated muscle. Our preferred technique for the neurorrhaphy is an end-to-end repair. In rare instances such as in the spinal accessory nerve to

suprascapular nerve transfer, we do perform a nerve transfer with an end-to-side neurorrhaphy using a partial neurotomy of the donor nerve.[25] While others have shown comparable results when using either end-to-end or end-to-side repair, there remains controversy over the effectiveness of the end-to-side repair. Our experimental studies show that while sensory nerves will spontaneously sprout from an epineural or perineural window, a motor nerve requires a partial neurectomy to facilitate end-to-side regeneration.[26] The more common nerve transfers with our preferred donor nerve can be seen in Table 6–4.

Planning of Nerve Transfer

A critical number of motor axons need to reach the target muscle and reinnervate the muscle fibers within a critical time period in order that motor function recovery can take place. At this time, that critical number is unknown; however, clinically we know that despite the nerve size discrepancy that exists in some of the transfers we use, such as in the anterior interosseous nerve (AIN) to ulnar motor nerve, the functional recovery is very good. The second limitation of nerve transfers at present is the constraints of distance and time. The time for muscle to become permanently denervation and unable to recover is not known; however, it is likely between 12 and 18 months in adults. Nerve growth in the clinical setting at present is limited to 1 in/month or 1 to 1.5 mm/day.[27] A nerve transfer closer to the motor end plate can significantly affect the distal component of an injury. The use of nerve transfers has considerably altered our concept of an absolute "window" of opportunity for reinnervation. This means that even late reconstructions (8 to 10 months) of high nerve injuries have the potential for successful reinnervation.

Operative Considerations

First and foremost, in all nerve transfer procedures, the entire affected limb is prepped and draped into the surgical field. This is essential in order to better determine

TABLE 6–4

List of Common Nerve Transfers

Injured Nerve	Donor Nerves	Recipient Nerves	Function Restored
Musculocutaneous	FCU fascicle of ulnar n. FCR fascicle of median n.	Biceps brachii br. Brachialis br.	Elbow flexion
Suprascapular	Spinal accessory n.	Suprascapular n.	Shoulder abduction, external rotation
Accessory	Medial pectoral br.	Spinal accessory n.	Shoulder elevation and abduction
Axillary	Triceps br. of radial n.	Deltoid br.	Shoulder abduction
Radial	FCR, FDS ± PL br. of median n.	Posterior interosseus n. ECRB br.	Wrist, finger extension
Median	FCU fascicle of ulnar n.	Anterior interosseus n.	Thumb opposition, finger flexion
Ulnar	Distal anterior interosseus n. of median n.	Ulnar motor br.	Hand intrinsics
Median (sensory)	Ulnar sensory n. Dorsal sensory n. of radial n.	1st web space common digital nerve	Sensation to key pinch area
Ulnar (sensory)	3rd web space common digital nerve (median n.)	4th web space common digital n. and ulnar digital n. of 5th digit	Sensation to 4th and 5th digits
Ulnar (sensory)	Lateral antebrachial cutaneous n.	Dorsal ulnar n.	Sensation to ulnar border of hand

br., branch; n., nerve.

the function of the fascicles being stimulated during the decision-making portion of the operation. The non-functioning nerve is exposed and stimulated with a hand-held nerve stimulator. In cases where there is some question that recovery is present but undetectable by electromyography (EMG) or nerve conduction studies, intraoperative nerve conduction studies may be obtained. Most often, if there is no evidence of recovery by preoperative EMG, our experience has been that the nerve is permanently injured.

We perform all nerve transfer surgery under general anesthesia. While depolarizing agents may be used for induction, only short-acting agents should be used, so that the effects of the medication have dissipated by the time the nerve in question needs to be stimulated. If a tourniquet is used during the exploration and dissection of more distal nerves, the length of time should be limited to less than 1 hour, as the compression of the tourniquet may cause first-degree conduction block, effectively preventing the uninjured donor nerve from stimulating appropriately. Additional time is added to the surgery to allow for the nerves to recover.

Once the injured nerve is identified and isolated, the donor nerve is selected based on its proximity to the injured nerve. An internal neurolysis is performed at a level along the nerve that will provide a suitable fascicle that will be able to be transposed to the injured nerve without tension and without the need for a nerve graft. Deciding where to start separating out a fascicle and for how long will depend on the particular plexus formation of the nerve itself. For example, the median nerve

in the forearm has fairly consistent interfascicular connections; however, even when the median nerve is explored at the same level each time, the cross-sectional area of the fascicle, the length before that particular fascicle being dissected "ends" because it intercalates with a neighboring fascicle, and the total length that can be mobilized is different in each individual. In addition, it is imperative that no more than 30% of the entire healthy nerve is sacrificed to restore function to the injured nerve. We have found that if more of the uninjured nerve is taken, the reinnervated nerve does not necessarily yield superior muscle strength as compared to a nerve innervated with a smaller caliber fascicle, and the possibility of deleterious effects to the healthy nerve from loss of strength and function is greater.

Once the fascicle is isolated, it is stimulated and compared to the remaining nerve. It is essential that the fascicle being sacrificed is one that supplies expendable function. We will abandon a seemly "perfect" fascicle that has the desired length and cross-sectional area if the function that it provides when stimulated with the nerve stimulator is clinically stronger than the residual nerve. In that situation, a different fascicle is explored and tested until the best fit is obtained. Ideally, the nerve transfer is performed with a primary repair without a nerve graft. The donor nerve is divided as far distal as possible and the recipient nerve is divided as far proximal as possible to facilitate the primary repair. If either nerve branch or fascicle cannot be mobilized to allow for primary repair without undue tension, a nerve graft is used to facilitate the transfer.

The next concern is what constitutes unnecessary tension. Excessive tension across a nerve coaptation site increases scarring and impairs regeneration. Mild tension, on the other hand, is actually believed to be beneficial to the repair by stimulating neurotropic growth factors; however, above a certain threshold value, nerve repair precipitously drops.[28] In clinical practice, we do not measure the tension across a neurorrhaphy, but rather rely on experience and clinical judgment. The nerve fascicles typically used in nerve transfers are between 1 and 3 mm in diameter. The donor and recipient nerves are sutured together with 9-0 nylon in an interrupted fashion. After the repair, the extremity is moved through a complete range of its usual motion. If the neurorrhaphy withstands the tension applied to it from passive movement, then a graft is not necessary. We use the same principle as for elongation of unscarred peripheral nerves, for which it is recommended that no more than 10% of the total length mobilized can be further stretched, after which the microvascular blood flow to the nerve is decreased by half.[29] Both the donor nerve and the recipient nerve can be stretched up to one-tenth of each respective length without risk for ischemia.[30] We have on occasion, performed a primary repair, knowing that the tension was slightly higher than desirable. In those instances, if the neurorrhaphy did not hold, a graft was interposed to allow for a tensionless repair.

The last important item to consider before dividing the chosen fascicle and performing the nerve transfer, is to carefully evaluate the donor nerve for any evidence of a secondary injury. Often, although the injury is at the level of the brachial plexus, and we are generally working at a distance from the original injury, the nerve under traction can be injured at a second site distal to the actual impact. We have observed a similar condition at locations where chronic compression can cause a double crush phenomenon.[31] For example, in shoulder traction injuries, the axillary nerve is presumable injured at the level of the clavicle, proximal to where it exits behind the shoulder. A second neuroma is usually present at the level of the quadrangular space. Care needs to be given when trying to perform the transfer without tension and without a graft, so that an internal neuroma is not inadvertently left in the proximal end of the recipient injured nerve, thereby decreasing the chance for optimal recovery.

Nerve transfers are always our first surgical option whenever possible. If the time of injury is significantly in the past, a free-functioning muscle graft is microsurgically anastomosed to the forearm. The gracilis muscle is our muscle of choice. It is easily harvested and anastomosed to a major artery and vein in the surgical field. Insertion of the tendon–muscle ends depends on the function being replaced and the obturator nerve is coapted to a noninjured nerve in the surgical field or a previously planned nerve graft. Tendon transfers and joint fusions remain part of the adjunct surgical procedures when multiple nerves need to be addressed.

MOTOR AND SENSORY TRANSFERS FOR ISOLATED NERVE INJURIES

Musculocutaneous Nerve: Elbow Flexion

Muscle transfers to restore elbow flexion include the pectoralis major, latissimus dorsi, triceps, and the Steindler flexorplasty using the flexor–pronator musculature.[32,33] Similarly, the nerves that innervate these muscles can be used to re-innervate the biceps brachii and brachialis muscles. Historically, the first nerve transfers were done to the musculocutaneous nerve using either several intercostal nerves with or without interposition nerve grafts or the spinal accessory nerve. In a meta-analysis of the English-language literature by Merrell et al.,[34] the use of the spinal accessory nerve was superior to the intercostal nerves for restoration of any function; however, in patients with grade-4 biceps strength, the intercostal nerves transfer was a more reliable transfer to restore strength. In 1993, we described our results with transferring the medial pectoral nerves branches to the musculocutaneous nerve.[35] We recognized that the critical portion of the musculocutaneous nerve to reinnervate was the motor fascicles to the biceps and brachialis muscles. This transfer moved the level of the repair more distal than previous reconstructions at the root or trunk level, and directed the motor axons to the musculocutaneous nerve distal to the coracobrachialis branch. In addition, the lateral antebrachial cutaneous (LABC) nerve was redirected into the biceps muscle to ensure that motor fibers were not directed toward cutaneous receptors.

In 1994, Oberlin et al.[36] moved the repair even further distal by coapting a fascicle of the ulnar nerve directly into the biceps branch of the musculocutaneous nerve. Leechavengvongs et al.[37] and Sungpet et al.[38] later reported excellent results in 32 and 36 cases, respectively, with rapid motor recovery of the biceps muscle without functional loss of the donor ulnar nerve. In these series, patients recovered between M3 and M4 biceps strength; however, some patients with poorer results needed additional reconstructive procedures. Therefore, given that the brachialis muscle is a stronger elbow flexor than the biceps brachii muscle, we have modified Oberlin's procedure to reinnervate both the biceps and the brachialis branches of the musculocutaneous nerve in order to maximize elbow flexion strength (Fig. 6–1).[22,39]

While there are several options to reinnervate the biceps and brachialis muscles, our preferred method is to use an expendable motor branch of the ulnar nerve

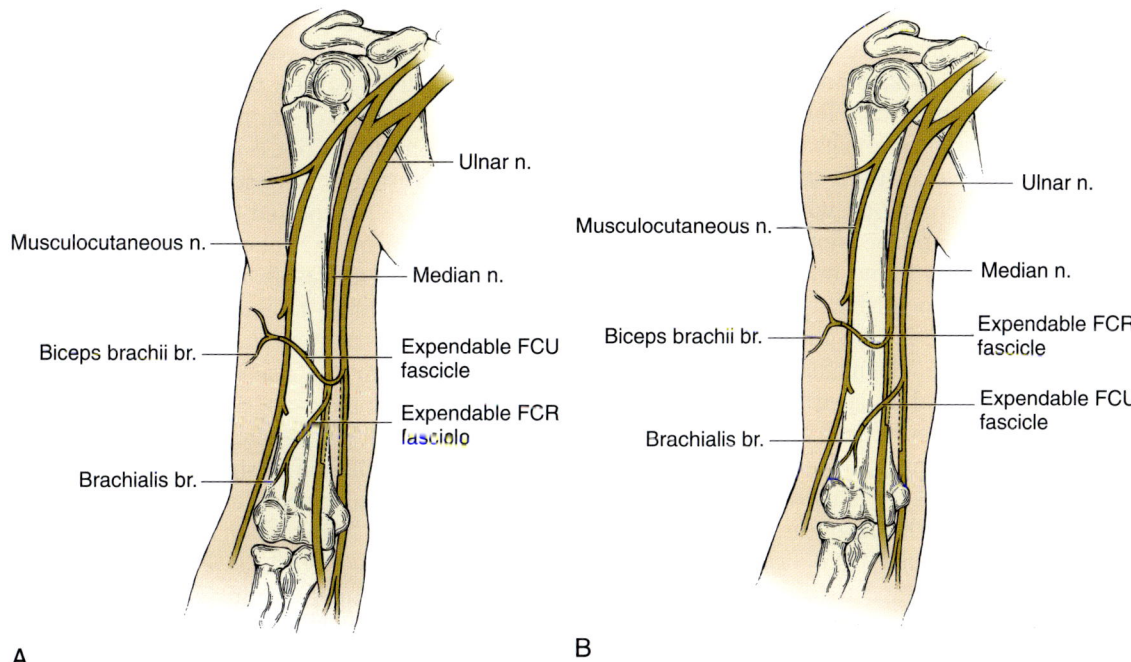

Musculocutaneous n.

Biceps brachii br.

Brachialis br.

Ulnar n.

Median n.

Expendable FCU fascicle

Expendable FCR fasciolo

Musculocutaneous n.

Biceps brachii br.

Brachialis br.

Ulnar n.

Median n.

Expendable FCR fascicle

Expendable FCU fascicle

A

B

Figure 6–1 To restore elbow flexion, both the biceps brachii and the brachialis are reinnervated using fascicles of median and ulnar nerve. **A:** Transfer of an expendable fascicle of the ulnar nerve to the biceps branch of the musculocutaneous nerve and an expendable fascicle of the median nerve to the brachialis branch of the musculocutaneous nerve. **B:** Transfer of an expendable fascicle of the median nerve to the biceps branch of the musculocutaneous nerve and an expendable fascicle of the ulnar nerve to the brachialis branch of the musculocutaneous nerve. (From Weber RV, Mackinnon SE. Nerve transfers in the upper extremity. J Am Soc Surg Hand 2004;4:200–13,[22] with permission.)

and an expendable motor branch of the median nerve to reinnervate both the biceps branch and the brachialis branch of the musculocutaneous nerve. Either donor nerve may be coapted to either recipient nerve. Recent studies have shown that fibers of a distinct fascicular group are located adjacent to each other, even in the proximal limb.[40] There is however, significant plexus interconnections at the midarm level, and the fascicle length and diameter vary considerably.[41,42] An intraoperative decision is made based on the ability to neurolize and approximate the nerves to each other, as well as match comparable size of the nerve fascicular diameter. When the median or ulnar nerves cannot be used, other successful nerve transfer donors include the medial pectoral, thoracodorsal, or intercostals nerves.

Authors' Preferred Surgical Procedure for Elbow Flexion

The patient is placed supine at the edge of the operating room table with the entire arm and a portion of the chest prepped into the field. An incision is made along the bicipital groove of the medial arm extending from about 4 cm distal to the axilla to approximately 4 cm proximal to the medial epicondyle (Fig. 6–2). The incision may be extended across the axilla if more proximal donor nerves are needed. The musculocutaneous nerve is identified, and the branches to the biceps muscle and

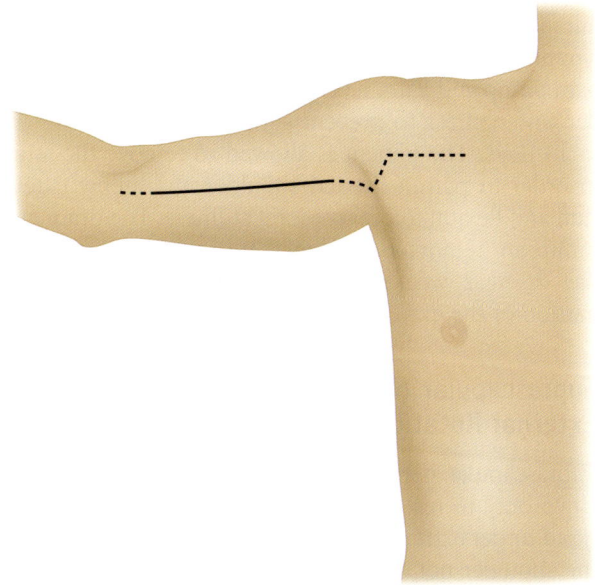

Figure 6–2 Incision to expose the musculocutaneous nerve is along the bicipital groove of the medial arm extending from about 4 cm distal to the axilla to approximately 4 cm proximal to the medial epicondyle. If more proximal nerves are used as donor nerves, the incision may be carried across the axilla as in a standard brachial plexus exploration incision *(dotted lines)*.

to the brachialis muscle are isolated. Both median and ulnar nerve fascicles transfer easily over to the biceps brachii branch. The brachialis branch, in some individuals, is a deeper dissection; therefore, the nerve transfer is first set up for the brachialis branch. Either the median or ulnar nerve is used as a donor to the brachialis branch, depending on which donor appears to be the easiest transfer. The motor fascicles on the median nerve are usually found on the medial side of the median nerve. The expendable motor branches from the ulnar are usually located on the lateral or central portion of the ulnar nerve. The median and ulnar nerves are likewise exposed and isolated. These nerves are examined and partially neurolyzed in order to find fascicles of proper caliber and adequate length for the transfer. The nerve stimulator is used to identify fascicles that innervate mostly the flexor carpi radialis (FCR), flexor digitorum superificialis (FDS), or palmaris longus (PL) of the median nerve, and the flexor carpi ulnaris (FCU) of the ulnar nerve. The residual median and ulnar nerves must still be able to provide wrist and finger flexion, pronation, and intrinsic motor function. It is the "redundant motor fascicles" that are expended and used for the transfer. The location of the neurolysis is planned so that the neurolyzed fascicles can be transferred to the biceps and brachialis branches without tension (Fig. 6–1 A and B). The repair is accessed to ensure that no tension exists through the complete range of motion of the arm. The coaptation is done with microscopic magnification using 9-0 nylon sutures. The wound is closed in layers, usually with a self-infusion pain pump and a drain. The patient is placed in a shoulder immobilizer to prevent shoulder abduction for 10 to 14 days. The patient is allowed to remove the strap in order to permit limited shoulder and elbow extension and flexion to prevent joint stiffness. The drain and pump are removed at the first postoperative check on day 2. At 2 weeks, the patient begins full range of motion of the extremity.

Suprascapular Nerve: Shoulder Abduction and External Rotation

Suprascapular nerve reinnervation is second in importance only to restoration of elbow flexion in the paralyzed upper extremity. A patient able to externally rotate the shoulder not only achieves better shoulder control, but also can flex the elbow through a more functional range. Originating from the upper trunk and passing across the posterior triangle of the neck, through the scapular notch, the suprascapular nerve innervates the supraspinatus and infraspinatus muscles, which control initial abduction and external rotation, as well as provide stabilization of the humeral head in the glenoid fossa. Tendon transfers used historically have been trapezius muscle, latissimus dorsi, teres major, long

head of the biceps, and the posterior deltoid muscle.[32,43] Nerve transfers that have been used in this situation include the distal portion of accessory nerve, the thoracodorsal nerve, intercostal nerves, and medial pectoral nerves. If a healthy C5–C6 root is available, the injury may be successfully reconstructed with a nerve graft. Motor recovery is expected to be good, as the distance from the donor nerve root or upper trunk to the recipient motor end plates is relatively short. The distal portion of the spinal accessory nerve after it has given off a branch to the trapezius is an excellent source of donor motor axons.[23] The trapezius controls scapular rotation with shoulder abduction. The accessory nerve transfer provides synergistic movement, making postoperative rehabilitation straightforward. The distal end of the suprascapular nerve can be coapted end to end (Fig. 6–3 A) to the proximal portion of the spinal accessory.

To decrease trapezius muscle morbidity associated with denervation of part of the trapezius muscle, a partial neurectomy in the accessory nerve can be made at the same level, and an end-to-side transfer or partial accessory nerve to suprascapular nerve transfer can be performed (Fig. 6–3 B). This principle is similar to the hemihypoglossal nerve to facial nerve transfer used for facial reanimation. When a proximal spinal accessory nerve is traumatized and not available as a donor nerve, the thoracodorsal[24] or medial pectoral[44] nerve can be the donor nerve for a transfer to the suprascapular nerve.

Authors' Preferred Surgical Procedure for Shoulder Abduction and External Rotation

With the patient in a supine position, a supraclavicular incision is used (Fig. 6–4). The suprascapular nerve is exposed through a supraclavicular approach by following the C5 root and upper trunk distally. The accessory nerve runs intimately with the trapezius muscle, and is most easily approached along the anterior border of the muscle and carried deep. A nerve stimulator is used to verify the accessory nerve, and is dissected distally to expose the branches to the trapezius muscle. The accessory nerve is divided as far distally as possible in order to leave some branches to the trapezius intact, yet still allow for the nerve transfer (Fig. 6–3 A). It is coapted to the supraclavicular nerve where the suprascapular nerve branches from the upper trunk, and is out of the zone of injury. When shoulder stability is compromised because of additional comorbidities, the trapezius muscle may be spared by coapting the suprascapular nerve in an end-to-side fashion to the spinal accessory (Fig. 6–3 B). This is currently our procedure of choice. This nerve transfer is augmented by creating a crush injury proximal to the neurotomy site in order to promote axonal sprouting. The benefit of this transfer is to allow innervation of the trapezius to remain intact.

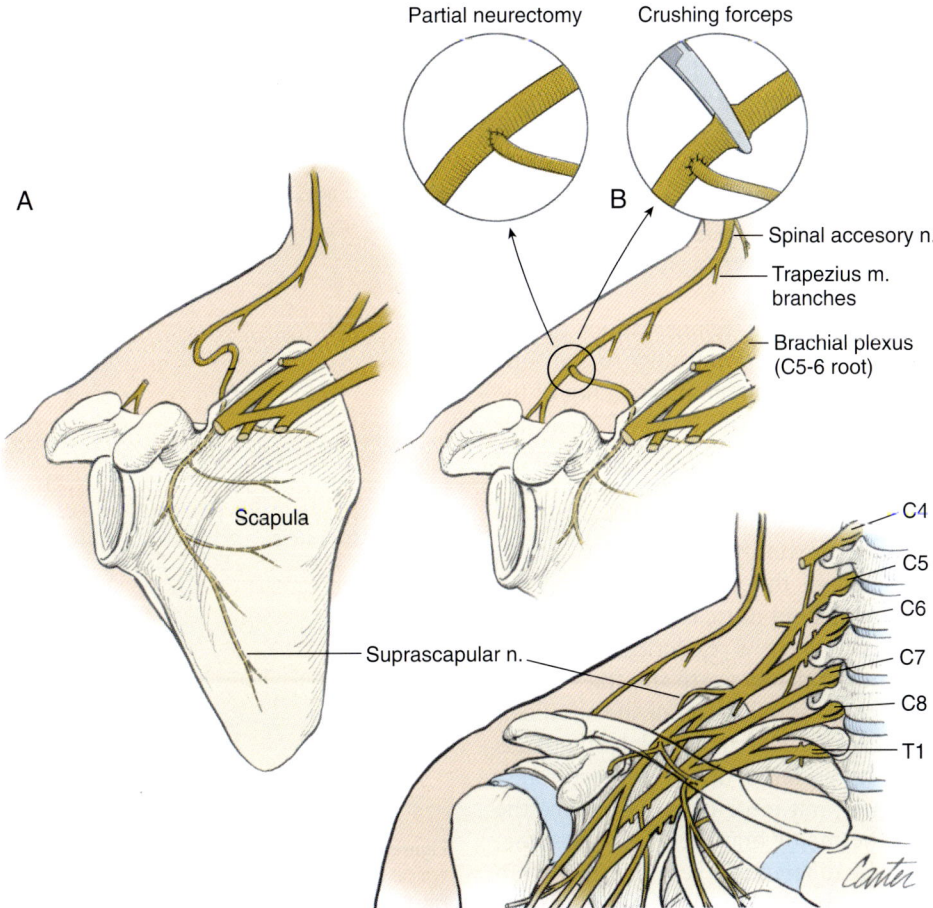

Figure 6–3   Distal spinal accessory nerve transfer to the suprascapular nerve for shoulder abduction. **A:** Direct transfer. **B:** End-to-side transfer with neurotization. (From Humphreys DB, Mackinnon SE. Nerve transfers. Operative Tech Plast Reconstr Surg 2002;9:89–99,[25] with permission.)

This repair is usually performed with loupe magnification because of the repair location. Frequently, a short nerve graft is needed. Patients who are obese or have a short neck are a definite operative challenge, and we have had to use a more traditional anterior approach in those instances in order to find the spinal accessory nerve (Fig. 6–4). We prefer the smaller incision for this particular procedure because of the minimal morbidity and better cosmetic result.

Postoperatively, the patients are placed in a shoulder immobilizer to prevent abduction; however, they are allowed to remove the strap in order to allow some flexion and extension of the shoulder and elbow to prevent stiffness. Drains and a pain pump are rarely used in this procedure, and the patient begins to range the extremity after 2 weeks.

Axillary Nerve: Shoulder Abduction

Originating from the posterior cord and passing posteriorly through the quadrangular space, the axillary nerve travels around the surgical neck of the humerus dividing into at least three branches distal to the quad-

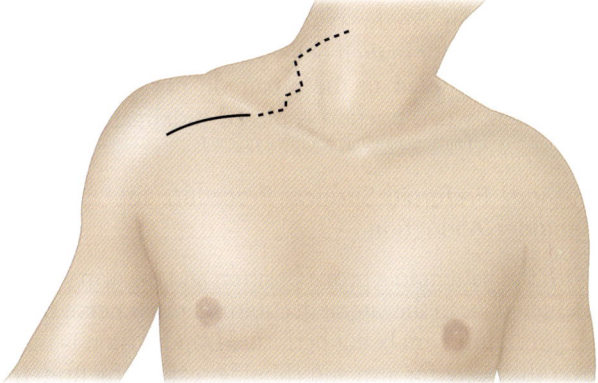

Figure 6–4   The limited incision for exposure of the suprascapular and spinal accessory nerves is usually through the supraclavicular incision as seen by the *solid line*; however, on occasion this needs to be extended into a more traditional incision *(dotted lines)*, such as for obese patient and patients with short necks.

rangular space to innervate the teres minor and deltoid muscles. The larger deltoid branch innervates the middle and anterior deltoid, while the smaller and most inferior branch innervates the posterior deltoid with a sensory component terminating as the superior lateral brachial cutaneous nerve. Injury can occur anywhere along its course, but is frequently localized to the quadrangular space. A direct nerve graft can be used to bridge the gap between a healthy proximal and distal stump. If a more proximal injury alone exists, then a nerve transfer is the preferable option. Nerve transfers using the medial pectoral nerves, triceps branch of the radial nerve, intercostal nerves, spinal accessory nerve, and the thoracodorsal nerves have been used to reconstruct the axillary nerve.[34,45]

Our preferred method for reinnervation of the deltoid muscle is to coapt the branch(es) to the long head of the triceps muscle to the motor branches of the axillary nerve using a posterior approach.[46] There are usually two to three branches of the radial nerve to the long head of the triceps. These branches are used rather than the branches to the lateral or deep head of the triceps because of their proximity to the axillary nerve, and the relative caliber of the nerve's diameter. Both motor branches to the deltoid muscle are reinnervated, while the cutaneous branch is excluded. We have recently begun including the nerve to the teres minor in order to provide better stabilization of the shoulder. Occasionally, the superior lateral brachial cutaneous nerve divides from the posterior deltoid motor branch proximal to the muscle, but more often will pierce the deltoid along with the motor branches. In either case, it is difficult to visually differentiate between the two to four branches entering the deltoid. A "tug test" is used to identify the sensory branch by placing gentle traction on the proximal end of the nerve, and observing for evidence of skin movement in the area of innervation. The cutaneous branch will have a positive "tug test," which denotes movement of skin in the upper lateral arm in this particular circumstance. The cutaneous branch is the most inferior branch of the axillary nerve. The motor branches included in the repair do not produce skin movement when traction is placed proximally.

Authors' Preferred Surgical Procedure for Shoulder Abduction

With the patient in a prone position and the arm slightly abducted, or in the lateral decubitus if other nerve transfer procedures are being performed, an incision is made over the posterior arm and shoulder extending from the level of the scapular spine to the midhumeral level (Fig. 6–5). The deltoid muscle is reflected cranially, and the axillary nerve and its branches are identified. The nerve is followed proximally toward the quadrangular space to provide adequate length for the transfer. Distal to the teres major muscle, the radial nerve emerges with the brachii profundus artery to supply the triceps muscle. The first branches dividing from the radial nerve after it emerges from the triangular space are to the long head of the triceps (Fig. 6–6). There are usually two to three

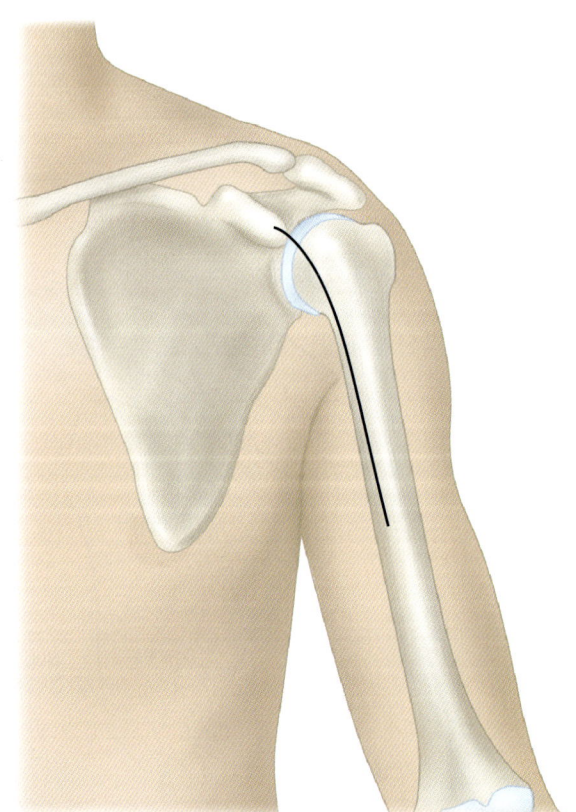

Figure 6–5 Incision for the radial nerve to axillary nerve transfer is typically through a posterior approach; an anterior approach similar to Fig. 6–2 is rarely used.

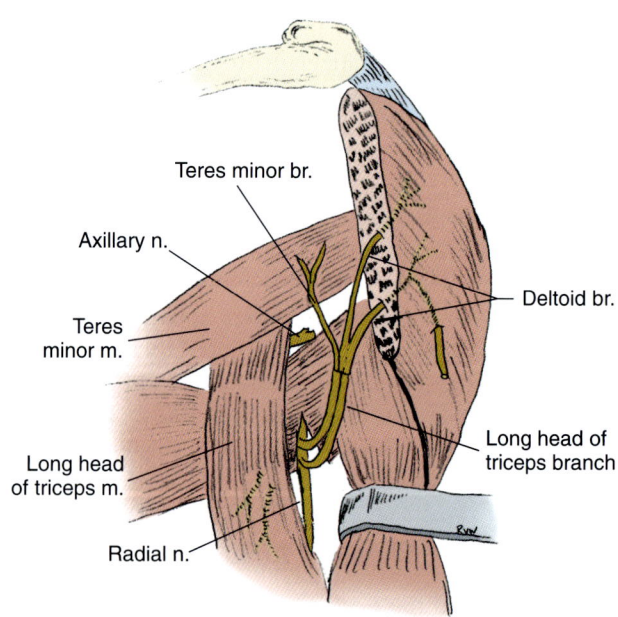

Figure 6–6 Transfer of long head of triceps branch of the radial nerve to the deltoid branch(es) and teres minor branch of the axillary nerve restores shoulder abduction and stability.

small branches. All branches to the long head of the triceps are divided distally before branching into the muscle and reflected cranially. The branches to the deltoid muscle and the teres minor muscle are divided as far proximally as needed to create a repair without tension. Furthermore, the tendinous distal edge of the teres major muscle is partially divided, allowing the triceps branches to be reflected proximally with less tension. A nerve stimulator is used to verify the presence or absence of muscular contraction of the deltoid and triceps nerves before division and repair. The incision is closed with a drain and pain pump, and the patient is placed in a shoulder immobilizer as in the other nerve transfers. Postoperative care is similar to the previous transfers.

Radial Nerve: Wrist and Finger Extension

Radial nerve palsies are typically reconstructed with direct nerve repair, nerve grafts or tendon transfers. For a high radial nerve injury, an "internal splint" is occasionally performed by transferring the pronator teres to the extensor carpi radialis brevis (ECRB) to provide wrist extension while the nerve is regenerating. In selected patients, we have used a nerve transfer to recover radial nerve function (Fig. 6–7). Redundant FCR fascicles of the median nerve are transferred to the ECRB branch of the radial and posterior interosseous nerves (PIN).[47] At the midforearm, the fascicles of the median nerve are well differentiated and consistent. The FDS has two nerve branches. Redundant nerve branches to the FDS, FCR, or PL may be transferred to the PIN. In addition, to restore sensation, the radial sensory branch can be coapted end to side to the median nerve at a location distal enough to prevent tension to the transfer. The FCU branch of the ulnar nerve may be used; however, this requires a second incision.[24]

Authors' Preferred Surgical Procedure for Wrist Extension

The radial and median nerves are exposed through a single volar incision from the proximal to midforearm level in a sinusoidal incision. The radial nerve is identified deep to the brachioradialis muscle where it divides into the superficial sensory and the PIN. The PIN is neurolyzed as far proximal as possible. The radial nerve branch to the ECRB is also dissected proximally, and both motor nerves are divided from the remaining radial nerve as far proximal as possible to provide the most length.

The median nerve is then isolated and the branches to the PL, the FCR, and the FDS identified. An internal neurolysis is not needed at this level, as the branches of the median nerve are distinct from the median nerve proper.[9] We use the PL and either the FDS or FCR

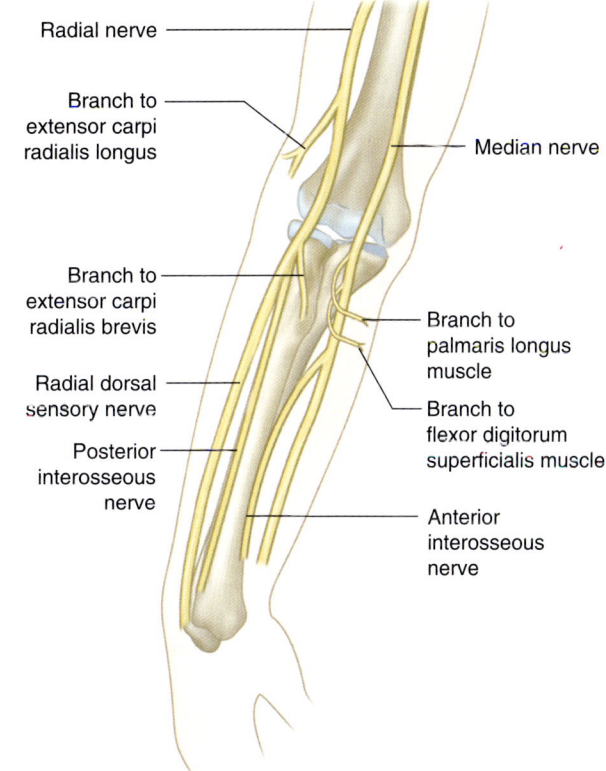

A

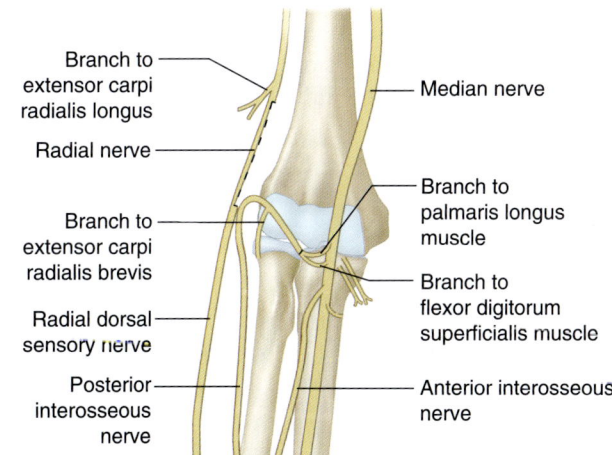

B

Figure 6–7 The PL and the FDS branches of the median nerve are transferred to the PIN and the ECRB branch of the radial nerve for restoration of wrist and finger extension.

branches as donors for the PIN and the ECRB branches (Fig. 6–7). The disposable handheld nerve stimulator is used to select the donor nerves. The strongest donor should be transferred to the ECRB to restore strong wrist rather than strong finger extension for maximum function.

The coaptation is done with the microscope using 9-0 or 10-0 nylon sutures. The repair is viewed in pronation and supination to check for tension. The wound is closed in layers usually with a pain pump and drain. The patient is placed in a posterior splint with the elbow at 90 degrees, and the shoulder, wrist, and fingers free. The splint, drain, and pump are removed at the first postoperative check on day 2, and the patient placed in a custom splint and sling for 2 more weeks.

Median Nerve: Forearm Pronation, Thumb Opposition, and Finger Flexion

We have used motor nerve transfers reliably for restoration of loss of pronation, thenar function, and flexor pollicis longus (FPL) function. If loss of pronation exists as an isolated finding, a branch from the ulnar nerve or an expendable branch from the median nerve itself may be used to innervate the pronator teres branches.[9] The two nonfunctioning branches to the pronator are found proximally at the level of the cubital fossa. Intraoperative simulation is used to locate the FDS branches of the median nerve. There are usually two branches to the FDS, and one or both can be transferred to the two non-functioning branches of the pronator teres muscle by direct repair (Fig. 6–8). The PL or FCR branches may also be used. If the entire median nerve is nonfunctional, then a redundant branch to the FCU from the ulnar nerve can be used.

In the case of combined lower ulnar and median nerve palsy with intact shoulder and elbow function, such as in C8–T1 avulsions, we have transferred the brachialis branch of the musculocutaneous nerve or the brachioradialis branch of the radial nerve with either a medial antebrachial cutaneous (MABC) or medial brachial cutaneous (MBC) nerve graft to the proximal AIN to restore some finger flexor function.

Thumb opposition can be corrected effectively with standard tendon transfers; however, transfer of the distal branch of the AIN to the pronator quadratus may be used to reinnervate the motor branch of the median nerve. The reconstruction will usually require a nerve graft to bridge the gap. In situations of isolated loss of FPL function in the proximal forearm, an expendable redundant motor branch of the same median nerve, such as the branch to the PL, FDS, or FCR may be used as donor axons for the FPL branch.

Authors' Preferred Surgical Procedure for Pronation

A sinusoidal longitudinal volar incision is used to expose the median nerve in a fashion similar to that above. The median nerve serves as its own donor nerve. The pronator teres nerve branches are identified as they course superficial to the muscle and are the most proximal branches from the median nerve. A nerve stimulator is used to verify lack of response to stimulation, and the pronator teres branches are divided as far proximally as possible before the nerve divides from the median nerve proper. The FDS or PL nerve branches are the preferred donor nerve to transfer to the nonfunctioning pronator teres branches, and these branches are dissected as far distally as possible into the muscle (Fig.

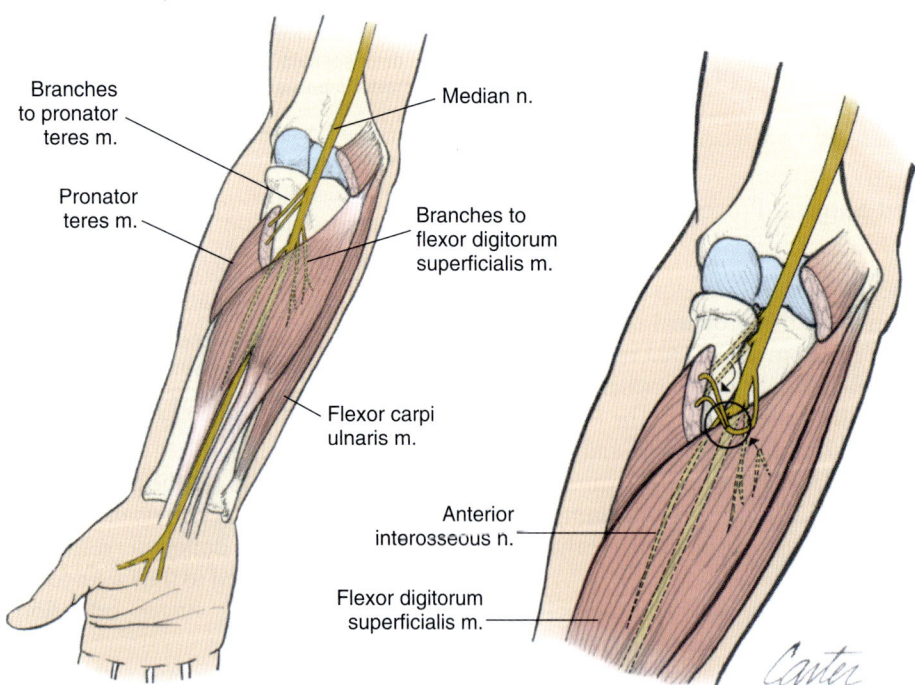

Figure 6–8 Transfer of expendable FDS branches of the median nerve to pronator teres branches of median nerve to restore pronation. (From Humphreys DB, Mackinnon SE. Nerve transfers. Operative Tech Plast Reconstr Surg 2002;9:89–99,[25] with permission.)

6–8). The forearm is pronated and supinated before the repair to confirm a tension-free repair. The wound is closed in layers, usually with a pain pump and drain. A posterior splint with the elbow flexed to 90 degrees is used, leaving the fingers, wrist, and shoulder free. On postoperative day 2, the splint, drains, and pain pump are removed, and the patient placed in a protective sling for an additional 2 weeks.

Ulnar Nerve: Intrinsic Muscle Function and Ulnar Sensory Loss

Recovery of intrinsic muscle function is uncommon following a high ulnar nerve injury, even with early repair.[48,49] Tendon transfers yield less than satisfactory results to correct these deficits.[32] Because the distance that the nerve needs to regenerate is excessively long, the purpose of the nerve transfer in this situation is to convert the high ulnar nerve injury to a low ulnar nerve injury. Patients with ulnar nerve palsy may have significant pinch and grip weakness as well as clawing of the

ulnar two digits. If the median nerve is available as a donor nerve, the distal branch of the AIN to the pronator quadratus may be transferred to the deep motor branch of the ulnar nerve (Fig. 6–9 A).[7,50] The disadvantage of this transfer is that it does not provide synergistic movement, and hand function is not normal. However, there is improvement such as to prevent clawing and provide pinch strength, and tendon transfers have not been necessary, except for one patient who required a secondary tendon transfer for persistent small finger abduction (Wartenberg's sign).[7] We further improve clawing and increase finger flexion by tenodesing the flexor digitorum profundus (FDP) tendons of the ring and small fingers side to side to the FDP tendons of the index and long.

Several nerve transfer options are available to restore ulnar nerve sensibility. Traditionally and end-to-end transfer of the third web-space nerves (median) to the main ulnar sensory nerve in the palm will divert sensation to the ulnar border of the hand. End-to-side transfer can also be used for recovery of some limited

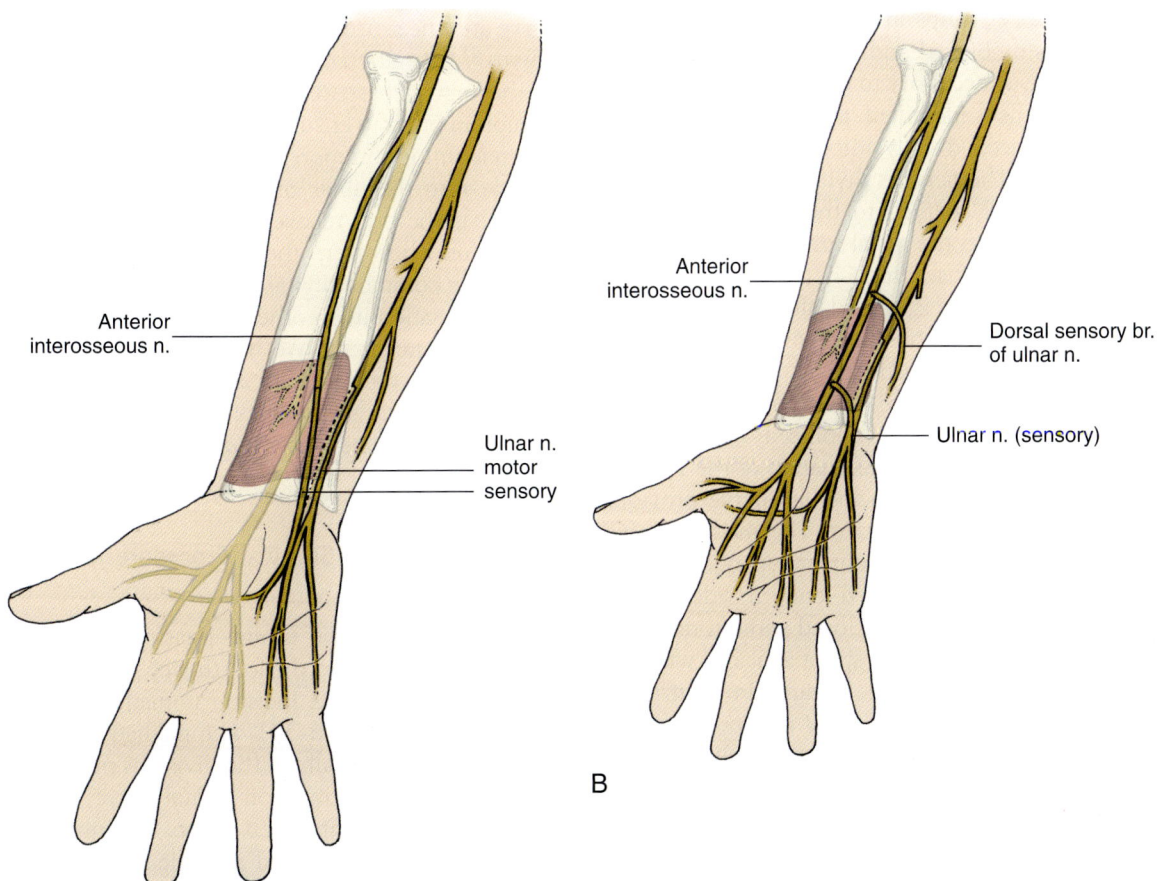

Anterior interosseous n.

Ulnar n. motor sensory

A

Anterior interosseous n.

Dorsal sensory br. of ulnar n.

Ulnar n. (sensory)

B

Figure 6–9   Nerve transfers to restore ulnar motor function. The distal branch of the AIN to the pronator quadratus is transferred to the deep motor branch of the ulnar nerve **(A).** The sensory portion of the ulnar nerve and the dorsal sensory ulnar nerves are transferred end to side to the median nerve in the distal forearm **(B).** (From Weber RV, Mackinnon SE. Nerve transfers in the upper extremity. J Am Soc Surg Hand 2004;4:200–13,[22] with permission.)

sensation. The sensory portion of the ulnar nerve can be reconstructed using an end-to-side repair of the ulnar sensory branch into the third web-space branch of the median nerve, or by transferring both the sensory component of the ulnar nerve and the dorsal cutaneous branch of the ulnar nerve to the main median nerve in the distal forearm (Fig. 6–9 B). When an end-to-side transfer is used to provide sensation, the perineurium is opened, as this maneuver produces limited and recoverable demyelination of the donor nerve. This allows increased sprouting from the sensory donor nerve without need for neurotomy.[51]

Authors' Preferred Surgical Procedure for Intrinsic Function and Ulnar Nerve Sensation

Using an extended carpal tunnel incision, the motor branch of the ulnar nerve is first identified in Guyon's canal, and traced proximally to the level of the distal forearm. Often, the motor branch can be identified without the need for an actual physical neurolysis to the level of the AIN by following the motor fascicles proximally under magnification. We call this a visual neurolysis. There is little plexus formation between the motor and sensory groups in the distal extremity. The proximal end is mobilized and transected as far proximally as possible or necessary to create the transfer. The pronator quadratus is identified, and the AIN branch to this muscle is traced distally into the muscle until it begins to branch. The nerve is divided just proximal to these branches, and coapted to the transected motor branch of the ulnar in the distal forearm (Fig. 6–9 A). A direct repair is easily accomplished despite the slight size mismatch. The arm is ranged after the nerves are juxtaposed to access for possible tension in both the pronated and supinated positions.

The ulnar sensory nerve and dorsal cutaneous branches of the ulnar nerve are mobilized, and the proximal ends are brought in approximation of the median nerve. The ulnar aspect of the median nerve provides sensation to the third web space. The median nerve epineurium is incised, the perineurium opened, and the two sensory nerves are coapted end to side to the median nerve. The wounds are closed without the need for drain or pain pump. A volar splint is placed with the elbow at 90 degrees and the forearm in neutral to prevent excessive forearm rotation. It is removed at the first postoperative visit, and the patient is splinted for 3 weeks to protect any tendon repair before active range of motion may begin.

First Web-Space Sensation: Median Nerve

Loss of sensation to the hand is a tremendous functional deficit. Proprioception is important for pinch and fine

motor movement. As with motor nerve deficits, nerve reconstruction should be attempted with direct repair or nerve grafts whenever possible. Unlike a motor nerve transfer, there is no limit from the time of injury that the repair needs to be performed to achieve sensory recovery. Attempts to restore sensation to the first web space have been made using expendable sensory branches of the ulnar and radial nerves as donors.[25] The goal is to direct sensation to the ulnar side of the thumb and radial side of the index finger. In the case of an upper-trunk brachial plexus injury, there will be sensation to the third web space from the intact cervical roots. The common digital nerve from the third or fourth web space is transferred to the first web-space nerves in a direct end-to-end manner. The distal ends of the terminal digital nerve in the third web space can be transferred end to side to the fourth web-space common digital nerve to restore sensation to the donor nerves. Alternatively, the common digital nerve to the second web space can be transferred more easily to the ulnar digital nerve to the small finger in the palm.

If the median nerve is injured, then the common digital nerve from the fourth web space supplied by the ulnar nerve, the dorsal sensory branch of the ulnar nerve and the sensory radial nerve can all serve as donor nerves.[25,52] In any combination of transfers, the repair to the first web space is performed in an end-to-end fashion in order to ensure the best result (Fig. 6–10).[53,54] The remaining common digital nerve(s) are coapted end to side into the ulnar or radial nerves. The first web space has the best recovery because of the end-to-end coaptation; however, the end-to-side repair of the remaining common digital nerves provides enough protective sensation in an otherwise insensate hand to give this procedure merit. We have no favorite transfer, as the possible combinations are many, and the optimal transfer depends on which nerves are injured, which nerves will serve as the best donor nerves, and patient preference.

Authors' Preferred Surgical Procedure for Median Nerve Sensation

Starting with a carpal tunnel incision, the incision is carried distally toward the fourth web space using a zig-zag pattern. A second incision is made to expose the first web space (Fig. 6–11). The median nerve is identified and traced distally to the divisions of the common digital nerves. The common digital nerve is mobilized to the level of the first web space. The ulnar nerve is identified in Guyon's canal and the sensory branch is traced distally to the level of the fourth web space. The common digital nerve to the fourth web space is divided at about the midmetacarpal distance. This allows for enough length of the proximal common digital nerve of

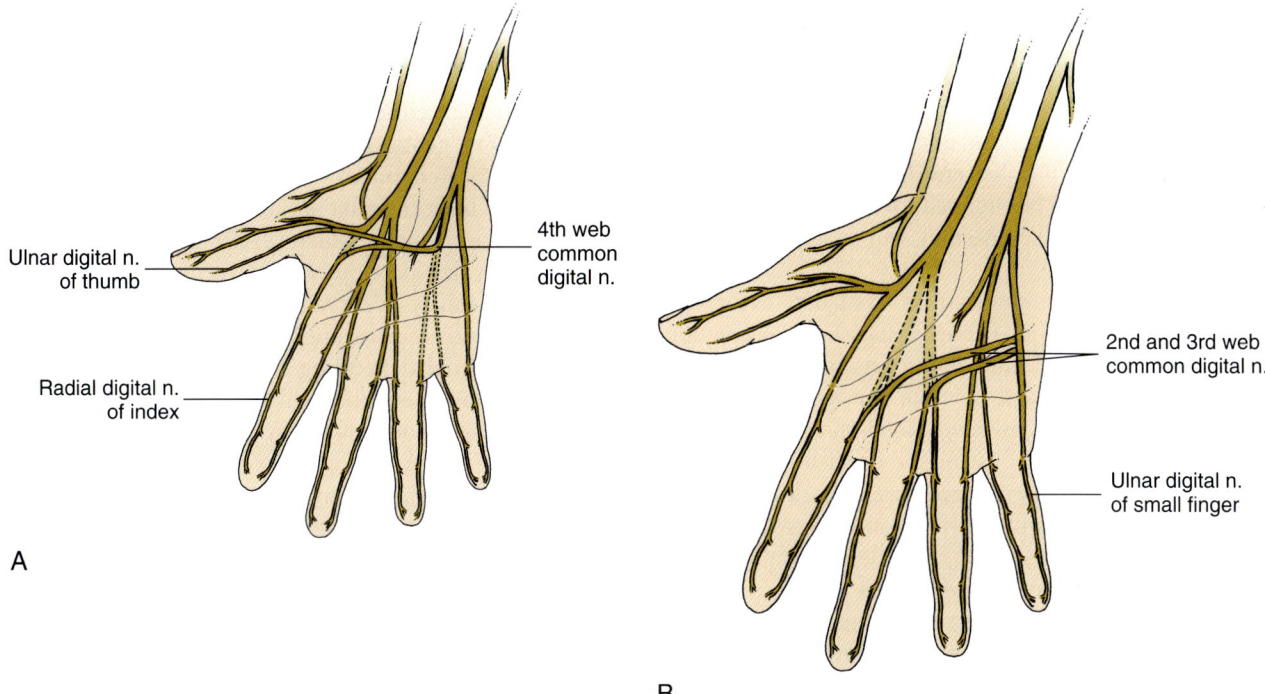

A

B

Figure 6–10 With complete median nerve injury, the common digital nerve from the fourth web space is transferred to the first web space nerve in a direct end-to-end manner **(A).** The distal ends of the terminal digital nerve of the second and third web spaces are transferred end to side to the ulnar small finger common digital nerve to restore protective sensation to the remaining median sensory distribution **(B).** (From Weber RV, Mackinnon SE. Nerve transfers in the upper extremity. J Am Soc Surg Hand 2004;4:200–13,[22] with permission.)

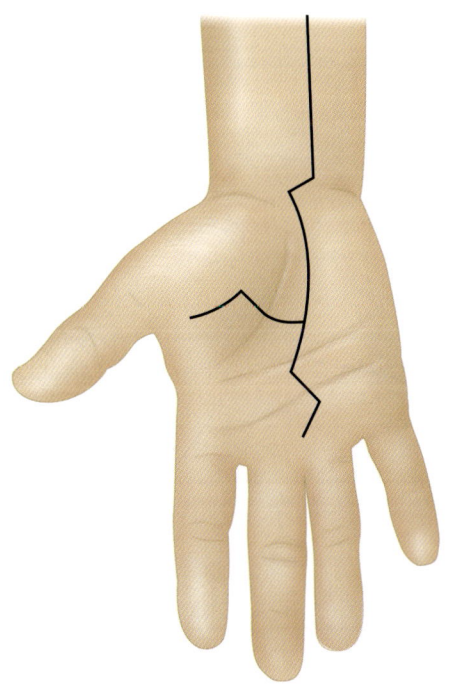

Figure 6–11 A distally extended carpal tunnel incision is used to expose the first and fourth webspace.

ulnar innervation to be transposed to the first web space. The proximal fourth web-space digital nerve is coapted primarily to the transected distal first web-space digital nerve. An epineural incision is created in the ulnar sensory branch leading to the ulnar border of the small finger. The distal portion of the fourth web-space digital nerve can be coapted end to side to the remaining innervated ulnar sensory nerve. The common digital nerve to the second and third web space can be dissected proximally to the takeoff just distal to the carpal tunnel. The distal segment is then coapted to the ulnar nerve to the ulnar border of the small finger as is the common digital nerve to the fourth web space in an end-to-side fashion. The wounds are closed without the need for a drain or pain pump. The patient is placed in a volar splint to prevent wrist movement, while the fingers remain free. Dressings are removed at the first postoperative visit, and the patient is splinted for 2 weeks to protect the repair, before active range of motion may begin.

MOTOR TRANSFERS FOR MULTIPLE NERVE INJURIES

In a multiple nerve injury, an algorithm of functional priority is followed, and all possible donor nerves are evaluated. The optimal transfers must be individualized for each patient. Once available nerves in the vicinity are selected and additional donor nerves are needed, we turn first to the chest for expendable nerves. These transfers will often require the use of a nerve graft. Depending on the number and length of the graft, the patient may need to be prepped for sural nerve harvest. When only one graft is needed, our first choice is the MABC nerve.

In addition to looking farther from the motor end plate for possible donor nerves, a staged reconstruction with a free functional muscle transfers may be required in patients who present too late for reinnervation of target muscles, after a previous failed reconstruction, or as an elective staged reconstruction consisting of a nerve graft followed by vascularized free muscle transfer.[55] The most common options for donor muscle are the gracilis, the latissimus dorsi, and the pectoralis major; however, we prefer to use the gracilis.

Tendon transfers may be required after all nerve transfer options have been exhausted. In addition, fusion of the shoulder or wrist may have a role. For patients in whom reconstruction of shoulder function is unsuccessful or not possible, a shoulder fusion will provide limited but useful amount of shoulder abduction and flexion from the trapezius muscle. Wrist fusion may also be considered in patients with no wrist function, or in those after recovery or reconstruction of finger and wrist flexion, but who still lack extension to stabilize the wrist when using the hand.

Nerve Grafts

Sural Nerve Graft

With the patient either prone or supine with the leg frog-legged, the sural nerve is identified lateral to the Achilles tendon. The easiest method for harvest of the sural nerve is to use a posterior midline incision. The closure is slightly lengthier and the resulting scar may be cosmetically undesirable. The alternative is to use a stepwise technique, which requires between four and six separate horizontal incisions along the back of the calf, each approximately 1 cm in length. The resulting scar is cosmetically more favorable, and the technique adds little additional operative time. More recently, we have been using an endoscopic approach to limit the scars even further. Approximately 25 to 30 cm of graft may be harvested from a typical adult patient.

Medial Antibrachial Nerve Graft

The medial antibrachial nerve is the most frequently used nerve graft in upper extremity nerve transfers. It is often in the operative field, and can be easily found coursing along side the basilic vein in the upper arm. Up to 25 cm of nerve graft may be obtained.

Distant Donor Nerves

Intercostal Nerve

With the patient either supine or in lateral decubitus, a 15- to 20-cm gentle sloping incision is made on the chest in the direction of the ribs at the lateral aspect between the midclavicular and the midaxial planes (Fig. 6–12). The decision on which ribs to use may be limited if the patient had previous rib fractures. In the absence of previous injury, we prefer to use three intercostal nerves from ribs four through six; however, will extend cranial or caudal depending on the situation. If more cranial ribs are used, the caliber of the nerve is often smaller and additional ribs may be needed. Lower ribs tend to have larger motor nerves, especially the intercostal nerve contribution to the rectus muscle; however, the need for longer nerve grafts may determine the limits of how low you can go.

Once the rib is exposed, an incision is made directly over the rib. The periosteum is elevated off the posterior aspect of the rib in order to expose the intercostals neurovascular bundle. The dissection begins in the midaxial plane, and the nerve is traced distally toward the ventrum. The larger branch encountered first is almost always the sensory branch. Tedious careful dissection and the use of a nerve stimulator are essential

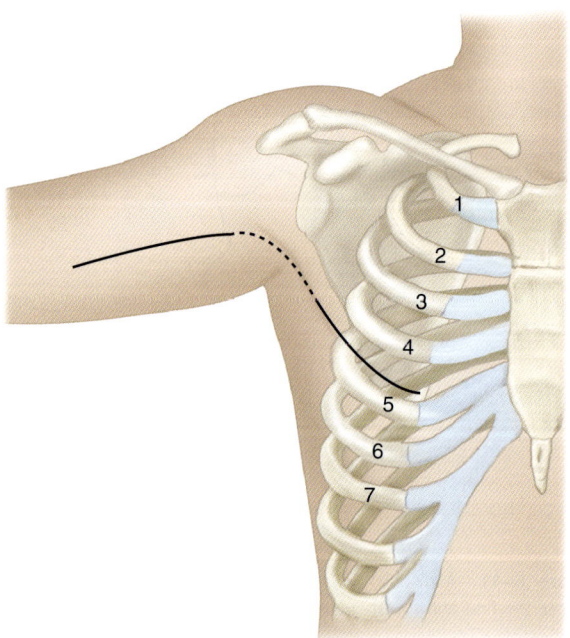

Figure 6–12   The incision is made on the chest in the direction of the ribs at the lateral aspect between the midclavicular and midaxial planes. A separate incision is made in the bicipital groove in order to expose the musculocutaneous nerve, leaving a skin bridge across the axilla.

for identifying and isolating the motor branch of the intercostal nerves. The intercostal nerves are divided as distally as possible and reflected posteriorly into the field. The average diameter of the intercostals nerves is 1 to 2 mm, and up to 10 to 12 cm of nerve can be neurolyzed.

The nerve graft is typically tunneled under the skin into position before coapting the graft to either the donor intercostals nerve or to the injured recipient nerve. The nerve graft is reversed, which not only prevents the loss of nerve fibers, but allows for better size match for the nerve graft to the intercostals nerve. Whenever possible, three intercostal nerves are coapted to one or two nerve grafts. The distal graft is then used to reinnervate the individual branches of the musculocutaneous nerve, or the main musculocutaneous nerve itself when the length of the graft is short. Ideally, we always prefer to be closer to the end plate of the target organ. The lateral brachial cutaneous nerve is essentially eliminated, and the nerve fibers crossing the coaptation site are channeled into a purely motor environment.

Medial and Lateral Pectoral Nerve

With the patient supine, an infraclavicular incision along the deltopectoral groove and extending across the axilla in a zig-zag fashion into the medial aspect of the arm is made to access the pectoral nerve branches as well as the musculocutaneous nerve. The pectoralis major muscle tendon is divided close to its insertion to the humerus, making sure to leave a 4- to 5-mm cuff of tendon to allow sufficient substance in order to repair the pectoralis muscle tendon. The pectoralis major tendon is repaired using 1 or 0 braided permanent suture. Branches piercing the pectoralis minor muscle and seen entering the deep portion of the pectoralis major muscle are identified. The pectoral nerves are easily located using a nerve stimulator on the undersurface of the pectoralis minor muscle. The lateral branches arise from the lateral cord and the medial branches come off the medial cord along with the MABC nerve. The medial branches supply the sternocostal head, while the lateral branches supply both the clavicular and part of the sternocostal heads. The medial branches, while a little harder to dissect, will result in a less functional defect than the lateral branches, and are the first choice when using pectoral nerve transfers. When the lateral branches are used, they can often be harvested without the need for dividing the pectoralis major muscle. In the case of nerve transfer to the axillary or very proximal radial nerve and its subdivision, the medial pectoral nerve branches may be coapted primarily, without need for an additional graft. For use in distal musculocutaneous branches, such as the biceps brachii and the brachialis, a nerve graft is necessary.

Less Commonly Used Nerves

Other possible donor nerves include the contralateral C7 root and the phrenic nerve, but their use is more controversial. The functional donor deficit from using the contralateral C7 root is minimal, but requires a very long nerve graft to the opposite upper extremity. In such cases, successful transfer depends on the use of a vascularized ulnar nerve graft. Functional outcome is hindered by the difficulty for adult patients to achieve completely independent movement from the donor extremity. The phrenic nerve is also a satisfactory donor nerve, but the potential long-term sequela on diaphragmatic function should be considered, particularly in a smoker who will have pulmonary compromise with age.[56]

MOTOR AND SENSORY RE-EDUCATION

Long-term rehabilitative goals focus on motor and/or sensory re-education. As in tendon transfers, the patient must be able to coordinate synchronized movement. With a nerve transfer, a new nerve is now innervating the muscle. The cortical command required to initiate movement is different from that of the preinjured period. The patient "relearns" motor control of the new muscle by trying to contract the donor muscle and the reinnervated muscle at the same time (Fig. 6–13).[24] This concept is similar to the re-education needed in tendon transfers. In addition, the ability to restore sensation can only improve recovery, but does not guarantee the return of good function. Sensory re-education usually begins as soon as the patient begins to perceive any input stimulus. Cortical remapping occurs from continued sensory input from the newly innervated areas.

OUTCOMES

The level of injury plays a significant role in the functional outcome of reconstruction. Proximal nerve injuries have longer distance to regenerate through before the target muscles are reached. Reinnervated and motor recovery of a more distal injury would be expected to have a more satisfactory outcome. Over the last 15 years, we have found that motor nerve transfers produce consistent results and are frequently superior to nerve grafts, particularly for a very proximal level of injury. For example, we find that we consistently achieve a functional recovery of elbow flexion with a greater than 4 MRC grade.[34,37,39,57]

A long-term patient-reported outcome study of surgical reconstruction after brachial plexus trauma verified that motor function and sensation remained

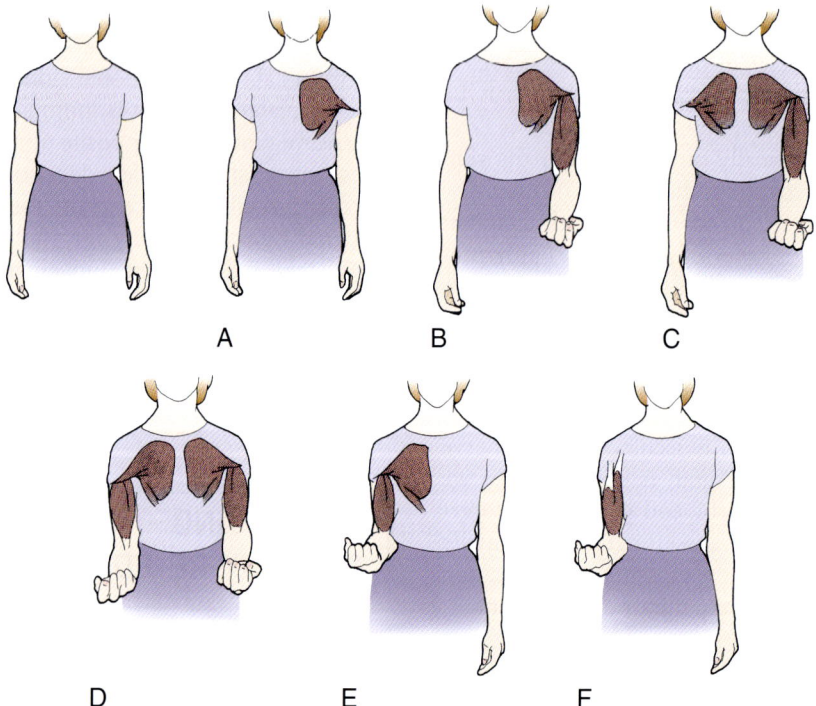

Figure 6–13   Motor reeducation after nerve transfer using medial pectoral branches to biceps brachii branch. To learn how to contract the rein-nervated right biceps muscle, the patient begins to exercise the pectoralis major muscle on the unaffected side **(A).** The patient then contracts both the pectoralis and the biceps muscles on the unaffected side **(B).** With the elbows flexed to 90 degrees, the patient is instructed to perform bilateral contractions of both pectoralis major muscles **(C).** The patient then attempts to contract both the pectoralis major and the biceps muscles bilaterally **(D).** Eventually, the patient progressed to unilateral contraction of the pectoralis and biceps muscles on the affected side **(E).** Once the patient is able to isolate biceps movement form pectoralis movement **(F),** strengthening of the biceps muscle can continue with elbow flexion exercises. (From Mackinnon SE, Novak CB. Nerve transfers: new options for reconstruction following nerve injury. Hand Clin 1999;15:643–66,[2] with permission.)

very abnormal and the majority of patients felt a negative impact on their work and career. Nevertheless, both employment status and overall satisfaction with quality of life did not seem to be significantly dependent on upper extremity function. Seventy-eight percent of these patients versus 90% of the general population were content with their quality of life on the whole. Among those patients who were employed at the time of injury, 54% had returned to work, and the majority of patients were able to do so by 1 year after injury. Seventy percent of the study group versus 85% of the general population described their job satisfaction as moderate to high. Most of those patients who were not able to return to work felt that their injury was responsible for their unemployment. So, even though these injuries produce significant long-term functional impairment, the majority of these patients maintain a high level of overall happiness and fulfillment from work. Thus, as the techniques for the reconstruction of severe brachial plexus injuries continue to evolve, a positive outlook for the functional outcomes achieved by surgical management is warranted.[12]

SUMMARY

Over the last century, significant advances in peripheral nerve surgery have been made. The introduction of microsurgery has transformed nerve surgery into a sophisticated specialty with procedures that generate fairly consistent results. The combined experience of brachial plexus surgery, tendon transfer surgery, and motor and sensory re-education has allowed for the introduction of nerve transfer techniques as a surgical option for reconstruction of nerve injuries. In the last decade, reconstruction of upper plexus injuries in our institution has progressed from the use of long nerve grafts to elegant nerve transfers. The need to expose and explore the brachial plexus is reserved to tumor cases and other special circumstances. Our use of nerve transfers far removed from the zone of injury, allows us to restore function and sensibility in shorter operative time, through smaller incisions, resulting in less morbidity and surprisingly better functional results than in the past. As our knowledge increases about internal anatomy of peripheral nerves, new nerve transfers will only increase and lead to improved outcomes.

REFERENCES

1. Harris W, Low VW. On the importance of accurate muscular analysis in lesions of the brachial plexus. BMJ 1903;2:1035.
2. Lurje A. Concerning surgical treatment of traumatic injury of the upper division of the brachial plexus (Erb's type). Ann Surg 1948;127:317–26.
3. Millesi H. Microsurgery of peripheral nerves. Hand 1973;5:157–60.
4. Millesi H, Berger A, Meissel G. Experimental study of healing of transected peripheral nerves. Chir Plast (Berl) 1972;1:174–206.
5. Millesi H, Meissel G, Berger A. The interfascicular nerve-grafting of the median and ulnar nerves. J Bones Joint Surg Am 1972;54:727–50.
6. Brandt KE, Mackinnon SE. A technique for maximizing biceps recovery in brachial plexus reconstruction. J Hand Surg Am 1993;18:726–33.
7. Novak CB, Mackinnon SE. Distal anterior interosseous nerve transfer to the deep motor branch of the ulnar nerve for reconstruction of high ulnar nerve injuries. J Reconstr Microsurg 2002;18:459–64.
8. Nath RK, Mackinnon SE. Nerve transfers in the upper extremity. Hand Clin 2000;16:131–9.
9. Tung TH, Mackinnon SE. Flexor digitorum superficialis nerve transfer to restore pronation: two case reports and anatomic study. J Hand Surg Am 2001;26:1065–72.
10. Midha R. Epidemiology of brachial plexus injuries in a multitrauma population. Neurosurgery 1997;40:1182–9.
11. Terzis JK, Papakonstantinou KC. The surgical treatment of brachial plexus injuries in adults. Plast Reconstr Surg 2000;106:1097–122.
12. Choi PD, Novak CB, Mackinnon SE, et al. Quality of life and functional outcome following brachial plexus injury. J Hand Surg Am 1997;22:605–12.
13. Mackinnon SE. New directions in peripheral nerve surgery. Ann Surg 1989;22:257–73.
14. Leffert RD. Clinical diagnosis, testing, and electromyographic study in brachial plexus traction injuries. Clin Orthop 1988;237:24–31.
15. Parry CBW. Thoughts on the rehabilitation of patients with brachial plexus lesions. Hand Clin 1995;11:657–75.
16. Dubuisson A, Kline DG. Indications for peripheral nerve and brachial plexus surgery. Neurol Clin 1992;10:935–51.
17. Panasci DJ, Holliday RA, Shpizner B. Advanced imaging techniques of the brachial plexus. Hand Clin 1995;11:545–53.
18. Berger A, Brenner P. Secondary surgery following brachial plexus injuries. Microsurgery 1995;16:43–7.
19. Gutowski KA, Orenstein HH. Restoration of elbow flexion after brachial plexus injury: the role of nerve and muscle transfers. Plast Reconstr Surg 2000;106:1348–57.
20. Guelinckx PJ, Faulkner JA. Parallel-fibered muscles transplanted with neurovascular repair into bipennate muscle sites in rabbits. Plast Reconstr Surg 1992;89:290–8.
21. Guelinckx PJ, Carlson BM, Faulkner JA. Morphologic characteristics of muscles grafted in rabbits with neurovascular repair. J Reconstr Microsurg 1992;8:481–9.
22. Weber RV, Mackinnon SE. Nerve transfers in the upper extremity. J Am Soc Surg Hand 2004;4:200–13.
23. Dvali L, Mackinnon S. Nerve repair, grafting, and nerve transfers. Clin Plast Surg 2003;30:203–21.
24. Mackinnon SE, Novak CB. Nerve transfers: new options for reconstruction following nerve injury. Hand Clin 1999;15:643–66.
25. Humphreys DB, Mackinnon SE. Nerve transfers. Operative Tech Plast Reconstr Surg 2002;9:89–99.
26. Goheen-Robillard B, Myckatyn TM, Mackinnon SE, et al. End-to-side neurorrhaphy and lateral axonal sprouting in a long graft rat model. Laryngoscope 2002;112:899–905.
27. Seddon HJ, Medawar PB, Smith H. Rate of regeneration of peripheral nerves in man. J Physiol 1943;102:191–201.
28. Sunderland IR, Brenner MJ, Singham J, et al. Effect of tension on nerve regeneration in rat sciatic nerve transection model. Ann Plast Surg 2004;53:382–7.
29. Trumble TE, McCallister WV. Repair of peripheral nerve defects in the upper extremity. Hand Clin 2000;16:37–52.
30. Allan CH, Trumble TE. Biomechanics of peripheral nerve repair. Operative Tech Orthop 2004;14:184–9.
31. Mackinnon SE. Double and multiple "crush" syndromes. Double and multiple entrapment neuropathies. Hand Clin 1992;8:369–90.
32. Leffert RD. Brachial plexus. In: Green DP, ed., Operative hand surgery, 4th ed. Philadelphia: Churchill-Livingstone, 1999:1557–87.
33. Tsuge K, Kanaujia RR, Steichen JB. Functional restoration in brachial plexus injury. In: Comprehensive atlas of hand surgery. Chicago: Year Book Medical Publishers, 1989:564–78.
34. Merrell GA, Barrie KA, Katz DL, et al. Results of nerve transfer techniques for restoration of shoulder and elbow function in the context of a meta-analysis of the English literature. J Hand Surg Am 2001;26:303–14.
35. Brandt KE, Mackinnon SE. A technique for maximizing biceps recovery in brachial plexus reconstruction. J Hand Surg 1993;18A:726–33.
36. Oberlin C, Béal D, Leechavengvongs S, et al. Nerve transfer to biceps muscle using a part of ulnar nerve for C5–C6 avulsion of the brachial plexus: anatomical study and report of four cases. J Hand Surg Am 1994;19:232–7.
37. Leechavengvongs S, Witoonchart K, Uerpairojkit C, et al. Nerve transfer to biceps muscle using a part of the ulnar nerve in brachial plexus injury (upper arm type): a report of 32 cases. J Hand Surg Am 1998;23:711–6.
38. Sungpet A, Suphachatwong C, Kawinwonggowit V, et al. Transfer of a single fascicle from the ulnar nerve to the biceps muscle after avulsions of upper roots of the brachial plexus. J Hand Surg Br 2000;25:325–8.
39. Tung TH, Novak CB, Mackinnon SE. Nerve transfers to the biceps and brachialis branches to improve elbow flexion strength after brachial plexus injuries. J Neurosurg 2003;98:313–8.
40. Brandt KE, Mackinnon SE. Microsurgical repair of peripheral nerves and nerve grafts. In: Aston SJ, Beasley RW, Thorne CHM, eds., Grabb and Smiths' Plastic Surgery, 5th ed. New York: Lippincott-Raven 1997:79–90.
41. Jabaley ME, Wallace WH, Heckler FR. Internal topography of major nerves of the forearm and hand: a current view. J Hand Surg Am 1980;5:1–18.
42. Watchmaker GP, Gumucio CA, Crandall RE, et al. Fascicular topography of the median nerve: a computer based study to identify branching patterns. J Hand Surg Am 1991;16:53–9.
43. Vallejo GI, Toh S, Arai H, et al. Results of the latissimus dorsi and teres major tendon transfer on to the rotator cuff for brachial plexus palsy at birth. Scand J Plast Reconstr Surg Hand Surg 2002;36:207–11.
44. Novak CB, Mackinnon SE. Treatment of a proximal accessory nerve injury with a nerve transfer. Laryngoscope 2004;114:1482–4.

45. El Gammal TA, Fathi NA. Outcomes of surgical treatment of brachial plexus injuries using nerve grafting and nerve transfers. J Reconstr Microsurg 2002;18:7–15.

46. Leechavengvongs S, Witoonchart K, Uerpairojkit C, et al. Nerve transfer to deltoid muscle using the nerve to the long head of the triceps, part II: a report of 7 cases. J Hand Surg Am 2003;28:633–8.

47. Lowe JB 3rd, Tung TR, Mackinnon SE. New surgical option for radial nerve paralysis. Plast Reconstr Surg 2002;110:836–43.

48. Stuebe AM, Novak CB, Mackinnon SE. Recovery of ulnar nerve innervated intrinsic muscles following anterior transposition of the ulnar nerve. Can J Plast Surg 2001;9:25–8.

49. Lester RL, Smith PJ, Mott G, et al. Intrinsic reinnervation—myth or reality? J Hand Surg Br 1993;18:454–60.

50. Wang Y, Zhu S. Transfer of a branch of the anterior interosseus nerve to the motor branch of the median nerve and ulnar nerve. Chin Med J 1997;110:216–9.

51. Steffensen I, Dulin MF, Walters ET, et al. Peripheral regeneration and central sprouting of sensory neurone axons in Aplysia californica following nerve injury. J Exp Biol 1995;198:2067–78.

52. Lesavoy MA, Dubrow TJ, Eisenhauer DM, et al. A new nerve pedicle for finger sensibility: the dorsal digital sensory nerve. Plast Reconstr Surg 1993;9:295–8.

53. Tarasidis G, Watanabe O, Mackinnon SE, et al. End-to-side neurorrhaphy: a long-term study of neural regeneration in a rat model. Otolaryngol Head Neck Surg 1998;119:337–41.

54. Tarasidis G, Watanabe O, Mackinnon SE, et al. End-to-side neurorrhaphy resulting in limited sensory axonal regeneration in a rat model. Ann Otol Rhinol Laryngol 1997;106:506–12.

55. Akasaka Y, Hara T, Takahashi M. Free muscle transplantation combined with intercostal nerve crossing for reconstruction of elbow flexion and wrist extension in brachial plexus injuries. Microsurgery 1991;12:346–51.

56. Chuang DC. Neurotization procedures for brachial plexus injuries. Hand Clin 1995;11:633–45.

57. Novak CB, Mackinnon SE, Tung TH. Patient outcome following a thoracodorsal to musculocutaneous nerve transfer for reconstruction of elbow flexion. Br J Plast Surg 2002;55:416–9.

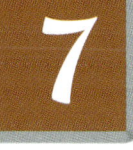

7

Treatment of Irreparable Nerve Damage in the Hand

Michael B. Wood

INTRODUCTION

The assessment of any patient who has suffered nerve injury to the hand should carefully consider whether surgery of any nature is indicated. Depending on the specific functional deficit, many patients may have adapted to their disability quite well by using eyesight or adjacent areas of tactile sensibility in place of sensory deficits. Moreover, in some patients loss of motor function may be well compensated for by various "trick maneuvers" or the use of an orthosis.

If a patient has not adequately compensated for the functional loss related to nerve injury, one should also consider the role of non-neural palliative surgical options. There is little in the way of non-neural palliative options for sensibility loss other than retraining by sensory re-education. However, for motor loss, a host of tendon transfers may be appropriate for consideration to reanimate the hand, and at times selected joint arthrodesis or tenodesis may be helpful to improve function.

For the purposes of this chapter, "irreparable nerve damage" is defined as that situation in which orthotopic nerve repair or reconstruction by nerve graft interposition is not a reasonably reliable option to restore lost function. Nerve injury in close proximity to the hand may result in loss of motor function or sensibility or both. This chapter will concentrate on heterotopic nerve transfer procedures that may be useful to restore motor or sensory function in the hand.

HETEROTOPIC MOTOR NERVE TRANSFER

For decades, heterotopic motor nerve transfers have been used to effectively reanimate the upper limb in patients with brachial plexus nerve root avulsions and extremely proximal nerve trunk ruptures.[1–5] Well known among these are the use of the spinal accessory, intercostal, medial pectoral, portion of ulnar, phrenic, and contralateral C7 nerves to reanimate the shoulder and elbow. Experience with such proximal heterotopic nerve transfers has taught that the following principles are the most important for successful reanimation: (1) use of an uninjured donor nerve; (2) use of a purely motor or predominantly motor donor nerve; (3) minimal functional loss resulting from transection of the donor nerve; (4) isolation of the recipient nerve into the fascicular groups that most directly leads to the intended muscle–motor end plates; (5) direct donor to recipient nerve coaptation (without the use of an intervening nerve graft) as close to the recipient muscle–motor end plates as is practical; (6) minimal period of recipient muscle denervation; in general, any heterotopic motor nerve transfer should be carried out within 6 months of injury and sooner if possible; and (7) reasonably close match between donor and recipient nerve caliber and motor axons counts. In theory, an additional principle is the ability for the successful cortical conversion by the patient from the donor nerve motor function to the recipient nerve motor function. Happily, this is rarely a problem with motor nerves even if the two functions are quite disparate, such as respiratory function with phrenic or intercostal nerves translated into elbow flexion. Motor nerves seem to be rather unsophisticated in terms of functional specificity, which stands in sharp contrast to sensory nerves[6] (to be discussed later).

For reanimation of the hand's intrinsic muscles, there is only one heterotopic donor nerve that fulfills the above seven principles—the distal anterior interosseous nerve. It may be used to neurotize either the thenar branch of the median nerve or the deep palmar branch of the ulnar nerve. It is fully expendable with minimal functional loss resulting from denervation of the pronator quadratus provided the pronator teres muscle is intact and functional. Except for conveying some sensory nerve fibers to the palmar wrist joint capsule, it is nearly a pure motor nerve. At the level of the pronator quadratus muscle, the anterior interosseous nerve contains an axon count that is about 75% that of the deep motor branch of the ulnar nerve and greater than this for the thenar branch of the median nerve.[7] With sufficient proximal interfascicular dissection of the distal median or ulnar nerves, direct coaptation of the transected distal anterior interosseous nerve to the fascicular origins of the thenar branch of the median nerve or the deep motor branch of the ulnar nerve is possible.

To our knowledge, Wang and Zhu were the first to report the use of the distal anterior interosseous nerve as a heterotopic nerve transfer.[8] The technique has subsequently been described by other authors.[9–11]

Indications

Median Nerve Injury

Transfer of the distal anterior interosseous nerve may be used only in those patients with median nerve loss distal to the origin of the anterior interosseous nerve, and with sparing of the entire anterior interosseous nerve branch. This technique should be considered in those patients who are unlikely to recover median innervated thenar motor function by a median nerve repair or reconstruction. Thus, it may be considered in those instances of median nerve laceration in the proximal or middle third of the forearm, and particularly when there is extensive loss of nerve substance. The injury should not be so distal as to obscure the precise identification of the median nerve fascicles giving rise to the thenar motor branch.

Ulnar Nerve Injury

Transfer of the distal anterior interosseous nerve should be considered in any patient with an ulnar nerve transsection at or proximal to the proximal forearm because in such patients recovery of intrinsic motor function with ulnar nerve repair or reconstruction is both poor and unpredictable. The indications are further heightened in patients with considerable loss of nerve substance. As was true for the median nerve, the level of injury should not be so distal as to obscure or damage the fascicular origins of the ulnar nerve deep motor branch.

With either ulnar or median nerve injury, the procedure should be carried out as soon as reasonably possibly, and certainly within 6 months from the date of injury.

Surgical Technique

Isolation of Distal Anterior Interosseous Nerve

A linear palmar incision is made in the distal forearm slightly ulnar to the midline. The dissection is deepened through the antebrachial fascia and the flexor digitorum superficialis and flexor digitorum profundus tendons and muscle bellies are retracted in a radial direction. The interosseous membrane, pronator quadratus muscle, and the anterior interosseous vessels and nerve are thus exposed. The nerve is isolated from the accompanying vessels 2 to 3 cm proximal to the proximal edge of the pronator quadratus muscle and then traced distally (Fig. 7–1). It is then further isolated within the proximal third

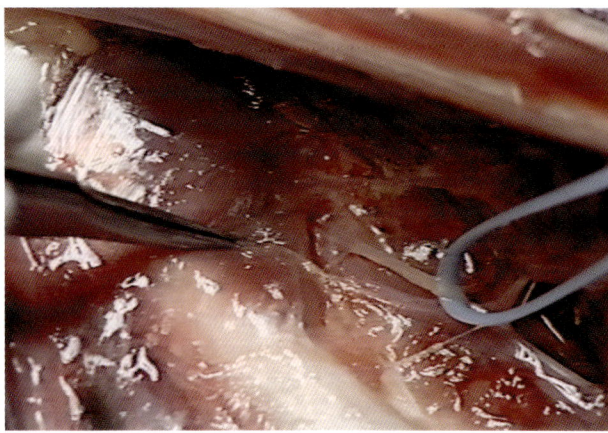

Figure 7–1 Isolated anterior interosseous nerve just proximal to entering the pronator quadratus muscle.

of the muscle, at which point it will branch. The nerve is then sharply transected 1 mm beyond the branch point.

Isolation of Median Nerve Thenar Branch

The forearm incision used to isolate the anterior interosseous nerve is lengthened distally to the midpalm crossing the flexor crease of the wrist in a zig-zag manner. The transverse carpal ligament is incised along its ulnar aspect and reflected, which exposes the median nerve. The thenar motor branch is precisely identified by sufficient exposure to visualize it penetrating the thenar muscles. It is then isolated in a proximal direction by interfascicular dissection for a sufficient distance (usually 8 to 10 cm) to permit a tension-free coaptation to the transected end of the anterior interosseous nerve (Fig. 7–2 A and B).

Isolation of Deep Motor Branch of Ulnar Nerve

The forearm incision used to isolate the anterior interosseous nerve is lengthened distally over and just distal to Guyon's canal crossing the flexor crease of the wrist in a zig-zag manner. The volar carpal ligament is incised and reflected in an ulnar direction, exposing the underlying ulnar artery and nerve. The deep motor branch of the ulnar nerve is precisely identified by sufficient exposure to visualize it coursing deep and in a radial direction into the palm. It is then isolated in a proximal direction by interfascicular dissection for a sufficient distance (usually 8 to 10 cm) to permit a tension-free coaptation to the transected end of the anterior interosseous nerve (Fig. 7–3).

Nerve coaptation is carried out using optical magnification and epineural sutures of 10-0 nylon. The coaptation site may be supplemented using fibrin adhesives. The wrist and fingers are immobilized with the wrist in a neutral position and the fingers in an intrinsic plus position for 2 to 3 weeks.

HETEROTOPIC SENSORY NERVE TRANSFER

Heterotopic sensory nerve transfer is perhaps less often carried out than motor nerve transfer because even proximal level nerve repair or graft reconstruction of large gaps in the median or ulnar nerves frequently result in an acceptable level of protective sensibility. Moreover, in contrast to the outcome of motor nerve transfers, sensory nerve transfers almost always retains the topographical sensibility characteristics of the donor nerve.[6] Thus, even years after the transfer, sensibility will be perceived in the donor nerve distribution as opposed to the recipient nerve distribution. Some patients may have difficulty adjusting to such sensory disorientation. Finally, as in the case with a great number of sensory neurorrhaphies, some degree of hypesthesia will result with sensory nerve transfer and this may diminish the quality of the functional result.

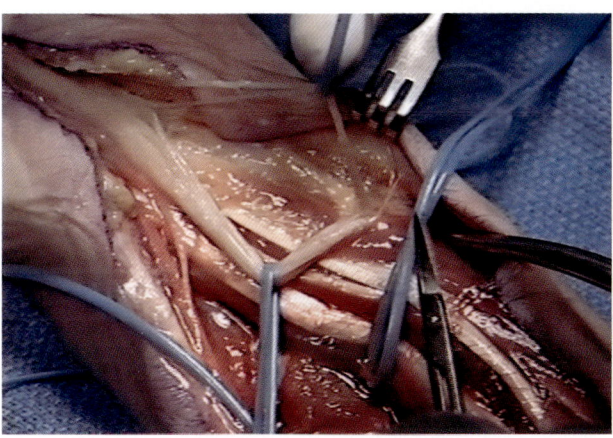

A

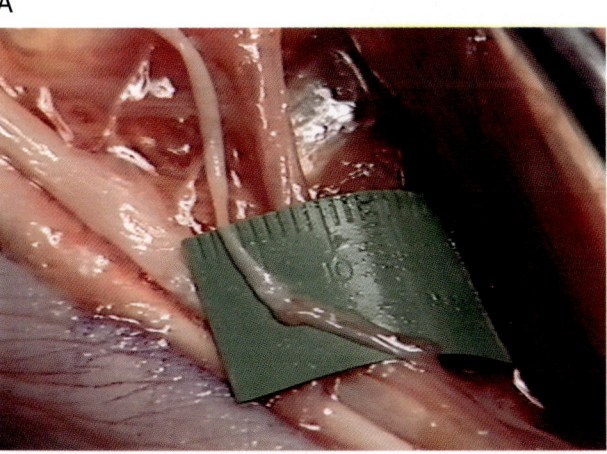

B

Figure 7–2 **A:** Isolated thenar motor branch with proximal isolation of fascicular origin. **B:** Coaptation of distal anterior interosseous nerve to fascicles contributing to median nerve thenar branch. (Note similar caliber of both nerve ends.)

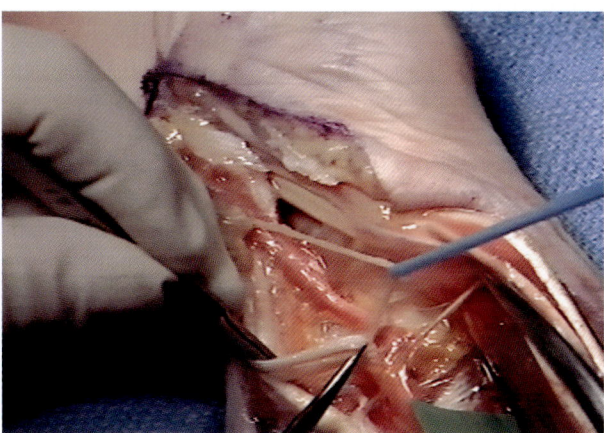

Figure 7–3 Isolated deep motor branch of ulnar nerve with proximal isolation of fascicular origin.

Indications

The most frequent indication for heterotopic sensory nerve transfer in the hand is for dense anesthesia of the thumb or total median nerve anesthesia. Rarely it may be indicated for restoration of protective sensibility along the ulnar border of the hand and fifth finger. The available donor nerves may be any source of sensory axons that are uninjured, and may be sacrificed without appreciably further impairing hand function. Most often, the preferred donor nerve for digital neurotization is a nearby normal digital nerve. For an anesthetic thumb with otherwise intact hand sensibility, a good choice is transfer of the long finger ulnar proper digital nerve. In the case of total median nerve distribution anesthesia with an intact ulnar nerve, the donor nerve should be the ring finger ulnar proper digital nerve. In the case of combined ulnar and median nerve loss, one may consider transfer of the superficial radial nerve or the dorsal sensory branch of the ulnar nerve (if uninjured) prolonged by an intercalated nerve autograft.

Surgical Technique

Transfer of Long Finger (or Ring Finger in Case of Complete Median Nerve Anesthesia) Ulnar Proper Digital Nerve to Thumb Ulnar Proper Digital Nerve

A zig-zag incision is made in the midpalm centered over the third web space (or fourth web space when using the ring finger as donor), and extending distally almost to the level of the web commissure. The dissection is deepened through the palmar aponeurosis and in the distal aspect of the wound, the ulnar proper digital nerve is identified. The nerve is then carefully isolated from the accompanying digital vessels, and then further mobilized proximally to the level of the superficial palmar arch by interfascicular dissection within the parent common digital nerve. This dissection should be meticulous with avoidance of injury to the fascicular contribution to the radial proper digital nerve of the adjacent finger (Fig. 7–4). The donor ulnar proper digital nerve is then sharply transected distally. A second zig-zag incision is then made over the palmar aspect of the thumb metacarpophalangeal joint flexor crease and distal aspect of the thenar eminence. It is deepened to expose the thumb ulnar proper digital nerve which is then carefully isolated and sharply transected proximally. Before transecting the nerve, one should ensure that the arc of rotation of the donor nerve is adequate to allow a tension-free coaptation to the recipient nerve (Fig. 7–5). A voluminous subcutaneous tunnel is then created by blunt dissection between the proximal aspects of both incisions. The mobilized long finger (or ring finger) ulnar proper digital nerve is then passed

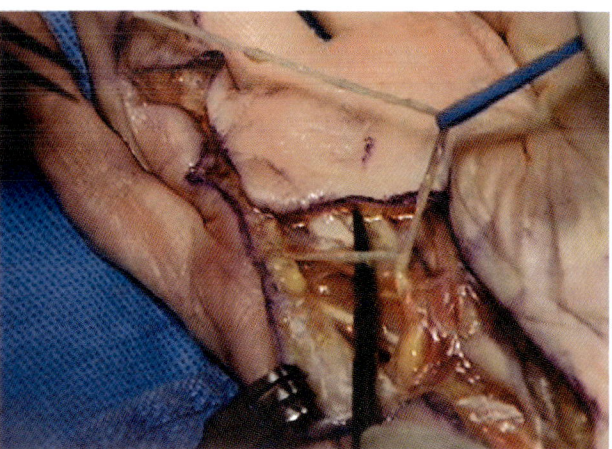

Figure 7–4 Isolated and proximally mobilized ulnar proper digital nerve of donor finger. (Note radial proper digital nerve of adjacent finger retracted by instrument.)

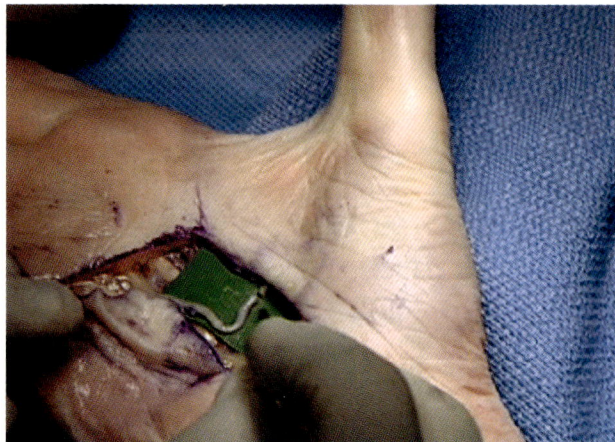

Figure 7–5 Approximation of donor finger ulnar proper digital nerve to thumb ulnar proper digital nerve just prior to suture coaptation.

through this tunnel to emerge near the base of the thumb. Care should be taken to prevent any kinking of the nerve or undue tension in this process. If doubt exists regarding the adequacy of the subcutaneous tunnel, the two incisions can be joined and the opposing skin margins undermined under direct vision. If the caliber of the donor digital nerve is significantly greater than that of the thumb ulnar proper digital nerve, the unsatisfied fascicular cross-sectional area of the donor nerve may be used as a source of sensory neurotization to additional recipient sites. For example, in patients with complete loss of the median nerve, the radial proper digital nerve of the index finger may be coapted to the unsatisfied cross-section of the donor nerve.

Nerve coaptation is carried out using optical magnification and epineural sutures of 10-0 nylon. The wrist and thumb are immobilized for 2 to 3 weeks.

Transfer of Superficial Radial Nerve or Dorsal Sensory Branch of Ulnar Nerve

When there is combined irreparable median and ulnar nerve loss, and thus no digital nerve is available as a donor nerve, one can consider using the superficial radial nerve at the level of the distal forearm as a source of sensory axons. Very rarely the dorsal sensory branch of the ulnar nerve may be similarly available in patients with destruction of the ulnar nerve distal to the origin of the dorsal sensory branch. Most patients in this situation, however, should be candidates for an orthotopic nerve reconstruction. If the superficial radial nerve is used as the donor nerve, an intercalated free nerve graft may be necessary as a conduit to bridge the superficial radial nerve to the thumb ulnar proper digital nerve. In such a case, the thumb digital nerve should be mobilized as far proximally as possible within the median nerve by interfascicular dissection in order to minimize the length of nerve graft needed.

NEUROVASCULAR ISLAND SKIN FLAP

An alternative to a heterotopic nerve transfer in patients with irreparable median nerve loss in the presence of an intact ulnar nerve is a neurovascular island skin flap transfer from the ulnar side of the ring finger to the palmar surface of the thumb tip. This procedure is technically more demanding than simple nerve transfer, and may be complicated by vascular insufficiency with necrosis of the skin flap. It also is somewhat disfiguring to the donor ring finger. However, restoration of thumb sensibility by neurovascular island flap transfer does have the advantage that the donor digital nerve remains completely intact and actual neurorrhaphy is not required. Thus, the quality of sensibility may be substantially better than that typically resulting from a repaired nerve.

Indications

The major indication for restoration of thumb sensibility by ring finger neurovascular island skin flap transfer is in those patients who have no identifiable recipient digital nerve. This may be the case with certain ring avulsion mechanism injuries to the thumb. A second important indication for this procedure would be to reconstruct a patient who requires skin coverage to the palmar surface of the thumb tip in addition to restoration of thumb sensibility.

Surgical Technique

A skin flap is designed over the ulnar side of the ring finger. The dimension and shape of the flap should be appropriate to fulfill the thumb requirements if skin coverage is deficient. In general, the dorsal and palmar skin flap margins should fall short of crossing the ring finger midline. The distal margin of the skin flap should not extend beyond the midpoint of the distal phalanx, and the proximal margin should not exceed the midpoint of the proximal phalanx. Initially, the skin flap is designed and marked but not elevated until later in the procedure. From the proximal margin of the so-designed skin flap, a zig-zag incision is made centered over the fourth intermetacarpal region and extending proximally to the level of the superficial palmar arch. The incision is deepened through the palmar aponeurosis exposing the fourth web common digital neurovascular bundle. The fourth web neurovascular bundle is then isolated with special care to include a generous cuff of surrounding tissue (Fig. 7–6). Preservation of a cuff of soft tissue is necessary to ensure maintaining the integrity of the accompanying venae comitantes. Once the fourth web common digital neurovascular bundle is isolated, the proper digital neurovascular bundle to the adjacent sides of the ring and small fingers are identified. The ulnar proper digital neurovascular bundle to the ring finger is then isolated to the level of the planned proximal margin of the skin flap together with a generous cuff of surrounding soft tissue. The proper digital artery to the radial side of the small finger is ligated and sectioned just distal to its origin from the common digital artery. The radial proper digital nerve to the small finger is then gently teased from the common digital nerve by interfascicular dissection back to the level of the superficial palmar arch.

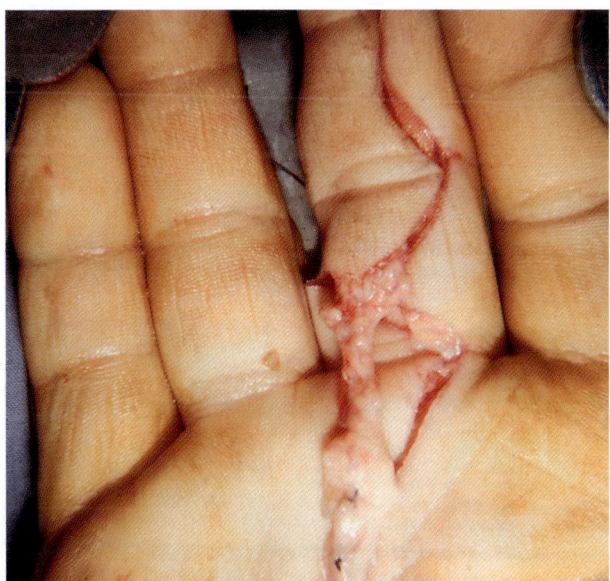

Figure 7–6   Isolated common digital neurovascular bundle with generous cuff of surrounding soft tissue.

In this process, the soft tissue cuff about the fourth web common digital neurovascular bundle should be disturbed as little as possible. At this point in the procedure, the previously designed skin flap margins are incised. Elevation of the skin flap together with the attached neurovascular bundle pedicle is accomplished by meticulous dissection proceeding from proximal to distal. Although it is essential to carry this dissection on a plane deep to the proper digital neurovascular bundle, care must be taken to leave a layer of adipose tissue and peritenon over the flexor tendon sheath and extensor tendon apparatus. Following complete elevation of the skin flap on its neurovascular pedicle, the tourniquet should be deflated and satisfactory perfusion of the skin flap confirmed (Fig. 7–7). The skin flap is then transposed across the palm to the thumb and positioned as far distally on the thumb as possible without creating undue tension on the neurovascular pedicle. The appropriate recipient location on the thumb palmar surface is then outlined and a matching skin defect created. This skin defect is then connected to the prox-imal region of the palmar skin incision either by creating a voluminous subcutaneous tunnel or by a joining zig-zag incision. The transposed skin flap is then inset into the thumb recipient skin defect with care to ensure that the neurovascular pedicle is free of kinking or undue tension. The resulting skin defect in the ring finger is closed using a defatted, full thickness skin graft taken from a hairless region of the patient. A tie-over stent is used over the skin graft. The hand and all fingers are immobilized in a mild intrinsic plus position for 2 weeks.

CONCLUSIONS

Most surgeons will seldom encounter patients with irreparable median and ulnar nerve injuries to the hand because most such injuries may be treated by nerve repair or orthotopic reconstruction. However, the application of heterotopic nerve transfers or of neurovascular skin island flaps should be part of the treatment option inventory of hand surgeons. These procedures may prove useful in certain desperate clinical situations for restoration or motor or sensory function when more conventional effective treatment options are lacking.

REFERENCES

1. Narakas AO, Hentz VR. Neurotization in brachial plexus injuries: indications and results. Clin Orthop 1988;237:43–56.
2. Krakhauer JD, Wood MB. Intercostal nerve transfer for brachial plexopathy. J Hand Surg Am 1994;19A:1–7.
3. Wood MB. Neurotization. In: Atlas of Reconstructive Microsurgery. Rockville MN: Aspen Publishers, 1990:29–34.
4. Chuang DC, Lee GW, Hashim F, et al. Restoration of shoulder abduction by nerve transfer in avulsed brachial plexus injury: evaluation in 99 patients with various nerve transfers. Plast Reconstr Surg 1995;96:122–8.
5. Mackinnon SE, Novak CB. Nerve transfers: new options for reconstruction following nerve injury. Hand Clin 1999;15:643–66.
6. Stice RC, Wood MB. Neurovascular island skin flaps in the hand: functional and sensibility evaluations. Microsurgery 1987;8:162–7.
7. Ustun ME, Ogun TC, Buyukmumcu M, et al. Selective restoration of motor function in the ulnar nerve by transfer of the anterior interosseous nerve. J Bone Joint Surg Am 2001;83:549–52.
8. Wang Y, Zhu S. Transfer of a branch of the anterior interosseous nerve to the motor branch of the median nerve and ulnar nerve. Chin Med J 1997;110:216–9.
9. Novak CB, Mackinnon SE. Distal anterior interosseous nerve transfer to the deep motor branch of the ulnar nerve for reconstruction of high ulnar nerve injuries. J Reconstr Microsurg 2002;18:459–64.
10. Haase SC, Chung KC. Anterior interosseous nerve transfer to the motor branch of the ulnar nerve for high ulnar nerve injuries. Ann Plast Surg 2002;49:285–90.
11. Wood MB. Hand intrinsic muscle reanimation by transfer of the distal portion of the anterior interosseous nerve. J Am Soc Surg Hand 2004;20:227–30.

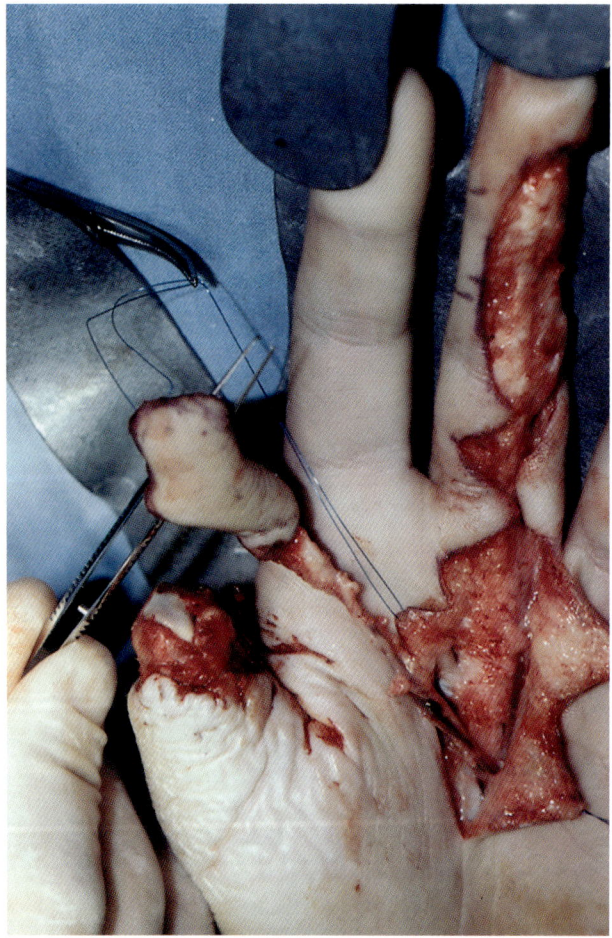

Figure 7–7 Mobilize neurovascular island skin flap with attached pedicle prior to transposition to thumb.

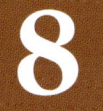

8

Vein Wrapping of Scarred Peripheral Nerves

Nickolaos A. Darlis and Dean G. Sotereanos

Life is short and the art is long; the occasion fleeting;
experience fallacious, and judgment difficult.

HIPPOCRATES

INTRODUCTION

Scarring of peripheral nerves can occur after trauma, but in everyday practice it is most commonly encountered after failed surgical decompression for entrapment neuropathies. Vein wrapping is a technique used to treat cicatrix formation around peripheral nerves by creating a barrier to adhesion in-growth from the surrounding tissues.

Carpal tunnel syndrome and cubital tunnel syndrome are the most common entrapment neuropathies of the upper extremity. Although surgical decompression is generally considered effective in both of these conditions, recurrence of symptoms is not uncommon. Rates of treatment failures or recurrence have been reported to be as high as 30%.[1-12] Results of revision surgery for entrapment neuropathies are less predictable.[1-4,13] Even after repeated decompression and neurolysis or transposition of the nerve, symptoms can recur because of scarring.

The etiology of persistent or recurrent pain following surgical decompression for entrapment neuropathies includes incomplete release, injury to the nerve trunk or its branches resulting in neuromas, reflex sympathetic dystrophy, and scarring of an intact nerve. Incomplete release can be addressed with repeated decompression. Neuromas may be partial or complete nerve injuries and are treated accordingly. The treatment of reflex sympathetic dystrophy must be individualized. Scarring of the nerve is by far the most difficult condition to treat, since attempts of repeated decompression and internal neurolysis further enhance scar tissue formation, and recurrence is inevitable.[13]

Postoperative epineural scarring leads to mechanical constriction, nerve ischemia, and impairment of nerve gliding on the adjacent tissues. Intraneural scarring is a common sequel. Pain can be caused by any of the above mechanisms. The term "traction neuropathy"[7] was used to describe chronic neuropathy secondary to nerve scarring. Although this term is clinically relevant (pain is usually exacerbated with motion of the adjacent joints), it describes only one of the mechanisms (lack of gliding) that lead to pain.

Soft tissue coverage of the scarred nerve is necessary to promote recovery of function. The ulnar nerve at the elbow is easier to cover by anterior transposition in the flexor–pronator musculature, but failures with this technique are not uncommon,[1,2,4] and it cannot be applied if submuscular transposition was used as the primary procedure. Soft tissue coverage for the median nerve at the wrist is scarce, and a number of flaps have been used in revision surgery. The hypothenar fat pad flap can produce good results, and is uncomplicated in most cases.[14] Pedicle or free flaps, including the groin flap, lateral arm flap, and posterior interosseous flap, provide excellent protection of the nerve, but the technique is complex and the result is not always satisfying.[14,15] Small local flaps, such as the abductor digiti minimi, the palmaris brevis, and the pronator quadratus, have also been described.[16–18] The dissection of these flaps, however, is not always easy, nerve coverage is sometimes inadequate, and skin closure problems may occur. A more conservative approach using implanted nerve stimulators or anesthetic reservoirs[19,20] has failed to consistently produce pain relief for these patients and was associated with complications.

BASIC SCIENCE

The first clinical report of vein wrapping of a scarred peripheral nerve is attributed to Masear.[21] Allograft vein wrapping with the use of allograft umbilical veins was tried clinically[22,23] before autogenous vein wrapping.[24] Ruch et al.[25] compared the femoral vein autografts with a glutaraldehyde-preserved allografts in an animal study, and found a significant increase in inflammatory cells and scar tissue associated with the allograft. Autologous vein grafts seemed to create fewer adhesions between the vein and the nerve compared with vein allografts. If the allograft vein adheres to the nerve the gliding between the nerve and vein might be impaired, which may have a negative effect on recovery.

The effect of wrapping scarred nerves with autogenous vein graft was studied by our group in the late 1990s.[26,27] The safety of the procedure was studied first by vein wrapping of intact sciatic nerves in 30 rats. No adverse effects on the nerve were recorded (no demyelination, nerve degeneration, or adhesion formation). An experimental chronic nerve compression model was then created in 100 rats. The sciatic nerve of rats was constricted with a silicone tube and nerve deficits were confirmed at 8 months. Animals were then randomly allocated in a vein wrapping or a control group. Assessment included walking track analysis, electrophysiologic testing concerning latency and amplitude, and histologic assessment using H&E, Trichrome, Silver, and Toluidine Blue stains. The sciatic nerves in the vein-wrapped group showed greater functional improvement than those in the non–vein-wrapped group. In electrophysiologic testing the latency was significantly shorter in the vein-wrapped group. Histologic evaluation showed marked nerve degeneration and scar tissue formation around the nerves in the

non–vein-wrapped group but not in the vein-wrapped group. These studies showed that autologous vein wrapping in a chronic nerve compression model could improve the functional recovery of the nerve and prevented scar in-growth.

The inhibition of scar formation with this technique has been verified by clinical observations from reexploration of vein-grafted nerves.[24,28–30] Biopsies obtained from re-explored vein grafts[28,29] showed very few adhesions between the adventitia of the vein and surrounding tissues, and no adhesions between the intimal surface of the vein and the nerve. Neovascularization of the vein graft and structural transformation of the vein endothelium, which is elevated into multiple papillary projections, was also observed.

In summary, vein wrapping seems to prevent both extrinsic and intrinsic scar formation. Although the exact mechanism is still unclear, basic research and clinical observations from re-explored nerves have revealed several factors that contribute to the good clinical results. These factors include prevention of epineurial adhesions, preservation or restoration of intrinsic epineurial vascularity, and formation of a gliding surface between the nerve and the surrounding tissues. Locally produced bioactive molecules may play a significant role in the structural changes observed.[29]

INDICATIONS

The primary indication for vein wrapping is significant epineurial scarring. Careful preoperative evaluation can guide patient selection for this technique, but intraoperative confirmation of nerve scarring is essential. In recurrent entrapment neuropathies, we usually reserve vein wrapping for the multiply operated patients and the ones with unrelenting symptoms following the initial surgical decompression. Patients who present for their first reoperation, with moderate pain and moderate scarring of the nerve on inspection, can be effectively treated with other soft tissue coverage procedures. Anterior transposition of the ulnar nerve with minimal medial epicondylectomy (if the nerve has not already been transposed) and hypothenar fat flap coverage for the median nerve are our choices in such instances. Vein wrapping can also be applied in recurrent radial tunnel and tarsal tunnel surgery and in cases of severe post traumatic scarring of peripheral nerves, but recurrent carpal tunnel and cubital tunnel are by far the most common indications. Small neuromas in continuity are sometimes found in association with scarring of the nerve. If the complaint is simply pain without motor or sensory deficit, vein wrapping may be indicated. If the neuroma is considerable in size or the patient's functional deficit is significant, the neuroma should be excised and nerve repaired with nerve grafts or conduits. In post-traumatic cases the presence of dense epineurial adhesions is the primary indication for the technique. If there is doubt about nerve continuity, internal neurolysis can be used to detect nerve fascicle continuity through the zone of injury. Intraoperative nerve simulation may also be helpful in such instances. This technique is most useful in covering superficially located nerve where soft tissue coverage by other means is difficult (e.g., the tibial nerve behind the medial malleolus) (Fig. 8–3 C).

The typical clinical presentation for a candidate for this technique in entrapment neuropathies is that of recurrent symptoms after an adequate primary decompression. The history of initial temporary relief after the primary decompression or a subsequent neurolysis is highly indicative of scar formation. The absence of even transient symptomatic relief after the initial surgery could signify inadequate decompression. With scar formation, the patients' complaints are usually that of pain worsening with activities and paresthesias. Severe pain (five or above in a visual analogue scale) is their chief complaint. A positive Tinel's sign is usually present, and most of the patients have abnormal two-point discrimination. Muscular atrophies are relatively uncommon, and when present they are indicative of more severe intrinsic scarring of the nerve. Electrodiagnostic testing often shows decreased electrical amplitude and sensory conduction after stimulation of the nerve; muscle denervation is seen less often. Nerve scarring can be present in the absence of two-point discrimination abnormalities and electrodiagnostic findings, but in that setting worker's compensation and litigation issues should be carefully taken into consideration.

An initial period of nonoperative treatment to reduce pain (especially in patients without a measurable sensory or motor deficit) is advisable. This can include splinting, injections, desensitization, scar massage, and nerve stimulation. Narcotic analgesics are avoided since these patients can easily become dependent.

Potential donor side morbidity must be also taken into consideration. The greater saphenus vein is harvested for this procedure. The length of vein graft taken is usually four times the length of the compressed segment of the nerve. Although this is well tolerated in most individuals, a vascular surgeon must be consulted in patients with peripheral vascular disease or deep venous thrombosis history. In patients with coronary heart disease, the saphenous vein is a major source of vein grafts for reconstruction and that should also be taken into consideration.

OPERATIVE TECHNIQUE

General anesthesia is used for this procedure because of the need to have two operating fields (one for nerve exploration and one for vein harvesting). A vein stripper (Codman, Johnson & Johnson, Raynham MA) is used for less invasive vein harvesting through two small incisions, and this has been our preference in recent years. No special instrumentation is needed for the procedure if the saphenous vein is to be harvested with a long incision or through several stab incisions using finger dissection. We do not routinely use nerve stimulation for recurrent compression neuropathies.

The affected nerve is surgically explored first. Vein harvesting is initiated only after the affected nerve is dissected and found to be severely scarred. Pre-existing incisions are typically used and are extended both proximally and distally to virgin tissues. The affected nerve should be identified in healthy tissues both proximally and distally, and then dissected toward the scarred section. Dissection is painstaking and is performed under loop or microscope magnification. All potential sites of nerve compression must be re-explored, and their release should be confirmed. If the structural continuity of the nerve is in doubt, the operating microscope is used to dissect fascicles from proximal to distal through the scarred segment. Internal neurolysis under the operating microscope is performed as necessary. Indications for internal neurolysis included severe compression and thinning of the nerve, lack of epineural vascularity, and muscle wasting. The length of the nerve that has to be vein wrapped is then measured. The required length of the vein is three to four times the scarred length of the nerve. It is advisable to vein wrap a 0.5- to 1-cm zone of healthy-appearing nerve at both ends of the scarred segment if the length of the graft is adequate. The vein length harvested is usually 20 to 30 cm.

The ipsilateral or contralateral lower extremity can be used for greater saphenous vein harvesting. The position of the great saphenous vein can be usually palpated, and is marked on the skin prior to tourniquet inflation. An incision is made 1 cm anterior to the medial malleolus, and the greater saphenous vein is identified (Fig. 8–1). Care is taken not to injure branches of the saphenous nerve. The vein is ligated distally and a small longitudinal phlebotomy is made. The vein stripper guide is introduced through the phlebotomy, and is advanced proximally to the predetermined length. The vein stripper guide can be usually palpated through the skin as it is advanced. A second 1-cm incision is made over the stripper proximally; the vein is ligated and cut. The vein stripper guide is advanced out of the vein through a second longitudinal phlebotomy and the appropriate size olive (usually 9F) is attached to the guide. The graft is retrieved by slowly pulling the stripper. The rupture of lateral vein branches can be felt while pulling. After vein harvesting, the skin is closed and a compressive dressing is applied to the leg prior to deflating the tourniquet to avoid hematoma formation. Alternatively,

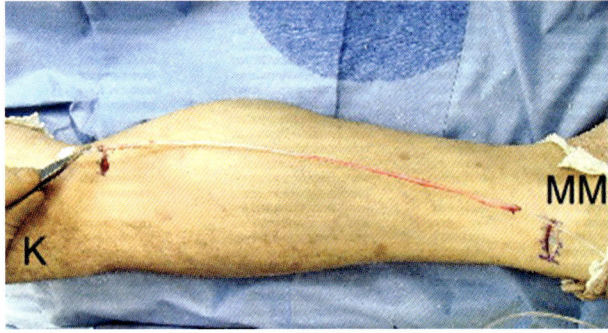

Figure 8–1 Incisions used in harvesting the predetermined length of greater saphenous vein in the lower extremity with a vein stripper. The required length of the vein is three to four times the scarred length of the nerve. MM, medial malleolus; K, knee.

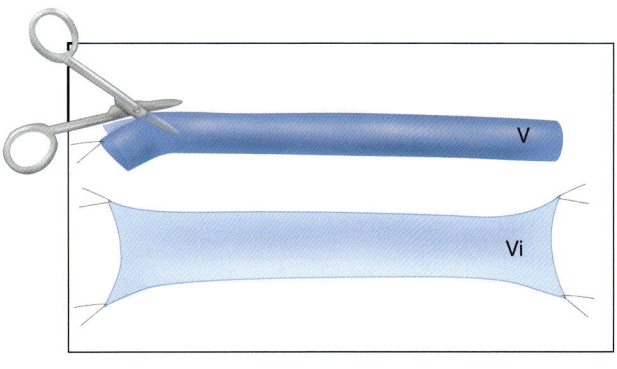

A

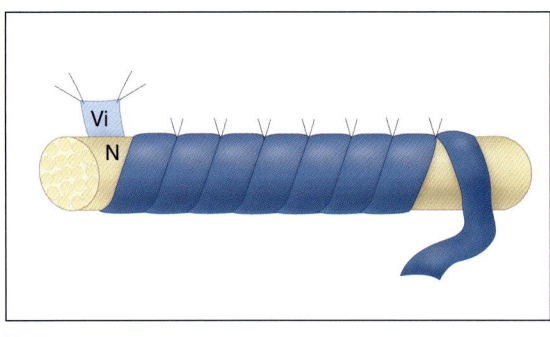

B

Figure 8–2 Schematic of technique used for vein wrapping of peripheral nerves. The saphenous vein is split longitudinally, and is opened to form a rectangle **(A).** The vein is then **(B)** tacked distal to the scarred portion of the nerve on a nonmobile tissue, and is wrapped around the scarred portion of the nerve in a spiral pattern with its intima apposed to the surface of the nerve. Each ring of the vein is secured to the adjacent rings with a stitch. N, nerve; V, vein; Vi, intimal.

the vein can be harvested through a continuous incision or interrupted incisions and dissection without the use of a vein stripper. After the saphenous vein is harvested, it is incised and opened longitudinally (Fig. 8–2 A). The adventitia of the vein graft is marked with a marking pen throughout its length, as the intimal side of the graft must come in contact with the scarred nerve.

One of the ends of the vein graft is tacked distally to the scarred portion of the nerve on a tissue that is not mobile, with the intima against the nerve, using a 7-0 or 8-0 nylon stitch. The wrapping proceeds circumferentially as described by Masear et al.[21] from distal to proximal, while care is taken not to make the wrap too snug and thus constrict the nerve (Fig. 8–2 B). After each complete circle on the nerve, the vein is stabilized with a loose 7-0 or 8-0 nylon stitch to the adjacent ring of vein (Fig. 8–2 B, Fig. 8–3 A to C). If enough vein graft length has been obtained, each loop of the vein graft around the nerve can partially overlap the previous loop. Ensuring that the intima of the vein graft is apposed to the nerve after each loop is important. Wrapping should not be too snug. The other end of the vein graft is tacked proximal to the scarred segment of the nerve on unscarred tissue. The coverage of the scarred nerve segment must be complete and must extend slightly to an unscarred segment to prevent recurrence. The tourniquet is the deflated, hemostasis is obtained, and routine loose closure is performed.

Postoperatively, for recurrent carpal tunnel cases the wrist is immobilized for 1 week in slight extension, and active and passive range of motion (ROM) exercises follow. For recurrent cubital tunnel, the elbow is mobilized the first postoperative day. In traumatic cases, immobilization is individualized with a trend toward early mobilization to avoid further adhesion formation.

PERSONAL SERIES

The results of autologous vein wrapping to treat recurrent compressive neuropathy using the aforementioned technique have been rewarding.[31,32] We reported 19 patients with recurrent compressive neuropathies (15 with recurrent carpal tunnel syndrome and 4 with recurrent cubital tunnel syndrome) treated with autologous saphenous vein wrapping between 1993 and 1997. The mean age was 53 years (range, 28 to 75 years). The mean number of previous procedures was three, with a minimum of two and a maximum of five for each patient. For the median nerve, these procedures included simple nerve decompression, tenosynovectomy, internal neurolysis, hypothenar fat pad flap, and local flaps. For the ulnar nerve, they included in situ decompression with or without medial epicondylectomy, and subcutaneous, submuscular, and intramuscular transposition of the ulnar nerve.

The average follow-up period was 43 months (range, 24 to 78 months). All patients reported pain relief. On a visual analogue scale, all patients rated their pain between two and six; their preoperative pain had been rated between six and nine. Sensation improved in all patients, although 16 of the 19 patients had residual numbness. Two-point discrimination improved from an

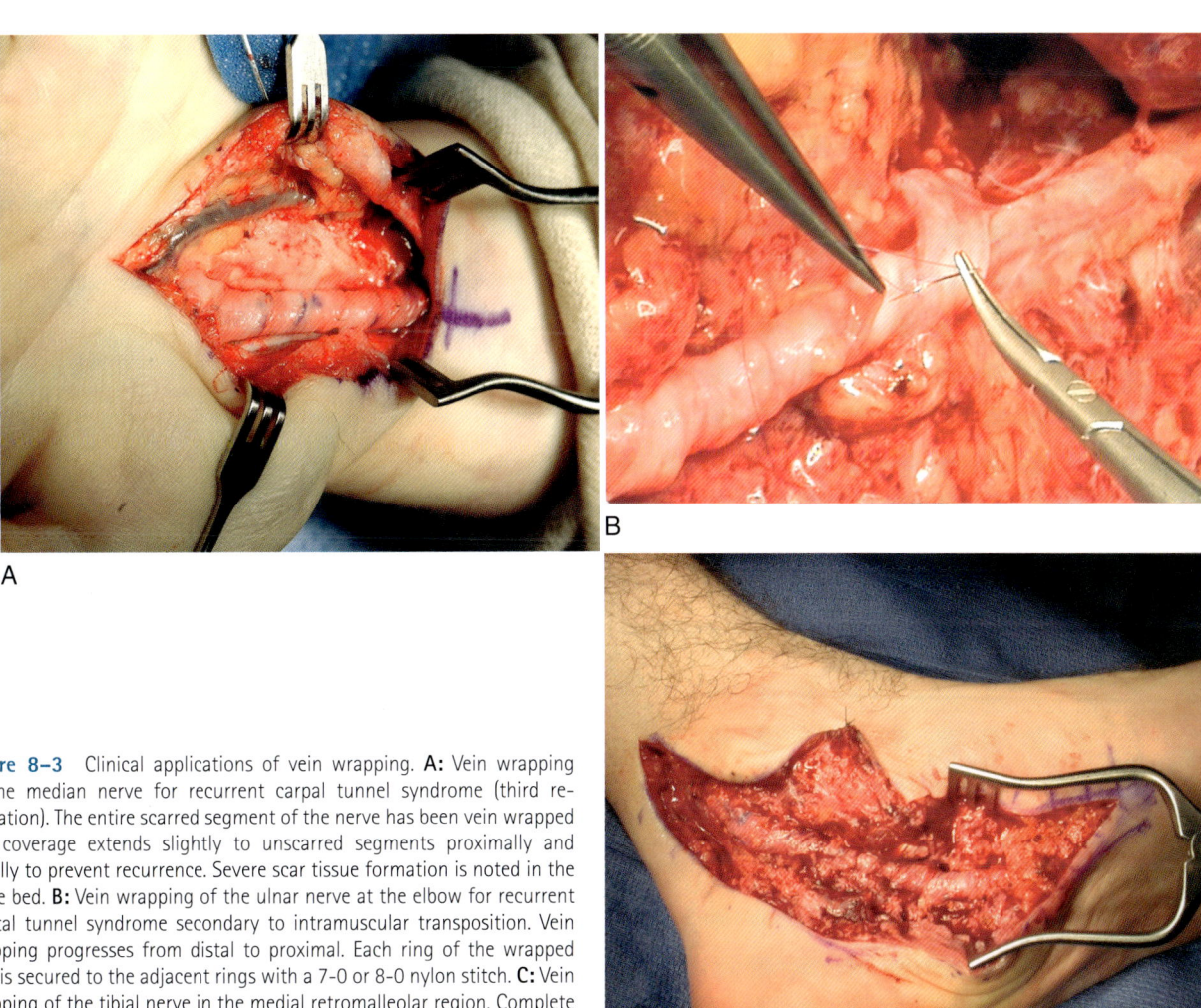

Figure 8–3 Clinical applications of vein wrapping. **A:** Vein wrapping of the median nerve for recurrent carpal tunnel syndrome (third re-operation). The entire scarred segment of the nerve has been vein wrapped and coverage extends slightly to unscarred segments proximally and distally to prevent recurrence. Severe scar tissue formation is noted in the nerve bed. **B:** Vein wrapping of the ulnar nerve at the elbow for recurrent cubital tunnel syndrome secondary to intramuscular transposition. Vein wrapping progresses from distal to proximal. Each ring of the wrapped vein is secured to the adjacent rings with a 7-0 or 8-0 nylon stitch. **C:** Vein wrapping of the tibial nerve in the medial retromalleolar region. Complete nerve block of the medial and lateral plantar nerves was diagnosed preoperatively secondary to a crushing injury 7 months prior. Intra-operatively the nerve was found to be in continuity with severe scarring. Internal neurolysis was performed and vein wrapping was used to cover the nerve. The patient recovered sensation on the sole of the foot.

average of 12 before surgery to 8 after surgery. Sixteen of the 19 patients demonstrated more than 2 mm of improvement in 2-point discrimination in comparison to preoperative values. Grip strength increased from an average of 27 kg before surgery to 38 kg after surgery. Abnormal nerve conduction velocities were found in all patients in their preoperative electrodiagnostic studies. The motor nerve conduction velocity improved from an average of 41 m/s before surgery to 43 m/s after surgery in the 10 patients who had both preoperative and post-operative values available. The sensory nerve conduction velocity improved from an average of 39 m/s before surgery to 43 m/s after surgery in the seven patients who had both preoperative and postoperative values available. Eighteen patients stated that they would undergo the procedure again if faced with a similar problem. No complications due to saphenous vein harvesting were noted other than mild discomfort and

swelling at the incision site that resolved in approximately 4 months.

The procedure has been performed numerous times, since the original series, for recurrent compressive neuropathies and severe post-traumatic nerve scarring both in the upper and in the lower extremity with consistently good results.

In summary, autologous vein wrapping of scarred nerves is an excellent option. In recurrent compressive neuropathies, the multiply operated patient with chronic nerve compression secondary to cicatrix formation is likely to benefit more from this procedure. It is a simple technique with minimal donor site morbidity. The donor vein is readily available and harvesting is easy. It consistently provides pain relief and improvement of sensation. Both experimental and clinical results support its use for recurrent compressive neuropathies.

Dedication

This chapter is dedicated to Donna, Alexis, and Stella, the loves of my life.

REFERENCES

1. Broudy AS, Leffert RD, Smith RJ. Technical problems with ulnar nerve transposition at the elbow: findings and results of reoperation. J Hand Surg Am 1978;3:85.
2. Rogers MR, Bergfield TG, Aulicino PL. The failed ulnar nerve transposition. Etiology and treatment. Clin Orthop 1991; 269:193.
3. Caputo AE, Watson HK. Subcutaneous anterior transposition of the ulnar nerve for failed decompression of cubital tunnel syndrome. J Hand Surg Am 2000;25:544.
4. Vogel RB, Nossaman BC, Rayan GM. Revision anterior submuscular transposition of the ulnar nerve for failed subcutaneous transposition. Br J Plast Surg 2004;57:311.
5. Cobb TK, Amadio PC, Leatherwood DF, et al. Outcome of reoperation for carpal tunnel syndrome, J Hand Surg Am 1996;21:347.
6. Gelberman RH, Pfeffer GB, Galbraith RT, et al. Results of treatment of severe carpal-tunnel syndrome without internal neurolysis of the median nerve. J Bone Joint Surg Am 1987;69:896.
7. Hunter JM. Recurrent carpal tunnel syndrome, epineural fibrous fixation, and traction neuropathy. Hand Clin 1991;7:491.
8. Yu G-Z, Firrell JC, Tsai T-M. Pre-operative factors and treatment outcome following carpal tunnel release. J Hand Surg Br 1992;17:646.
9. Haupt WF, Wintzer G, Schop A, et al. Long-term results of carpal tunnel decompression: assessment of 60 cases. J Hand Surg 1993;18:471.
10. Mackinnon SE. Secondary carpal tunnel surgery. Neurosurg Clin N Am 1991;2:75.
11. Gelberman RH, Eaton R, Urbaniak JR. Peripheral nerve compression. J Bone Joint Surg Am 1993;7A:1854.
12. Kessler FB. Complications of the management of carpal tunnel syndrome. Hand Clin 1986;2:401.
13. Rhoades CE, Mowery CA, Gelberman RH. Results of internal neurolysis of the median nerve for severe carpal-tunnel syndrome. J Bone Joint Surg Am 1985;67:253.
14. Urbaniak JR. Complications of treatment of carpal tunnel syndrome. In: Gelberman RH, ed., Operative Nerve Repair and Reconstruction. Philadelphia: J.B. Lippincott, 1991:937–79.
15. Gould JS. Treatment of the painful injured nerve in-continuity. In: Gelberman RH, ed., Operative Nerve Repair and Reconstruction. Philadelphia: J.B. Lippincott, 1991:1541–9.
16. Botte MJ, von Schroeder HP, Abrams RA, et al. Recurrent carpal tunnel syndrome. Hand Clin 1996;12:731.
17. Rose EH, Norris MS, Kowalski TA, et al. Palmaris brevis turnover flap as an adjunct to internal neurolysis of the chronically scarred median nerve in recurrent carpal tunnel syndrome. J Hand Surg Am 1991;16:191.
18. Jones NF. Treatment of chronic pain by "wrapping" intact nerves with pedicle and free flaps. Hand Clin 1996;12:765.
19. Nashold BS, Goldner JL, Mullen JB, et al. Long-term pain control by direct peripheral-nerve stimulation. J Bone Joint Surg Am 1982;64:1.
20. Monsivais JJ, Monsivais DB. Managing chronic neuropathic pain with implanted anesthetic reservoirs. Hand Clin 1996;12:781.
21. Masear VR, Tullos JR, St Mary E, et al. Venous wrapping of nerve to prevent scarring. J Hand Surg Am 1990;15:817.
22. Koman LA, Neal B, Santichen J. Management of the postoperative painful median nerve at the wrist. Orthop Trans 1995;18: 765.
23. Masear VR, Colgin S. The treatment of epineural scarring with allograft vein wrapping. Hand Clin 1996;12:773.
24. Sotereanos DG, Giannakopoulos PN, Mitsionis GI, et al. Vein-graft wrapping for the treatment of recurrent compression of the median nerve. Microsurgery 1995;16:752.
25. Ruch DS, Spinner RM, Koman LA. The histologic effect of barrier vein wrapping of peripheral nerves. J Reconstr Microsurg 1996;12:291.
26. Xu J, Sotereanos DG, Moller AR. Nerve wrapping with vein grafts in a rat model: a safe technique for the treatment of recurrent chronic compressive neuropathy. J Reconstr Microsurg 1998; 14:323.
27. Xu J, Varitimidis SE, Fisher KJ, et al. The effect of wrapping scarred nerves with autogenous vein graft to treat recurrent chronic nerve compression. J Hand Surg Am 2000;25:93.
28. Vardakas DG, Varitimidis SE, Sotereanos DG. Findings of exploration of a vein-wrapped ulnar nerve: report of a case. J Hand Surg Am 2001;26:60.
29. Campbell JT, Schon LC, Burkhardt LD. Histopathologic findings in autogenous saphenous vein graft wrapping for recurrent tarsal tunnel syndrome: a case report. Foot Ankle Int 1998;19: 766.
30. Chou KH, Papadimitriou NG, Sarris I, et al. Neovascularization and other histopathologic findings in an autogenous saphenous vein wrap used for recalcitrant carpal tunnel syndrome: a case report. J Hand Surg Am 2003;28:262.
31. Varitimidis SE, Vardakas DG, Goebel F, et al. Treatment of recurrent compressive neuropathy of peripheral nerves in the upper extremity with an autologous vein insulator. J Hand Surg Am 2001;26:296.
32. Varitimidis SE, Riano F, Vardacas DG, et al. Recurrent compressive neuropathy of the median nerve at the wrist: treatment with autogenous saphenous vein wrapping. J Hand Surg Br 2000; 25:271.

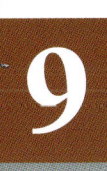

A SYNTHETIC NERVE CONDUITS

Thomas E. Trumble, Debra Parisi, Simon Archibald, and Christopher H. Allan

INTRODUCTION

A number of growth factors and cytokines have been investigated in order to improve the accuracy of nerve repair. Trophic (growth-promoting) factors studied include nerve growth factor (NGF), brain-derived neurotrophic factor (BDNF), fibroblastic growth factors (FGFs), ciliary neurotrophic factor (CNTF), and interleukin-6 (IL-6), among many others.[1–3] The roles of these factors and cytokines are only partially understood, with some having greater effects on the regeneration of sympathetic and sensory axons,[3,4] whereas others such as BDNF or CNTF have a greater effect on motor neuron regeneration.[2,5] Many of the growth factors and other cytokines are released into the surrounding tissues following nerve injury. The key clinical questions follow: In what scenarios will they help? Over what time period must they be delivered to promote nerve regeneration in the setting of acute versus delayed repair? Although a gap at the nerve repair site would theoretically allow budding nerve axons to correctly identify the target end organ, investigations have shown that optimal nerve regeneration requires tightly coapted nerves with no gap and with accurate alignment.[6] Finally, the ability of certain axon membrane glycoproteins to preferentially attract either motor or sensory axons has been investigated as a method of guiding nerve regeneration.[7]

Bioengineering of nerve grafts has focused on the ability to attract nerve axons with a number of different materials, including polylactic acid (PLA), polyglycolic acid (PGA), and collagen.[8,9] These have been combined with techniques or agents that may speed nerve regeneration or increase the window of opportunity for nerve regeneration, such as trophic factors, factors to inhibit the degeneration and reabsorption of motor end plates, antibodies that block inhibitory proteins, and electrical stimulation.[10,11] Studies have investigated whether there are specific factors that enhance motor versus sensory recovery. Timing of the delivery of nerve growth factors is a key factor in the success of nerve regeneration.[3,12] Work on synthetic nerve conduits or tubes has included analysis of ideal porosity, substrate, and embedded growth factors. Although earlier studies did not suggest a benefit with electrical stimulation, new studies indicate that electromagnetic fields can enhance the rate of nerve regeneration.[11] As part of the quest for a bioengineered nerve graft, certain factors that may inhibit the reabsorption of motor end plates have been investigated. Finally, the ability to incorporate allogeneic tissues into bioengineered grafts may be a key factor in replacing the cellular functions provided by autonomous nerve grafts. The ability of allogeneic cells to survive transplantation depends on the major histocompatibility complexes (MHC) types I and II. Our ability to use tissue typing and, perhaps in the future, tissues derived from embryonic stem cells may help to overcome the problems of nerve rejection.[13–17] Peripheral nerve tissue can be easily stored using cryoprotection to facilitate banking and tissue typing.[18,19] The goal

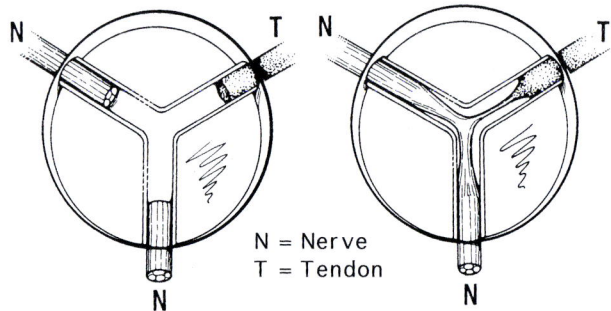

Figure 9A–1 A Y-shaped chamber was used to determine the specificity for nerve regeneration. Tropic (directional) factors allowed regenerating axons to selectively target nerve rather than tendon in downstream limbs of the chamber.

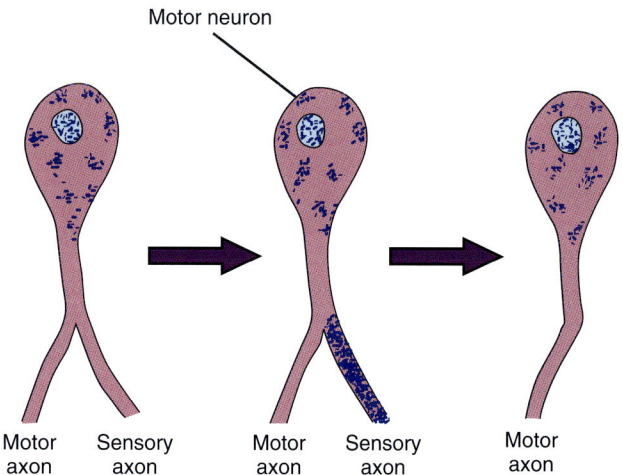

Figure 9A–2 Cutting back (pruning) of incorrect collateral projections. The neuron on the left has regenerated after transection of its axon. Collateral sprouts have formed with one entering the motor branch and one entering the sensory branch. Subsequently, the axonal collateral to the motor branch matures while its counterpart, the sensory branch, degenerates. This reflects tropic support to the collateral with the motor branch that is not available to the sensory axonal sprout. At the end of the process, on the right, the only projection remaining is the one to the correct motor pathway. (From Trumble T. Physiology and repair of peripheral nerves. In: Trumble T, ed., Principles of Hand Surgery and Therapy. Philadelphia: Elsevier Sciences, 2000:279–96,[1] with permission.)

is to avoid the need for chronic immunosuppression with toxic chemotherapy such as cyclosporin or FK506.[16,20] Finally, new methods of evaluating clinical recovery after grafting will allow us to compare methods of nerve repair and identify areas of even incremental improvement.[21–23]

NEUROTROPHISM VERSUS NEUROTROPISM

Neurotrophism is the ability of chemotactic hormonal or growth factors to enhance the rate of nerve regeneration, and neurotropism describes the directional accuracy of regeneration based on the alignment of the nerve at the time of repair. In early studies of neurotropism, the proximal end of a transected nerve was given the choice of two targets, one being a tendon stump and the other being a nerve stump (Fig. 9A–1).[24,25] This work demonstrated that the cut nerve end will preferentially grow toward the nerve stump rather than non-nerve tissue.

Elegant studies with double labels including different fluorescent markers for motor neurons (in the spinal cord) versus sensory neurons (in the dorsal root ganglion) showed that regenerating axons cannot differentiate between target motor versus sensory neurons (Fig. 9A–2).[26,27] In a parallel experiment using prelabeled sensory neurons in the dorsal root ganglion, it was shown that the sensory nerve axon sprouts and regenerates with the same random pattern as motor nerve axons (Fig. 9A–3).[28]

It has been further shown that a nerve gap at the repair site will result in greater dispersion of the regenerating axons, and studies using the adjacent peroneal and tibial branches of the sciatic nerve in a rat model have demonstrated that regenerating axons will target the largest and closest fascicle rather than the correct

distal nerve branch (Fig. 9A–4).[6] Based on this research, a surgeon would not want to use nerve chambers that leave a gap for the regenerating axons to cross because the axonal sprouts cannot make corrections in alignment. There is evidence that basement membrane glycoproteins such as L2/HNK-1 (uniquely expressed in the sheath of motor nerve axons) can selectively direct regenerating motor axonal sprouts.[7] In contrast, Ng-CAM/L1, N-CAM, and N-cadherin (CAD) are expressed by both motor and sensory nerve axons, and so would not likely lead to selective neurotropism of regenerating axons.

Bioengineering of Nerve Guides

Early studies of nerve guides evaluated hollow versus spun fiber guides. In a study of PLA spun guides, the guides with the lowest packing density of filaments allowed for the best axonal regeneration (Fig. 9A–5).[29]

In order to control the invasion of fibroblasts, a double-walled PLA guide was fashioned. An outer porous wall allowed for vascular ingrowth with diffusion of nutrients, while a less porous inner wall (coated with FGF to promote regeneration) prevented the invasion of fibroblasts (Fig. 9A–6 A).[30] The experimental groups with FGF demonstrated superior nerve regeneration.

In tests of another regeneration-promoting cytokine, a subcutaneous reservoir providing sustained delivery

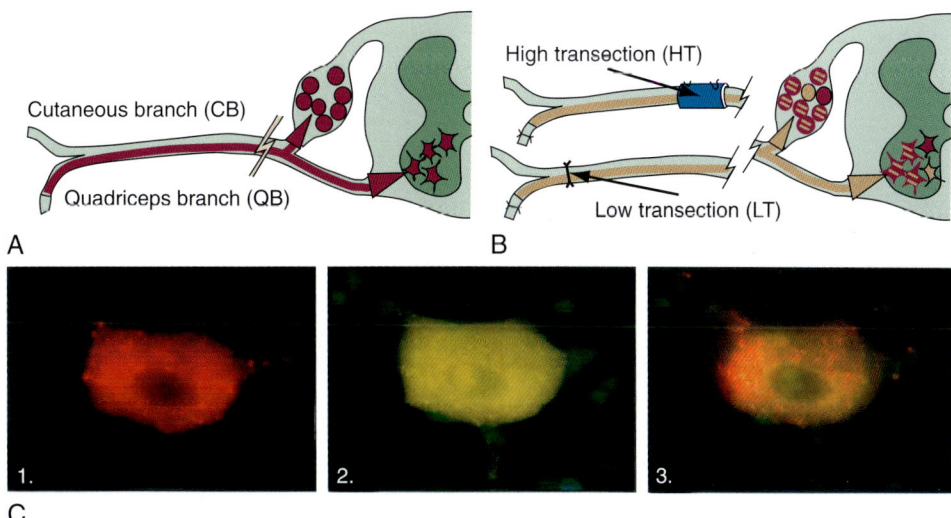

Figure 9A–3   Femoral nerve model for determining regeneration specificity. **A:** Initial retrograde labeling with DiI (Molecular Probes, Eugene OR) of the motor and sensory neuron pools innervating the terminal branch of the femoral nerve to the QB (quadriceps branch) before any experimental manipulation of the femoral nerve. **B:** Secondary retrograde labeling with fluorogold (FG) of the motor and sensory neurons that regenerate axons into the QB 4 weeks after transection and repair of the parent femoral nerve. One of two repair procedures was used: entubulation repair of a high femoral nerve transection *(HT)*, or a direct suture repair of a low femoral nerve transection *(LT)*. The suture marks distal to the FG application site indicate the location of the previous exposure to DiI (Molecular Probes, Eugene OR). **C:** Photomicrographs of a regenerated motor neuron label with both tracers: (1) rhodamine optics (DiI) (Molecular Probes, Eugene OR); (2) fluorogold *(FG)* (Fluorochrome, Inglewood, CO) optics; and (3) a double exposure using successive fluorogold rhodamine filter sets. (From Madison RD, Archibald SJ, Brushart TM. Reinnervation accuracy of the rat femoral nerve by motor and sensory neurons. J Neurosci 1996;16:5698–703,[28] with permission.)

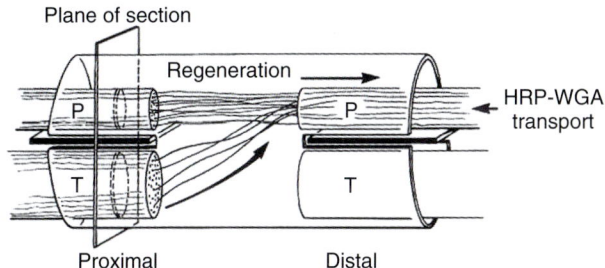

Figure 9A–4   Using a rat model with peroneal *(P)* and tibial *(T)* nerves, axons specifically targeted the closest nerve axon whether they were correctly aligned, as shown in this figure, or whether the alignment was reversed. There appears to be no directionality for a nerve axon to target the correct distal nerve stump. HRP-WGA, horseradish peroxidase-wheat germ agglutinin. (From Brushart TM, Mathur V, Sood R, et al. Boyes Award. Dispersion of regenerating axons across enclosed neural gaps. J Hand Surg Am 1995;20:557–64,[6] with permission.)

of NGF was studied in a rat model.[12] Animals receiving the sustained NGF dosing (to help overcome the short half-life of the growth factor) showed superior nerve regeneration across an implanted guide tube (Fig. 9A–6 B).

In contrast, some growth factors, such as insulin-derived growth factor (IGF), have not enhanced nerve regeneration through nerve guides.[31] Other substrates such as fibronectin and laminin have been used, but to date there has been no large-scale comparison trial to determine the most effective nerve guide and the best combination of growth factors and substrate.[32,33]

Comparison of Collagen Conduits versus Polyglycolic Acid Conduits

We have recently performed a comparison of collagen nerve conduits (Integra Neurosciences, Plainsboro, NJ), polyglycolic acid (PGA) conduits (Synovis, Birmingham, AL), and standard nerve grafting to bridge a 1.0-cm defect in the rat sciatic nerve (Fig. 9A–7 A) (Parisi et al., unpublished data). Twelve weeks after the surgery, the animals were sacrificed and the tissues harvested for axonal counts within and distal to the conduit and muscle weights of the tibialis anterior muscle. The collagen conduit resulted in significantly higher muscle weights (Fig. 9A–7 B) and axonal counts (Fig. 9A–7 C) than for either PGA conduit or nerve graft groups.

In an unpublished clinical series at our institution, nine patients with lesions of the radial sensory nerve or lateral antebrachial cutaneous nerve and gaps of under 1.0 cm were treated with synthetic nerve guides, with four patients randomized to receive polyglycolic acid tubes and five receiving collagen tubes. The conduits were sutured in place using horizontal mattress suture to pull the nerve end 2 to 3 mm into the conduit (Figs. 9A–8 and 9A–9). The conduit is filled with saline before completing the attachment of the conduit, to minimize risk of clotting the conduit. All regained protective sensibility, and avoided another sensory deficit and the donor site morbidity risk seen with nerve grafting. Two of four patients with PGA tubes experienced skin problems over the tube, while none of the five patients with collagen tubes had such problems.

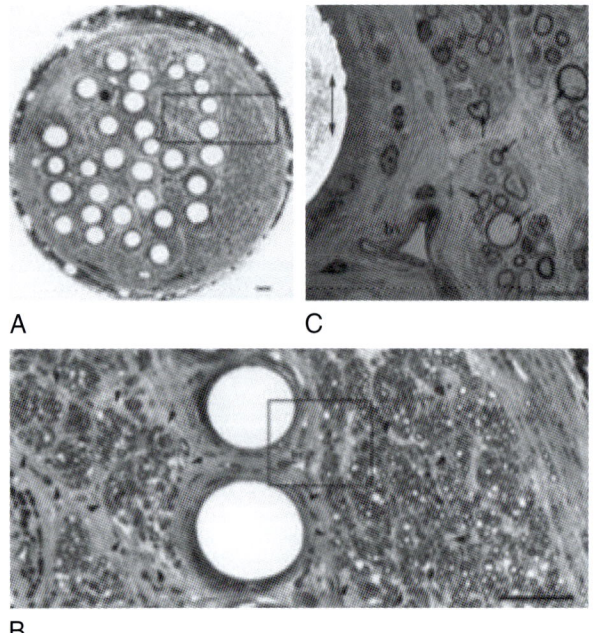

B

Figure 9A–5 Nerve guide of spun polylactic acid using different densities of microfilaments within the guide. The guide with the lowest density of microfilaments allowed the greatest regeneration of axons. Photomicrographs of regeneration across 1.0-cm lesioned gap of sciatic nerve in rats. **A:** Transverse cross-section of the distal end of a reconstituted nerve 10 weeks after implantation showing many well-defined fascicles. **B:** High magnification of one of the fascicles (box in **A**) showed bundles of myelinated axons surrounded by well-delineated perineurium *(arrowheads)*. **C:** Further examination of the nerve region (box in **B**) by TEM showed a number of unmyelinated axons (*) present within the endoneurial sheaths of Schwann cells as well as blood vessels *(bv)*. Myelinated axons *(arrows)* could also be seen a few microns away from the filament edge *(double-headed arrow)*, which was surrounded by thin layers of cells. Scale bars = 50 μm **(A, B)**; 10 μm **(C).** (From Ngo TT, Waggoner PJ, Romero AA, et al. Poly(L-Lactide) microfilaments enhance peripheral nerve regeneration across extended nerve lesions. J Neurosci Res 2003;72:227–38,[29] with permission.)

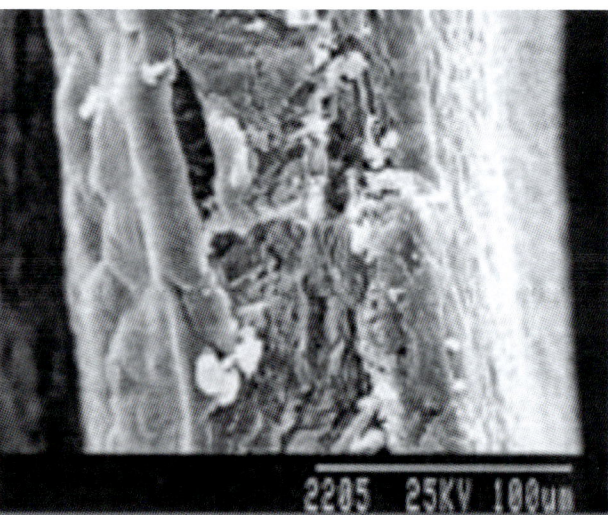

Figure 9A–6 Two-ply structure of a nerve guide made of poly (D,L-lactide). Outer layer is at *left,* inner layer at *right.* Original magnification ×500. (From Wang S, Cai Q, Hou J, et al. Acceleration effect of basic fibroblast growth factor on the regeneration of peripheral nerve through a 15-mm gap. J Biomed Mater Res 2003;66:522–31,[30] with permission.)

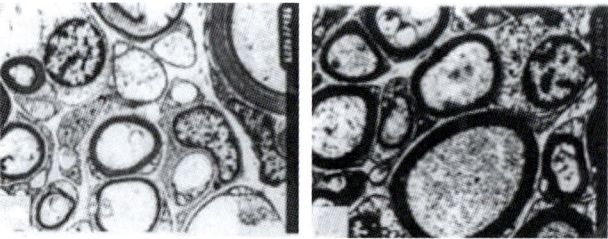

Figure 9A–7 SEM photos of regeneration of myelinated nerve fibers of rats in various groups: *left,* Group a, PDLLA tube without bFGF; *right,* Group b, PDLLA tube containing bFGF. Original magnification ×500. (From Wang S, et al., Center for Molecular Sciences, Institute of Chemistry, Chinese Academy of Sciences, Beijing, China, Nov. 2002, Fig. 8,[43] with permission.)

Assessing clinical cases at our trauma center that have been managed with synthetic nerve guide tubes, we have observed that limiting their use to shorter defects (<2 cm) and ensuring adequate soft-tissue coverage over the guide tube are crucial components of this technique in our hands (Figs. 9A–10 and 9A–11), and that (as others have reported)[34] the somewhat firmer, corrugated PGA tubes (as compared with the softer, but more expensive, collagen tubes) have been prone to irritate overlying skin, often resulting in delayed wound healing.

In summary, research into the ideal nerve conduit will need to determine the best substrate, the ideal porosity and density, and the optimal combination of incorporated growth factors—and perhaps even allogeneic Schwann or other cells. The ability to block the invasion of scar tissue and to release growth factors in the correct sequence may be important to optimize nerve regeneration.

Can Allograft Tissue Be Used in Nerve Grafts and Conduits?

Studies of nerve graft incorporation have demonstrated significant vascular in-growth preceding the regeneration axons traveling from proximal to distal. In fluorescent labeling studies, the label began to penetrate the graft within 3 days (Fig. 9A–12), and by 45 days the label had completely penetrated the 2.0-cm graft (Fig. 9A–13).

Nerve allografts will support nerve regeneration if immunosuppression is maintained. Without immunosuppression, the cells in the allograft are rejected, as shown by similar labeling studies[14,15,35] (Fig. 9A–14). Because of the toxicity of immunosuppressive chemotherapy, tissue typing to avoid rejection may be desirable—especially since banking nerve allografts is fairly practical.[15]

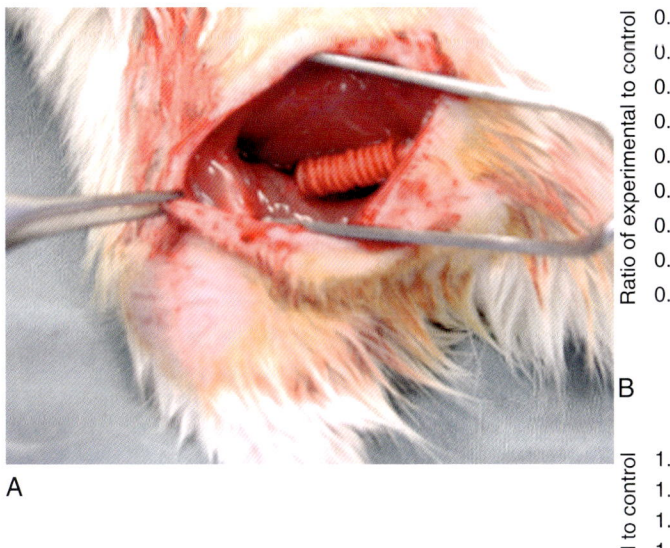

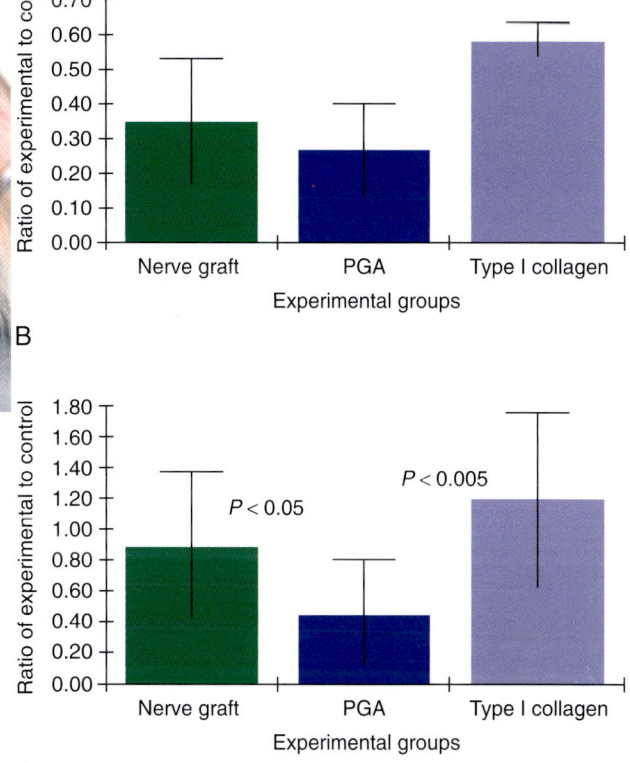

Figure 9A–8 **A:** This photograph demonstrates the polyglycolic acid (PGA) tube (Neurotube™, Secant Medical, Perkasie, PA) used to bridge a defect in the sciatic nerve in a rat model. **B:** This graph demonstrates greater muscle weights indicating improved nerve regeneration in the collagen tube as compared to the PGA tube. There is no significant difference between the control nerve autograft group and the collagen nerve tube. **C:** This graph demonstrates great axonal regeneration in the collagen conduit and the control nerve autograft as compared to the PGA tube.

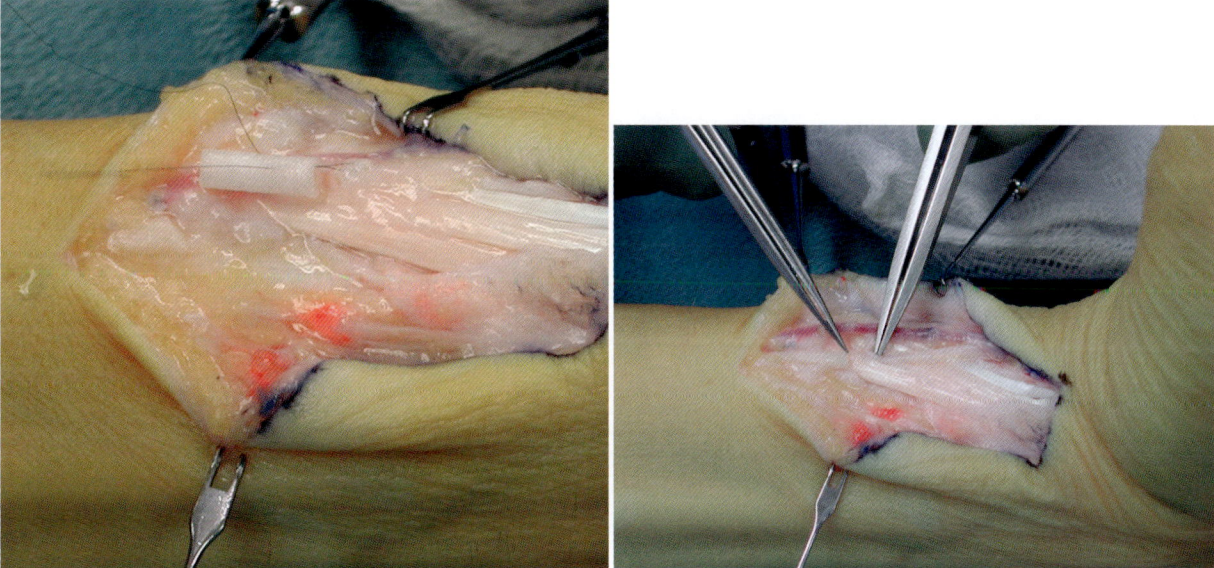

Figure 9A–9 Horizontal mattress suture from tube into nerve (epineurium) and back to tube allows fit of nerve end several millimeters into guide tube.

The chief barriers to allograft tissue usage are the major histocompatibility complex (MHC) markers. Class I markers are found on all cells and they involve the standard ABO blood typing, but MHC class II markers are highly variable and are associated with lymphocytes and special dendritic cells that populate skin and endothelium. The presence of MHC class II markers makes the use of vascularized grafts impossible without constant immunosuppression. Using special inbred strains of mice that only vary in either MHC class I or

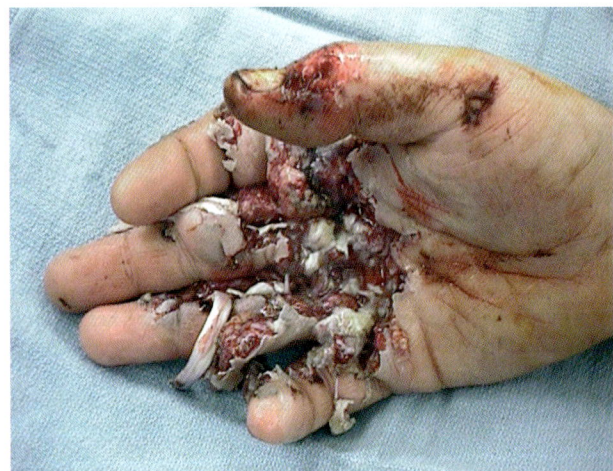

Figure 9A–10 Palmar avulsion of skin and nerves as a result of a motor vehicle injury with hand out window, abraded on road surface.

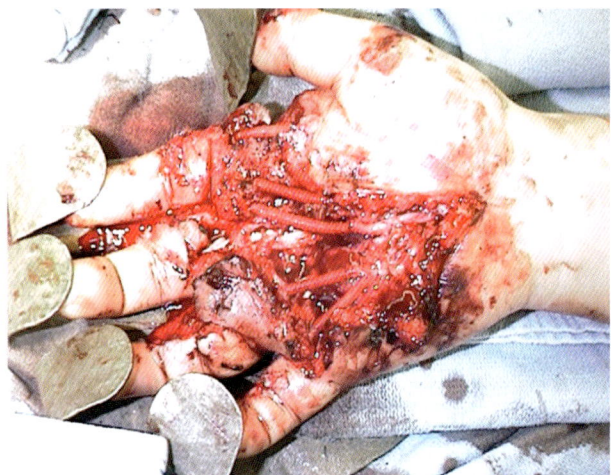

Figure 9A–11 Large gaps and poor soft tissue coverage yield poor results with the use of nerve tubes.

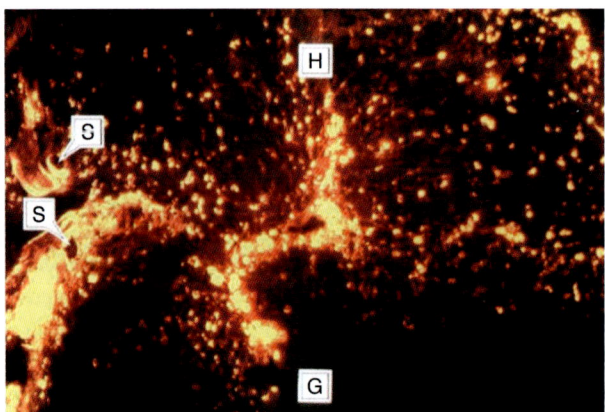

Figure 9A–12 This is a longitudinal section (magnification ×200) with the proximal or host nerve end *(H)* at the top and the distal or graft end *(G)* below. The suture line is marked. This section was taken 3 days after repair with a graft. The label is now penetrating the graft from the coapted nerve end along the lines of vascular ingrowth. S, sutures.

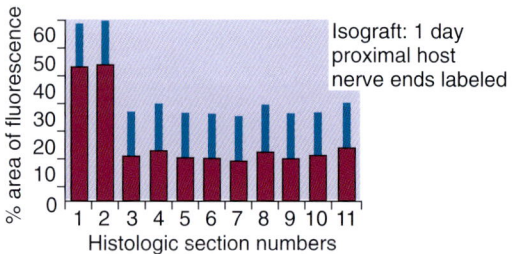

Isograft: 1 day
proximal host
nerve ends labeled

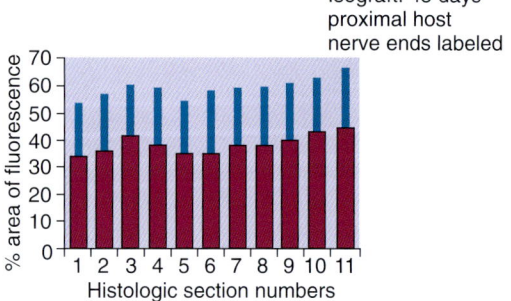

Isograft: 45 days
proximal host
nerve ends labeled

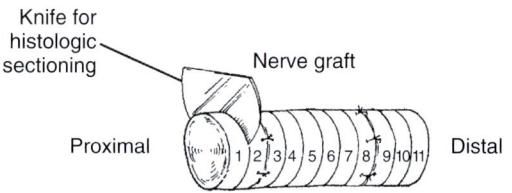

Nerve sections for histologic analysis

Figure 9A–13 Uptake of the fluorescent label at each of the histological sections along the course of the host nerve proximally, the intercalary nerve graft, and at the distal end of the host nerve as shown at the bottom of the figure. At day 1 there is only fluorescent label present at the proximal end of the nerve. By day 45, the label has penetrated all the way to the distal end of the graft.

Allograft: 45 days
nerve graft labeled

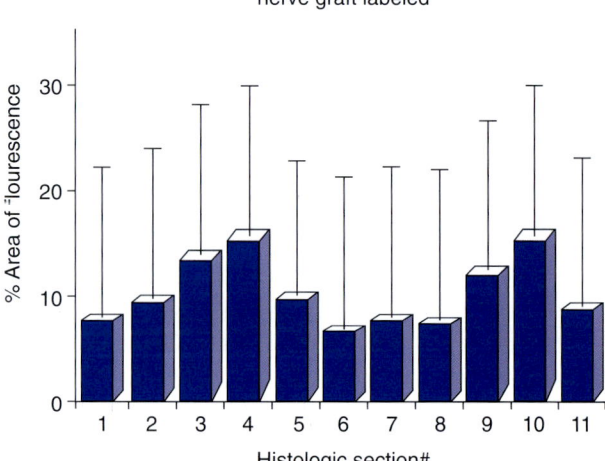

Figure 9A–14 Initially, the label is taken up by the allograft in a similar fashion, and by 45 days there is a substantial loss of label within the body of the graft indicating rejection when immunosuppression is not maintained. (From Trumble T. Physiology and repair of peripheral nerves. In: Trumble T, ed., Principles of Hand Surgery and Therapy. Philadelphia: Elsevier Sciences, 2000:279–96,[1] with permission.)

II, the effects of tissue typing for either MHC I or II or both have been evaluated.

Only a mismatch at both MHC I and II sites produced a significant rejection response[16] (Figs. 9A–15 and 9A–16). The prospect of tissue typing and the even more exciting opportunities for using embryonic stem cells means that the lattice of future bioengineered nerve conduits might be populated with stromal cells that can support regeneration.

Role of Vein Conduits for Nerve Gaps

Although some historical reports of vein conduits for nerve grafts can be identified dating back to 1891,[36] the modern use of these grafts began with the identification of regenerating axons in blood vessels by Chumasov and Chalisova.[37]

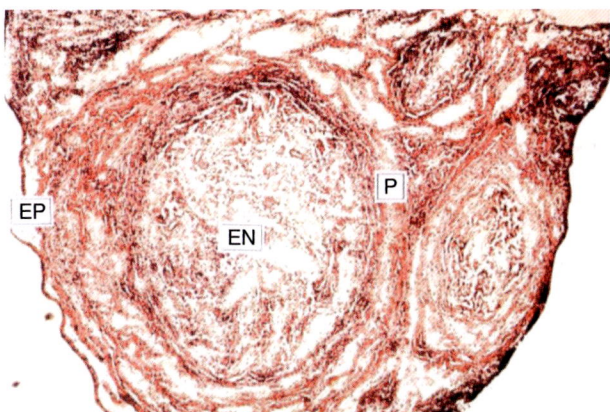

Figure 9A–15 Nerve cross-section (magnification ×200) of a nerve allograft with cross-match for MHC Class I antigens. No rejection is seen, and there is normal architecture of the nerve fascicles. EP, epineurium; EN, endoneurium; P, perineurium.

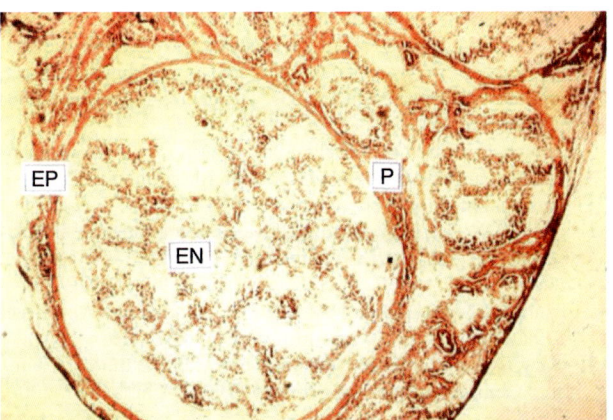

Figure 9A–16 This is a cross-section (magnification ×200) of an allogeneic nerve graft with mismatches at both MHC Class I and II sites. Rejection is underway, with lymphocytic infiltration into the structure of the nerve invading throughout the fascicles.

In a series of experiments by Chiu et al.,[38,39] nerve defects of 1.0 to 6.0 cm were evaluated. Although the use of nerve growth factors did improve the distance that the graft could support regeneration for up to 3.0 centimeters, the vein grafts did not perform as well as nerve autografts for distances over 1.0 cm. No regeneration was noted for distances over 3.0 cm.[40] The technique for the vein conduits includes suturing the reversed vein graft in place distally so that the valves in the vein cannot collapse and block axonal migration. The proximal repair is performed after filling the vein with saline to prevent clot formation that will produce scarring which can obstruct the axons.[41]

CONCLUSION

The quest to improve nerve regeneration is still one of the greatest challenges to surgeons and scientists. The ongoing improvements in our understanding of the complex interactions among the neuron, regenerating axons, and end organ have helped to guide research efforts. At this point we can at least envision the goals of designing nerve conduits with structural components that accurately match the nerve anatomy, and delivering the correct physiologic sequence of growth factors and cytokines in a sustained fashion over the entire period of regeneration. Accurate methods of assessing nerve regeneration and function recovery are very important in designing clinical trials. In a clinical evaluation of nerve grafts, the length of the graft and the delay to nerve grafting were key factors in success of the surgery.

A coordinated effort will be necessary to thoroughly evaluate the best graft design and to apply the grafts in multicentered trials.[22,23,42]

Dedication

To Sir Sidney Sunderland, M.D., and to Paul Brand, M.D. We recognize Sir Sidney Sunderland for his brilliant work on nerve repair and for his lifelong efforts to bring together the best clinicians and scientists to improve the science and surgery for nerve repair. Dr. Paul Brand set an example to all physicians by taking risks to treat patients with nerve injuries and nerve palsies due to leprosy with a special blend of compassion and science.—Thomas Trumble

To Nancy and Emily Anne, with thanks for your patience.—Chris Allan

REFERENCES

1. Trumble T. Physiology and repair of peripheral nerves. In: Trumble T, ed., Principles of Hand Surgery and Therapy. Philadelphia: Elsevier Sciences, 2000:279–96.

2. McCallister WV, Tang P, Smith J, et al. Axonal regeneration stimulated by the combination of nerve growth factor and ciliary neurotrophic factor in an end-to-side model. J Hand Surg Am 2001;26:478–88.

3. Bothwell M. Functional interactions of neurotrophins and neurotrophin receptors. Annu Rev Neurosci 1995;18:223–53.

4. Schatteman GC, Langer T, Lanahan AA, et al. Distribution of the 75-kD low-affinity nerve growth factor receptor in the primate peripheral nervous system. Somatosens Mot Res 1993;10: 415–32.

5. Al-Majed AA, Brushart TM, Gordon T. Electrical stimulation accelerates and increases expression of BDNF and trkB mRNA in regenerating rat femoral motoneurons. Eur J Neurosci 2000;12:4381–90.

6. Brushart TM, Mathur V, Sood R, et al. Boyes Award. Dispersion of regenerating axons across enclosed neural gaps. J Hand Surg Am 1995;20:557–64.

7. Martini R, Schachner M, Brushart TM. The L2/HNK-1 carbohydrate is preferentially expressed by previously motor axon-associated Schwann cells in reinnervated peripheral nerves. J Neurosci 1994;14:7180–91.

8. Nyilas E, Chiu TH, Sidman RL, et al. Peripheral nerve repair with bioresorbable prosthesis. Trans Am Soc Artifial Int Organs 1983;29:307–13.

9. Archibald SJ, Shefner J, Krarup C, et al. Monkey median nerve repaired by nerve graft or collagen nerve guide tube. J Neurosci 1995;15:4109–23.

10. Mears S, Schachner M, Brushart TM. Antibodies to myelin-associated glycoprotein accelerate preferential motor reinnervation. J Peripher Nerv Syst 2003;8:91–9.

11. Brushart TM, Hoffman PN, Royall RM, et al. Electrical stimulation promotes motoneuron regeneration without increasing its speed or conditioning the neuron. J Neurosci 2002;22:6631–8.

12. Santos X, Rodrigo J, Hontanilla B, et al. Evaluation of peripheral nerve regeneration by nerve growth factor locally administered with a novel system. J Neurosci Methods 1998;85:119–27.

13. Easterling KJ, Trumble TE. The treatment of peripheral nerve injuries using irradiated allografts and temporary host immunosuppression (in a rat model). J Reconstr Microsurg 1990; 6:301–10.

14. Trumble T, Gunlikson R, Parvin D. A comparison of immune response to nerve and skin allografts. J Reconstr Microsurg 1993;9:367–72.

15. Trumble TE, Parvin D. Cell viability and migration in nerve isografts and allografts. J Reconstr Microsurg 1994;10:27–34.

16. Trumble TE, Gunlikson R, Parvin D. Systemic immune response to peripheral nerve transplants across major histocompatibility class-I and class-II barriers. J Orthop Res 1994;12:844–52.

17. Trumble TE, Shon FG. The physiology of nerve transplantation. Hand Clin 2000;16:105–22.

18. Trumble TE, Whalen JT. The effects of cryosurgery and cryoprotectants on peripheral nerve function. J Reconstr Microsurg 1992;8:53–60.

19. Ruwe PA, Trumble TE. A functional evaluation of cryopreserved peripheral nerve autografts. J Reconstr Microsurg 1990;6: 239–44.

20. Doolabh VB, Mackinnon SE. FK506 accelerates functional recovery following nerve grafting in a rat model. Plast Reconstr Surg 1999;103:1928–36.

21. Trumble TE, Kahn U, Vanderhooft E, et al. A technique to quantitate motor recovery following nerve grafting. J Hand Surg Am 1995;20:367–72.

22. Trumble TE, Vanderhooft E, Khan U. Sural nerve grafting for lower extremity nerve injuries. J Orthop Trauma 1995;9:158–63.

23. Trumble T, Vanderhooft E. Nerve grafting for lower-extremity injuries. J Pediatr Orthop 1994;14:161–5.

24. Lundborg G, Dahlin LB, Danielsen N, et al. Nerve regeneration in silicone chambers: influence of gap length and of distal stump components. Exp Neurol 1982;76:361–75.

25. Lundborg G, Dahlin LB, Danielsen N, et al. Nerve regeneration across an extended gap: a neurobiological view of nerve repair and the possible involvement of neuronotrophic factors. J Hand Surg Am 1982;7:580–7.

26. Brushart TM, Seiler WD. Selective reinnervation of distal motor stumps by peripheral motor axons. Exp Neurol 1987;97:289–300.

27. Brushart TM. Preferential reinnervation of motor nerves by regenerating motor axons. J Neurosci 1988;8:1026–31.

28. Madison RD, Archibald SJ, Brushart TM. Reinnervation accuracy of the rat femoral nerve by motor and sensory neurons. J Neurosci 1996;16:5698–703.

29. Ngo TT, Waggoner PJ, Romero AA, et al. Poly(L-Lactide) microfilaments enhance peripheral nerve regeneration across extended nerve lesions. J Neurosci Res 2003;72:227–38.

30. Wang S, Cai Q, Hou J, et al. Acceleration effect of basic fibroblast growth factor on the regeneration of peripheral nerve through a 15-mm gap. J Biomed Mater Res 2003;66:522–31.

31. Fansa H, Schneider W, Wolf G, et al. Influence of insulin-like growth factor-I (IGF-I) on nerve autografts and tissue-engineered nerve grafts. Muscle Nerve 2002;26:87–93.

32. Yu X, Dillon GP, Bellamkonda RB. A laminin and nerve growth factor-laden three-dimensional scaffold for enhanced neurite extension. Tissue Eng 1999;5:291–304.

33. Ahmed Z, Underwood S, Brown RA. Nerve guide material made from fibronectin: assessment of in vitro properties. Tissue Eng 2003;9:219–31.

34. Weber RA, Breidenbach WC, Brown RE, et al. A randomized prospective study of polyglycolic acid conduits for digital nerve reconstruction in humans. Plast Reconstr Surg 2000; 106:1036–45, discussion 1046–8.

35. Trumble TE, Parvin D. Physiology of peripheral nerve graft incorporation. J Hand Surg Am 1994;19:420–7.

36. Buengner OV. Ueber die Degerations-und Regenerationsvorgaenge am Nerven nach Verletzungen. Beitr Pathol Anat 1891;10:321.

37. Chumasov E, Chalisova NI. Peripheral nerve regeneration in the lumen of implanted blood vessels. Bull Eksp Bio Med 1983;96:104–7.

38. Chiu DTW, Janecka I, Krizek TJ. Autogenous vein graft as a conduit for regeneration. Surgery 1982;91:226–33.

39. Chiu DTW, Lovelace RE, Yu LT. Comparative electrophysiologic evaluation of nerve grafts and autogenous vein grafts as nerve conduits: an experimental study. J Reconstr Microsurg 1988; 4:303–9.

40. Strauch B, Ferder M, Lovelle-Allan S. Determing the maximal length of a vein conduit used as an interposition graft for nerve regeneration. J Reconstr Microsurg 1996;12:521–7.

41. Chiu DTW, Strauch B. A prospective clinical evaluation of autologous vein grafts used as a nerve conduit for distal sensory nerve defects of 3 cm or less. Plast Reconstr Surg 1990;82:928–34.

42. Trumble TE, McCallister WV. Repair of peripheral nerve defects in the upper extremity. Hand Clin 2000;16:37–52.

43. Wang S, et al. Center for Molecular Sciences, Institute of Chemistry, Chinese Academy of Sciences, Beijing, China, Nov. 2002, Fig. 8.

CLINICAL RESULTS WITH THE POLYGLYCOLIC ACID NEUROTUBE™ FOR NERVE REPAIR AND RECONSTRUCTION

A. Lee Dellon

INTRODUCTION

When I was involved in my first research with peripheral nerve evaluation in medical school at Johns Hopkins University, Hanno Millesi was perfecting his technique for interfascicular interposition nerve grafting.[1] Raymond Curtis, who began Hand Surgery in Baltimore, was a friend of Millesi, and so I was aware of this technique in the early years of my interest in plastic surgery. Millesi's pioneering adventures in this area are described well in his chapter in this book. By 1978, when I had finished my hand surgery fellowship with Curtis and my plastic surgery residency at Johns Hopkins Hospital, I was a firm believer in nerve grafting for any length defect in any peripheral nerve, and, with one caveat, I still am committed to nerve reconstruction with nerve grafts. As with all surgical techniques, there are potential complications; the implications of nerve grafting include a nerve graft donor site scar, donor nerve sensory loss, and the possibility of a painful neuroma forming at the harvesting site. Interfascicular nerve grafting carried another theoretical, and sometimes practical problem: there were two sets of suture lines, and thus two regions to form a painful in-continuity neuroma.[2]

While these risks were acceptable to the surgeon, and usually to the patient, the possibility existed that there might be a way to reconstruct relatively small peripheral nerve defects with a technique that was being investigated in the laboratory; a technique called "entubulation."[3–5] This technique employed some form of nerve wrapping or conduit. Wrapping the nerve repair site, attempting to confine the axonal sprouting, and guiding the sprouts along the conduit, held the promise of permitting more axons to reach their target destination guided by neurobiological events rather than the microsurgical placement of sutures in the interfascicular epineurium and perineurium. A problem that I noted with the laboratory models being used was that the nerves would only regenerate 10 mm in the rat sciatic nerve model when silicone tubes were used. Silicone tubes were favored over other materials because fluids could be harvested from within these nonporous tubes for evaluation of neurotrophic substances, such as nerve growth factor. In addition, various substances could be added to the tube to examine their effect on neural regeneration.[6]

In 1981, Susan Mackinnon did her hand surgery fellowship with us in Baltimore. Mackinnon and I developed a model for chronic nerve compression that utilized a nonconstricting silicone tube to create the site of nerve compression.[7] I thus became aware of a second problem with the use of silicone as the conduit for neural regeneration; in time it would cause nerve compression and have to be removed.

During this time period, Goran Lundborg, in Sweden, had pioneered the use of a vascularized pseudosheath for nerve regeneration.[8] He also demonstrated that the peripheral nerve in the rat, given a choice, would regenerate preferentially toward a nerve rather than toward non-neural tissues.[9] Mackinnon and I, utilizing Lundborg's concept created a 30-mm long vascularized pseudosheath that we used to reconstruct a 3-cm ulnar nerve defect at the elbow in a subhuman primate (i.e., a baboon). To our surprise, by 7 months, there was a conducted compound nerve action potential.[10] We then collaborated with Lundborg in repeating his work on neurotropism in a monkey model. We showed that the primate peripheral nerve, would also preferentially grow toward neural tissue rather than non-neural tissue, and, more so toward an intact nerve with a distal target as compared to an isolated piece of nerve.[11] In order for this technique to have clinical applications in a hand surgery practice, one requirement would include a tube that could be placed once, without the need for removal. Mackinnon and I chose to create a tube from absorbable sutures. Polyglycolic acid was already used as an absorbable suture[12] and was available as a sheet.[13] We thus began to "roll our own" tubes from these polyglycolic acid (PGA) sheets to form PGA tubes.

At present, silicone tubes are being employed in clinical practice.[14–16] Because the nerve will only regenerate a short distance through this type of tube, a silicone tube is indicated only for a primary or secondary nerve repair, and cannot be used to reconstruct a nerve defect. As we predicted, many patients required a second operation to remove the silicone tube as it created a site of chronic nerve compression after the nerve had regenerated.[17–19]

Mackinnon and I went on to peform a series of inter-fascicular interposition sural nerve grafts to reconstruct a 3-cm ulnar nerve defect at the elbow in monkeys, and compared the results to those obtained following the use of a 3-cm bioabsorbable PGA tube. One year later, both the sural nerve graft and the PGA tube had comparable results by electrodiagnostic evaluation and histomorphometric analysis: In other words, the degree of nerve regeneration following reconstruction of a 3-cm nerve gap with the PGA tube compared favorably to the gold standard of sural nerve grafting. We also noted electromyographic (EMG) evidence of intrinsic muscle reinnervation, which would be unlikely following reconstruction of a similar proximal ulnar nerve defect in humans.[20] It was time to proceed with our first clinical use of the PGA tube, which we now call the Neurotube™.

EARLY CLINICAL RESULTS WITH THE NEUROTUBE™

The first use of the Neurotube™ was for reconstruction of failed digital nerve repairs and failed median nerve repairs. The results of the first clinical series was reported in 1990.[21] In each patient, the previous failed nerve repair was resected, and replaced with a piece of PGA mesh that had been rolled and heat welded to form a tube. The initial primate experimental data demonstrated that a 3.0-cm gap could be crossed. Subsequent primate experiments showed that reinnervation was incomplete across a 5.0-cm gap. This prompted us to restrict the clinical use of the Neurotube™ to those patients[22] with a nerve gap of less than 3.0 cm.

Sixteen patients who underwent digital nerve reconstruction, with a mean gap of 1.7 cm. Of the four patients who underwent median nerve reconstruction, the mean gap was 2.4 cm. The surgical technique for insertion of the Neurotube™ is illustrated in Fig. 9B–1. A clinical example of the current version of the 2.3-mm-diameter Neurotube™ used to reconstruct a common volar digital nerve is provided in Fig. 9B–2. Each patient received sensory re-education[23] postoperatively and was assessed at final follow-up with static and moving two-point discrimination.[24] The results of this study are given in Tables 9B–1 and 9B–2. In comparison to the historic results achieved with nerve grafts, whereby only 10% of adult patients were expected to achieve excel-

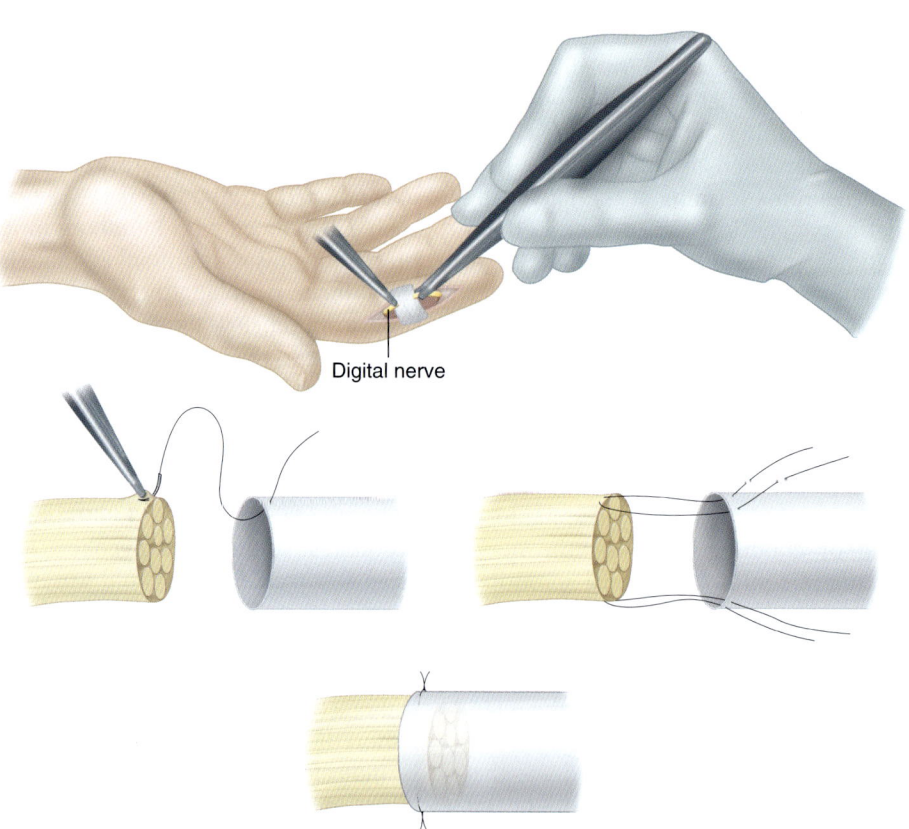

Digital nerve

Figure 9B–1 Technique for connection of nerve to Neurotube™. An 8-0 nylon suture is placed from outside the conduit into the inside, then horizontally through the epineurium, and then back again into the tube, and then out to the outside of the tube. This completes a horizontal suture that pulls the nerve 5 mm into the inside of the tube. An additional suture can be placed at 180 degrees to this just from the edge of the conduit to the epineurium.

TABLE 9B–1					
Results of First Clinical Neurotube™ Study, Digital Nerves					
	Normal		**Reconstructed Finger**		
	Autonomous	*Tip*	*Autonomous Reconstructed*	*Tip*	*Autonomous Normal*
Moving 2pd (mm)	2.7	2.6	3.3	3.1	2.9
Static 2pd (mm)	3.4	3.2	4.6	3.8	4.0

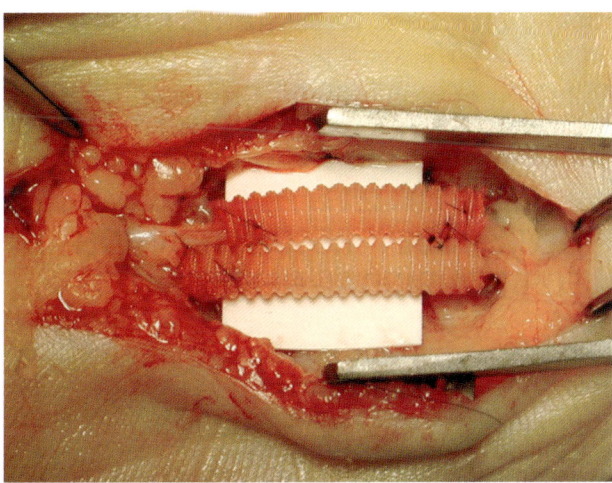

Figure 9B–2 Intraoperative example of two Neurotubes™ in place for reconstruction of a common volar digital nerve defect in the distal palm.

TABLE 9B–2			
Results of First Clinical Neurotube™ Study, Median Nerves			
	Thumb	**Index**	**Middle**
Moving 2pd (mm)	3.7	4.0	3.3
Static 2pd (mm)	5.7	5.0	5.3

lent results at 5 years following digital nerve grafting, and only 1% following median nerve grafting, the results of our first study demonstrated that 80% of the patients achieved excellent results following nerve tube reconstruction of digital nerve defects, with 75% achieving excellent results following the median nerve reconstruction at 1 year.

About this time, an opportunity arose to reconstruct a cranial nerve with a Neurotube™. A patient had the inferior alveolar nerve (mandibular branch of the fifth cranial nerve) avulsed during extraction of a third molar. The patient had jaw pain and a numb lip. A groove was fashioned in the mandible, and the inferior alveolar nerve was put into the tube proximally, and the mental nerve placed into the tube distally. At 6 months, neurosensory testing demonstrated sensory recovery in the lower lip, which by 1 year was approximating normal sensation in the lip.[25]

RANDOMIZED PROSPECTIVE MULTICENTER STUDY USING THE NEUROTUBE™ FOR THE FEDERAL DRUG ADMINISTRATION

The first ever randomized, prospective, multicenter, blinded study of the use of a nerve conduit for reconstruction of a sensory nerve defect in the hand was reported in 2000 by Weber et al.[26] The conduit used was the Neurotube™, formerly distributed by NeuroRegen LLC (Bel Air, MD), and, as of December 2004, by Synovis Microsystems (Synovis, Birmingham, AL). This study, conducted at the University of Chicago (orthopedics and plastic surgery), the Louisville Hand Surgery Group (Jackson, MS, principal investigator, Michael E. Jabaley, and San Antonio, TX, principal investigator, David Green), and Southern Illinois University (principal investigators, Richard Brown and Robert Russel). Inclusion criteria included any patient who underwent surgical exploration for a potential digital nerve injury in the hand, and that the nerve tissue defect if any was 3 cm or less. If there was a nerve injury, the treatment was randomized to either a standard nerve repair if the gap was less than 4 mm, or a nerve graft for larger defects, or a Neurotube™. Each therapist who provided the postoperative sensory re-education and who made the final measurement was blinded as to the surgical technique used to reconstruct the defect. All surgeons at each institution received the same surgical training regarding the nerve repair and the use of the conduit by David Seiler, and who also served as the clinical monitor for the multicenter study. Robert Weber, a plastic surgeon and hand surgeon from the Scott and White Clinic in Temple, TX, analyzed the results and wrote the paper for the study group. Neither Mackinnon nor myself participated in that study. The study took about 4 years from start to finish. The study included 136 injured nerves in 98 patients, with sharp injuries accounting for 72%. The mean follow-up was 10.5 months, with 77 patients being followed for 1 year.

The results of that study were that the Neurotube™ resulted in a statistically significant better recovery of sensation for digital nerve gaps of less than 4 mm as compared to an end-to-end nerve repair, and a statistically significantly better recovery of sensation for digital nerve gaps greater than 8 mm when compared to a nerve graft. Excellent results (moving two-point discrimination less than 4 mm or static two-point discrimination less than 6 mm) were obtained in 10 of 11 patients (91%) with nerve repairs performed with use of the PGA tube, with a group average moving two-point discrimination of 3.7 ± 1.4 mm, whereas only 19 of 39 patients (49%) whose nerves were repaired by the end-to-end method achieved excellent results and had an average two-point discrimination of 6.1 ± 3.3 mm ($p = 0.02$ and 0.03, respectively). A comparison of the eight nerve-grafted repairs with the 17 conduit repairs showed that the conduit group achieved significantly better sensory recovery. In the greater than 8-mm nerve gap group, there were 0% excellent results in the control group and 42% excellent results in the Neurotube™ group ($p < 0.06$), with the mean static two-point discrimination being 12.9 mm in the control group and 6.8 mm in the Neurotube™ group ($p < 0.001$).[26] This study suggests that one should consider the use of a nerve conduit for primary digital nerve repairs with gaps of up to 30 mm. Based on this study, the U.S. Food and Drug Administration approved the Neurotube™ for clinical use in 1997. Seventeen years from the time Mackinnon and I began working on reconstructing nerve injuries with a bio-absorbable, one-stage PGA conduit, it was approved for human use in the United States.

Another series of digital nerve injuries reconstructed with the Neurotube™ was published in 2003.[27] A prospective study was carried out in which all patients requiring primary or secondary digital nerve reconstruction in the palm or finger were reconstructed using the same technique in two different centers. Rehabilitation was deferred in that in one center the patients were not always available for sensory re-education. A total of 24 patients had 28 nerves reconstructed. Age ranged from 15 to 73, with a mean of 44 years. Follow-up ranged from 6 to 74 months, with a mean of 26 months. The nerve gap ranged from 1.0 to 4.0, with a mean of 2.1 cm. Overall, there were 11 with an excellent result (39%), 11 with a very good result (39%), 4 with a good result (13%), and 2 with a poor result (7%). The two poor results and one good result were all in a single patient with a severe crush injury, including the single gap of 4 cm. Of the 19 nerves for which sensory re-education was given, there were 11 excellent (58%) and 8 very good (42%) results, compared with the 9 nerves for which no sensory re-education was given, for which there were no excellent results, 3 very good results (33%), 4 good results (44%), and 2 poor results (23%). Significantly better results were achieved in the group that received sensory re-education ($p < 0.001$). It was

concluded that digital sensory nerve reconstruction with the Neurotube™ provided good to excellent recovery of two-point discrimination following nerve injury in 78% of patients, and that the success rate can be increased to 100% good to excellent results when sensory re-education is added, providing that crush injuries that extend beyond the 3-cm zone of reconstruction are excluded. This study added to the literature in that it permitted a comparison of patients who did not have sensory re-education to those that did have this rehabilitation, with the patients who had the sensory re-education having statistically significantly better results. The typical postoperative range of motion for a digit is demonstrated in Fig. 9B–3. This patient is a dentist and a guitar player with an ulnar digital nerve injury in the little finger after a crush injury.

NEUROTUBE™ RECONSTRUCTION FOR NONDIGITAL NERVES

Table 9B–3 outlines current clinical reports that have used the Neurotube™ to reconstruct nerve defects. The *plantar digital nerve* is analogous to the palmar digital nerve, and is subject to trauma as well.[28] Fig. 9B–4 demonstrates the reconstruction of a painful neuroma of the digital nerve to the medial side of the big toe in an 11-year-old boy who sustained a glass injury at age 6. He had walked on the lateral aspect of his foot due to pain, and was immobilized for 4 weeks. Then he began water walking. Eight weeks after the Neurotube™ construction, he could walk normally, and at 12 weeks resume gym activities in school. By 8 months, he had regained normal moving and static two-point discrimination in his big toe, and remained without pain. I have a second patient, an adult, with a similar result after a riding lawnmower injury, who, at 1 year after the reconstruction of the painful interdigital neuroma to the big

TABLE 9B–3	
Clinical Reports for Neurotube™	
Peripheral Nerve Reconstructed	**Date of Report**
Ulnar nerve at elbow (monkey)[20]	1988
Sensory nerve: upper extremity	
Digital and median at the wrist[21]	1990
Digital[25]	2000
Digital[27]	2003
Sensory nerve: foot[28]	2001
Cranial nerves: sensory	
V (inferior alveoloar)[26]	1992
Cranial nerve: motor	
VII (facial)[29]	2005
XI (spinal accessory)[30]	2005
Median nerve in the forearm[31]	2005
Median and ulnar nerves in brachium[32]	2005
Distal ulnar motor, forearm[32]	2005

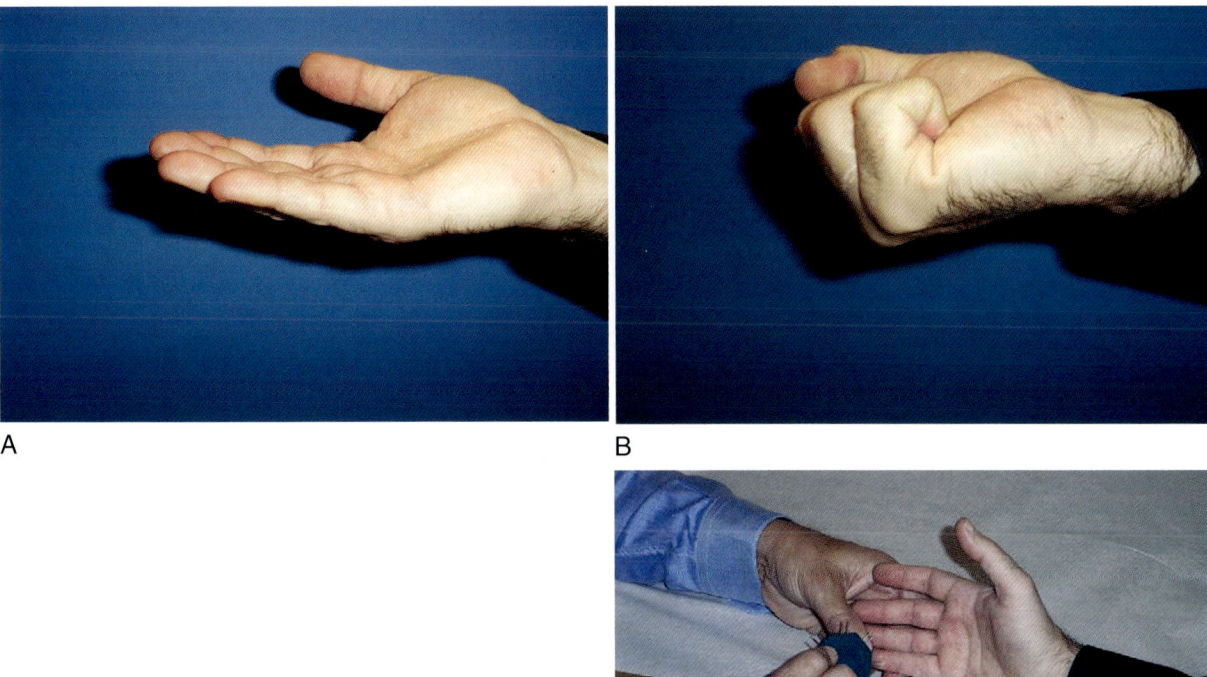

A   B

C

Figure 9B–3   Postoperative illustration of range of motion and sensibility achieved 6 months after placement of Neurotube™ into ulnar digital nerve defect of the little finger at the proximal phalangeal level. **A:** Full extension. **B:** Full flexion of finger. **C:** Static two-point discrimination with the Disk-Criminator is 4 mm in the autonomous zone of the digit.

toe, returned to work wearing normal footwear. This patient has not been separately reported.

The *facial nerve* is a cranial (VII) motor nerve. The microsurgery team at the University of Turino, Italy, is in the process of reporting a series of seven patients with acute injury to the facial nerve who have had the nerve gap reconstructed with a Neurotube™.[29] Facial motor function was restored in each of these patients.

The *spinal accessory nerve,* the XI cranial nerve, is a motor nerve. A woman who had her spinal accessory nerve injured during a lymph node biopsy was reconstructed at 3 months from the time of her injury (Fig. 9B–5). Instead of using the greater auricular nerve as a graft to reconstruct the 2.5-cm defect, a Neurotube™ was used. By 4 months after the reconstruction, she had EMG evidence of reinnervation of the trapezius, and by 6 months could hold her arm over her head.[30]

The *median nerve in the forearm* has been reconstructed with four interposition interfascicular Neurotubes™ in four patients. The first two patients were presented to the American Society for Peripheral Nerve Surgery in 2002, and now have 4-year follow-ups.[31] An example of one of these reconstructions is given in Fig. 9B–6. This man had division of his median nerve in the forearm during an open carpal tunnel decompression. He is 63 years old, and was reconstructed at 10 months after the injury. His motor branch was separately iden-

tified on the radial volar aspect of the median nerve, and reconstructed with a separate tube. He received sensory re-education postoperatively. By 1 year, he had excellent localization in his palm, thumb, index, and middle finger. At 4 years after the reconstruction, he has regained 5-mm static two-point discrimination in his thumb and index finger, and has regained thenar motor function (Fig. 9B–6).

Median and ulnar nerve reconstruction in the brachium was required for a 53-year-old man after a glass laceration in the right axilla. The brachial artery was repaired primarily. At 3 months, reconstruction of the divided ulnar nerve was done with two 2.3 mm, and the median nerve with three 2.3-mm Neurotubes™. At 18 months, forearm muscle bulk is evident (Fig. 9B–7), and EMG documented reinnervation of these muscles. With intensive sensory re-education, he had excellent localization to each fingertip by 24 months.

The *larger diameter Neurotube™* is now available. A damaged median nerve in a 71-year-old woman was reconstructed 3 years after it was injured in an open carpal tunnel decompression (Fig. 9B–8 A). The defect was 3.5 cm. The 4.0 mm diameter tube at present is only available in 2.0-cm lengths (Fig. 9A–8 B). For this reconstruction, two of these tubes were sutured end to end with 7-0 nylon, and because the gap length was greater than 3.0 cm, a source of nerve growth factor, a

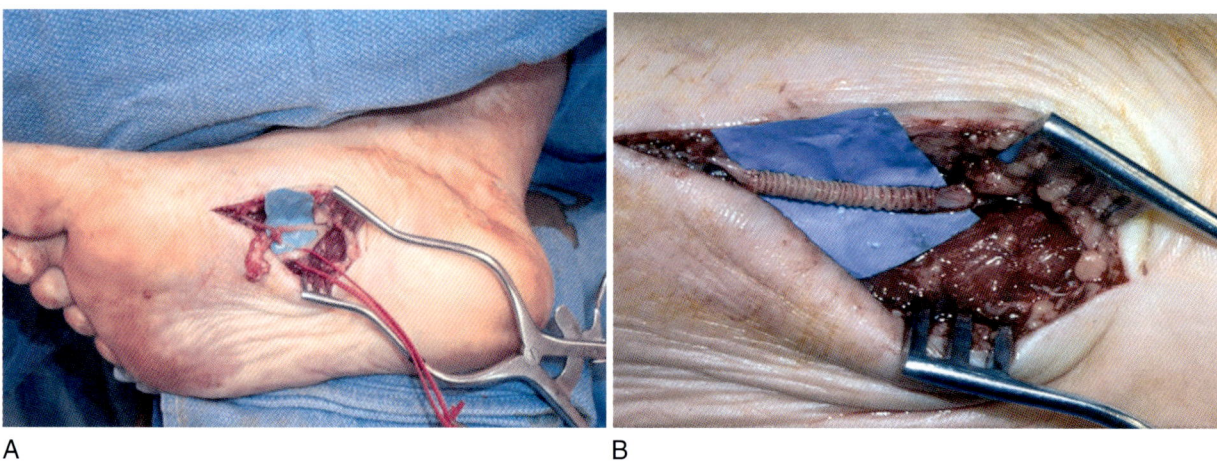

A   B

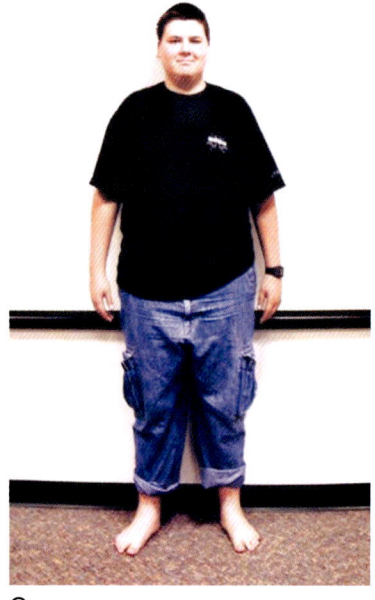

C

Figure 9B–4 Intraoperative demonstration of a painful neuroma-in-continuity 5 years after a glass injury to the foot in a 6-year-old boy. **A:** The neuroma in-continuity of the medial digital nerve to the big toe with an intact interdigital nerve to the first web space. **B:** The Neurotube™ reconstruction. **C:** One-year postoperative result.

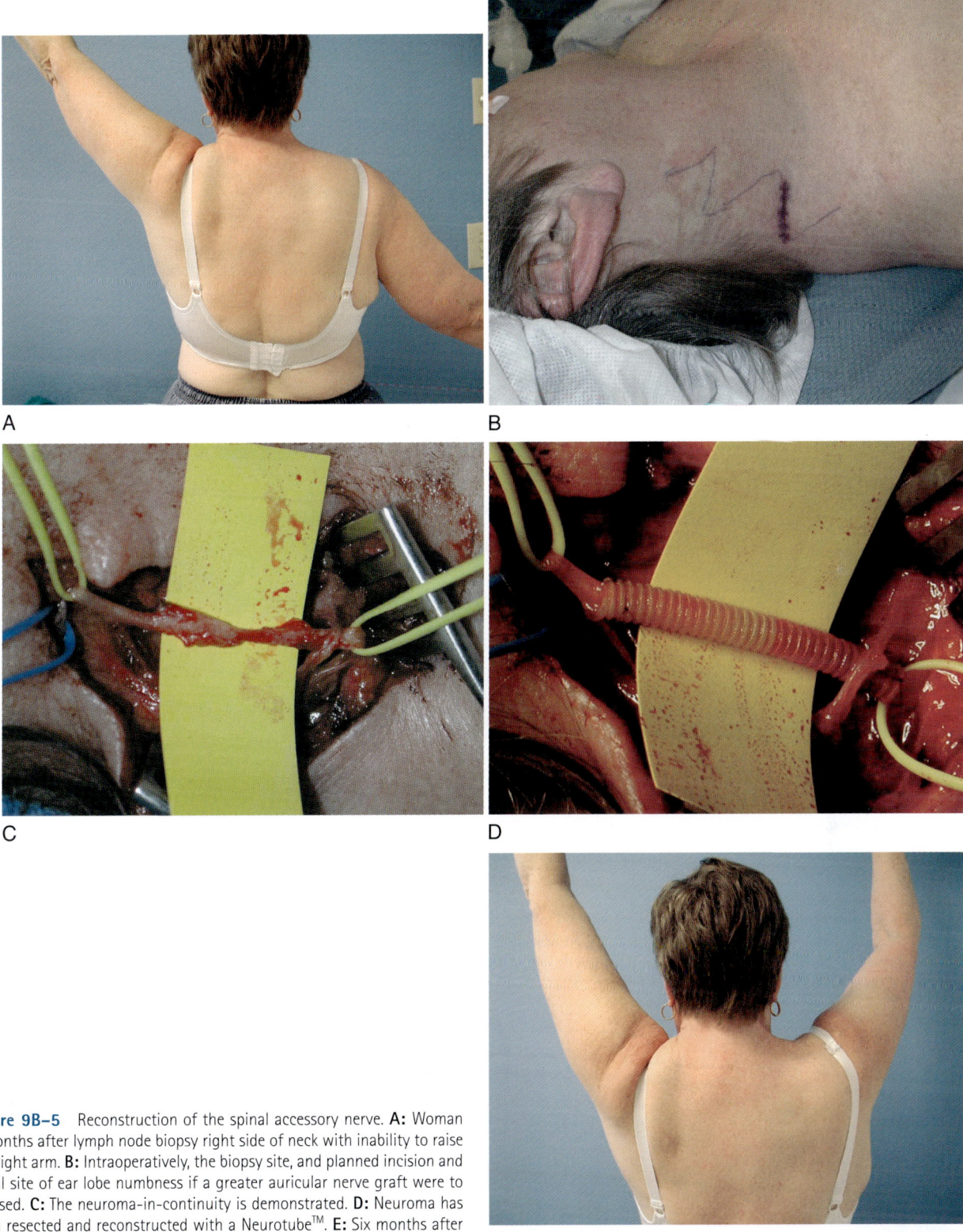

Figure 9B–5 Reconstruction of the spinal accessory nerve. **A:** Woman 3 months after lymph node biopsy right side of neck with inability to raise the right arm. **B:** Intraoperatively, the biopsy site, and planned incision and usual site of ear lobe numbness if a greater auricular nerve graft were to be used. **C:** The neuroma-in-continuity is demonstrated. **D:** Neuroma has been resected and reconstructed with a Neurotube™. **E:** Six months after the surgery, complete trapezius muscle restoration of function.[30]

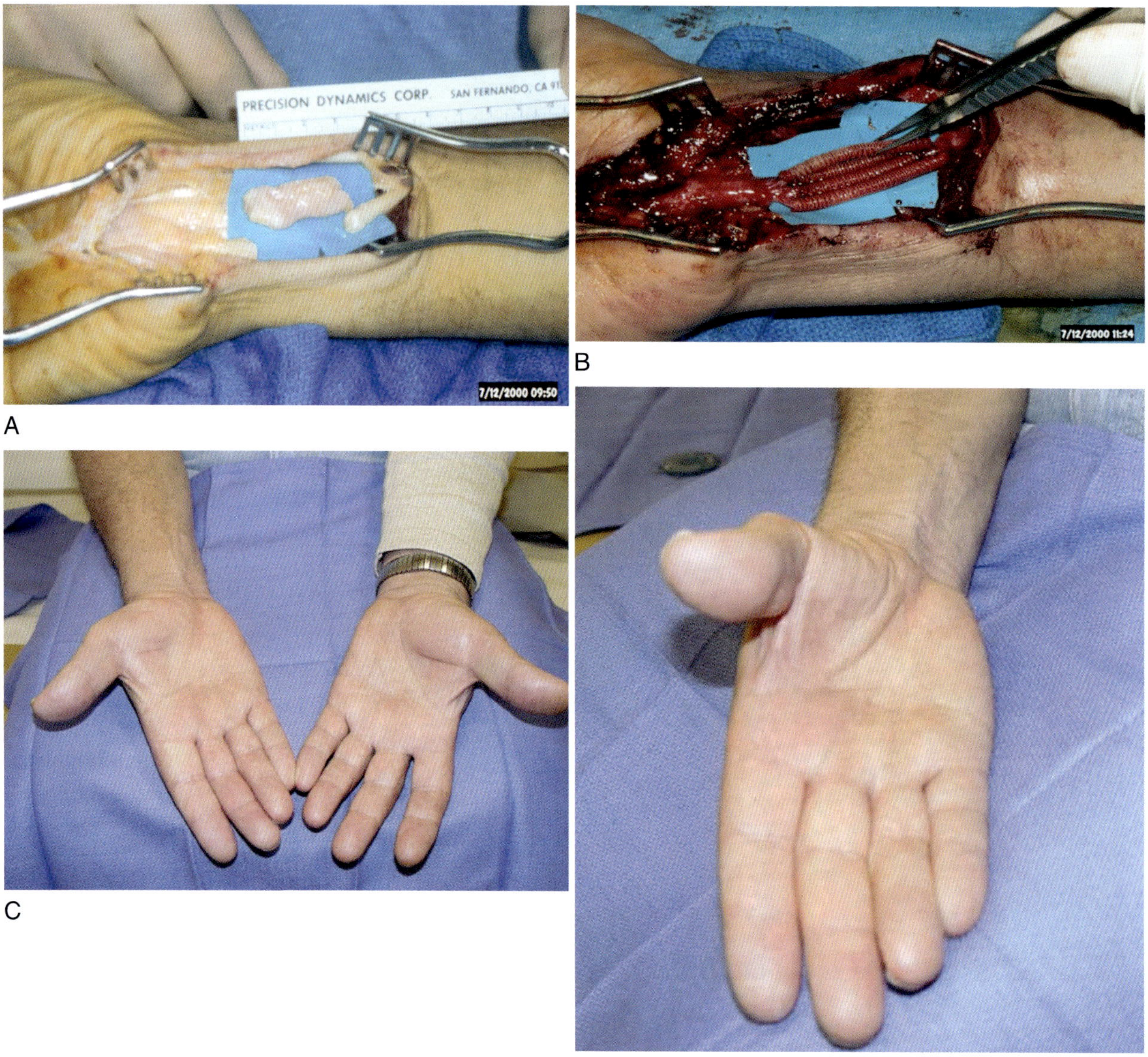

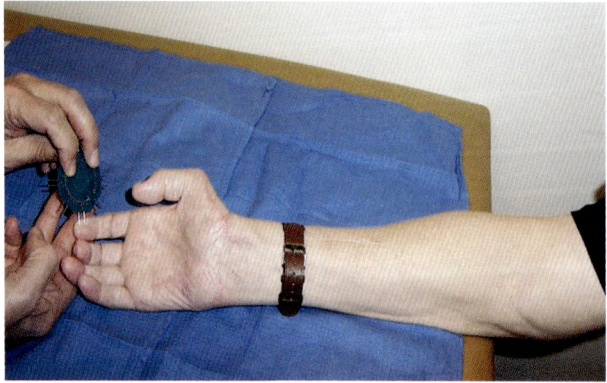

Figure 9B–6   Reconstruction of the neuroma-in-continuity of the right median nerve in the forearm of a 63-year-old man who had an injury to the median nerve during an open carpal tunnel surgery. **A:** Resection of the neuroma demonstrating the 3 cm gap in the median nerve. Tournique inflated. **B:** Interfascicular reconstruction of the defect with four 2.3-mm diameter Neurotubes™, each 4 cm in length. **C:** At 4 years following the reconstruction, good thenar bulk. **D:** At 4 years postreconstruction, EMG demonstrated median nerve motor function.[31]

Figure 9B–7   Reconstruction of the median and ulnar nerve at the level of the brachium, 18 months ago postsurgery in a 53-year-old man injured with glass. Note the recovered bulk of the forearm muscles. Electromyographic evidence of reinnervation of the flexor carpi radialis, flexor profundus, flexor superficialis, pronator, and flexor carpi ulnaris was obtained. Sensation was recovered in the fingertips with two-point discrimination and good localization by 24 months after the Neurotube™ reconstruction. Two tubes were placed for the ulnar nerve and three for the median nerve.[32]

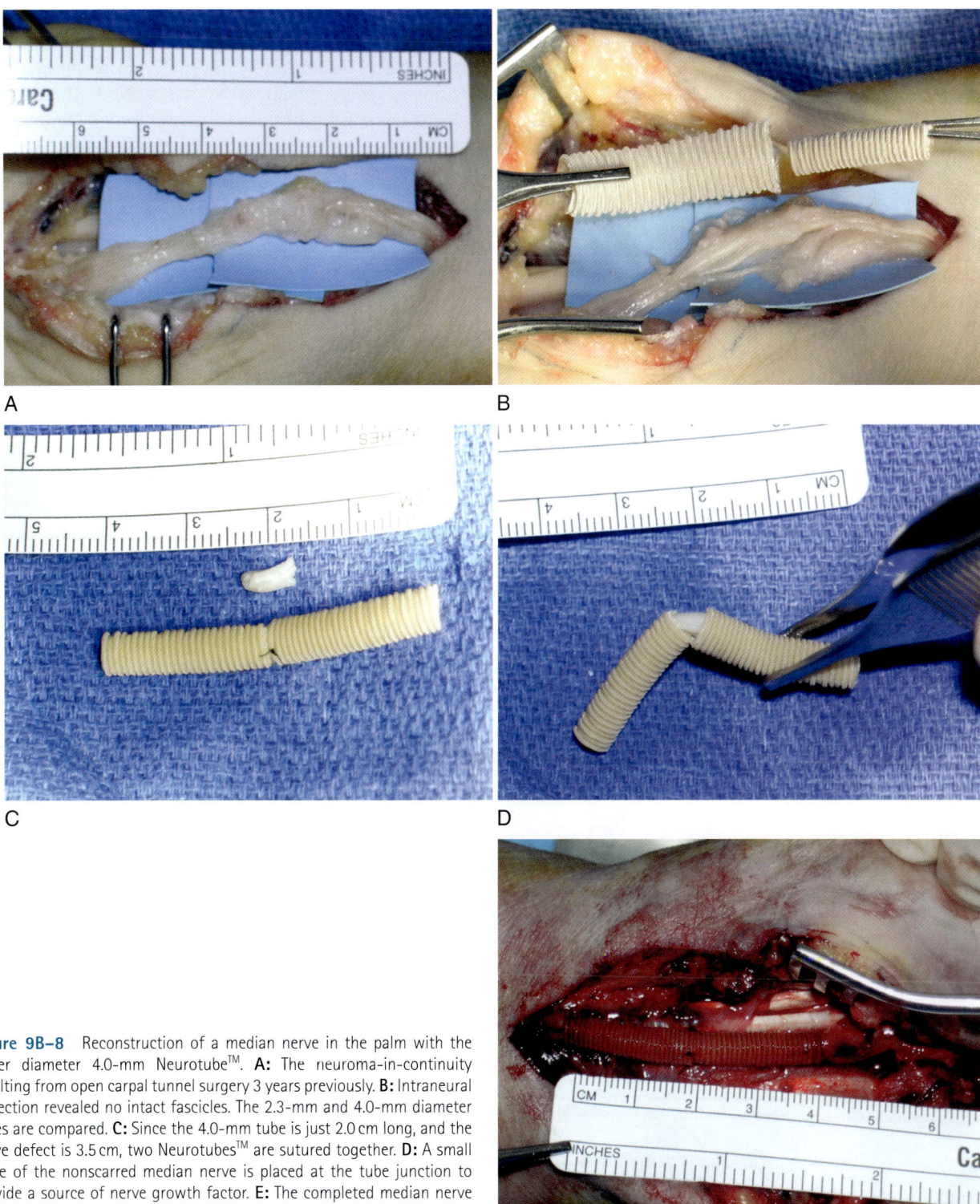

Figure 9B–8 Reconstruction of a median nerve in the palm with the larger diameter 4.0-mm Neurotube™. **A:** The neuroma-in-continuity resulting from open carpal tunnel surgery 3 years previously. **B:** Intraneural dissection revealed no intact fascicles. The 2.3-mm and 4.0-mm diameter tubes are compared. **C:** Since the 4.0-mm tube is just 2.0 cm long, and the nerve defect is 3.5 cm, two Neurotubes™ are sutured together. **D:** A small piece of the nonscarred median nerve is placed at the tube junction to provide a source of nerve growth factor. **E:** The completed median nerve reconstruction. (Photographs courtesy of Virginia H. Hung, MD, and A. Lee Dellon, MD, Dellon Institute for Peripheral Nerve Surgery, Boston, 2005.)

piece of median nerve, was placed between the two Neurotubes™ (Fig. 9B–8 C and D). A similar "stepping stone" concept has worked favorably in a silicone tube model experimentally[32] (Fig. 9B–8 E).

Peripheral nerve tumor resection and nerve reconstruction constitute other uses of the Neurotube™. An example of this is given in Fig. 9B–9, in which a neurofibroma of the superficial peroneal nerve is resected and that fascicle is reconstructed. This preserves function and minimizes risk of the proximal end of the tumor resection from forming a painful neuroma.

Ulnar nerve motor function in the distal forearm was recovered in this 9-year-old boy who had a dog bite. The injury created an in-continuity neuroma of the motor branch of the ulnar nerve 6 cm proximal to the wrist. The sensory branch was not injured. The 2.7-cm nerve defect was reconstructed with one 2.3-mm diameter Neurotube™. At 3 years after reconstruction, hypothenar bulk is demonstrated, first dorsal interosseous has recovered, although not completely, and he demonstrates his violin playing (Fig. 9B–10).

TECHNICAL DETAILS

The results of the randomized prospective study with the Neurotube™ demonstrated that the results with this conduit give statistically better results than does a primary nerve repair (in digital nerves when the defect is <3 cm).[26] Accordingly, my preferred technique for a primary nerve repair is to use a Neurotube™. The logical extension of this is that in elective surgery—for example, a neurovascular free flap—the nerve connection should be done with a Neurotube™. Another example is a cross-facial nerve graft, where the Neurotube™ is an ideal coupler between the larger sural nerve graft and the smaller facial nerve. To emphasize the advantage of the bioabsorbable PGA conduit over the silicone conduit, even the most recent article, with a 5-year follow-up of silicone tubes for primary repairs concluded that there was no advantage in terms of functional recovery when the silicone tube was used, except perhaps for some difference in cold intolerance. Some of those silicone tubes required a secondary operation for removal. In contrast, a Neurotube™ has not had to be removed for complaints of pain, and, as indicated above, has statistically significant better results than a primary nerve, at least in digital nerves.

Should the Neurotube™ be filled with something? It should not be filled with clot, since that discourages neural regeneration. For this reason, the initial dissection is done with the tourniquet inflated, and then the tourniquet is let down and hemostasis is obtained. Either serum or heparinized saline (1,000 U in 100 cc

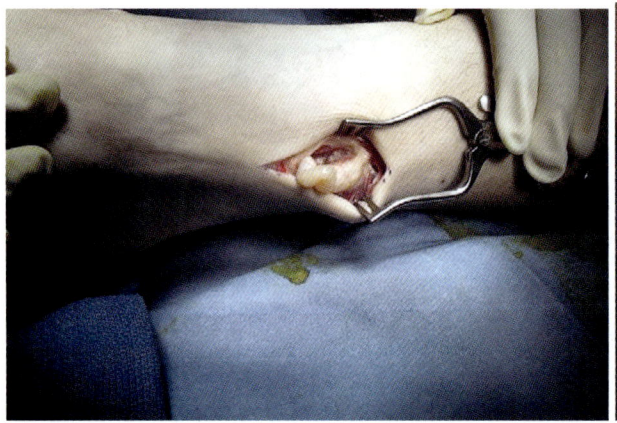

A

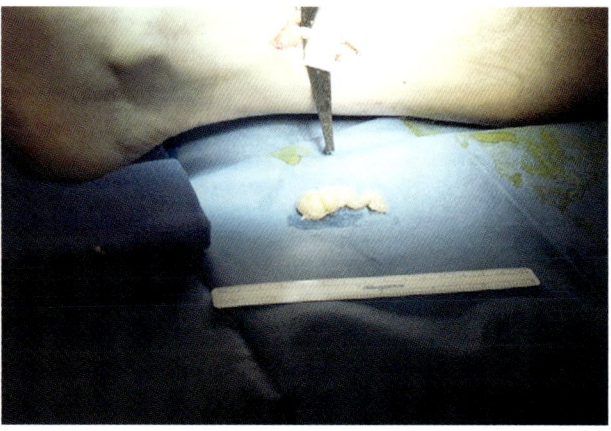

B

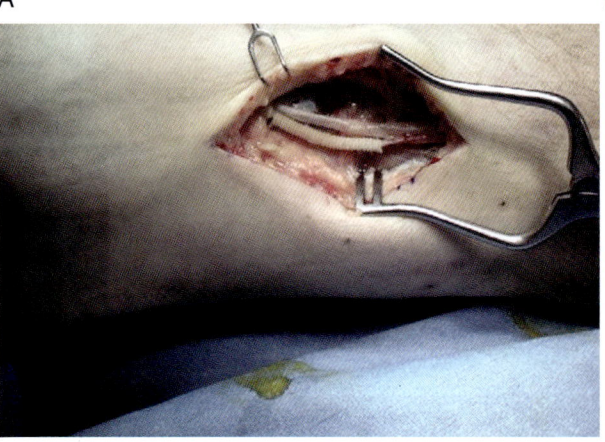

C

Figure 9B–9 Use of Neurotube™ in peripheral nerve tumor reconstruction. **A:** Demonstrated for a neurofibroma of the superficial peroneal nerve. **B:** Resection of the tumor. **C:** Resected fascicle is reconstructed, preventing painful neuroma and restoring function.

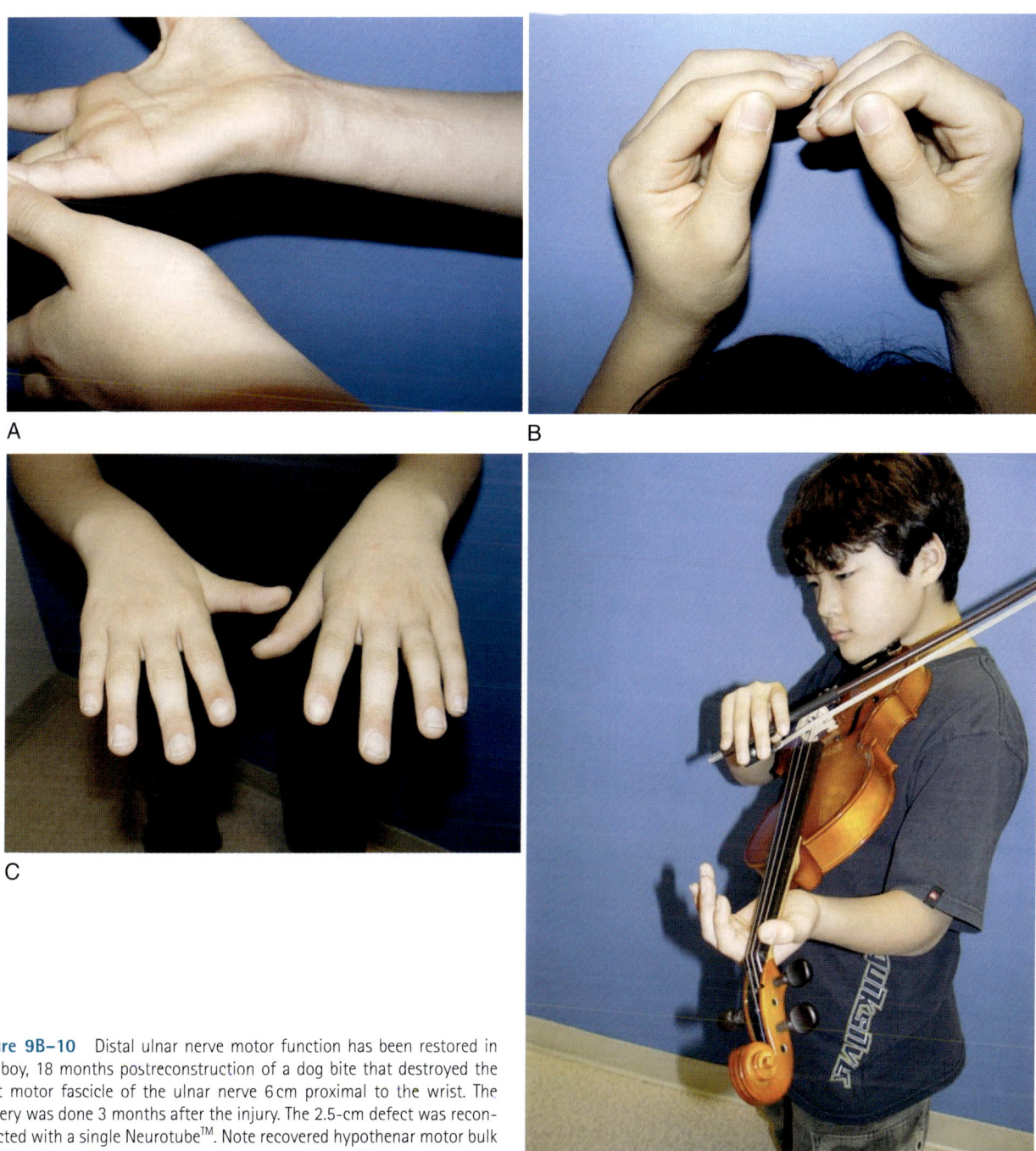

Figure 9B–10   Distal ulnar nerve motor function has been restored in this boy, 18 months postreconstruction of a dog bite that destroyed the right motor fascicle of the ulnar nerve 6 cm proximal to the wrist. The surgery was done 3 months after the injury. The 2.5-cm defect was reconstructed with a single Neurotube™. Note recovered hypothenar motor bulk **(A)**, first dorsal interosseous muscle recovered but without normal bulk **(B)**, absence of clawing **(C)**, and he now plays the violin in school **(D)**.

of normal saline) should be injected into the lumen of the tube to prevent clot from forming. Nerve growth factors are not needed for a gap of up to 3.0 cm. Axons will grow through a PGA tube (Maxxon) for distances of up to 5 cm, but the number of axons is quite small as compared to the number of axons with a 3.0-cm gap. For gaps beyond 3.0 cm, it remains to be proven that placing a small piece of nerve with Schwann cells into the lumen of the tube at its midway point will facilitate the growth of axons past this 3.0 cm distance.

Acknowledgment

The author has a proprietary interest in the Neurotube™.

REFERENCES

1. Millesi H. Interfascicular nerve grafting. Orthop Clin N Am 1970;2:419–26.
2. Mackinnon S, Dellon AL, eds. Nerve repair and nerve grafting. In: Surgery of the Peripheral Nerve. New York: Thieme Medical Publishers, 1988.
3. Lundborg G, Dahlin LB, Danielsen N, et al. Nerve regeneration in silicone chambers. Influence of gap length and distal stump contents. Exp Neurol 1982;76:361–75.
4. Seckel BR, Chiu TH, Nyilas E, et al. Nerve regeneration through synthetic biodegradable nerve guides: regulation by the target organ. Plast Reconstr Surg 1984;74:173–81.
5. Suematsu N. Tubulation for peripheral nerve gap: its history and possibility. Microsurgery 1989;10:71–4.
6. Longo FM, Manthorpe M, Skaper SD, et al. Neuronotrophic activities accumulate in vivo within silicone nerve regeneration chambers. Brain Res 1983;261:109–17.
7. Mackinnon SE, Dellon AL, Hudson AR, et al. A primate model for chronic nerve compression. J Reconstr Microsurg 1985;1:185–94.
8. Lundborg G, Dahlin LB, Danielsen NP, et al. Reorganization and orientation of regenerating nerve fibers, perineurium and epineurium in preformed mesothelial tubes. An experimental study on the sciatic nerve of rats. J Neurosci Res 1981;6:265–81.
9. Lundborg G, Dahlin LB, Danileson N, et al. Tissue specificity in nerve regeneration, Scand J Plast Reconstr Surg 1986;20:279–83.
10. Mackinnon SE, Dellon AL, Hudson AR, et al. Nerve regeneration through a pseudosynovial sheath in a primate model. Plast Reconstr Surg 1985;75:833–9.
11. Mackinnon SE, Dellon AL, Lundborg G, et al. A study of neurotropism in a primate model. J Hand Surg Am 1986;11:888–94.
12. Herman JB, Kelly RJ, Higgins GA. Polyglycolic acid sutures. Laboratory and clinical evaluation of a new absorbable suture material. Arch Surg 1970;100:486–90.
13. Marmon LM, Vinocur CD, Standiford SB, et al. Evaluation of absorbable polyglycolic acid mesh as a wound support. J Pediatr Surg 1984;20:737–42.
14. Lundborg G, Rosen B, Dahlin L, et al. Tubular repair of the median or ulnar nerve in the human forearm: a 5-year follow-up. J Hand Surg Br 2004;29:100–7.
15. Lundborg G, Rosen B, Dahlin L, et al. Tubular versus conventional repair of median and ulnar nerves in the human forearm: early results from a prospective, randomized, clinical study. J Hand Surg Am 1997;22:99–106.
16. Braga-Silver J. The use of silicone tubing in the late repair of the median and ulnar nerves in the forearm. J Hand Surg Br 1999;24:703–6.
17. Merle M, Dellon AL, Campbell J, et al. Clinical complications of silicon-polymer entubulation of nerve. Microsurgery 1989;10:130–3.
18. Johnston B, Zachary LS, Dellon AL, et al. Neural regeneration through a distal site of nerve compression. J Reconstr Microsurg 1993;9:271–4.
19. Dellon AL. Tube or not tube... J Hand Surg Br 1994;19:271–2.
20. Dellon AL, Mackinnon SE. An alternative to the classical nerve graft for the management of the short nerve gap. Plast Reconstr Surg 1988;82:849–56.
21. Mackinnon SE, Dellon AL. Clinical nerve reconstruction with a bioabsorbable polyglycolic acid tube. Plast Reconstr Surg 1990;85:419–24.
22. Mackinnon S, Dellon AL. A study of nerve regeneration across synthetic (maxon) and biologic (collagen) nerve conduits for nerve gaps up to 5 cm in the primate. J Reconstr Microsurg 1990;6:117–21.
23. Dellon AL. Evaluation of Sensibility and Re-Education of Sensation in the Hand. Baltimore: Williams & Wilkens, 1981.
24. Dellon AL. The moving two-point discrimination test: clinical evaluation of the quickly-adapting fiber/receptor. J Hand Surg Am 1978;3:478–81.
25. Crawley WA, Dellon AL. Inferior alveolar nerve reconstruction with a polyglycolic acid, bioabsorbable nerve conduit: a case report. Plast Reconstr Surg 1992;90:300–2.
26. Weber RA, Breidenbach WC, Brown RE, et al. A randomized prospective study of polyglycolic acid conduits for digital nerve reconstruction in humans. Plast Reconstr Surg 2000;106:1036–45.
27. Laroas G, Battiston G, Sard A, et al. Digital nerve reconstruction with the bioabsorbable Neurotube. Clin Exp Plast Surg 2003;35:125–8.
28. Kim J, Dellon AL. Reconstruction of a painful post-traumatic medial plantar neuroma with a bioabsorbable nerve conduit: a case report. J Foot Ankle Surg 2001;40:318–23.
29. Navissano M, Malan F, Carnino R, Battiston B. Neurotube for facial nerve repair. Microsurgery 2005;25(4):268–71.
30. Ducic I, Maloney CT, Dellon AL: Reconstruction of the spinal accessory nerve: autograft or Neurotube? Two case reports. J Reconstr Microsurg 2005;21:29–33.
31. Rosson GD, Swier P, Kim J, et al. Reconstruction of forearm median nerve deficit with four interfascicular interposition Neurotube™ reconstructions. J Bone Joint Surg. In press.
32. Rosson GD, Dellon AL. Reconstruction of the motor function with the Neurotube™. Report of a case and review of the literature. J Reconstr Microsurg. In press.
33. Francel PC, Francel TJ, Mackinnon SE, et al. Enhancing nerve regeneration across a silicone tube conduit by using interposed short-segment nerve grafts. J Neurosurg 1997;87:887–92.
34. Lundborg G, Rosen B, Dahlin L, et al. Tubular repair of the median and ulnar nerve in the human forearm: a five year follow-up. J Hand Surg Br 2004;29:100–7.

Pedicled Neurosensory Flaps for Hand Coverage

David J. Slutsky

10

INTRODUCTION

"Neurosensory" can be defined as being of or relating to afferent nerves.[1] A neurosensory flap can therefore be considered to be an innervated flap that provides sensory feedback, either immediately or following a neurorrhaphy. Incorporating a cutaneous nerve in a skin flap provides a means for sensory innervation, and may also aid the flap circulation since the skin vascularity partly depends on the vessels around these nerves.[2] Noninnervated flaps may also acquire some degree of sensibility through peripheral innervation, but often to a lesser degree. Neurosensory flaps have special application to hand injuries.[3,4] Protective sensibility is desirable when providing soft tissue coverage of the dorsum of the hand and palm, but critical sensibility of the digits is important for functional hand use.[5] Moberg stated that precision sensory grip or tactile gnosis requires two-point discrimination of less than 6 mm, whereas gross sensory grip would be possible at 6 to 15 mm.[6]

Pedicled neurosensory flaps have a number of advantages in comparison to free neurosensory transfers. The arterial supply is often more reliable, which simplifies postoperative monitoring and lends itself to outpatient procedures. Most of these flaps can be dissected under loupe magnification and permit early active motion, which is desirable in acute injuries. Microvascular technique may be of use, but it is not an absolute prerequisite. Finger flaps may be harvested from the same finger (homodigital) or an adjacent finger (heterodigital). Pedicled flaps may be antegrade or retrograde (reversed flow).

Caveats

It is good practice to add 10% to 15% more to both the length and size of the flap. Incorporating a small skin island along the vascular pedicle simplifies insetting and aids in avoiding skin bridges. Methods of salvaging a failing flap may include suture removal, leech therapy, or even conversion to a free flap. Some general contraindications to pedicled flaps include any cause of massive hand swelling such as crush-avulsion and wringer injuries, high-energy trauma, or prior arterial injury. Some pitfalls common to pedicled flaps include an inadequate arc of rotation, a short pedicle, and vascular insufficiency due to tunneling or inadequate flap size.

There are myriad pedicled neurosensory flaps described for fingertip and thumb coverage. Flap selection will ultimately be based on the size of the defect, the requirements for sensibility, the surgeon's comfort level, and the patient profile such as gender, age, or systemic disease. A knowledge of the skin topography and flap anatomy is integral to the success of any flap.

THE HUESTON FLAP

This is a local transposition flap for fingertip skin loss that is pedicled on one neurovascular bundle. It was described by Hueston in 1966,[7] and subsequently modified by Souquet in 1986 to include both neurovascular bundles.[8]

Anatomy

The flap is an asymmetric arterial advancement flap based upon either the radial or ulnar neurovascular bundle. It relies on cutaneous perforators from the digital artery. The flap is drained by the venae comitantes as well as the intact subdermal venous plexus. It receives its innervation from the proper digital nerve. The advancing free edge of the flap is initially insensate but regains sensibility with time, and has a range of advancement of 12 to 18 mm.

Indications

The flap is used to cover a loss of the pulp tissue of the fingers and thumb. It is indicated in situations where it is important to preserve bone length to diminish the risks of a hook nail deformity, and where there is no possibility of distal replantation.

Advantages

The flap is homodigital and provides satisfactory texture for resurfacing fingertips. It is simple, reliable, and allows immediate finger motion.

Limitations

The flap cannot be used with injury to a neurovascular bundle. It is not indicated when more than 18 mm of transposition are required.

Surgical Technique

The skin is advanced on the side of relatively less functional importance, such as the radial pulp of the thumb and small finger or the ulnar border of the middle digits. An L-shaped incision is made proximal to the fingertip defect. The longitudinal limb extends along the midlateral line while the transverse limb is placed in the metacarpophalangeal (MP) or proximal interphalangeal (PIP) flexion crease. The plane of dissection passes superficial to the neurovascular bundle that is closest to the midlateral incision. The contralateral neurovascular bundle is incorporated into the base of the flap, which is then advanced obliquely to cover the amputation stump. A proximally based triangle of skin raised along

the longitudinal border of the flap can be rotated transversely to cover the donor site.[9]

Variations

The flap can be modified by including both neurovascular bundles (Fig. 10–1 A to C). This was thought to preserve the sensibility of the flap at the expense of restricting some distal advancement.[8] The longitudinal incision is made in the same manner as above, while the transverse incision is extended to the opposite midlateral line, ending with a back cut. The plane of dissection proceeds deep to both neurovascular bundles, which are incorporated into the skin flap. The flap is then advanced and inset as above.

Sensory Recovery

In Foucher's series of 43 flaps, two-point discrimination averaged 7 mm in the standard Hueston flap (31 cases) and 6 mm with the modified flap (12 cases).[9]

Complications

The palmar tension pulls on the nail matrix, which causes a tendency toward a parrot-beak nail deformity. This can be minimized by skewering the tip of the flap with a transfixing needle. The free edge of the flap can lead to a dog-ear deformity, which can be corrected by excising a segment of dorsal skin. Cold intolerance is common during the first year, and correlates with poor return of sensation. Persistent fingertip sensitivity may occur due to neuroma formation. A contracture of the distal or proximal interphalangeal joint may result if there is excessive joint flexion during flap insetting.

INNERVATED CROSS-FINGER FLAP

More than 50 years after its description, the cross-finger flap is still widely in use.[10] In cases where the dorsal digital networks cannot be used or when elaborate microsurgical procedures are not available, cross-finger flaps are still useful for finger coverage distal to the PIP joint. Sensory return, however, is unpredictable, and can mar the ultimate functional result. The innervated cross-finger flap was developed to improve upon this by transferring the dorsal skin over the middle phalanx along with its sensory nerve.[11] A neurorrhaphy is performed between this nerve and one of the severed digital nerve ends of the injured finger.

Anatomy

The initial blood supply of this random pattern flap comes from one of the paired dorsal branches arising

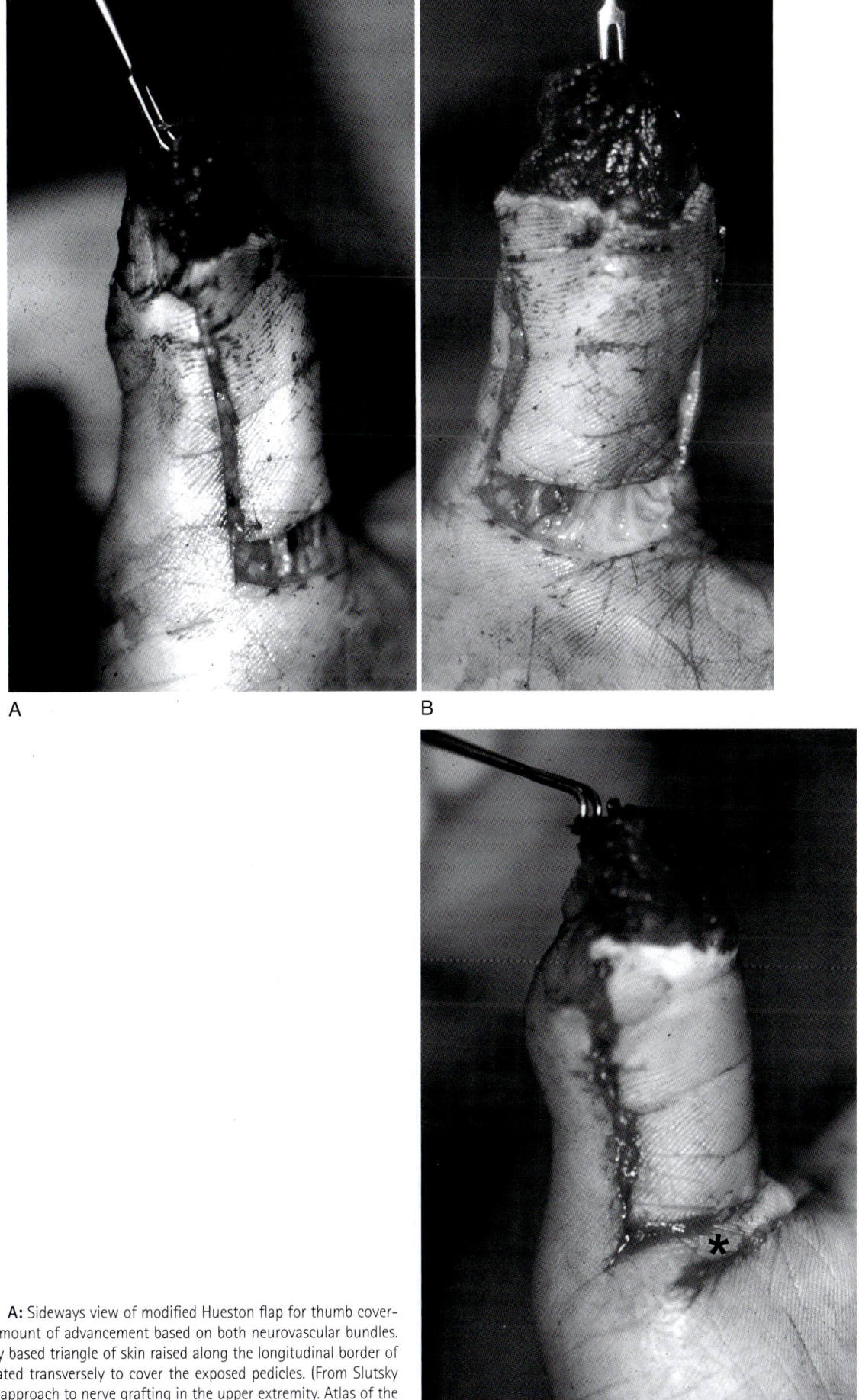

Figure 10–1 **A:** Sideways view of modified Hueston flap for thumb coverage. **B:** Note amount of advancement based on both neurovascular bundles. **C:** A proximally based triangle of skin raised along the longitudinal border of the flap is rotated transversely to cover the exposed pedicles. (From Slutsky DJ. A practical approach to nerve grafting in the upper extremity. Atlas of the Hand Clinics. Nerve Repair and Reconstruction: A Practical Guide, Vol. 10, No. 1. Philadelphia: W.B. Saunders, 2005:73–92, with permission.)

from the palmer digital artery at the proximal one-third of the middle phalanx.[12] The venous drainage is initially from the venae comitantes and subdermal veins. The major dorsal branch of the superficial radial nerve (SRN) and the dorsal cutaneous branch of the ulnar nerve innervate the dorsum of the hand up to the level of the PIP joints. Distal to this, the dorsal skin is innervated by a dorsal sensory branch that arises from the proper digital nerve. This branch most commonly arises proximal to the PIP flexion crease (Fig. 10–6). It then crosses superficial or deep to the digital artery to lie just above the extensor mechanism, innervating the dorsum of the middle phalanx.[13,14]

The arc of rotation of the cross-finger flap is short, since the skin is pedicled on the midlateral line of the finger. The flap is left attached to the donor finger until sufficient peripheral arterial and venous anastomoses have occurred, and then divided.

Indications

The innervated cross-finger flap is indicated in cases of full thickness loss of the entire pulp of an adjacent finger, especially with exposed bone or tendon. The long finger is used for coverage of the thumb pulp.

Advantages

The cross-finger flap is extremely reliable and easy to perform. It can be used for larger defects that may not be suitable for homodigital flaps. With the innervated flap, no additional donor finger denervation occurs because the dorsal sensory branch is ordinarily transected when elevating the standard cross-finger flap. Suturing this branch to the transected digital nerve in the recipient finger allows reinnervation without any need for cortical reorientation.

Limitations

The innervated cross-finger flap cannot be used when there is concomitant injury to adjacent digits. Flap innervation is not possible if there has been damage to either the dorsal sensory branch or the proximal digital nerve. Patient age greater than 40 years is a relative contraindication, due to the finger stiffness that results from 2 weeks of immobilization to an another digit.[15]

Surgical Technique

The dissection is performed under tourniquet control.[16] A pattern of the defect is outlined over the dorsum of the middle phalanx of an adjacent finger. Two transverse incisions delineate the proximal and distal extent of the flap. A longitudinal incision is then made on the side opposite the injured finger. The incision should not extend volar to the midlateral line to prevent a scar contracture. The dorsal sensory branch is isolated through a separate proximal incision that extends to the edge of the flap. The nerve is sectioned proximally, leaving a 1.5- to 2-cm tail. The flap is then elevated along with the nerve branch. The plane of dissection proceeds superficial to the paratenon of the extensor mechanism. The flap is dissected laterally to the opposite midlateral line, until it can be transposed without acute angulation.

Next, the digital nerve end is isolated along the opposite border of the injured digit. The tourniquet is released ensuring flap viability. A full-thickness skin graft is placed over the donor site and secured with a tie-over bolster. The flap is transposed and inset so that the deep surface of the flap lies against the finger defect (Fig. 10–2 A and B). An epineurial repair between the dorsal sensory nerve branch and the digital nerve is performed with 9-0 nylon. A finger spica splint or bulky dressing is applied to prevent tension on the suture sites. At the time of flap division 2 weeks later, no special care for the nerve repair is necessary since the nerve junction is on the side opposite the flap base.

Variations

Lassner et al.[17] have used a bilaterally innervated sensory cross-finger flap. First, the contralateral dorsal sensory branch is elevated with the flap at the PIP joint level, and sutured to the digital nerve end on the far side of the injured finger. After 3 weeks when the pedicle is dissected, the remaining dorsal sensory branch is dissected and sutured to the remaining digital nerve of the injured finger. Because the regenerative distance is only 1.5 to 2 cm, there is excellent sensory reinnervation, with two-point discrimination ranging from 2 to 6 mm.

Gaul described an innervated cross-finger flap from the index that provides immediate sensation for resurfacing volar defects of the thumb.[18] The flap is transferred along with the dorsoradial digital nerve to the index, which is a continuation of the major dorsal branch of the superficial radial nerve.[19] This sensory branch is mobilized at the same time that the cross-finger flap is transposed, and transferred subcutaneously to lie under the volar skin envelope of the thumb.

In an effort to improve the ultimate sensibility, Hastings modified this index finger flap by turning it into a dual innervated flap (Fig. 10–3 A to E). The superficial radial sensory nerve is mobilized and transposed as above. The dorsal sensory branch of the proper radial digital nerve of the index is then sutured to the severed end of the radial digital nerve of the thumb. Sensory reinnervation is reported to be rapid, and does not require cortical reorientation.[20]

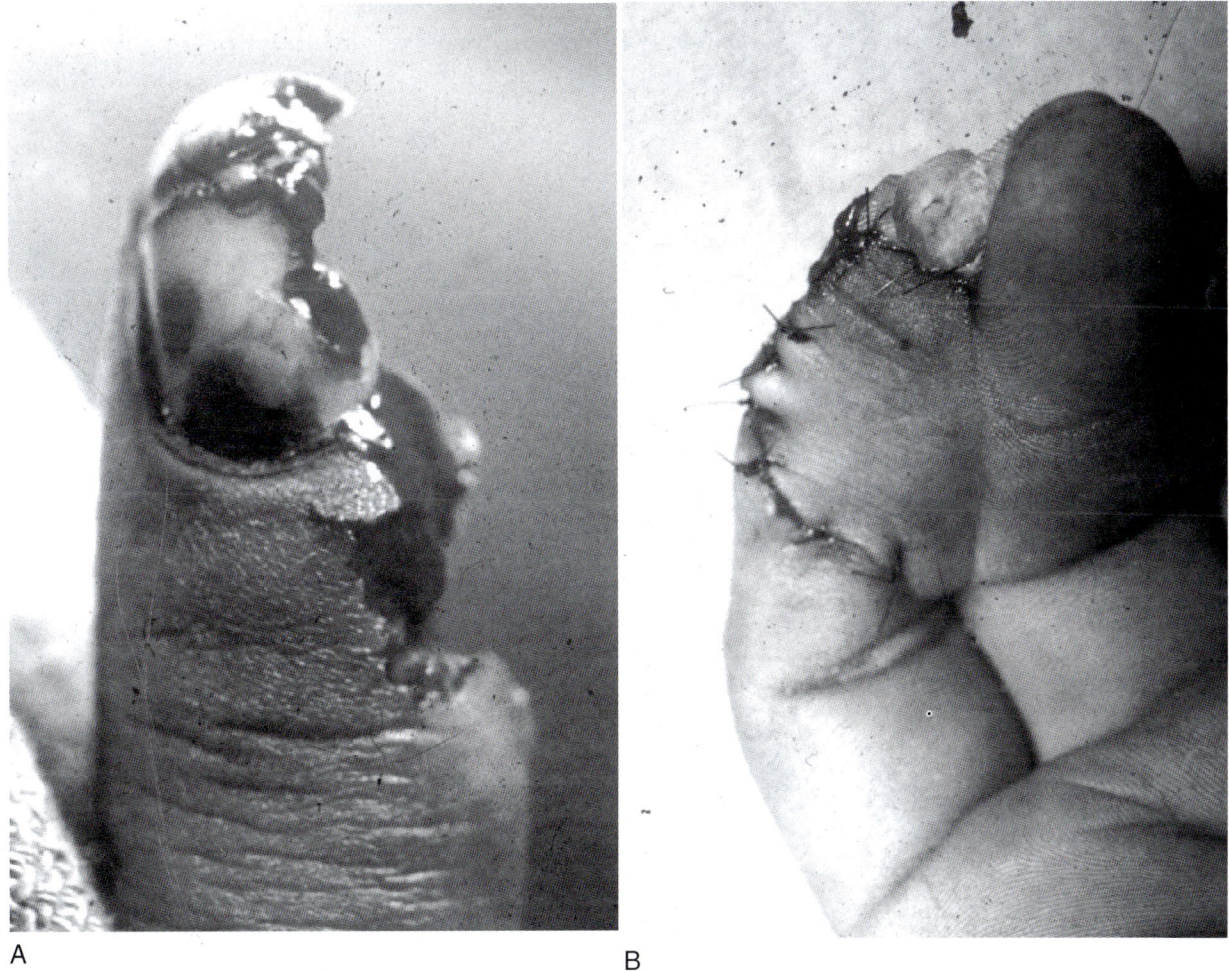

A   B

Figure 10–2   **A:** Fingertip saw injury. **B:** Pedicled cross finger flap. (From Slutsky DJ. A practical approach to nerve grafting in the upper extremity. Atlas of the Hand Clinics. Nerve Repair and Reconstruction: A Practical Guide, Vol. 10, No. 1. Philadelphia: W.B. Saunders, 2005:73–92, with permission.)

Sensory Recovery

In one series of innervated cross-finger flaps, seven of eight patients achieved an average two-point discrimination of 4.8 mm, as compared to noninnervated cross-finger flaps in whom patients achieved a mean value of 9 mm.[16]

Complications

Joint stiffness is common. The flap may be hair bearing. Donor finger morbidity includes poor skin graft color match and a visible contour deformity. If only one digital nerve anastomosis is performed, a painful neuroma may develop from the unrepaired digital nerve stump.

The functional outcome of the radial sensory innervated cross-finger flap is compromised in some patients by double sensitivity. In this case, sensation from the ulnar side of the flap is interpreted as arising from the dorsum of the index finger, whereas sensation on the radial side of the flap is interpreted as coming from the thumb. Sensory testing shows that after transfer to the thumb, the ulnar side of the flap still receives its innervation from the superficial sensory branch of the radial nerve.[21]

REVERSED DIGITAL ARTERY FLAP

The reversed digital artery (RDA) flap described in 1986 by Kojima et al.[22] is used for one-stage reconstruction of finger pulp defects. The flap can be innervated by including the dorsal sensory nerve branch.

Anatomy

The RDA flap is harvested from the dorsolateral skin of the proximal phalanx, which derives its blood supply from the opposite digital artery through abundant communicating branches. There are three transverse palmar

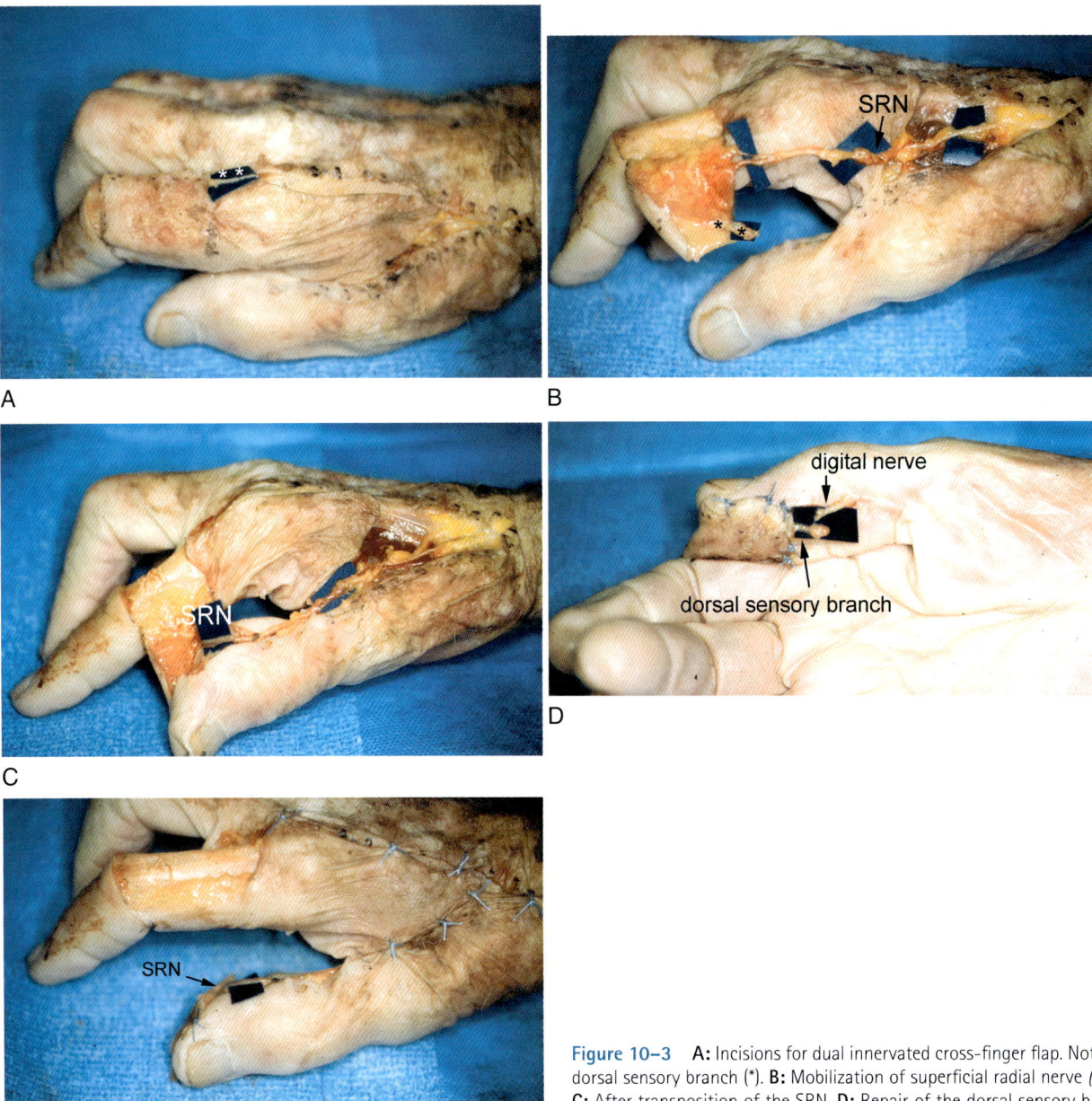

Figure 10–3   **A:** Incisions for dual innervated cross-finger flap. Note the dorsal sensory branch (*). **B:** Mobilization of superficial radial nerve *(SRN)*. **C:** After transposition of the SRN. **D:** Repair of the dorsal sensory branch to the thumb radial digital nerve. **E:** After division of the flap pedicle.

arches connecting the radial and ulnar digital arteries. The proximal and middle arches are always in association with the limbs of the C1 and C3 pulleys. The distal arch lies just beyond the insertion of the profundus tendon.[23]

When the proximal digital artery is ligated, the blood crosses over from the opposite digital artery through the middle and distal transverse palmar arches. The blood then flows down the ligated artery in a retrograde fashion (Fig. 10–4). The RDA flap is designed over the dorsolateral area of the proximal phalanx, which is nourished by a proximal dorsal cutaneous branch. This small branch, 0.3 mm to 0.6 mm in size, arises from the palmar digital artery at the midpoint of the proximal phalanx (Fig. 10–5).[12] It passes through Cleland's

ligament, running close to the bone and emerges on the dorsal aspect of the finger. Histologic studies have revealed the presence of venules and capillaries in the perivascular fat tissue that appear to represent adequate channels for venous drainage.[13]

The dorsal sensory nerve branch is harvested with the skin flap (Fig. 10–6). In the border digits, the terminal branches of the superficial radial nerve or dorsal cutaneous branch of the ulnar nerve can also be transferred. The arc of rotation is around the midpoint of the middle phalanx, which allows the flap to easily reach the fingertip. The digital artery cannot be elevated beyond the middle phalanx for fear of disrupting the distal transverse arch.

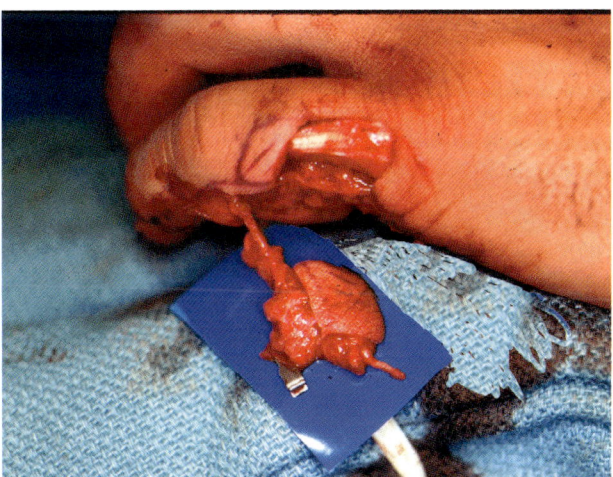

Figure 10–4   Retrograde blood flow down the ligated artery (clamp). Note the dorsal sensory nerve branch. (From Slutsky DJ. A practical approach to nerve grafting in the upper extremity. Atlas of the Hand Clinics. Nerve Repair and Reconstruction: A Practical Guide, Vol. 10, No. 1. Philadelphia: W.B. Saunders, 2005:73–92, with permission.)

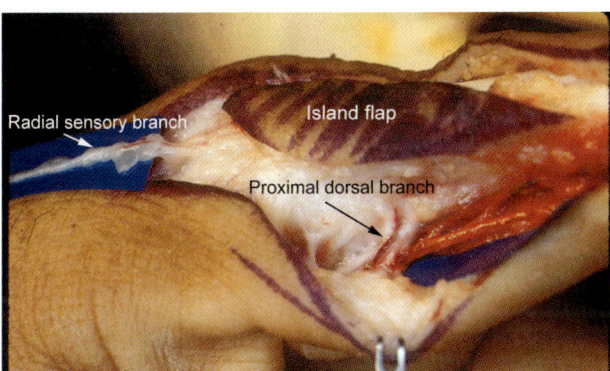

Figure 10–5   Proximal dorsal branch supplying a skin island flap of the index finger. Note the proximal tail on the skin flap and terminal branch of the superficial radial sensory nerve. (From Slutsky DJ. A practical approach to nerve grafting in the upper extremity. Atlas of the Hand Clinics. Nerve Repair and Reconstruction: A Practical Guide, Vol. 10, No. 1. Philadelphia: W.B. Saunders, 2005:73–92, with permission.)

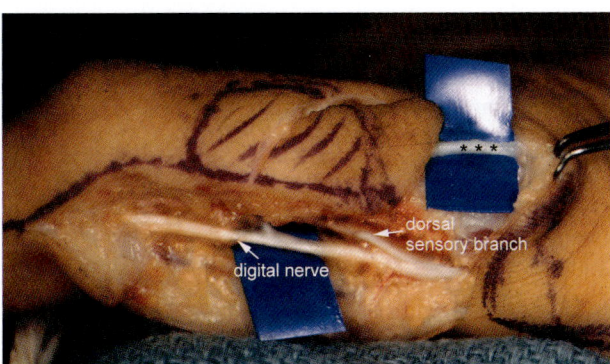

Figure 10–6   Dorsal sensory branch arising from the proper digital nerve of the small finger. DCBUN (*) = dorsal cutaneous branch of the ulnar nerve. (From Slutsky DJ. A practical approach to nerve grafting in the upper extremity. Atlas of the Hand Clinics. Nerve Repair and Reconstruction: A Practical Guide, Vol. 10, No. 1. Philadelphia: W.B. Saunders, 2005:73–92, with permission.)

Indications

This flap is indicated for coverage of acute and chronic fingertip defects. It can be used for fingertip reconstruction to correct a hook nail deformity (Fig. 10–7 A to D). Some authors recommend the RDA flap for coverage of large defects of the dorsal aspects of the middle and distal phalanx that cannot be covered with other local digital sensory flaps (Fig. 10–8 A to C).[24] It may also be useful following release of volar scar contractures of the fingers.

Advantages

This procedure provides a method for a one-stage reconstruction of finger pulp defects. It restores sensation with a good color match, while allowing early finger motion. The RDA flap has great mobility and transfers to the pulp defect without any tension when based on a reverse vascular pedicle. Neurorrhaphy between the dorsal sensory branch and the terminal digital nerve allows for flap innervation through the normal anatomic pathway, so that cortical misinterpretation can be avoided.[13]

Limitations

A disadvantage of this procedure is that it sacrifices a digital artery, and a nerve repair is required. The RDA flap cannot be used if there is only one patent digital artery, or if there has been an injury to the distal transverse palmar arch.

Surgical Technique

A digital Allen's test with or without doppler is used to ascertain that both digital arteries are intact.[25] Under tourniquet control, the injured tip is debrided and a pattern of the defect is outlined over the proximal phalanx. The flap margins are incised and elevated, including the subcutaneous tissue and the digital artery. The dorsal sensory branch is identified and divided 10 mm proximal to the flap margin. A midlateral incision is then made from the distal flap margin, as far as the midpoint of the middle phalanx. The artery is separated from the digital nerve, leaving as much surrounding fat as possible for venous drainage.

A microvascular clamp is applied to the digital artery proximal to the skin flap while the tourniquet is released to check the circulation of both the finger and the flap. The proximal artery is then divided and elevated to the midportion of the middle phalanx.

The skin island is rotated 180 degrees into the fingertip defect, taking care to avoid kinking the pedicle. Leaving a tail on the flap or skin grafting the pedicle can avoid arterial compression. The dorsal sensory nerve

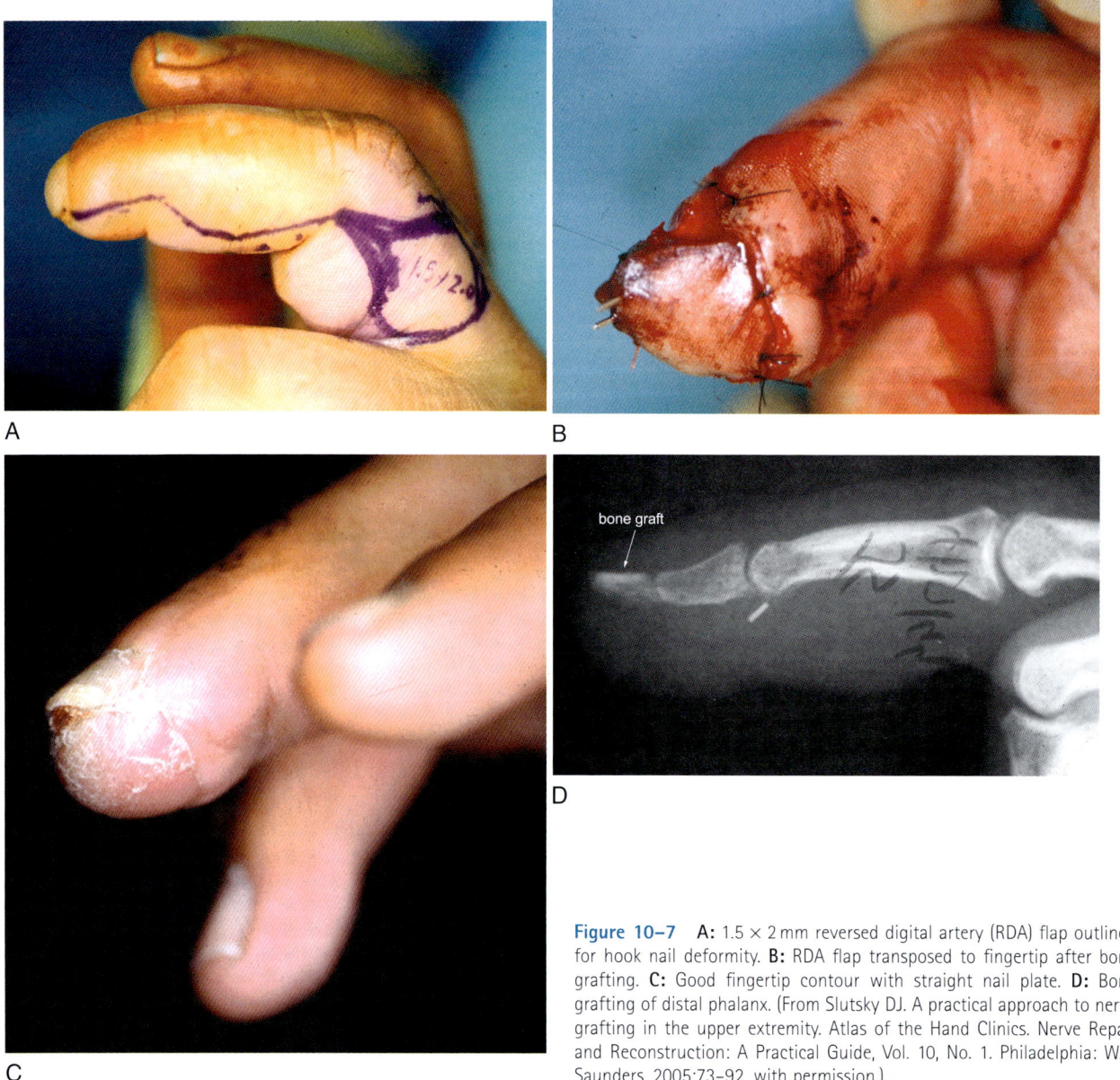

A

B

C

D

Figure 10–7   A: 1.5 × 2 mm reversed digital artery (RDA) flap outlined for hook nail deformity. **B:** RDA flap transposed to fingertip after bone grafting. **C:** Good fingertip contour with straight nail plate. **D:** Bone grafting of distal phalanx. (From Slutsky DJ. A practical approach to nerve grafting in the upper extremity. Atlas of the Hand Clinics. Nerve Repair and Reconstruction: A Practical Guide, Vol. 10, No. 1. Philadelphia: W.B. Saunders, 2005:73–92, with permission.)

branch is sutured to the recipient nerve prior to insetting. Donor site defects up to 2 × 3 cm can be closed primarily. Flaps up to 5 × 2 cm can be harvested.

Variations

Lai et al.[26] described an extended RDA flap in which the dorsal skin over the metacarpophalangeal (MP) joint may be included. This skin extension is a fasciocutaneous flap that survives on the rich anastomosis between the first dorsal metacarpal artery and the digital artery near the metacarpal head.[27] Lai et al.[26] noted that the sensory recovery of this skin extension was relatively poor. In an effort to overcome this, both the dorsal

sensory branch from the proper digital nerve and the superficial sensory branch from the corresponding radial or ulnar nerve are sectioned at their proximal ends and included with the RDA flap (Fig. 10–6).[26] For bilaterally innervated flaps, these branches are sutured to both digital nerve ends. Static two-point discrimination of 5 mm was obtained in a series of 3 patients.[26]

In cases where one of the digital arteries has been injured, an innervated RDA cross-finger flap harvested from the proximal phalanx of the adjacent finger can be used to cover defects of the middle and distal phalanges. A piece of skin graft is placed over the pedicle, which is divided at 2 weeks.[28]

In situations in which the fingertip pulp is lost completely, some authors have included the proper digital nerve in the pedicle, which is then sutured to the stump of the opposite proper digital nerve.[29]

Sensory Recovery

Mean values for two-point discrimination range between 6 and 10 mm.[30] Noninnervated flaps have also been reported to regain less than 10 mm of two-point discrimination sensation.[31]

Complications

Flap edema secondary to impaired venous drainage from kinking of the pedicle, or due to an inadequate amount of perivascular fat for venous drainage is common. The flap tends to be bulky if applied over subcutaneous tissue rather than bone (Fig. 10–9). Skin grafting the pedicle at the distal interphalangeal joint may be necessary. Inadequate finger perfusion occurring when the digital artery proximal to the island flap is clamped may preclude use of this flap. Numbness over the dorsum of the middle phalanx due to transection of the dorsal sensory branch may be bothersome. If the margin of the flap extends volar to the midaxial line a PIP flexion contracture can develop. Cold intolerance is a risk, especially for outdoor workers in cold climates.

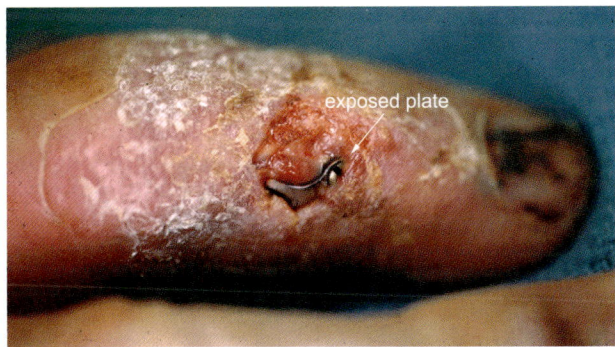
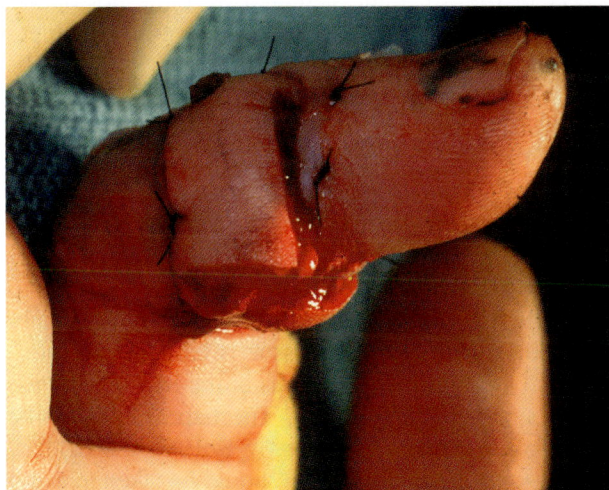
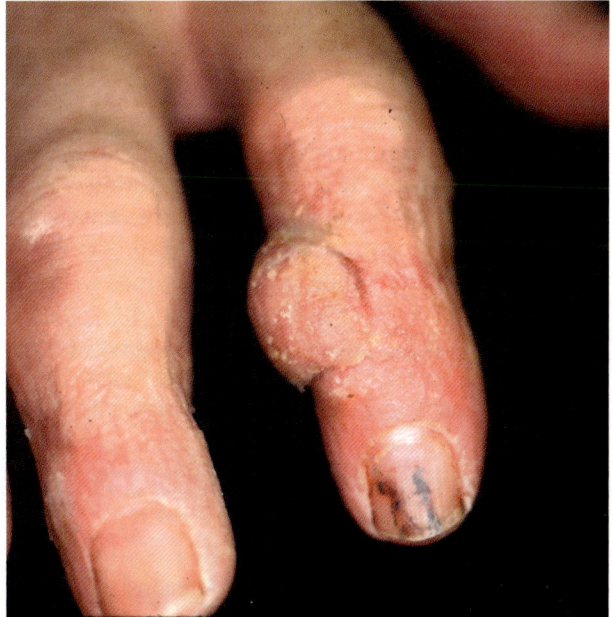

Figure 10–8 **A:** Status post-ORIF (open reduction and internal fixation) of open fracture with exposed plate along ulnar side of index, 56-year-old male. **B:** RDA flap raised from radial side of the index finger. **C:** Flap insetting. (From Slutsky DJ. A practical approach to nerve grafting in the upper extremity. Atlas of the Hand Clinics. Nerve Repair and Reconstruction: A Practical Guide, Vol. 10, No. 1. Philadelphia: W.B. Saunders, 2005:73–92, with permission.)

Figure 10–9 Note bulkiness of flap when applied directly over bone. (From Slutsky DJ. A practical approach to nerve grafting in the upper extremity. Atlas of the Hand Clinics. Nerve Repair and Reconstruction: A Practical Guide, Vol. 10, No. 1. Philadelphia: W.B. Saunders, 2005:73–92, with permission.)

DORSOULNAR FLAP OF THE THUMB

The arterial supply of the thumb is quite different from that of the fingers. The direct- or reverse-flow volar island flaps centered on only one arterial pedicle that have been described for the fingers are not possible for the thumb.

Through their anatomical studies, Brunelli et al.[32] discovered a consistent artery along the dorsoulnar aspect of the thumb that they used as the basis for a reverse pedicled skin flap. The flap can be innervated by incorporating the terminal branches of the superficial radial nerve and can be used for coverage of distal thumb defects.

Anatomy

The princeps pollicus artery divides into two palmer digital arteries at the level of the MP flexion crease. As a consequence, any pedicled flap of the thumb that is based upon the palmar arteries has a short pedicle. This would require marked IP joint flexion in order to prevent undue tension on the princeps pollicus. The dorsal arteries of the fingers are extremely segmental, inconstant, and dependent on palmar anastomoses. In the thumb, there is a constant dorsoulnar artery that originates from the palmar arteries at the neck of the thumb metacarpal and runs along the dorsoulnar side of the thumb. It may be as large as 1 mm and travels superficially within the subcutaneous tissue, above the aponeurosis. A similar but less constant and smaller artery may be found 72% of the time along the dorsoradial aspect of the thumb.[33]

The dorsoulnar artery is reinforced by an anastomosis with the palmer digital artery at the neck of the proximal phalanx, approximately 2.3 cm from the nail fold. The artery terminates in a dorsal arcade within 0.7 cm of the nail. Venae comitantes can be present when the artery is of a large size (about 50% of cases). In the remaining cases venous drainage is mostly based on tiny venules in the perivascular fatty tissue (Francesco Brunelli, personal communication, 2004). The terminal sensory branch of the superficial radial nerve is located 1 to 2 cm from the median axis of the thumb.

Indications

The dorsoulnar flap is indicated for reconstruction of extensive loss of the thumb pulp. It can be used for coverage of amputation stumps at the IP joint level or for coverage of dorsal skin loss over the proximal and distal phalanx.

Advantages

The flap provides satisfactory texture for resurfacing fingertips, and is homodigital, which allows immediate thumb motion. Because of the distal nature of its pedicle, the flap can easily reach the tip of the thumb. Primary closure of the donor site is possible for smaller flaps.

Limitations

The flap cannot be used with injury to the princeps pollicus or ulnar digital artery. It is also contraindicated when there is a significant soft tissue injury at the base of the thumb.

Surgical Technique

The following points are first marked on the skin: (1) the dorsal arcade of the proximal nail fold, 0.9 cm proximal to the nail base; (2) the palmar anastomosis at the level of the neck of the proximal phalanx, 2.5 cm proximally; and (3) the course of the dorsoulnar artery, 1 cm from the median axis of the thumb at the level of the neck of the proximal phalanx (Fig. 10–10 A to D).[34] The flap dimensions are then marked out on the dorsoulnar aspect of the MP joint, centered over the dorsoulnar artery. The flap is raised in a proximal to distal direction. The terminal sensory branch of the radial nerve is located and divided 2 cm from the proximal flap edge. A midlateral incision is then extended along the ulnar side of the thumb connecting to the distal area of soft tissue loss. This incision is very superficial in order to avoid damaging the arterial pedicle. Two dermoepidermis skin flaps are raised in a dorsal and palmar direction starting from the ulnar incision, taking care not to harm the subcutaneous tissue. A 1-cm wide, full thickness strip of subcutaneous tissue is harvested en bloc, centered around the arterial axis of the flap, leaving the extensor aponeurosis in situ. The flap artery may be quite small[34] and is not directly isolated during harvesting to avoid damage. Care should be taken to avoid any tension or compression where the subcutaneous pedicle is reflected on itself.

The flap can be pedicled distally at two levels, which determines the arc of rotation. It can be pedicled at the dorsal nail fold arcade for cases of distal amputation, or for loss of palmar or dorsal tissue. Dissection of the pedicle must be limited to 1 cm from the nail base. When used for more proximal amputation stumps, it is pedicled on the palmar anastomosis at the neck of the proximal phalanx. In this case, the dissection should be limited to 2.5 cm from the nail base.

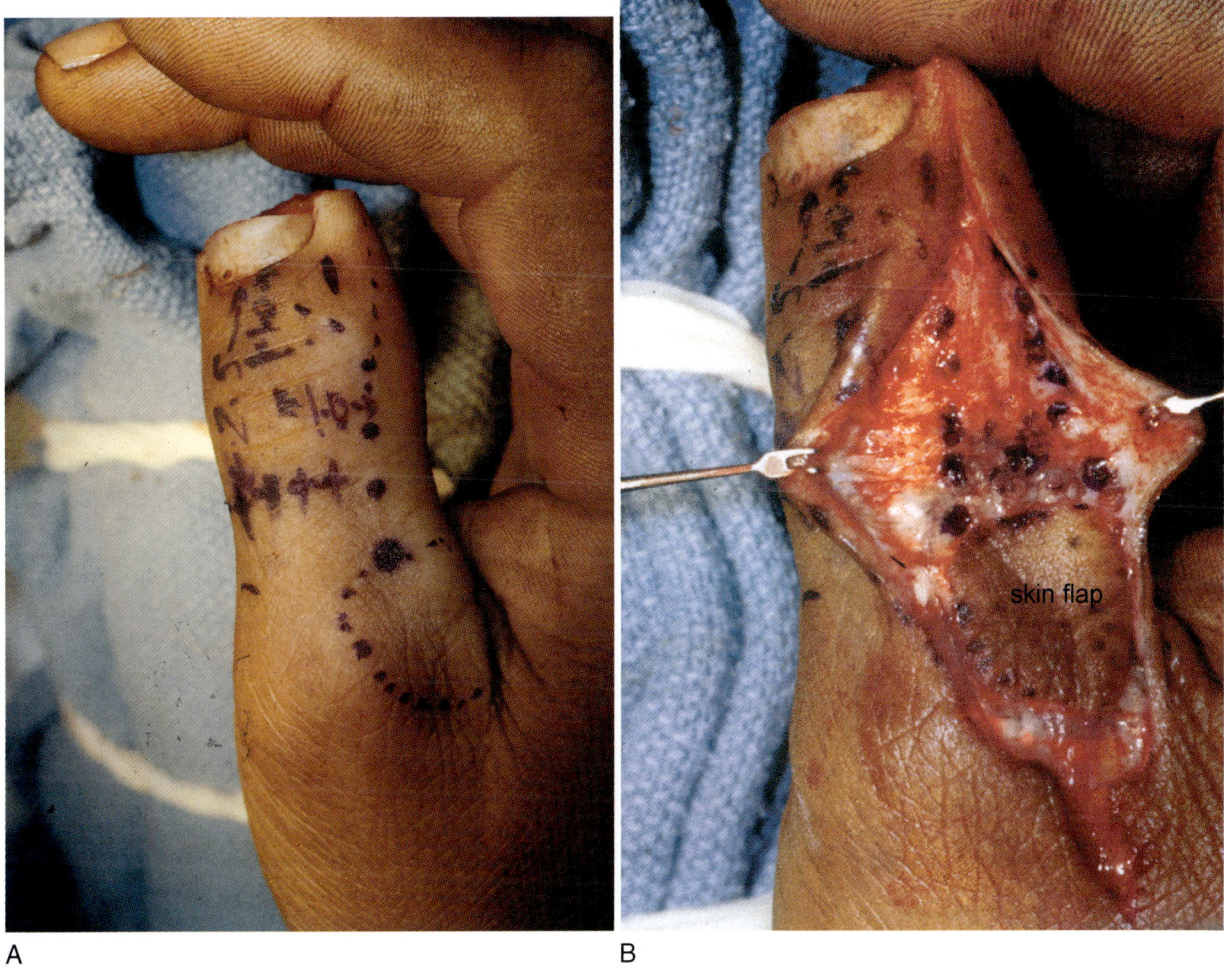

A   B

Figure 10–10   **A:** Skin markings for dorsoulnar thumb flap. **B:** Flap elevated on dorsoulnar artery.

Variations

The flap can be used as a cross-finger variant for coverage of skin loss of the fingers. Any part of the hand is accessible to this flap based on the distal end of a mobile thumb.[35] The temporary pedicle, composed of a 1-cm wide band of skin and subcutaneous tissue, is divided at 15 days after a clamping test confirms that the flap has become autonomous.

The dorsoulnar artery sends several periosteal and osseous branches to the neck of the first metacarpal. Vascularized bone from the metacarpal neck can be harvested with a reversed pedicled dorsoulnar skin flap for reconstruction of combined skin and bone defects of the distal phalanx.[36]

Sensory Recovery

Sensory recovery is disappointing, ranging from 10 mm to protective sensibility. In Brunelli's series, there was no significant difference in sensibility between innervated and noninnervated flaps.

Complications

Raising the flap proximal to the MP joint may exclude the nutrient artery, resulting in flap failure. Harvesting the terminal radial sensory nerve branch of the thumb leads to sensory loss over the dorsum of the thumb, and could result in neuroma formation. Harvesting the skin from the dorsoulnar aspect of the thumb MP can result in a restriction of MP motion along with a decrease in the first web space span. The donor area is hair bearing and debulking of the flap may be necessary due to overlap of the pedicle.

FIRST DORSAL METACARPAL ARTERY FLAP

This is a fasciocutaneous flap first described by Holevich in 1963.[37] It was modified and used as a neurosensory island flap by Foucher and Braun in 1979.[38] It is based on the first dorsal metacarpal artery

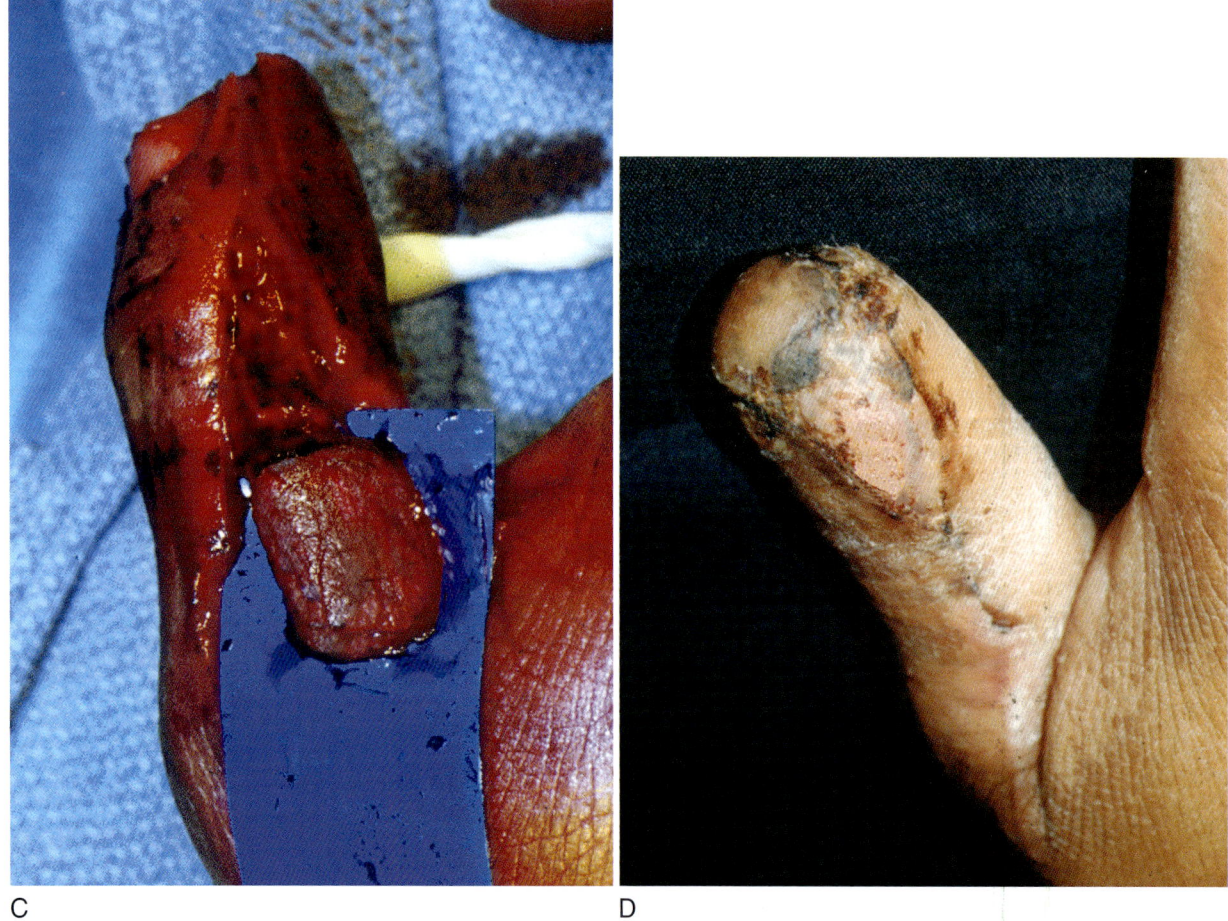

C

D

Figure 10–10—Cont'd **C:** Skin flap elevated. **D:** Good color match and contour of distal thumb. (From Slutsky DJ. A practical approach to nerve grafting in the upper extremity. Atlas of the Hand Clinics. Nerve Repair and Reconstruction: A Practical Guide, Vol. 10, No. 1. Philadelphia: W.B. Saunders, 2005:73–92, with permission.)

(FDMA) or its dorsal digital branches. It is innervated by terminal sensory branches of the superficial radial nerve.

Anatomy

The FDMA arises from the radial artery just distal to the extensor pollicus longus tendon, before the artery dives between the two heads of the first dorsal interosseous (FDI) muscle (Fig. 10–11 A). The FDMA typically measures 1.2 to 1.5 mm in diameter. There is usually more than one accompanying vein. The artery runs superficial to the FDI fascia and divides into three terminal branches: radial (FDMAr), ulnar (FDMAu), and intermediate. The radial branch runs along the thumb metacarpal and becomes or anastomoses with the dorsoulnar artery. The ulnar branch runs along the index metacarpal up to the MP joint, giving branches to the periosteum and adjacent extensor tendons. It terminates in a plexus over the dorsal fascia of the index (Fig. 10–11 B). The intermediate branch runs toward the first web space and anastomoses with branches from the other two. The flap is based on either the radial or ulnar branch of the FDMA. A proximally based flap is rotated around the point of origin of the artery at the base of the first dorsal interosseous space. The arc of rotation can include the palmar or dorsal thumb, wrist, and palm to the third metacarpal.

The venous drainage is that of the accompanying superficial veins. The superficial branch of the radial nerve becomes subcutaneous after it leaves the brachioradialis, and then bifurcates into two major branches 4 cm proximal to the styloid (Fig. 10–12).[39] Both branches pass radially to Lister's tubercle. The major palmar branch passes over the first dorsal wrist compartment, and then continues distally to become the dorsoradial digital nerve of the thumb. The major dorsal branch also bifurcates into the dorsoulnar digital nerve to the thumb and the dorsoradial digital nerve to the index, which supplies the adjacent sides of the second web space.[19]

Indications

The FDMA is indicated for resurfacing either volar or dorsal defects of the distal thumb as far distal as the IP joint (Fig. 10–13 A to D). It can be used to cover the

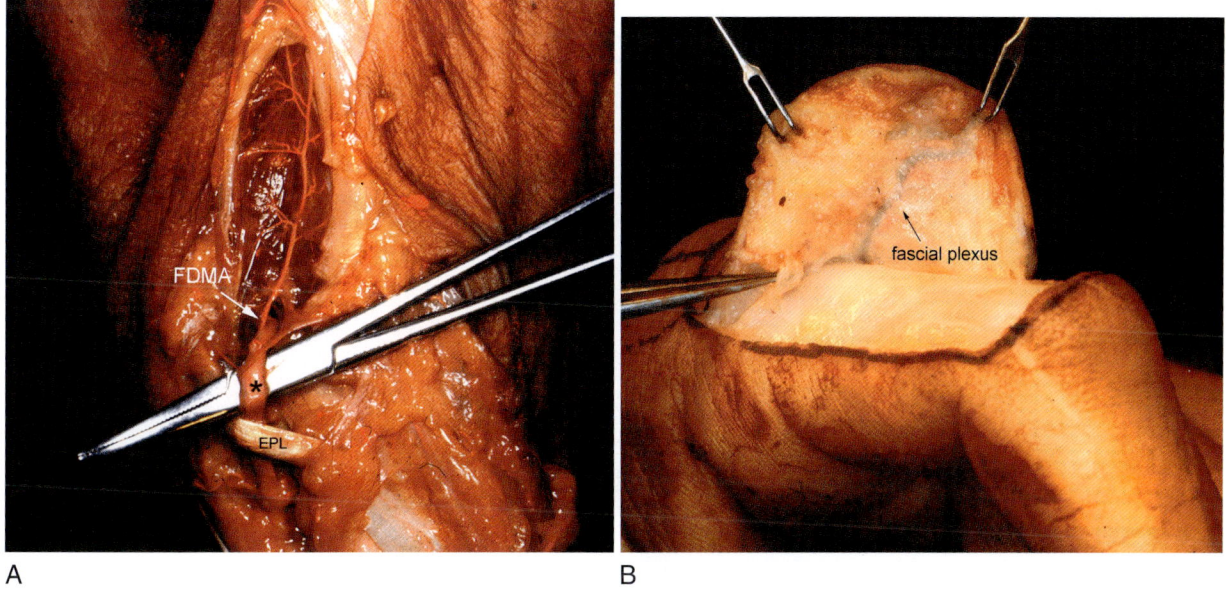

A   B

Figure 10–11   A: Cadaver injection studies demonstrating the origin of the first dorsal metacarpal artery *(FDMA)* from the radial artery (*). **B:** Demonstration of the FDMAu, which terminates in a plexus over the dorsal fascia of the index. (From Slutsky DJ. A practical approach to nerve grafting in the upper extremity. Atlas of the Hand Clinics. Nerve Repair and Reconstruction: A Practical Guide, Vol. 10, No. 1. Philadelphia: W.B. Saunders, 2005:73–92, with permission.)

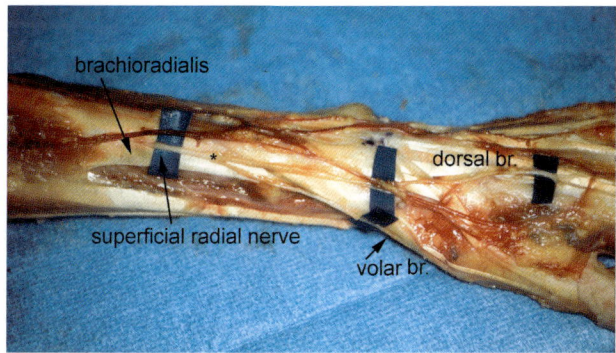

Figure 10–12   Superficial radial nerve arising from underneath the brachioradialis. Note the bifurcation (*) into a major dorsal and volar branch.)

ulnar surface of the dorsum of the hand and the wrist, or the palm up to the third metacarpal. The FDMA flap is useful for first web-space reconstruction following contracture, and it can provide soft tissue coverage of the index finger up to the level of the proximal phalanx (Fig. 13 A to C).

Advantages

Some of the advantages of this flap are its variable size, stability, and pliability. It provides innervated skin with no major donor site morbidity. Its elevation does not sacrifice a major artery. It can be transferred as a pedicled flap or an island flap. The innervated FDMA flap allows immediate postoperative mobilization and the avoidance of a nerve repair. It restores sensibility,

particularly in the older patient, in whom nerve repairs of a pedicle or a free flap yields poorer results than in younger patients.[40]

Limitations

The flap cannot be used with radial artery injury in the snuffbox. If the skin overlying the first web space is included in the flap, skin grafting the donor site defect may lead to a secondary contracture. The arterial pedicle is difficult to dissect. The flap is at risk of partial necrosis if pedicled on a nondominant branch.

Surgical Technique

Pedicled Flap

A doppler probe may be used to check the pulse of the FDMAr and FDMAu against the first and second metacarpals. The flap is drawn over the dorsum of the index, thumb or back of the hand according to the skin defect. Under tourniquet the flap is raised from distal to proximal, in the areolar plane over the extensor paratenon. The skin incision is continued along the radial aspect of the index metacarpal to include a large subcutaneous vein in the pedicle. At the second metacarpal neck a large perforator is consistently present and should be ligated. The entire interosseous fascia over the FDI is included to avoid a meticulous dissection of the pedicle, and to avoid raising the flap on a nondominant branch. A small cuff of muscle of the FDI may be included to ensure the artery is included in

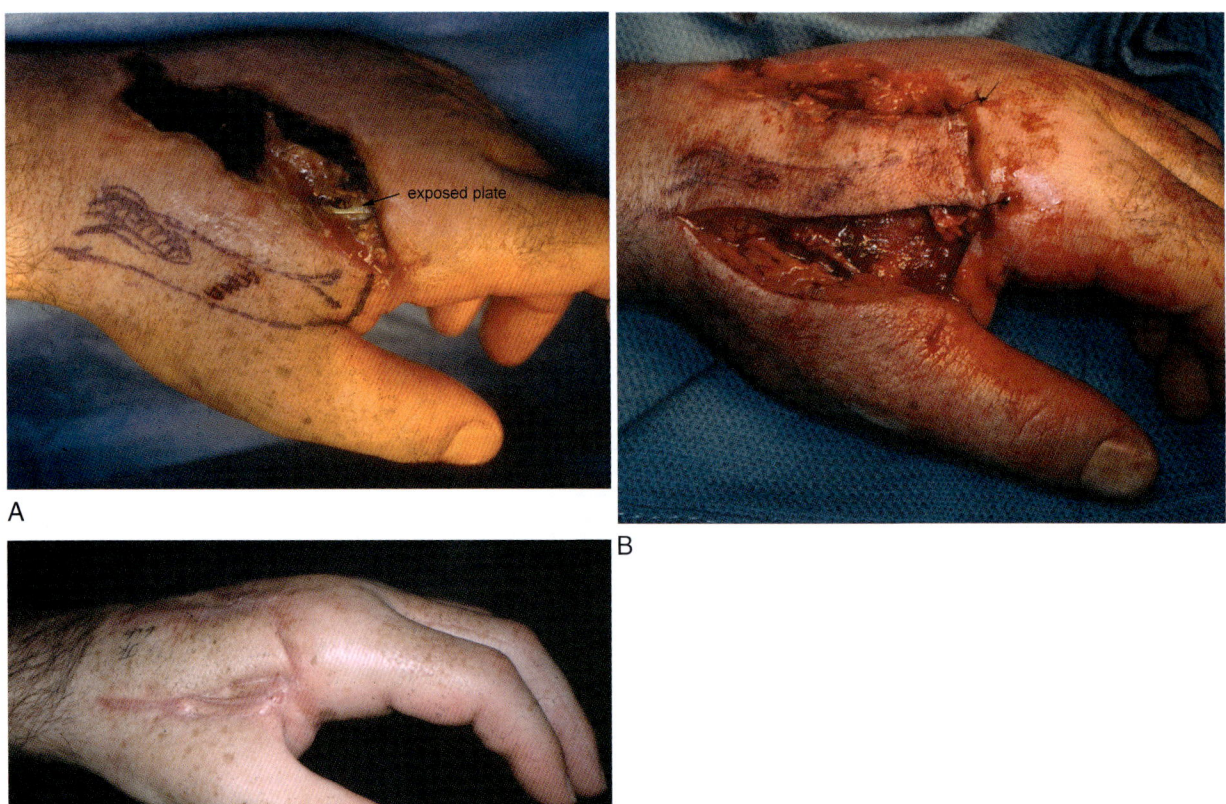

exposed plate

C

Figure 10–13 **A:** Exposed plate following revascularization for partial hand amputation. **B:** Flap based upon the FDMAr. **C:** Long-term result. (From Slutsky DJ. A practical approach to nerve grafting in the upper extremity. Atlas of the Hand Clinics. Nerve Repair and Reconstruction: A Practical Guide, Vol. 10, No. 1. Philadelphia: W.B. Saunders, 2005:73–92, with permission.)

the pedicle. Either the major palmar or dorsal branch of the SRN is incorporated into the flap. The fascia is released from the metacarpal until the flap can reach the defect. If the flap is used for first web reconstruction the interosseous fascia is released from both the thumb and index metacarpals. The flap is enlarged ulnarly toward the third metacarpal so that the skin extension lies on the first web space, avoiding a first web contracture.[41]

Island Flaps

The flap is pedicled on the FDMAu when used to cover defects over the volar surface of the distal thumb[42] (Fig. 10–14 A to D). Alternatively, the dorsal skin over the proximal phalanx of the thumb, which is supplied by the FDMAr can resurface the radial side of the index. The flap is outlined over the dorsum of the index proximal phalanx. A proximal longitudinal incision is made over the FDI muscle. The flap is elevated starting distally, developing the plane between the subcutaneous tissue and the extensor tendon paratenon up to the level of the MP joint. The dorsoradial branch of the SRN is harvested with the skin island. The subdermal fascia can

be quite thin; hence, care is taken to preserve its continuity with the FDI fascia. Inclusion of a small strip of extensor hood along the radial aspect of the extensor hood is recommended to protect the vascular connection from the pedicle to the skin island.[43] Flap dimensions extend from the base of the proximal phalanx to the PIP extension crease, and can be up to 4 × 2 cm. The pedicle can be up to 9 cm in length.

The proximally based flap is rotated around the origin of the FDMA at the base of the first web space. It can be rotated and passed through a subcutaneous tunnel, taking care not to compress the pedicle at the thumb IP joint. Harvesting a proximal tail with the island flap simplifies insetting, and avoids the need for tunneling (see Fig. 10–5). The donor site is skin grafted.

Variations

Harvesting the dorsal skin over the middle phalanx of the index as a random extension allows coverage of larger defects than a standard FDMA flap, in a normal-length thumb.[44] Composite flaps can include the extensor indicis proprius or communis tendon, which can be

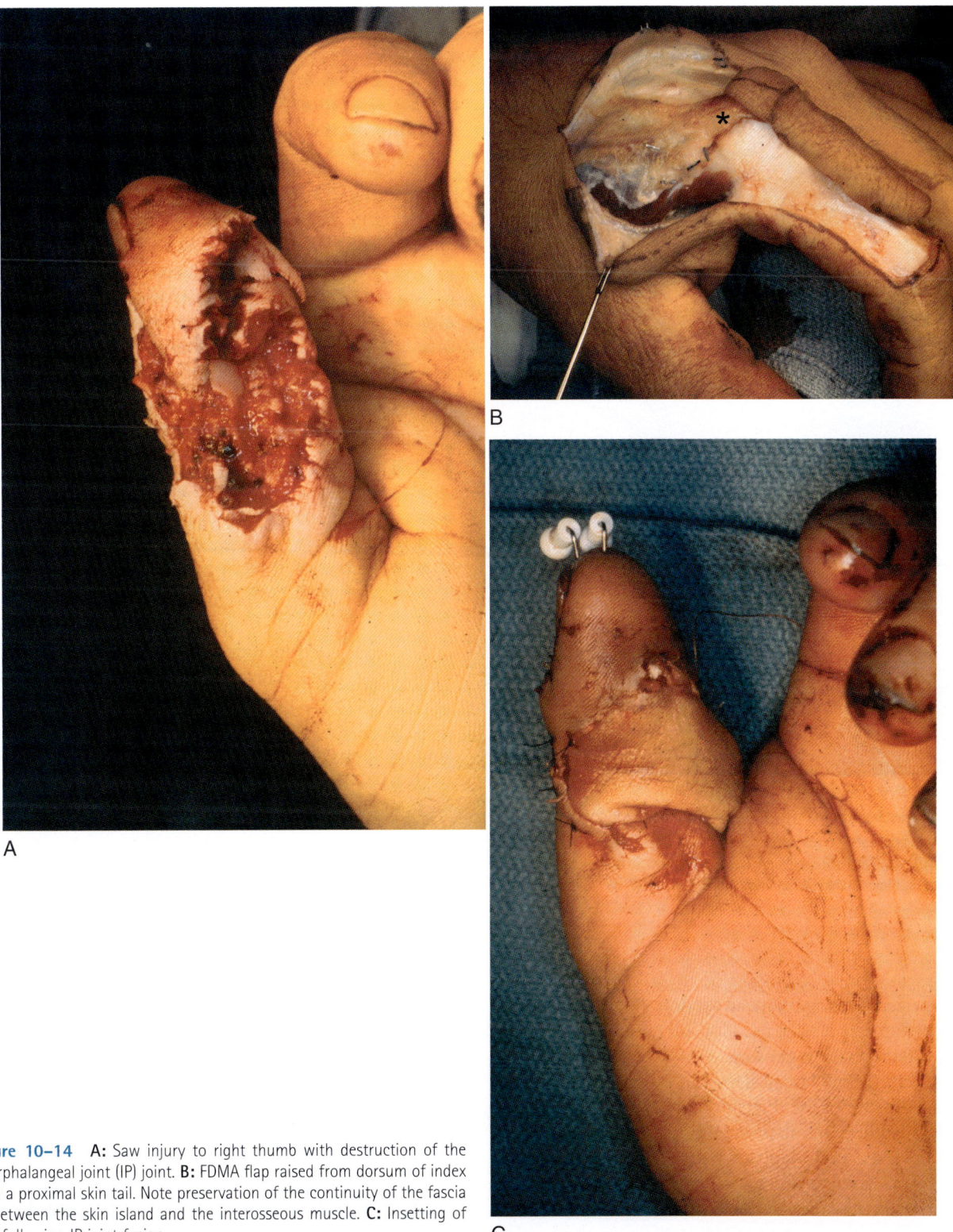

Figure 10–14 **A:** Saw injury to right thumb with destruction of the interphalangeal joint (IP) joint. **B:** FDMA flap raised from dorsum of index with a proximal skin tail. Note preservation of the continuity of the fascia (*) between the skin island and the interosseous muscle. **C:** Insetting of flap following IP joint fusion.

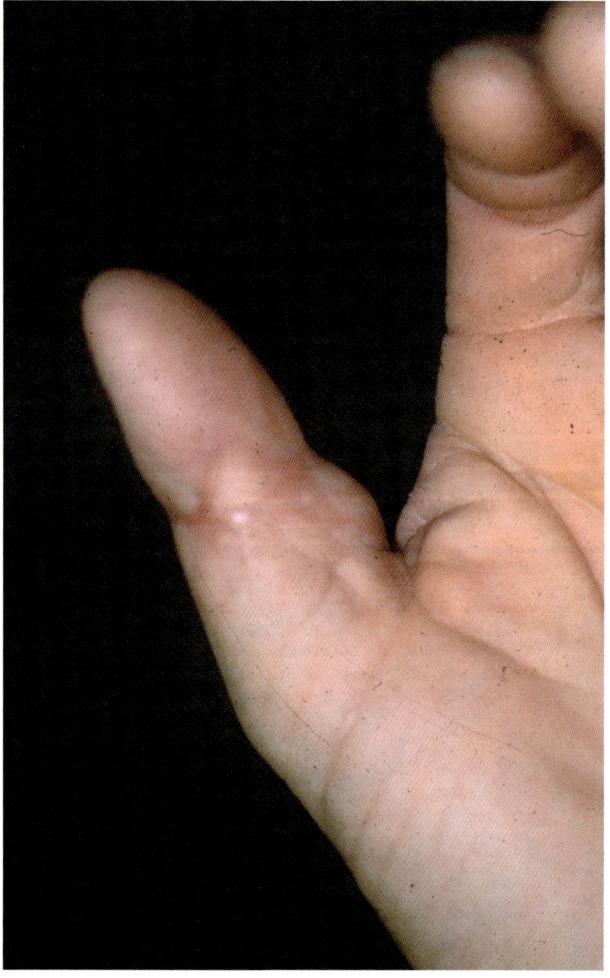

D

Figure 10–14–Cont'd **D:** Long-term result. (From Slutsky DJ. A practical approach to nerve grafting in the upper extremity. Atlas of the Hand Clinics. Nerve Repair and Reconstruction: A Practical Guide, Vol. 10, No. 1. Philadelphia: W.B. Saunders, 2005:73–92, with permission.)

transferred as a vascularized tendon graft. An insensate fascial flap may also be used for soft tissue coverage only, but it requires skin grafting.

Reversed flow fascial flaps can be used for coverage of the dorsum of the digits proximal to the PIP joints.[41] Unfortunately, this flap variant cannot be innervated. The reversed flow flap can reach as far ulnarly as the fifth metacarpal head. In this variation, the FDMA is ligated at its origin from the radial artery. The interosseous fascia is then elevated up to the level of the metacarpal neck. The donor site is skin grafted if primary closure is not possible.

Sensory Recovery

In one large series, the average two-point discrimination was 10.8 mm (range, 4 to 15 mm). There was no differ-

ence in patients younger or older than 50 years. The average loss of two-point discrimination over the flap area compared with the donor area was 2.7 mm.[43]

Complications

Postoperative complications may include flap edema from kinking of the pedicle. Flap necrosis can occur with injury to the thin fascial extension between the index island flaps and the FDI. Numbness over the dorsum of the middle phalanx of the index or hair growth over the volar aspect of the thumb may be an irritation. Loss of index finger motion, poor take of the skin graft over the index extensor tendon, or both is possible. Cold intolerance and dysesthesia can occur in up to 30% of patients.[45]

PEDICLED RADIAL FOREARM FLAP

The radial forearm flap is a useful and versatile fasciocutaneous flap designed on the radial artery. It was initially developed as a free flap in 1978 by Goufang and coworkers.[46] It was subsequently described as a pedicled flap using either antegrade or retrograde blood flow.[47,48] The flap includes the volar forearm skin, the underlying antebrachial fascia, and the intermuscular fascia, which contains the radial artery and its cutaneous branches. It can be innervated by the medial and lateral antebrachial cutaneous nerves. With retrograde flaps, neurorrhaphy to the local nerves is required.

Anatomy

The skin of the forearm flexor surface does not have any truly axial artery. An axial pattern flap is effectively created by raising a flap, including the fascial and subcutaneous vessels with their longitudinal orientation and interconnections.[49] The entire radial artery from its brachial artery origin to the wrist can be transferred. For most of its course, the radial artery lies under the brachioradialis. The pronator teres, flexor pollicus longus, and pronator quadratus lie deep to the artery. The SRN is lateral to the artery under the brachioradialis. After giving off the radial recurrent artery near its origin, the radial artery has no named branches until it reaches the wrist. Here it gives off a superficial palmar branch and a palmar carpal branch. Cadaver studies have demonstrated between 9 to 17 branches from the radial artery to the fascia along the flexor surface of the forearm. The branches supplying the skin are contained in an intermuscular septum between the brachioradialis and the flexor carpi radialis (Fig. 10–15). These branches are arranged into a proximal and distal group with corresponding zones of perfusion.[50] In the distal half of the forearm, there are branches every 1 to 2 cm. As

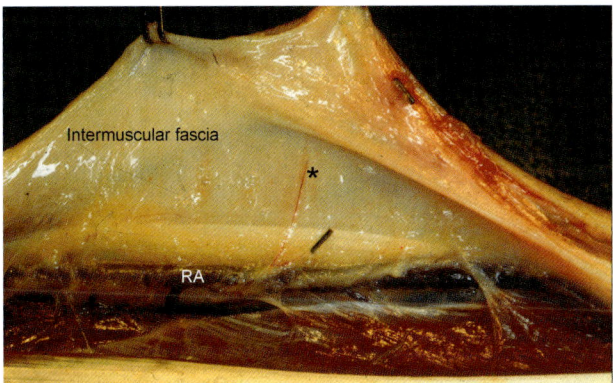

Figure 10–15 Demonstration of cutaneous branches (*) arising from radial artery *(RA)* coursing through the intermuscular septum. (From Slutsky DJ. A practical approach to nerve grafting in the upper extremity. Atlas of the Hand Clinics. Nerve Repair and Reconstruction: A Practical Guide, Vol. 10, No. 1. Philadelphia: W.B. Saunders, 2005:73–92, with permission.)

elsewhere, one vascular zone can be extended into another. The distal zone vessels can perfuse a fasciocutaneous flap as far proximal as the elbow. In a reverse pedicled flap, the skin blood supply is dependent on retrograde flow from the ulnar artery through the deep palmar arch.

Venous drainage of the radial forearm flap is by means of both the superficial and deep veins. There are three subcutaneous veins including the cephalic, basilic, and the median forearm vein, as well as the paired deep venae comitantes of the radial artery. A reverse pedicled flap is drained by means of retrograde flow through the venae comitantes. Normally, the venous valves prevent backflow. When a distally based flap is raised, the veins are denervated. The veins are kept filled by blood from the wrist and hand, which leads to an increased venous pressure after ligation of their proximal ends. The combination of these factors allows reverse flow through the venous valves.[50]

The SRN, the brachioradialis, flexor carpi radialis, and palmaris longus tendons are each supplied by direct branches and branches off cutaneous vessels. The medial and lateral antebrachial cutaneous nerves enter the proximal margin of the flap, and supply sensibility to the volar forearm.

The radial artery gives off at least two periosteal branches of 0.2 mm to 0.5 mm in size along the lateral aspect of the radius, immediately distal to the pronator teres insertion. These branches are accompanied by two small venae comitantes and pass along the fascial layer deep to the extensors carpi radialis longus and brevis. Musculoperiosteal vessels form a constant source of blood supply over the anterior aspect of the distal shaft. They are in turn fed by branches of the radial artery supplying the flexor pollicus longus and pronator quadratus.[51]

Over the distal volar forearm the flap is thin with little fat, but it leaves a poor bed for skin grafting, consisting of tendons covered only by paratenon. A proximal flap is hair bearing and thicker since it has more subcutaneous fat. The donor site contains muscle bellies, which is more favorable for skin grafting. The skin can be innervated by including the medial or lateral antebrachial cutaneous nerve. The flap can include the entire volar forearm skin from the subcutaneous border of the ulna around to the radial dorsum of the forearm, extending as far proximal as the antecubital fossa. Forearm flaps as large as 35 × 15 cm have been reported.

Indications

The flap is useful for thumb reconstruction (Fig. 10–16 A to F). It can be used for coverage of the palm or extensor surface of the carpus, with or without vascularized tendon (Fig. 10–17 A to C). It provides a durable surface for coverage of amputation stumps (Fig. 10–18 A to C).

Advantages

Distally based radial forearm flaps designed on the proximal forearm can easily reach the dorsal and palmar surfaces of the hand. They can include vascularized tendon and bone. Pedicle lengths up to 15 cm are possible. If the flap is less than 6 cm in width, the donor site can be closed primarily.

The flap arc of rotation can be increased by freeing the radial artery in the snuff box and passing the flap underneath the thumb extensors. This allows the flap to reach as far as the thumb tip.[38] The forearm flap permits postoperative elevation and early mobilization of the injured limb. Proximally based flaps can be used to resurface defects well above the elbow joint.[20] These flaps are directly innervated by including the medial or lateral cutaneous nerve of the forearm.

Limitations

Underdevelopment of the radial artery or injury to the superficial and deep palmar arches would preclude the use of this flap, as would the absence of a connection between the radial and ulnar arteries. In Coleman and Anson's dissection of 650 cadaver arms,[53] only 3.2% had no communication between the radial and ulnar artery, and 3% had an incomplete deep arch. If both of these variations are present, the thumb will be dependent on the radial artery (approximately 1 in 1,100). This can be identified by a preoperative Allen's test.[54] Vein graft reconstruction of the radial artery would be necessary in these cases. Care should be exercised in acute trauma when hematoma extends to the snuff box.

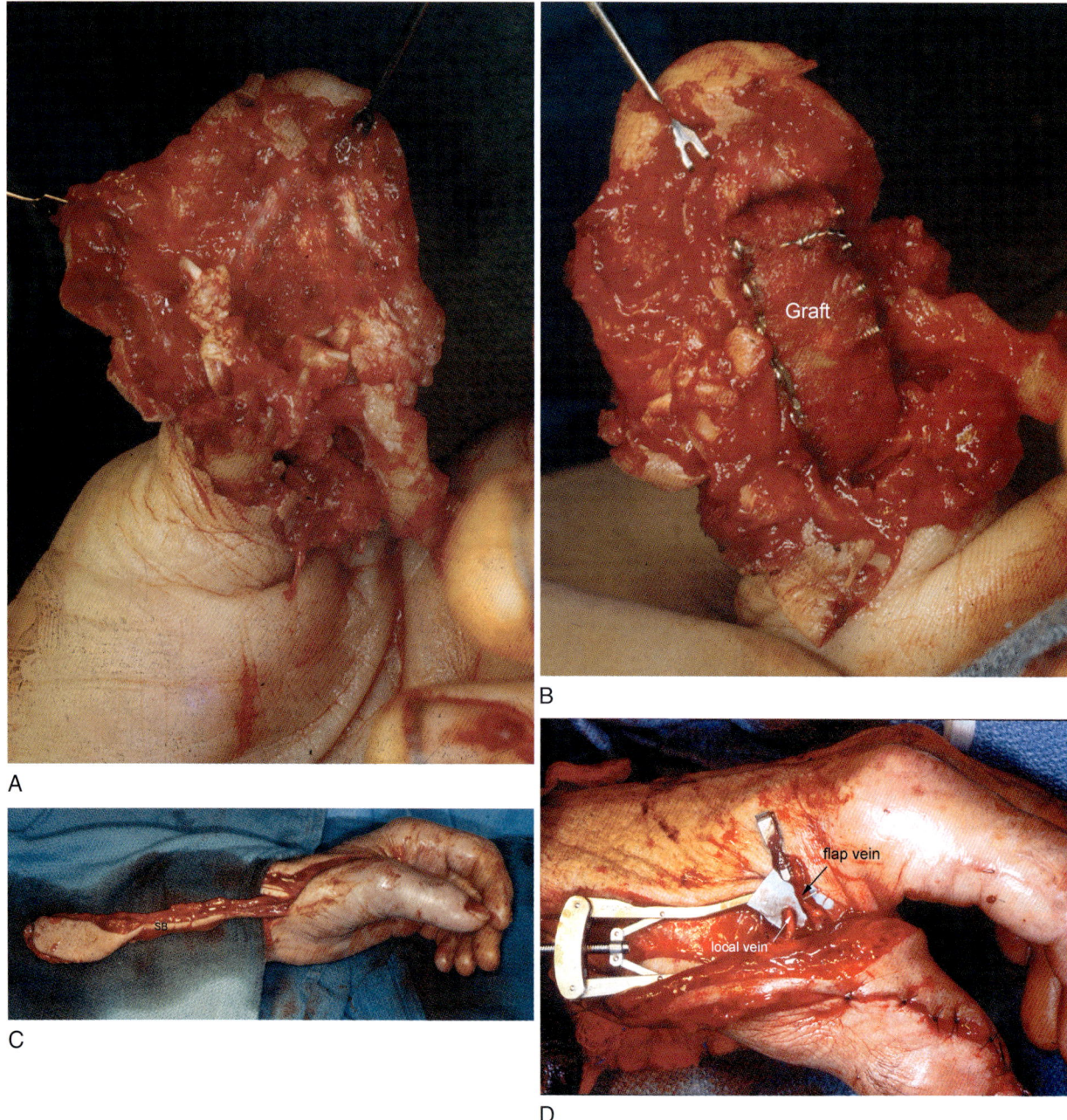

Figure 10–16   **A:** Saw injury with skin and bone loss of distal thumb. **B:** Bone reconstruction using iliac crest graft and minicondylar plate. **C:** Pedicle reversed-flow radial forearm flap. Note skin bridge (SB) over the pedicle. **D:** Supplemental venous anastomosis.

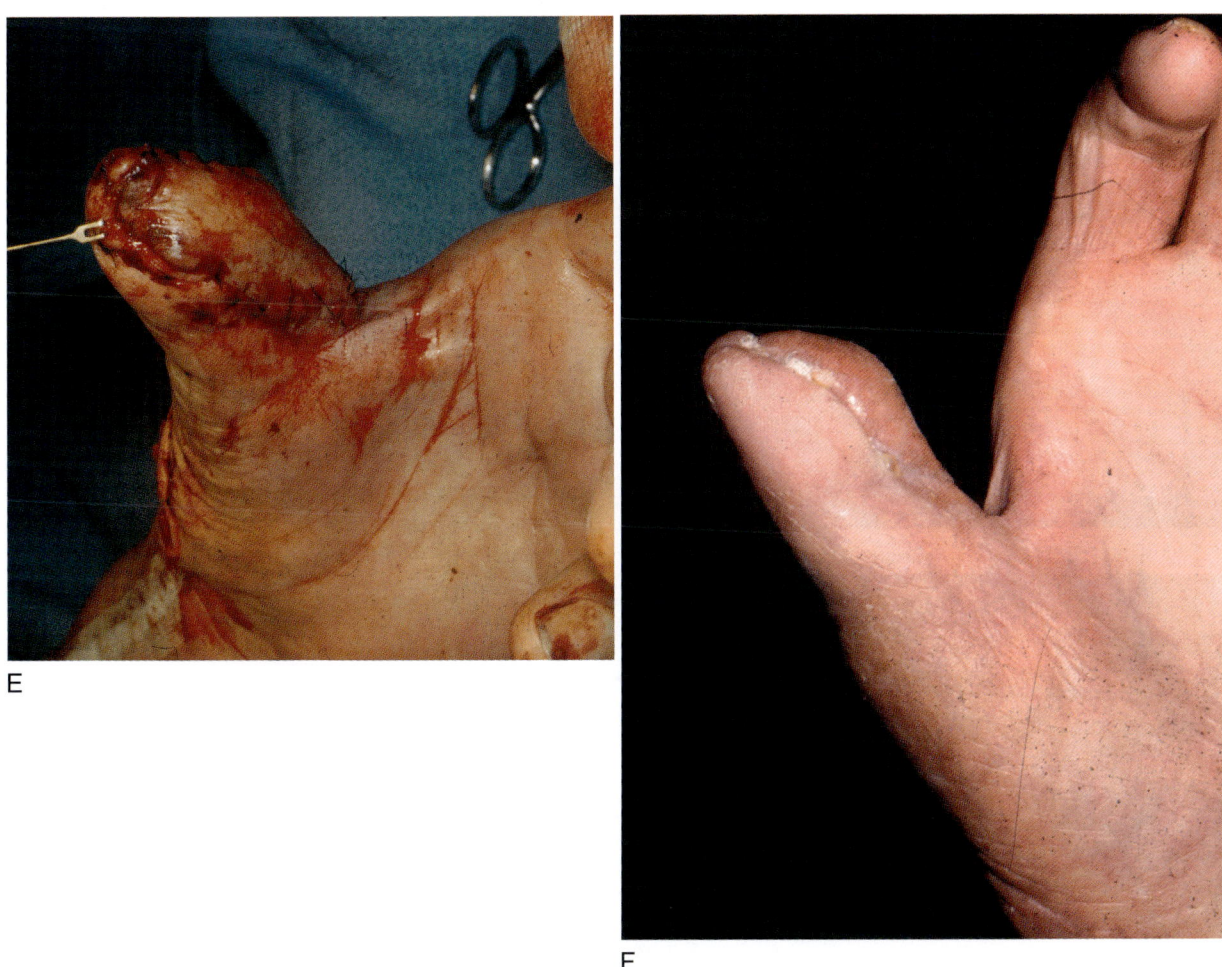

E

F

Figure 10–16–Cont'd E: Insetting of flap. **F:** Long-term result. (From Slutsky DJ. A practical approach to nerve grafting in the upper extremity. Atlas of the Hand Clinics. Nerve Repair and Reconstruction: A Practical Guide, Vol. 10, No. 1. Philadelphia: W.B. Saunders, 2005:73–92, with permission.)

Surgical Technique

The course of the radial artery is marked. Using a pattern from the recipient site, outline the size of the defect on the proximal forearm. If the flap is outlined over the proximal ulnar forearm, it will be thinner and less hair bearing. A thin skin island can be left over the course of the radial artery to prevent the need for skin grafting the pedicle later on and to avoid an overlying skin bridge. Incise the flap down to the deep fascia. Harvest veins along the proximal medial border of the flap. This allows an easier anastomosis with local veins once the flap has been rotated 180 degrees. Identify the medial or lateral antebrachial cutaneous nerve, and then make a proximal extensile incision for a longer nerve pedicle. The SRN should be protected to preserve sensation to the radial aspect of the hand.[25]

Develop a plane deep to the radial artery at the wrist and find the intermuscular septum between the flexor carpi radialis (FCR) and the brachioradialis. Incise the deep fascia over the FCR muscle belly, well medial to the intermuscular septum. Dissect the interval between the deep fascia and the muscle. Suture the deep fascia to the skin flap to minimize shear on the septocutaneous perforators. Continue the dissection deep to the radial artery on both side of the septum. The fascia superficial to the radial artery is left undisturbed since it contains the septocutanous perforators that supply the skin flap. After the flap dissection is complete, apply a microvascular clamp to the proximal radial artery prior to releasing the tourniquet. If there is adequate perfusion to the flap and the thumb, then the artery is divided. Raise the flap, ligating all the perforators deep to the artery. Transpose the flap to the dorsum of the hand. If desired, perform a venous anastomosis prior to insetting the flap (see Fig. 10–16 D).

Variations

The radial forearm flap can be raised as a composite skin flap, including vascularized bone and tendon for thumb

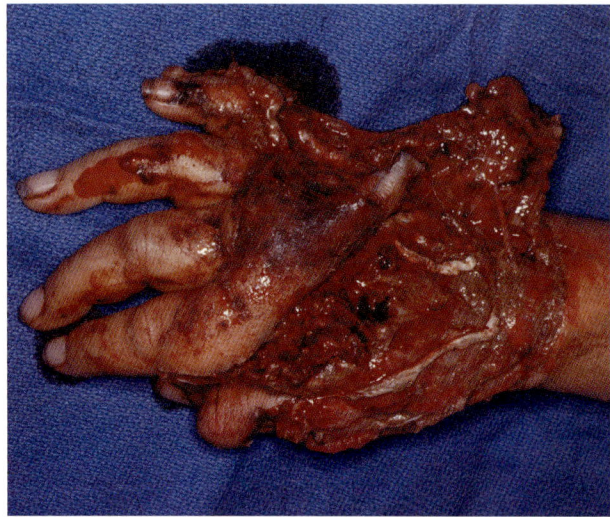

A

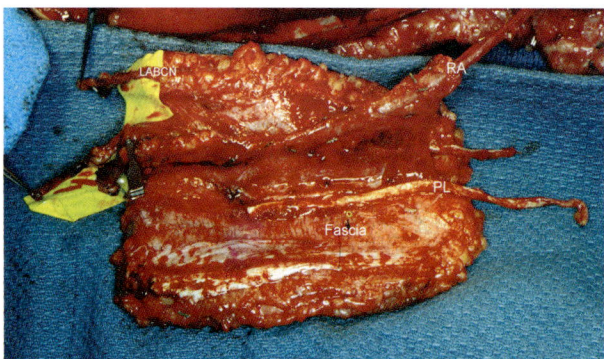

B

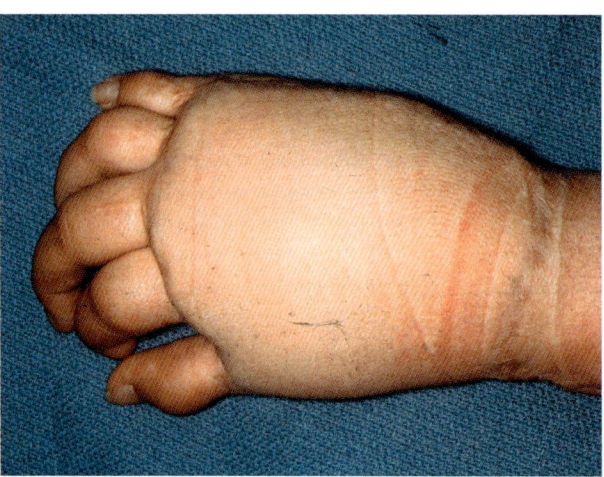

C

Figure 10–17 **A:** Rollover crush injury with devitalized skin, extensor tendon loss, and multiple open fractures. **B:** Pedicled retrograde flap based on the radial artery (RA). Note the vascularized palmaris longus tendon (PL) and the lateral antebrachial cutaneous nerve (LABCN). **C:** Long-term result. (From Slutsky DJ. A practical approach to nerve grafting in the upper extremity. Atlas of the Hand Clinics. Nerve Repair and Reconstruction: A Practical Guide, Vol. 10, No. 1. Philadelphia: W.B. Saunders, 2005:73–92, with permission.)

reconstruction.[55] A purely fascial radial forearm flap can be used to cover exposed tendons on the dorsum of the hand, but it has to be skin grafted and innervation is not possible.[56] A reverse radial fascial-fat flap preserves the radial artery, and has been used to cover a scarred median nerve.[57,58]

Vascularized Bone Dissection

The vascularized bone graft does not carry an intact blood endosteal supply, but instead survives on the perisoteal branches. The lateral half of the radius from the insertion of the pronator teres to the metaphyseal flare of the distal radius can be harvested. Up to 10 cm of slightly curved, mostly cortical bone, that comprises half the circumference of a circle is obtained. Preserve the perforators deep in the radial artery along the length of the desired bone graft. Dissect medial to the intermuscular fascia over the radius. Divide the pronator teres, sublimus muscle, and flexor pollicus longus muscle directly on top of the midline of the bone. This preserves the musculoperiosteal branches to the bone graft. Predrill the osteotomy site prior to performing the osteotomy. Bevel the proximal and distal corners to decrease stress risers and to diminish the risk of postoperative fracture.

Fascial Flap Dissection

A purely fascial flap is raised in a similar manner to the fasciocutaneous flap. The plane of dissection, however, proceeds between the deep fascia and the skin, which divides all the cutaneous branches.

The reverse radial fascial-fat flap survives on retrograde blood flow through perforating vessels coming off the radial artery. These perforators are found within 1.5 to 7 cm from the radial styloid and run directly upward from the radial artery into the fascia (Fig. 10–19). The fascia thus serves as a viable supporting membrane for perfusion of the fat on its surface.[57] The most proximal perforators are sacrificed for retrograde orientation of this flap. The fat and deep fascia are developed as a long, distally based rectangular flap. The interval between the fat and fascia is not violated. The lateral antebrachial cutaneous nerve and SRN are preserved. After elevation, the flap is turned distally 180 degrees and simultaneously twisted 90 degrees to place the vascularized fat layer directly over the median nerve (Fig. 10–20). The donor site is closed primarily.

Sensory Recovery

In one series, the moving two-point discrimination averaged 13.2 mm. This was more sensitive than the donor forearm; hence, it was postulated that the sensory return was more dependent on the recipient nerve than on the donor nerve.[59]

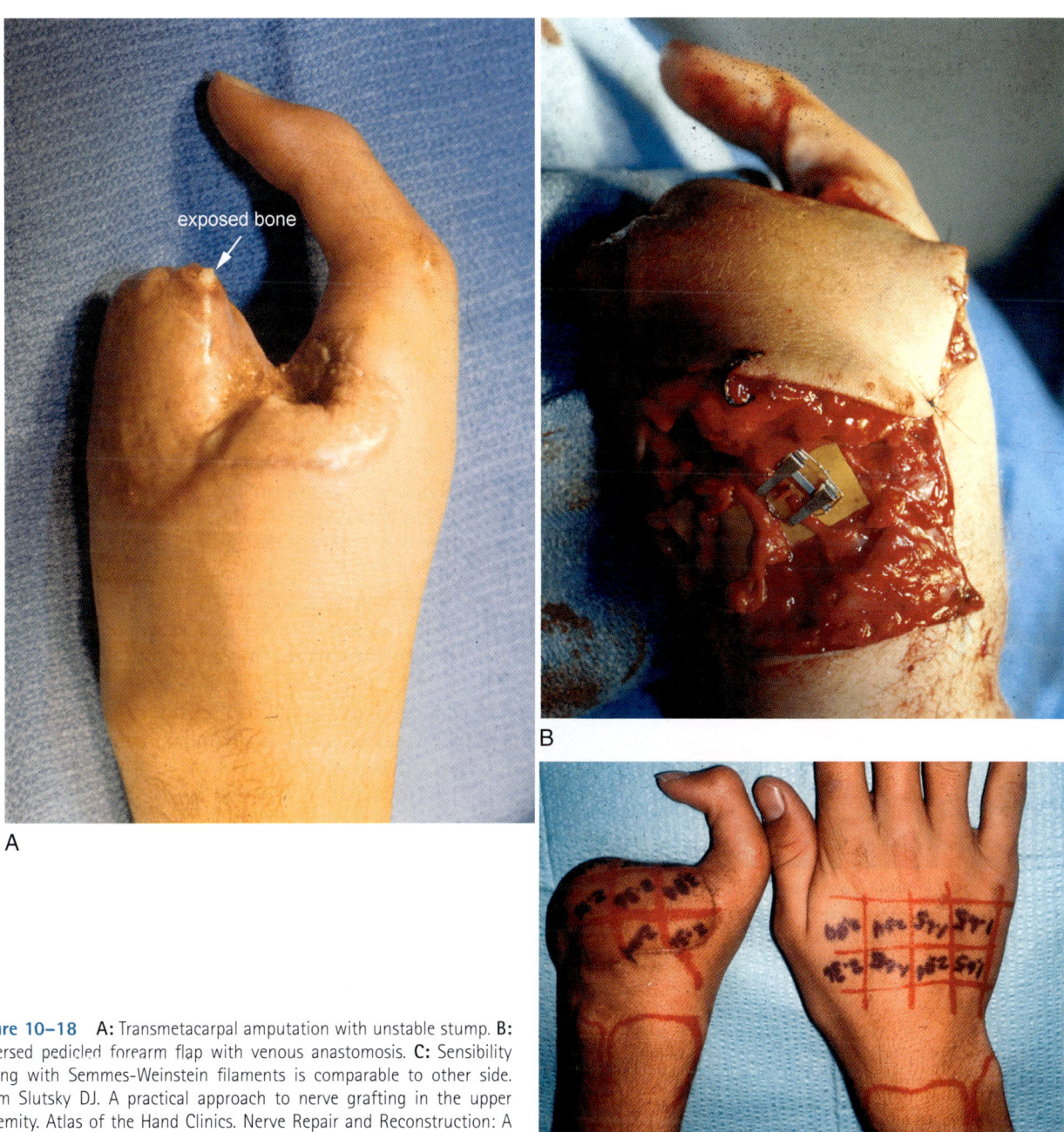

Figure 10–18 **A:** Transmetacarpal amputation with unstable stump. **B:** Reversed pedicled forearm flap with venous anastomosis. **C:** Sensibility testing with Semmes-Weinstein filaments is comparable to other side. (From Slutsky DJ. A practical approach to nerve grafting in the upper extremity. Atlas of the Hand Clinics. Nerve Repair and Reconstruction: A Practical Guide, Vol. 10, No. 1. Philadelphia: W.B. Saunders, 2005:73–92, with permission.)

Complications

Postoperative complications include flap edema, unstable skin graft over tendons, hand swelling, and superficial radial nerve injury. Flap edema is common due to associated forearm injury or impaired venous drainage. Additional venous anastomoses will help minimize this. Skin graft failure is most likely to occur over tendons, especially the FCR. Even when they have successfully taken on tendons, skin grafts may suffer recurrent breakdown. Avoidance of the distal forearm as a donor site and covering the tendons with adjacent muscle fibers from portions of the brachioradialis, flexor digitorum superficialis, and flexor carpi ulnaris provide a better skin graft bed. Unmeshed skin grafts can be used to maximize the bridging phenomenon. Preoperative tissue expansion can also be used.[60]

The donor site defect is quite noticeable. The flap is hair bearing and often bulky. A radial shaft fracture can occur following harvest of vascularized one; hence, above elbow casting or splinting for up to 8 weeks is recommended. Although digital temperature com-

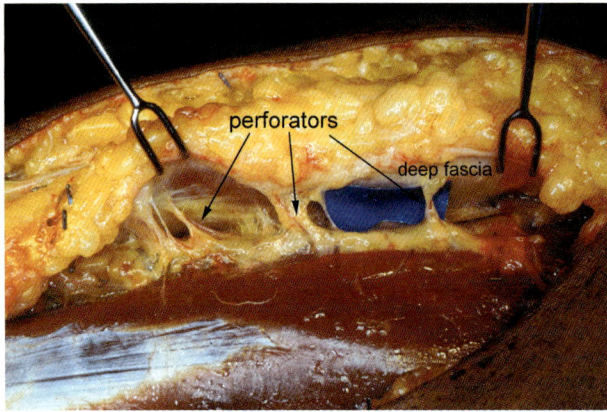

Figure 10-19 Demonstration of perforating vessels supplying the deep fascia. (From Slutsky DJ. A practical approach to nerve grafting in the upper extremity. Atlas of the Hand Clinics. Nerve Repair and Reconstruction: A Practical Guide, Vol. 10, No. 1. Philadelphia: W.B. Saunders, 2005:73–92, with permission.)

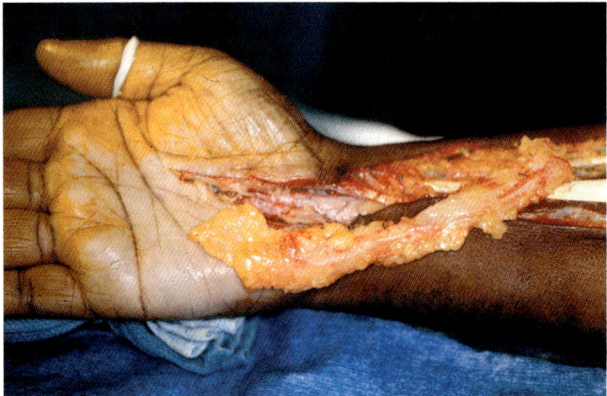

Figure 10-20 Pedicled fascial forearm flap used to cover median nerve following neurolysis. (From Slutsky DJ. A practical approach to nerve grafting in the upper extremity. Atlas of the Hand Clinics. Nerve Repair and Reconstruction: A Practical Guide, Vol. 10, No. 1. Philadelphia: W.B. Saunders, 2005:73–92, with permission.)

parisons show an average 2.5% decrease following the use of the radial forearm flap, cold intolerance is often transient.[61]

INNERVATED GROIN FLAP

The groin flap, introduced by McGregor and Jackson in 1972, was one of the first axial pattern flaps.[62] It was revolutionary because it allowed greater potential for reconstruction of difficult upper extremity wounds. Despite the wide variety of pedicle flaps, the groin flap still has a place in cases where there are inadequate vessels for a free flap or where there has been an injury to the carpal arch, which precludes the use of a pedicled forearm flap. Joshi[63] modified the flap to include branches of the lateral cutaneous branch of the subcostal nerve (12th thoracic nerve). This facilitates sensory innervation of the flap after neurorrhaphy to local donor nerves.

Anatomy

The groin flap is supplied by either the superficial circumflex iliac artery (SCIA) or the superficial epigastric artery (SEA). Taylor and Daniel found the SCIA to be present and greater than 1 mm in diameter, 98% of the time.[64] The SCIA and SEA usually arise separately off the femoral artery, although a common arterial trunk was found in 29% of specimens in one series.[65] Either the common trunk or the SCIA is used as the pedicle unless the SEA is larger.

The SCIA arises from the anterolateral aspect of the femoral artery, 2 to 3 cm below the inguinal ligament. It runs laterally in a line parallel to the inguinal ligament superficial to the iliacus fascia, enveloped by the fatty lymphatic tissue in the femoral triangle. At the medial border of the sartorius muscle, it usually divides into a superficial and deep branch. The superficial branch continues laterally, above the sartorius fascia to supply the skin surrounding the anterior superior iliac spine (ASIS). The deep branch runs underneath the sartorius fascia. It pierces the fascia at the lateral border of the sartorius, 1 to 4 cm below the ASIS, giving off cutaneous and muscular branches. If a long groin flap is required, the deep branch must be included in the pedicle. The vascular network lateral to the ASIS is quite extensive, allowing elevation of a large random pattern skin extension of the flap.

The SEA arises in a similar fashion to the SCIA, and then runs laterally, superficial and superior, to the inguinal ligament. It remains medial to the ASIS to supply an area of skin above the territory of the SCIA. The territories of these vessels overlap.

The venous drainage is quite variable. The groin area is drained by the superficial epigastric vein (SEV), the superficial circumflex iliac vein (SCIV), and the associated venae comitantes. These veins drain into either the saphenous bulb or the femoral vein. The SEV and SCIV lie superficial to their respective arteries and to Scarpa's fascia. They frequently form a common trunk measuring more than 2mm.[66]

The sensory supply of the lateral half of the groin flap corresponds to nearly the entire distribution of the lateral cutaneous branch of the subcostal nerve. This branch exits between the internal and external oblique muscles. It descends over the iliac crest about 5 cm behind the ASIS, before supplying the skin over the front part of the buttocks. This nerve branch is separate from the lateral cutaneous nerve of the thigh, which arises from the lumbar plexus (L2 and L3) and then travels behind the inguinal ligament.

Indications

The groin flap is indicated for cases requiring massive soft tissue coverage of the hand. It provides a means for the resurfacing of very large soft tissue defects, up to 15 cm × 30 cm. This flap may be used for thumb reconstruction or for limb salvage after a failed free or pedicled flap. It may be useful in selected pediatric cases where the donor site defect from other pedicled or free flaps may be substantial.

Advantages

The flap anatomy is reliable, and microvascular technique is not a prerequisite to raising the flap. It can be used in situations where inadequate vessels, or patient factors (age, systemic illness, atherosclerotic vessels) preclude the use of a free flap. It may be useful when

where there is an injury to the superficial and deep palmar arch that precludes the use of a reversed pedicled radial forearm flap (Fig. 10–21 A to C). The donor site scar can be closed primarily, and is hidden by a bathing suit. Since regional nerves are utilized, there is no problem with cortical reorientation.

Limitations

A history of lymphadenitis or previous surgery in the groin including hernia repairs, lymph node biopsies[57] or vein stripping may preclude use of this flap for fear of prior injury to the vascular pedicle. Patients with marked limb edema, or shoulder or elbow contractures[57]

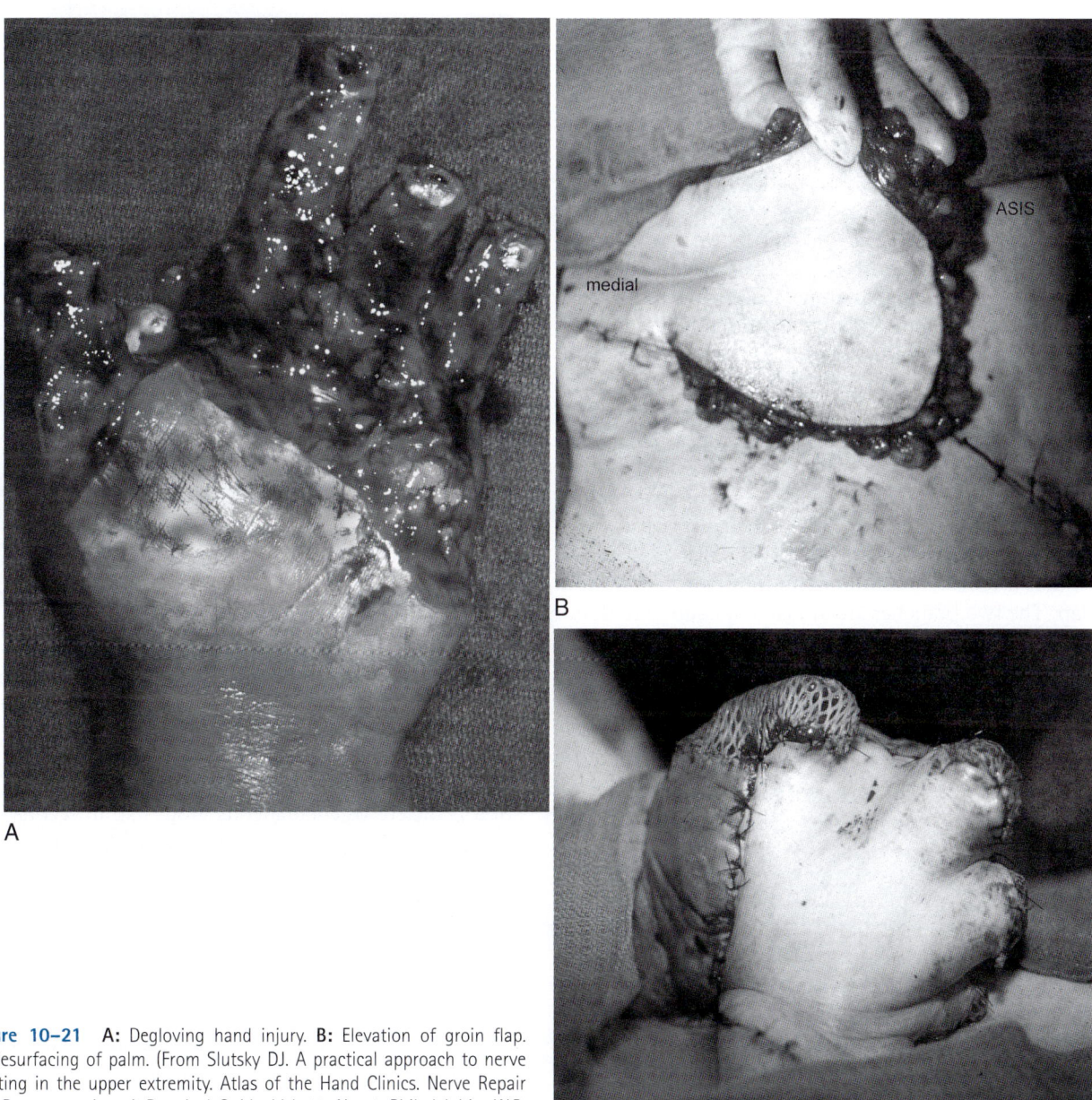

Figure 10–21   A: Degloving hand injury. **B:** Elevation of groin flap. **C:** Resurfacing of palm. (From Slutsky DJ. A practical approach to nerve grafting in the upper extremity. Atlas of the Hand Clinics. Nerve Repair and Reconstruction: A Practical Guide, Vol. 10, No. 1. Philadelphia: W.B. Saunders, 2005:73–92, with permission.)

or patients who cannot tolerate prolonged upper extremity immobilization for psychological reasons, may not be appropriate candidates.

Surgical Technique

The patient is positioned supine with a sand bag under the ipsilateral buttock. The amount of skin that can be removed while still allowing direct closure can be estimated by flexing the hip and approximating the skin edges manually. The pubic tubercle, inguinal ligament, and ASIS are drawn along with a pattern taken from the tissue defect. The most dependable approach is to approximate the flap axis through the center of both vascular territories by drawing a line 2 cm distal to the inguinal ligament that extends past the ASIS.

The flap is elevated from lateral to medial to allow identification of the SCIA or SEA. The flap is then based upon the larger of the two arteries at the time of dissection. A thin layer of subcutaneous fat is harvested with the skin lateral to the ASIS, since this represents a random pattern flap extension of the flap. Once the ASIS is encountered, however, the entire width of the subcutaneous fat must be harvested in order to include the arterial pedicle. The interval between the tensor fascia lata and the sartorius is delineated. The deep branch of SCIA courses from a deep to a superficial plane as it passes through the sartorius fascia to reach the subcutaneous tissue. Both the fascia and the subcutaneous tissue are carefully elevated from the lateral border of the muscle to prevent injury to the SCIA. If the SCIA is not visible, transilluminating the flap may be of some help.

The subcostal nerve emerges from the oblique muscles and spreads into two branches just below the iliac crest. The nerve is divided at the iliac crest region so that it remains ensheathed in the layers of the groin flap. The two branches are available for suture to donor nerves in the hand, with the pedicle entering on one end and the nerve exiting the other end of the flap.[63] The hand is placed in the groin and the flap is sewn over the soft tissue defect. Shoulder range of motion exercises are emphasized until the flap is divided at 3 to 4 weeks.

Variations

If the flap is tubed for thumb reconstruction (Fig. 10–22), one side of the flap is cut longer than the other, and diagonal closure of the donor site and the flap is performed. This diagonal closure increases the circumference of the tube at the base of the flap, thereby reducing the risk of vascular compression. Diagonal closure also produces a spiral in the tube. The direction of the spiral can be controlled to facilitate closure of defects on the palm or dorsum of the hand.[67] The use

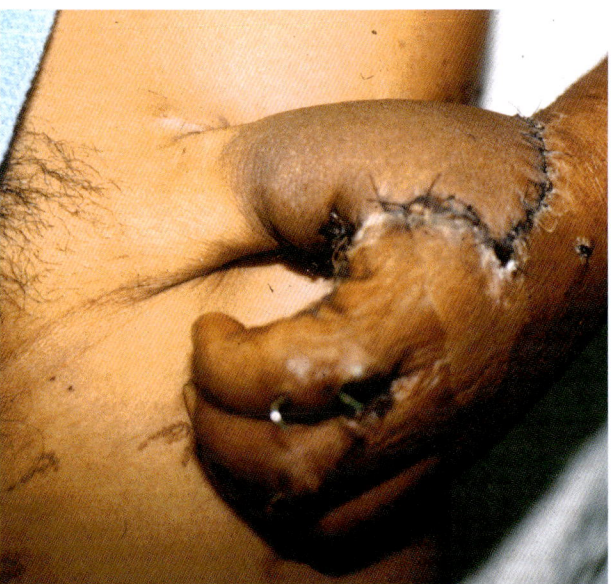

Figure 10–22 Tubed groin flap for thumb reconstruction. (From Slutsky DJ. A practical approach to nerve grafting in the upper extremity. Atlas of the Hand Clinics. Nerve Repair and Reconstruction: A Practical Guide, Vol. 10, No. 1. Philadelphia: W.B. Saunders, 2005:73–92, with permission.)

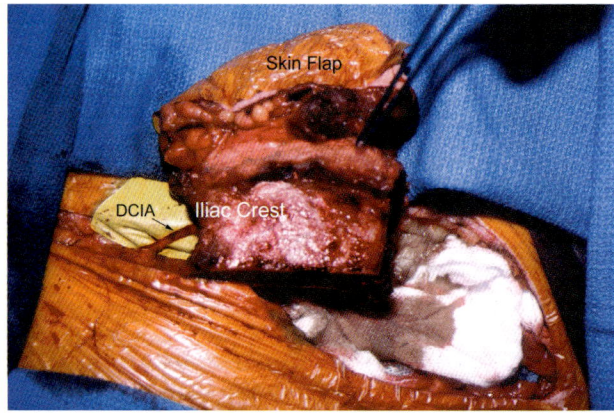

Figure 10–23 Osteocutaneous groin flap pedicled on the deep circumflex iliac artery *(DCIA)*. (From Slutsky DJ. A practical approach to nerve grafting in the upper extremity. Atlas of the Hand Clinics. Nerve Repair and Reconstruction: A Practical Guide, Vol. 10, No. 1. Philadelphia: W.B. Saunders, 2005:73–92, with permission.)

of a pedicled, osteocutaneous groin flap to reconstruct composite interpositional bone loss of the thumb has been described (Fig. 10–23).[68] Taylor has demonstrated the superiority of the deep circumflex iliac vessels when harvesting vascularized bone with the groin flap.[69]

Sensory Recovery

In Joshi's series of four patients,[63] the innervated groin flap provided protective sensation or better. The maximum return of sensation occurred by 4 months, as compared to 1-1/2 years for a noninnervated flap.

Complications

The flap carries pubic hair on its medial aspect. The flap is bulky and a secondary procedure for defatting may be necessary. Shoulder stiffness is common, especially in elderly patients. Partial fat necrosis, seroma, and infection, as well as complications related to bed rest can complicate the results.

SUMMARY

It is apparent that any particular soft tissue defect of the hand can be managed in a variety of ways. Oftentimes the simplest procedure with the fewest potential complications will suffice. Soft tissue coverage is merely one component in the management of complex hand injuries, which may also require bony stabilization, neurovascular repair, and tendon reconstruction. Although not specifically addressed, the role of aggressive hand therapy with edema control, early active motion, and functional retraining cannot be overemphasized. Providing stable soft tissue coverage with the potential for sensibility, however, expands the subsequent reconstructive options and enhances the ultimate functional result.

REFERENCES

1. Merriam-Webster's Collegiate Dictionary, 10th ed. Spring field, MA, 1999.
2. Bertelli JA, Catarina S. Neurocutaneous island flaps in upper limb coverage: experience with 44 clinical cases. J Hand Surg Am 22:515, 1997.
3. Slutsky DJ. Vascularized Pedicled Flaps of the Forearm and Hand. Instruction course presented at American Society for Surgery of the Hand, 53rd annual meeting, Minneapolis MN, September 1998.
4. Slutsky DJ. Vascularized Pedicled Flaps of the Forearm and Hand. Skills course with cadaver demonstration at American Society for Surgery of the Hand, 54th annual meeting, Boston, September 1999.
5. Swartz WM. Restoration of sensibility in mutilating hand injuries. Clin Plast Surg 16:515, 1989.
6. Moberg E. Aspects of sensation in reconstructive surgery of the upper extremity. J Bone Joint Surg Am 46:817, 1964.
7. Hueston J. Local flap repair of fingertip injuries. Plast Reconstr Surg 37:349, 1966.
8. Souquet R, Souquet JR. The actual indications of cross finger flaps in finger injuries. Ann Chir Main 5:43, 1986.
9. Foucher G, Dallaserra M, Tilquin B, et al. The Hueston flap in reconstruction of fingertip skin loss: results in a series of 41 patients. J Hand Surg Am 19:508, 1994.
10. Cronin TD. The cross finger flap: a new method of repair. Am Surg 17:419, 1951.
11. Berger A, Meissl G. [Reestablishment of sensation in the distal phalanges using innervated flaps or grafts]. Handchirurgie 7:169, 1975.
12. Endo T, Kojima T, Hirase Y. Vascular anatomy of the finger dorsum and a new idea for coverage of the finger pulp defect that restores sensation. J Hand Surg Am 17:927, 1992.
13. Lai CS, Lin SD, Chou CK, et al. A versatile method for reconstruction of finger defects: reverse digital artery flap. Br J Plast Surg 45:443, 1992.
14. Tellioglu AT, Sensoz O. The dorsal branch of the digital nerve: an anatomic study and clinical applications. Ann Plast Surg 40:145, 1998.
15. Kleinert HE, McAlister CG, MacDonald CJ, et al. A critical evaluation of cross finger flaps. J Trauma 14:756, 1974.
16. Cohen BE, Cronin ED. An innervated cross-finger flap for fingertip reconstruction. Plast Reconstr Surg 72:688, 1983.
17. Lassner F, Becker M, Berger A, et al. Sensory reconstruction of the fingertip using the bilaterally innervated sensory cross-finger flap. Plast Reconstr Surg 109:988, 2002.
18. Gaul JS Jr. Radial-innervated cross-finger flap from index to provide sensory pulp to injured thumb. J Bone Joint Surg Am 51:1257, 1969.
19. Abrams RA, Brown RA, Botte MJ. The superficial branch of the radial nerve: an anatomic study with surgical implications. J Hand Surg Am 17:1037, 1992.
20. Hastings H 2nd. Dual innervated index to thumb cross finger or island flap reconstruction. Microsurgery 8:168, 1987.
21. Walker MA, Hurley CB, May JW Jr. Radial nerve cross-finger flap differential nerve contribution in thumb reconstruction. J Hand Surg Am 11:881, 1986.
22. Kojima T, Hirase Y, Sakurai N, et al. Eleven cases of vascular pedicle island flap for difficult skin defects on the hand. J Jpn Soc Surg Hand :350, 1986.
23. Strauch B, de Moura W. Arterial system of the fingers. J Hand Surg Am 15:148, 1990.
24. Oberlin C. A reversed digital artery island flap for the treatment of fingertip injuries. J Hand Surg Am 19:342, 1994.
25. Slutsky DJ. Cadaver Dissections: Vascularized Pedicled Flaps of the Forearm and Hand. Presented in videotape theater at American Society for Surgery of the Hand, 53rd annual meeting, Minneapolis MN, September 1998, and 54th annual meeting, Boston, September 1999.
26. Lai CS, Lin SD, Chou CK, et al. Innervated reverse digital artery flap through bilateral neurorrhaphy for pulp defects. Br J Plast Surg 46:483, 1993.
27. Earley MJ, Milner RH. Dorsal metacarpal flaps. Br J Plast Surg 40:333, 1987.
28. Lai CS, Lin SD, Tsai CC, et al. Reverse digital artery neurovascular cross-finger flap. J Hand Surg Am 20:397, 1995.
29. Karacalar A, Sen C, Ozcan M. A modified reversed digital island flap incorporating the proper digital nerve. Ann Plast Surg 45:67, 2000.
30. Han SK, Lee BI, Kim WK. The reverse digital artery island flap: clinical experience in 120 fingers. Plast Reconstr Surg 101:1006, 1998.
31. Sapp JW, Allen RJ, Dupin C. A reversed digital artery island flap for the treatment of fingertip injuries. J Hand Surg Am 18:528, 1993.
32. Brunelli F, Pegin Z, Cabral J. Dorsal arterial supply to the thumb. New surgical possibilities for palmar skin coverage. Surg Radiol Anat 13:240, 1991.
33. Pistre V, Pelissier P, Martin D, et al. Vascular blood supply of the dorsal side of the thumb, first web and index finger: anatomical study. J Hand Surg Br 26:98, 2001.
34. Brunelli F, Vigasio A, Valenti P, et al. Arterial anatomy and clinical application of the dorsoulnar flap of the thumb. J Hand Surg Am 24:803, 1999.
35. Kumar VP, Satku K, Liu J. The Brunelli reversed flow pedicle flap from the thumb. Plast Reconstr Surg 98:1298, 1996.
36. Cavadas PC. Reverse osteocutaneous dorsoulnar thumb flap. Plast Reconstr Surg 111:326, 2003.
37. Holevich J. A New Method of Restoring Sensibility to the Thumb. J Bone Joint Surg Br 45:496, 1963.

38. Foucher G, Braun JB. A new island flap transfer from the dorsum of the index to the thumb. Plast Reconstr Surg 63:344, 1979.

39. Steinberg BD, Plancher KD, Idler RS. Percutaneous Kirschner wire fixation through the snuff box: an anatomic study. J Hand Surg Am 20:57, 1995.

40. Chiu HY, Shieh SJ, Hsu HY. Multivariate analysis of factors influencing the functional recovery after finger replantation or revascularization. Microsurgery 16:713, 1995.

41. Sherif MM. First dorsal metacarpal artery flap in hand reconstruction. II. Clinical application. J Hand Surg Am 19:32, 1994.

42. Slutsky DJ. The first dorsal metacarpal artery flap. In: Wrist Arthroscopy 2000 Course Videotapes. Chicago: American Society for Surgery of the Hand, 2000.

43. Trankle M, Sauerbier M, Heitmann C, et al. Restoration of thumb sensibility with the innervated first dorsal metacarpal artery island flap. J Hand Surg Am 28:758, 2003.

44. El-Khatib HA. Clinical experiences with the extended first dorsal metacarpal artery island flap for thumb reconstruction. J Hand Surg Am 23:647, 1998.

45. Ege A, Tuncay I, Ercetin O. Foucher's first dorsal metacarpal artery flap for thumb reconstruction: evaluation of 21 cases. Isr Med Assoc J 4:421, 2002.

46. Yang G, Chen B, Gao Y, et al. Forearm free skin flap transplantation. Natl Med J China 61:139, 1981.

47. Muhlbauer W, Herndl E, Stock W. The forearm flap. Plast Reconstr Surg 70:336, 1982.

48. Song R, Gao Y, Song Y, et al. The forearm flap. Clin Plast Surg 9:21, 1982.

49. Cormack GC, Lamberty BG. A classification of fascio-cutaneous flaps according to their patterns of vascularisation. Br J Plast Surg 37:80, 1984.

50. Timmons MJ. The vascular basis of the radial forearm flap. Plast Reconstr Surg 77:80, 1986.

51. Cormack GC, Duncan MJ, Lamberty BG. The blood supply of the bone component of the compound osteo-cutaneous radial artery forearm flap—an anatomical study. Br J Plast Surg 39:173, 1986.

52. Fatah MF, Davies DM. The radial forearm island flap in upper limb reconstruction. J Hand Surg Br 9:234, 1984.

53. Coleman SS, Anson BJ. Arterial patterns in the hand based upon a study of 650 specimens. Suvr Med (Sofiia) 113:409, 1961.

54. Gelberman RH, Blasingame JP. The timed Allen test. J Trauma 21:477, 1981.

55. Biemer E, Stock W. Total thumb reconstruction: a one-stage reconstruction using an osteo-cutaneous forearm flap. Br J Plast Surg 36:52, 1983.

56. Reyes FA, Burkhalter WE. The fascial radial flap. J Hand Surg Am 13:432, 1988.

57. Braun RM, Rechnic M, Neill-Cage DJ, et al. The retrograde radial fascial forearm flap: surgical rationale, technique, and clinical application. J Hand Surg Am 20:915, 1995.

58. Tham SK, Ireland DC, Riccio M, et al. Reverse radial artery fascial flap: a treatment for the chronically scarred median nerve in recurrent carpal tunnel syndrome. J Hand Surg Am 21:849, 1996.

59. Yamauchi T, Yajima H, Kizaki K, et al. Sensory reconstruction in sensate radial forearm flap transfer. J Reconstr Microsurg 16:593, 2000.

60. Liang MD, Swartz WM, Jones NF. Local full-thickness skin-graft coverage for the radial forearm flap donor site. Plast Reconstr Surg 93:621, 1994.

61. Kleinman WB, O'Connell SJ. Effects of the fasciocutaneous radial forearm flap on vascularity of the hand. J Hand Surg Am 18:953, 1993.

62. McGregor IA, Jackson IT. The groin flap. Br J Plast Surg 25:3, 1972.

63. Joshi BB. Neural repair for sensory restoration in a groin flap. Hand 9:221, 1977.

64. Taylor GI, Daniel RK. The anatomy of several free flap donor sites. Plast Reconstr Surg 56:243, 1975.

65. Harii K, Omori K, Torii S, et al. Free groin skin flaps. Br J Plast Surg 28:225, 1975.

66. Harii K, Ohmori K, Torii S, et al. Microvascular free skin flap transfer. Clin Plast Surg 5:239, 1978.

67. Schlenker JD. Important considerations in the design and construction of groin flaps. Ann Plast Surg 5:353, 1980.

68. Button M, Stone EJ. Segmental bony reconstruction of the thumb by composite groin flap: a case report. J Hand Surg Am 5:488, 1980.

69. Taylor GI, Townsend P, Corlett R. Superiority of the deep circumflex iliac vessels as the supply for free groin flaps. Plast Reconstr Surg 64:595, 1979.

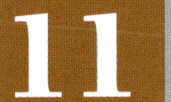

11 A NEUROSENSORY FREE FLAPS FOR HAND RECONSTRUCTION: THE FIRST WEB–SPACE FLAP

Ziv M. Peled, Jonathan M. Winograd, and James W. May, Jr.

INTRODUCTION

Since the beginnings of microsurgery nearly 4 decades ago,[1] hand surgery has experienced continued growth in the understanding and reconstruction of hand defects. Nowhere are these capabilities more obvious than in free tissue transfer to the hand. Composite tissue transfer (e.g., digital replantation, pollicization, toe-to-thumb transfer) has received much of the spotlight in this regard. In this chapter, we discuss neurosensory free flaps and their application in hand surgery. As much as any of the abovementioned procedures, these flaps epitomize the pinnacle of functional hand restoration.

When discussing free tissue transfer of any kind, the goals of reconstruction must be kept clearly in mind. In the case of a hand defect, there are several objectives that must be achieved. First and foremost, any wound must be closed. Second, it is critical to minimize functional impairment. For example, transferred tissues must be stable and durable enough to allow tendons to glide freely and should not be overly bulky or inflexible so as to interfere with joint movement or object grasp. Third, the hand is the most important tactile sensory organ through which we experience the world; hence, sensory restoration is critical. At a minimum, protective sensation is required to prevent further injury, but ideally tactile precision is the goal. Our understanding of this concept must be credited to Moberg who first used the term tactile gnosis or "knowing touch" to describe the functional value of sensibility in the hand.[2] After all, a healed wound with supple joints and mobile tendons means little if we are unable to sense the objects we are meant to manipulate. Fourth, donor site defects must be kept to a minimum, and finally, since the hand is a conspicuous part of our anatomy, appearance becomes an important reconstructive goal.

Neurosensory flaps in hand surgery began, not surprisingly, with the Moberg flap for sensate reconstruction of the thumb.[3] This flap was the first volar advancement flap described for the hand and paved the way for others such as Littler, who took Moberg's contributions a step further in designing a neurovascular, *heterodigital* island flap, now appropriately known as the Littler flap.[4,5] Unlike the Moberg flap, the Littler flap allowed sensate tissue from one digit to be used in sensory restoration of another digit. Neurosensory *free* flaps for hand reconstruction were first described in 1976.[6,7] This achievement led to the development of other neurosensory free flaps for use in reconstructing hand defects.[8–10] In spite of these many options, we believe that the gold standard for wound coverage with durable, pliable, and sensate soft tissue for the hand remains the first web-space flap from the foot.[9] JWM first used this flap in 1976, and long-term follow-up of the same patient is presented here.[9] Compared with the flap originally described by Daniel et al.,[6] this flap has the advantage of transferring sensate tissue with better native two-point discrimination (2PD) and significantly less donor site morbidity. Although the foot first web-space flap is smaller than the dorsalis pedis flap, fine sensibility is only necessary in relatively small areas of the hand, a concept that we elaborate upon when considering the indications for this flap. We also describe a more recent patient in whom we had occasion to utilize the first web-space flap. Our reasoning in considering this flap as the first choice in neurovascular reconstruction for the hand rests on several key principles of flap surgery.

The first web-space flap fulfills many of the above-stated criteria for an ideal tissue transfer. This flap can be elevated to encompass both the skin overlying the lateral aspect of the great toe as well as the medial aspect of the second toe and so functions well in terms of coverage. Concurrently, the skin of the first web space of the foot is also thin and glabrous, with 2PD just over 11 mm,[9] thus matching the anatomy and approaching critical sensation of the native hand soft tissues. From a technical standpoint, the flap comes with a dual arterial blood supply and dual venous outflow sources that allow considerable flexibility in flap design. Arterial inflow comes from either the first dorsal metatarsal artery (FDMA) or the common plantar digital artery. The branching pattern of the FDMA can be somewhat variable.[9] Approximately 78% of the time, it arises superficially from the dorsalis pedis artery (DPA), and courses in the subcutaneous tissues under the extensor hallucis brevis tendon. The other 22% of the time, the FDMA arises from the DPA as it descends to join with the plantar arterial tree and travels distally plantar to the mid metatarsal axis before ascending in the first metatarsal space (Fig. 11A–1). The two potential venous outflow sources are the venae comitantes accompanying the FDMA and the superficial dorsal venous system

that ultimately drains into the saphenous system (Fig. 11A–2).

From a sensory standpoint, the dorsal and plantar neural supply to the first web-space flap comes predominantly from the deep peroneal nerve (dorsally) and the medial plantar nerve.[11] Testing of normal individual donor tissues revealed considerably better 2PD over the foot first web space (mean 11.3 mm) compared with the skin on the medial dorsal aspect of the foot (mean 32 mm).[9] It follows then, that for sensate thumb reconstruction, the radial sensory nerve ends would ideally be coapted to the deep peroneal nerve branches within the flap and the median nerve branches of the hand would be repaired to the plantar digital nerve. Two-point discrimination under 10 mm has been described when using this or very similar flaps for sensate hand reconstruction.[12,13] While the exact mechanism for such a precise return of sensory function is not completely understood, three factors may be involved. The first factor is an increase in the representation of the injured hand or digit within the somatosensory cortex.[14,15] For

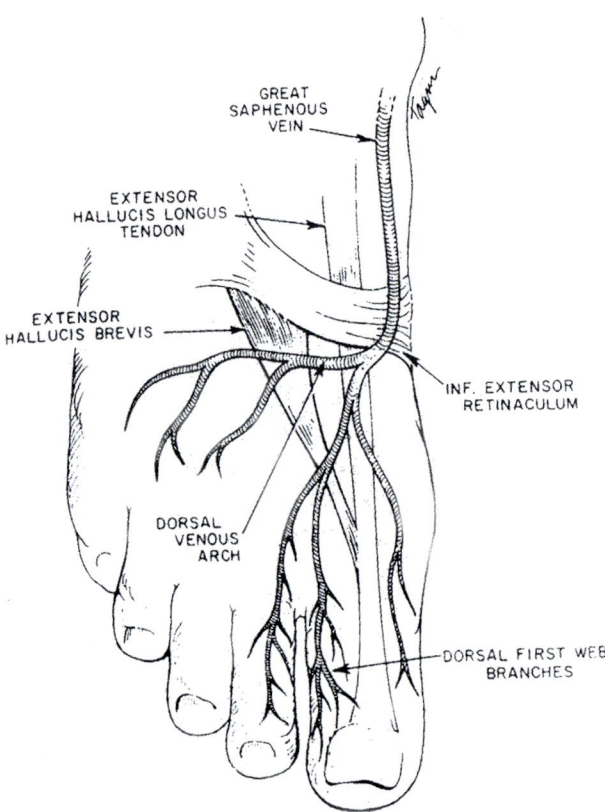

Figure 11A–2   Predominant venous outflow to the foot, first web-space flap, which ultimately drains into the saphenous system (From May JW Jr, Chait LA, Cohen BE, et al. Free neurosensory vascular flap from the first web of the foot in hand reconstruction. J Hand Surg 1977;2:387–93,[9] with permission.)

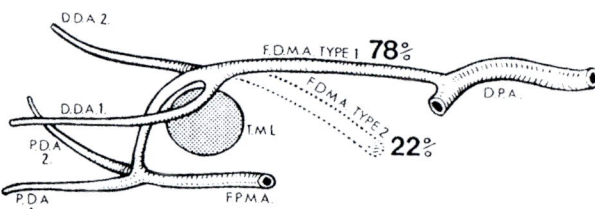

Figure 11A–1   Two anatomic variations of the first dorsal metatarsal artery as it passes distally into the foot. (From May JW Jr, Chait LA, Cohen BE, et al. Free neurosensory vascular flap from the first web of the foot in hand reconstruction. J Hand Surg 1977;2:387–93,[9] with permission.)

example, string musicians have digital cortical representations that are larger than their nonmusician counterparts, and furthermore, this representation increases commensurate with years of playing experience.[16] Second, cortical plasticity can occur through a process known as sensory re-education. In this process, areas of the body which are deprived of a particular sensory input (e.g., as a result of blindness, nerve injury, or neurovascular free flap surgery) are systematically exposed to a similar stimulus. Results have demonstrated improved moving and static 2PD in the re-educated patients as seen, for example, in blind Braille readers who are able to discriminate dots separated by as little as 1.5 mm or in patients who have better postoperative sensation following median nerve repair.[11,17] Third, good sensory recovery may also be a function of the relatively large area of cortical representation of the *recipient* site. Finally, the donor site for the first web-space flap is a relatively inconspicuous one that can usually be covered adequately with a skin graft that results in little functional disturbance to the foot.

Because the sensory function of neurovascular free flaps to the hand is so important, it is critical to recognize what factors affect the ultimate result after sensory nerve repair. While specific information is lacking with regard to the first web-space flap (presumably due to the lack of large series), there is information on similar flaps and in series of primary digital nerve repairs, to which this experience is analogous. In a recent study of several types of sensory free flaps from the toes to the fingers, Kato et al.[18] analyzed the factors affecting final sensory outcomes. He concluded that younger age (<12 years) and lack of vascular complications perioperatively were associated with superior sensory restoration. More specifically, children younger than 12 years typically had static 2PD less than 6 mm, whereas the corresponding value in adults aged over 18 years was typically 6 to 16 mm.[18] Similarly, those patients who did not have a perioperative vascular complication had static 2PD results ranging from 6 to 16 mm, while over half of those who did have a perioperative vascular complication could not perceive more than one point on postoperative testing.[18] No trend towards improved sensory restoration was noted when neurorrhaphies were performed between digital nerves of the donor toe and recipient finger or between deep peroneal nerve branches of the toe and radial sensory nerve branches on the recipient finger.[18] In primary digital nerve repairs, better sensory restoration is usually seen in younger people, nonsmokers, and simple lacerations, as compared with lacerations involving a crush component or concomitant fractures or tendon injuries.[19]

Despite the advent of other neurovascular free flaps to reconstruct hand defects, the first web-space free flap remains the first choice for many.[20] In the future, this belief may change. Several authors have applied the technique of perforator free flaps to the hand.[21,22] At the moment, these flaps are primarily being used to provide stable soft tissue coverage and currently, no other nonhand neurosensory free flaps are available which have glabrous skin and as good native 2PD as the first web-space free flap. However, as experience with them increases, the ability to incorporate peripheral sensory nerve territories into perforator flap design may expand our donor site options for neurosensory free flap reconstruction. Perforator flaps that encompass peripheral sensory nerve territories into neurovascular free flaps may also help to elucidate the role of the recipient site in sensory restoration for even if the sensory territory of the donor tissue is not densely innervated, it remains to be seen whether the more densely innervated recipient site could compensate for this.

INDICATIONS AND CONTRAINDICATIONS

Although the ability of neurosensory free flaps to accomplish a variety of reconstructive goals simultaneously is considerable, the actual indications for such a reconstruction are quite stringent. First and foremost, the defect must be stable with respect to infection and vascularity. Therefore, neurovascular free flap reconstruction is never undertaken in an acute setting when these aspects of a defect are still unclear. Second, the patient must have an otherwise functional hand or limb so that the precise sensation which is restored will be useful for the fine motor grasp functions it enables. The defect must include a location within the hand that requires fine tactile gnosis. In our opinion, the tips of the digits are the only locations that meet this qualification, as other areas such as the first web-space and the palm, while normally sensate, do not require fine sensation for adequate function. Additionally, local innervated flaps such as the radial nerve innervated cross-finger flap[23] must be ruled out as possible reconstructive options before attempting a more complicated free tissue transfer. Finally, the patient must be compliant with postoperative rehabilitation since, after a successful surgical procedure, this factor is the ultimate determinant of a successful functional outcome.

PROCEDURE

In preparation for this procedure, we find it useful to obtain an angiogram of both feet and the recipient hand. This imaging study complements the physical exam and allows a more precise delineation of the arterial

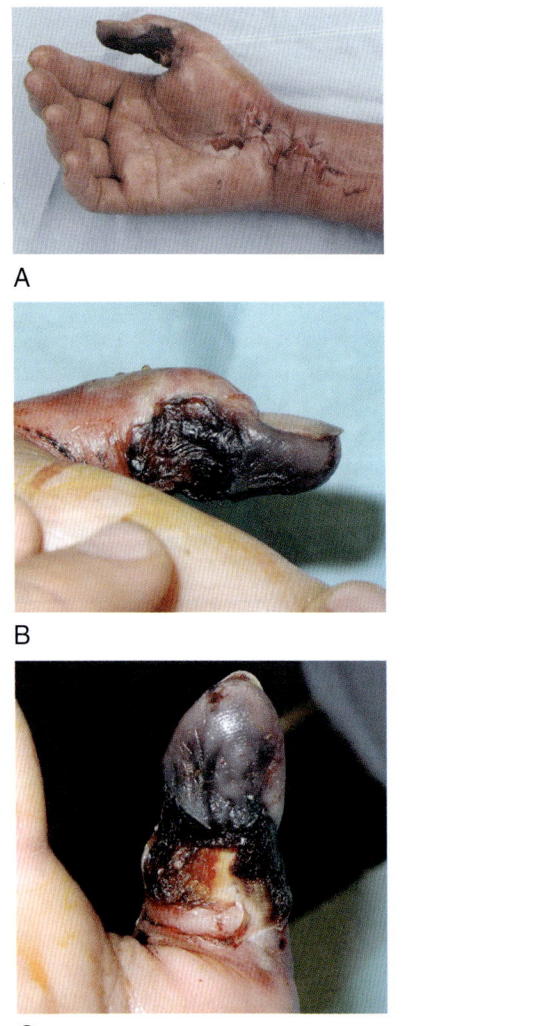

A

B

C

Figure 11A–3   Three different views (**A** to **C**) of the right volar thumb belonging to patient J.C. Full thickness necrosis was present down to the tendon and bone.

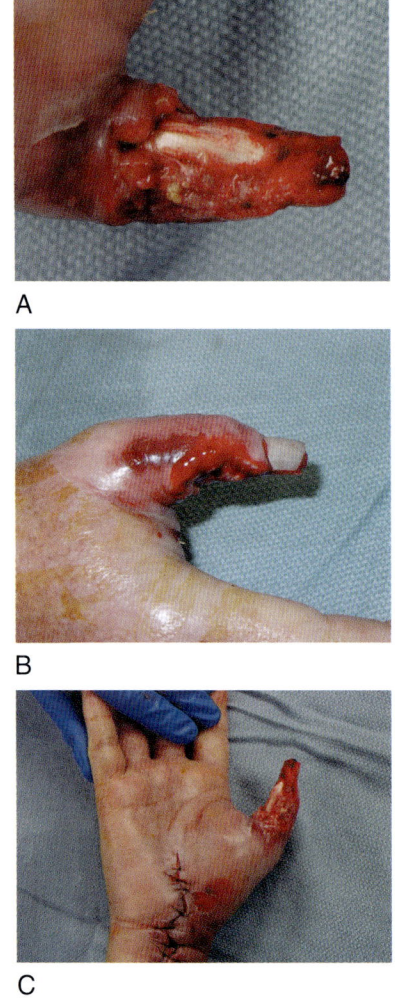

A

B

C

Figure 11A–4   Three different views (**A** to **C**) of the right volar thumb belonging to patient J.C. after debridement. Exposed bone and flexor tendon are visualized.

anatomy. Consequently, the surgeon is able to choose a donor side based on the more favorable anatomy. Moreover, the preoperative physical exam should include a Tinel's test so as to determine the length of the neural pedicle required from the donor site and to be able to consistently monitor the postoperative neurological recovery. A representative example of this type of flap is described below.

J.C. is a 63-year-old female who suffered a necrotizing soft tissue infection of her right thumb pad. She was treated conservatively at an outside hospital unsuccessfully and subsequently presented to us for definitive management (Fig. 11A–3). The wound was serially debrided until all necrotic tissue was removed and the infection was no longer present (Fig. 11A–4). The flexor tendon became necrotic and was debrided as well, and the defect was initially successfully covered with a split-

thickness skin graft directly applied to periosteum (Fig. 11A–5). In postoperative follow-up, the patient expressed a desire for more extensive reconstruction given her active lifestyle as a semi-pro golfer. She subsequently underwent thumb reconstruction with an innervated foot first web-space flap. Her case illustrates many of the technical aspects of this surgery:

1. Preoperatively, an angiogram of both the donor foot and the recipient hand is obtained to rule out the possibility of any unusual anatomic variations in vascularity (Figs. 11A–6 and 11A–7).
2. The Tinel's sign is located at the end of the digital nerves to help determine the length of neural pedicle that will be required.
3. In the operating room, the patient is placed in a supine position on the operating table, and the size

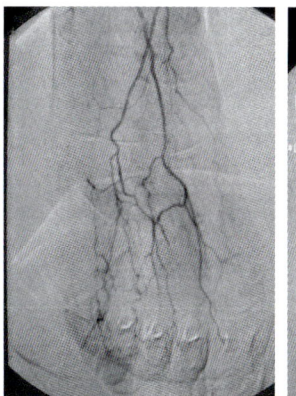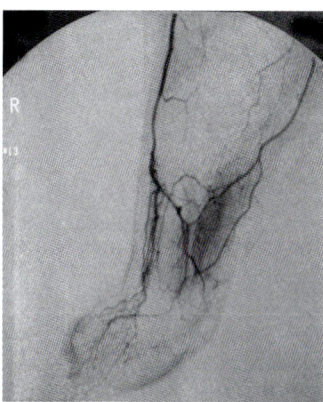

Figure 11A–7 This image shows the angiogram of patient J.C.'s right foot. Note the presence of the more common variation of the first dorsal metacarpal artery (arising directly from the dorsalis pedis artery) as it passes distally into the foot.

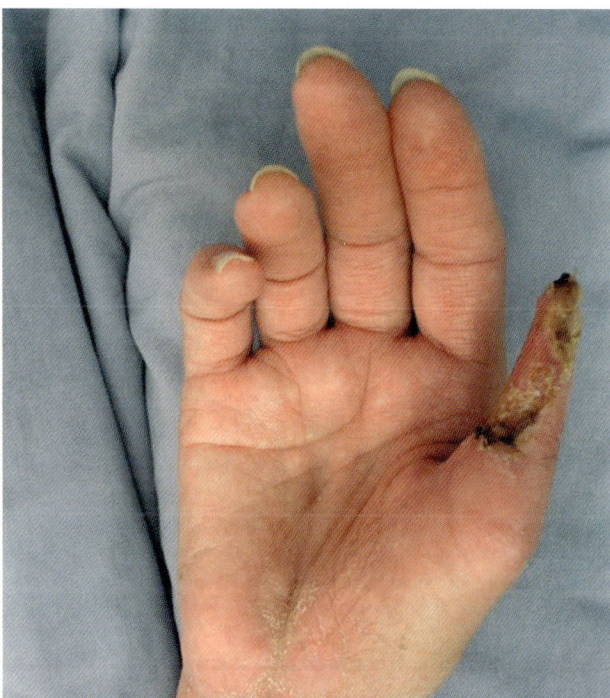

Figure 11A–5 This figure demonstrates patient J.C.'s right thumb approximately 3 weeks after successful split thickness skin grafting. Some dessication is noted at the periphery of the graft margins, but graft take was essentially 100%.

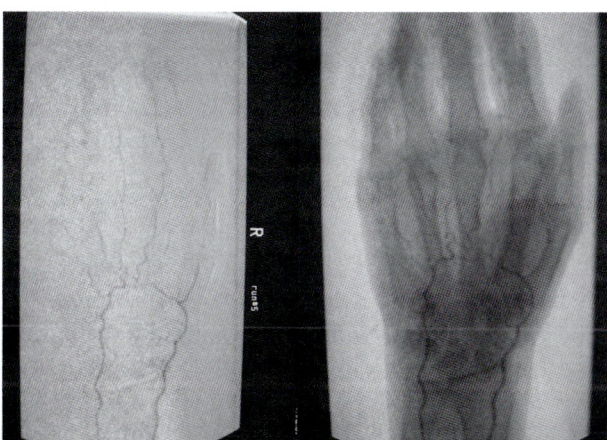

Figure 11A–6 This image shows the angiogram of patient J.C.'s right hand. Note the presence of a complete palmar arch.

of skin defect required on the hand is measured and marked on the first web space of the foot; the position of the saphenous vein branches to the foot along with the dorsalis pedis artery are marked as well.

4. As this is a somewhat lengthy operation with two dissection fields, general anesthesia is always used and a Foley catheter is placed. We have no preference as to the type of general anesthetic given and muscle relaxants may be used at the anesthesiologist's discretion.

5. Nonsterile tourniquets are placed on the arm and thighs to be used as the recipient and donor sites, respectively. Ideally, *once a workable flap is established,* two surgical teams should be used—one to prepare the recipient site and the other to harvest the flap from the foot.

6. Attention is first turned to the foot that is mapped to locate the saphenous vein tributaries with a venous tourniquet followed by exsanguination and inflation of the thigh tourniquet to 300 mm Hg.

7. Dissection begins by exposure of the saphenous vein branches to the foot just distal to the ankle crease. These branches are traced distally to the proximal portion of the flap and teased from the subcutaneous fat of the skin flaps raised as part of the exposure outside of the flap skin.

8. The extensor pollicis brevis tendon is then identified and sharply divided, and the underlying fascia opened to expose the dorsalis pedis artery.

9. Using a bipolar cautery, the dorsalis pedis artery and venae comitantes as well as the deep peroneal nerve are dissected from the forefoot to the proximal portion of the flap.

10. The flap itself is then raised from distally to proximally taking care to remain superficial to the extensor apparati including the paratenon of the first and second toes as well as the plantar circulation, unless this is included in the flap design (Fig. 11A–8).

11. During dissection, anastomotic branches between the dorsal and plantar circulation are divided with the bipolar cautery and hemoclips, until the flap is elevated in its entirety. Caution must be taken during this dissection to preserve the continuity of the dorsal circulation.

12. Papaverine-soaked neural pledgets are placed on the pedicle of the flap to allow for vasodilatation, and the tourniquet is released.

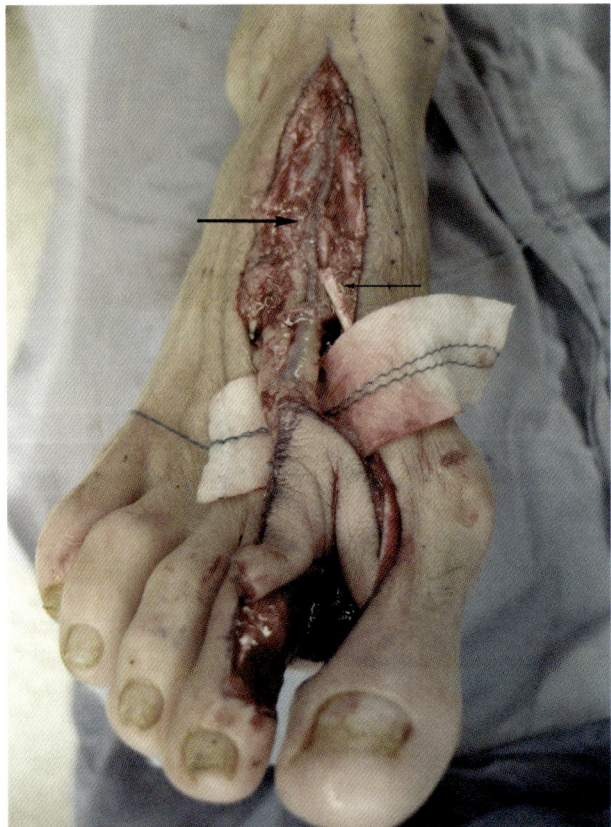

Figure 11A–8 Dissected foot first web-space flap. Note the more common variation of the first dorsal metacarpal artery *(large arrow)* arising directly from the dorsalis pedis artery and the presence of the divided extensor hallicus brevis tendon *(little arrow)*.

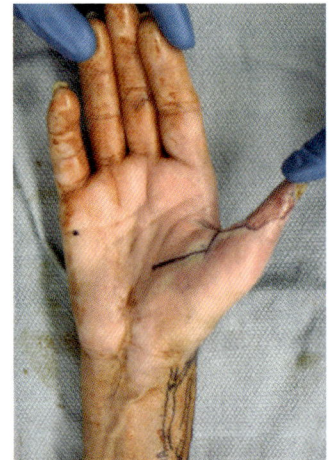 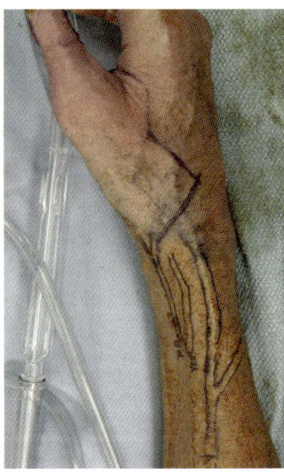

A   B

Figure 11A–9 Antero-posterior **(A)** and lateral **(B)** views of patient J.C.'s right hand with the planned incision lines for inset of the foot first web-space flap. Also note the markings delineating the location of the radial artery and two dorsal veins.

13. Once the foot first web-space flap is dissected and found to have an adequate neurovascular pedicle, attention is turned to the hand where the dorsal branch of the radial artery as well as one or more dorsal veins are identified by ultrasound and by palpation (Fig. 11A–9). Venous mapping can be performed prior to this dissection with a venous tourniquet if the venous anatomy is not otherwise easily visualized.

14. The hand is exsanguinated and the tourniquet inflated to 250 mm Hg.

15. Any temporary tissue coverage (e.g., skin graft in this case) or granulation tissue is excised sharply with a #15 blade.

16. An incision is then extended into the volar aspect of the thumb and palm if necessary to expose the digital nerves, and then dorsally to open the anatomic snuff box, thereby exposing the arterial inflow branches.

17. Once the recipient vessels and nerves are identified, papaverine-soaked neural pledgets are placed over the blood vessels, and saline-soaked gauze is placed over the nerves. The arm tourniquet is then released.

18. The operating microscope is brought into the room and set up on the hand.

19. The hand vessels and digital nerves are further prepared under the microscope.

20. Using hemoclips, the flap pedicle is divided and transferred to the hand.

21. In the foot, hemostasis is achieved with the bipolar cautery, and the extensor pollicis brevis tendon is repaired with 3-0 Ethibond horizontal mattress sutures.

22. The skin of the proximal foot is then closed with interrupted 3-0 Vicryl in the deep dermal layer followed by a running 4-0 nylon suture.

23. A thick split thickness skin graft is harvested from the ipsilateral anterior thigh and sutured onto the first web-space with a running 4-0 chromic suture and multiple 4-0 nylon interrupted sutures for the bolster. The skin graft is covered with a xeroform dressing followed by a cotton bolster soaked with mineral oil (Fig. 11A–10). If two operative teams are unavailable, and should the cutaneous portion of the flap require a large skin graft, it is acceptable to leave this step until after inset of the flap into the hand so as to minimize the ischemic insult to the flap.

24. The foot is then splinted in dorsiflexion with a 6-in plaster posterior splint to the calf.

25. Attention is now turned back to the hand where the flap is provisionally tacked into place so as to orient the vessels and nerves appropriately.

26. The hand is elevated for 3 minutes to exsanguinate it and the arm tourniquet reinflated.

27. The recipient vessels in the hand are clamped proximally and ligated distally, and then irrigated with heparinized saline solution to remove any debris or clot.

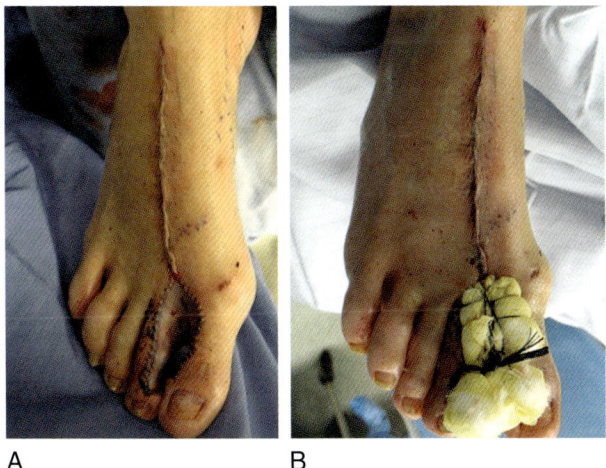

A   **B**

Figure 11A–10 Donor site defect from the foot first web-space flap with the split thickness skin graft sewn into place **(A)** and after dressing with a bolster **(B).**

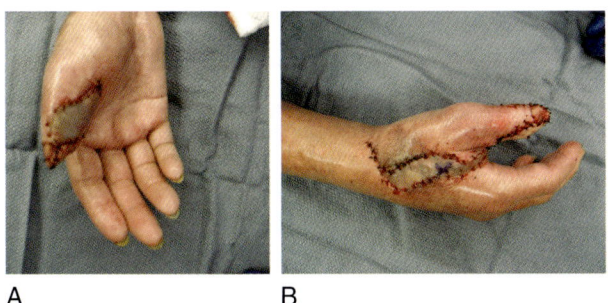

A   **B**

Figure 11A–11 Antero-posterior **(A)** and lateral **(B)** views of patient J.C.'s right hand after inset of the foot first web-space flap. Note the presence of a split thickness skin graft dorsally over the first web-space **(B)**, which was necessary for closure so as to avoid compression of the flap pedicle.

28. An end-to-end anastomosis between a dorsal branch of the radial artery and the dorsalis pedis artery is accomplished with interrupted 8-0 nylon sutures.

29. Similarly, anastomoses between the venae comitantes of the dorsalis pedis artery are anastomosed to dorsal venous branches in the hand.

30. The vessel clamps are released proximally followed by release of the tourniquet.

31. Attention is then turned to the neurorrhaphy between the deep peroneal nerve and the ulnar digital nerve of the thumb, which is completed with interrupted 9-0 nylon sutures. The radial sensory nerve innervation to the dorsum of the thumb was intact in this case and was not disturbed.

32. The flap is then inset with interrupted 5-0 nylon sutures.

33. In this particular case, a small gap in the dorsal first web space was split skin grafted as primary closure would have compressed the pedicle in a highly scarred first web-space (Fig. 11A–11).

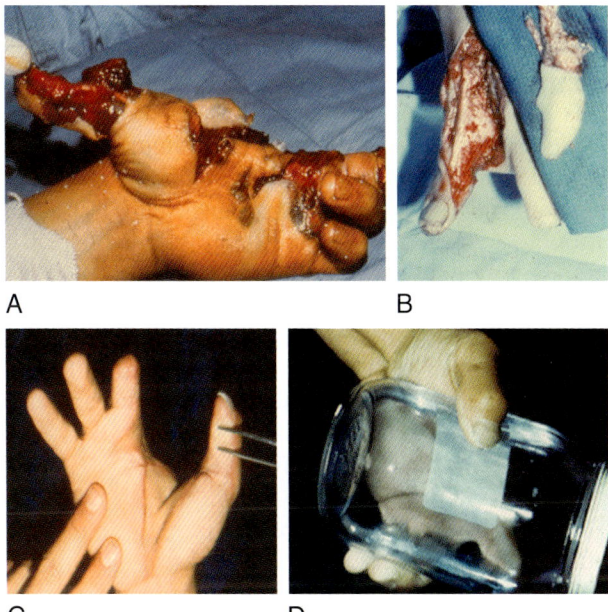

A   **B**

C   **D**

Figure 11A–12 First foot web-space flap performed by JWM 28 years ago. **A:** Severity of the initial injury, including loss of the volar thumb soft tissues, is clearly seen. **B:** Foot first web-space flap and the donor site. **C:** Results of the foot first web-space flap 6 months postsurgery demonstrating excellent healing of the soft tissues and two-point discrimination of 10 mm. **D:** Same patient demonstrating the tactile sensation necessary to pick up large objects.

34. The hand is then dressed by placing xeroform gauze over the incision lines, followed by fluff gauze in the second, third, and fourth web spaces. A Jones soft cotton dressing was then applied followed by splinting of the hand in functional position with 4-in plaster. The hand dressing must allow for monitoring of the viability of the flap; the flap skin should be left visible for surveillance purposes and a doppler signal can be marked within the skin paddle using a superficially placed 6-0 prolene suture.

RESULTS

In addition to the above patient, JMW had occasion to use this flap for a hand defect in 1976. D.T. was a 16-year-old male who was injured in a homemade bomb accident. The severity of the injuries necessitated amputations of the index and middle fingers, and demonstrated an open fracture of the thumb metacarpophalangeal joint as well as obliteration of the soft tissues of the left volar thumb from the metacarpal level distally (Fig. 11A–12 A). The wounds were debrided, the fractures stabilized, and the volar thumb covered with a split skin graft. Eighteen weeks after the injury, the patient was reconstructed using a foot first web-space flap (Fig. 11A–12 B). Several weeks after this procedure, the hand demonstrated good healing of all flaps, and by 6 months, 2PD was noted to be 10 mm at the volar thumb pad (Fig. 11A–12 C). In addition, the patient was able to hold large objects in his hand (Fig. 11A–12 D). This patient was recently seen in our office for follow-up, 28 years after the initial injury. His hand remains supple with maintenance of a large web space between the thumb and remaining digits, and no atrophy or breakdown of the neurovascular free flap representing the new volar thumb pad (Fig. 11A–13 A and B). Furthermore, his donor site is barely perceptible, and the patient ambulates normally (Fig. 11A–13 C). These results highlight the durability of this flap.

Patient J.C. continues to follow up with us, and also has had a good result from surgery. The flap is well healed, as is the donor site (Fig. 11A–14 A to C). She reports no alteration in her gait as a result of the foot donor site. Finally, while the patient is not yet 6 months out of surgery, she has had return of sensation to the thumb pad at 4 months postsurgery, and is able to pick up and hold a pen (Fig. 11A–15). Her interphalangeal joint, which was involved in the original infection, continued to drain intermittently from beneath her flap, and has recently been debrided and fused.

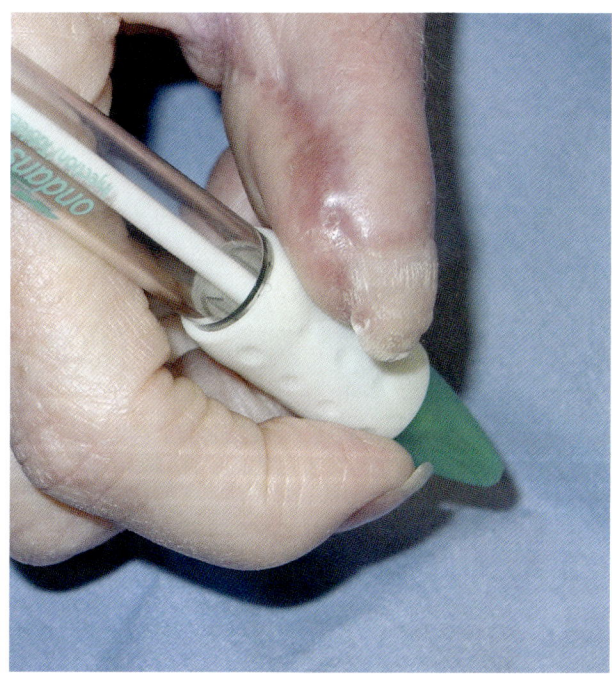

Figure 11A–15 Patient J.C.'s ability for fine grasp demonstrated in holding a pen as she would have preoperatively. Her sensation has returned at 4 months postoperatively, although she does note occasional parasthesias in the thumb pad.

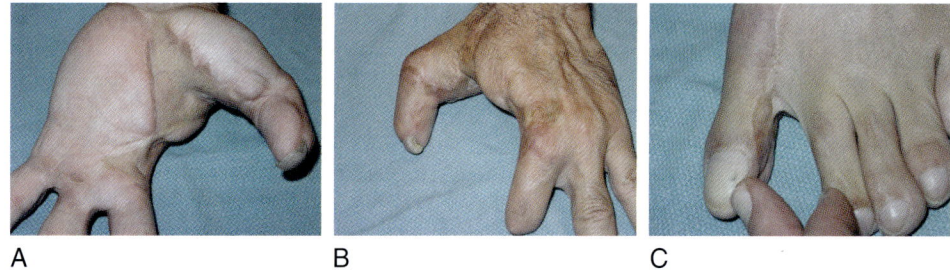

A B C

Figure 11A–13 Results of the foot first web-space flap 28 years postsurgery. **A** and **B:** Volar and dorsal views of the patient's right hand demonstrate intact soft tissues of the foot first web-space flap despite many years of use. **C:** The flap donor site is nearly imperceptible, and the patient enjoys normal ambulation.

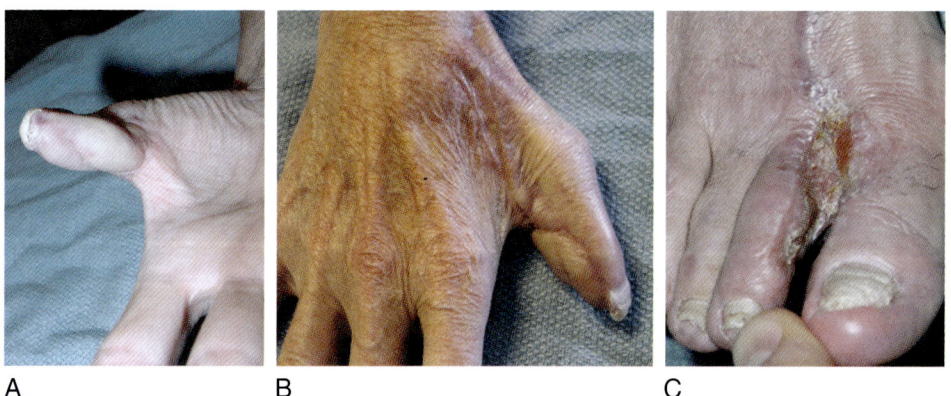

A B C

Figure 11A–14 Results of patient J.C. postsurgery. Volar **(A)** and dorsal **(B)** views of the hand demonstrate good healing and viability of the foot first web-space flap soft tissues. The donor site in the foot **(C)** is also healing well, despite a small amount of dessication at the distal end of the incision.

Dedication

To my wife Beth and my sons Joshua and Adam, my true inspiration.—Jonathan M. Winograd

REFERENCES

1. Buncke HJ Jr, Schulz WP. Total ear reimplantation in the rabbit utilising microminiature vascular anastomoses. Br J Plast Surg 1966;19:15–22.
2. Moberg E. Objective methods for determining the functional value of sensibility in the hand. J Bone Joint Surg Br 1958;40:454–76.
3. Moberg E. Aspects of sensation in reconstructive surgery of the upper extremity. J Bone Joint Surg Am 1964;46:817–25.
4. Dellon AL. The sensational contributions of Erik Moberg. J Hand Surg Br 1990;15:14–24.
5. Littler JW. Neurovascular pedicle transfer of tissue in reconstructive surgery of the hand. J Bone Joint Surg Am 1956;38:917.
6. Daniel RK, Terzis J, Midgley RD. Restoration of sensation to an anesthetic hand by a free neurovascular flap from the foot. Plast Reconstr Surg 1976;57:275–80.
7. Ohmori K, Harii K. Free dorsalis pedis sensory flap to the hand, with microneurovascular anastomoses. Plast Reconstr Surg 1976;58:546–54.
8. Lee WP, May JW Jr. Neurosensory free flaps to the hand. Indications and donor selection. Hand Clin 1992;8:465–77.
9. May JW Jr., Chait LA, Cohen BE, et al. Free neurovascular flap from the first web of the foot in hand reconstruction. J Hand Surg Am 1977;2:387–93.
10. Wechselberger G, Schoeller T, Pulzl P, et al. [Free tissue transplantation for defect coverage of the dorsum of the hand: aesthetic and functional aspects]. Handchir Mikrochir Plast Chir 2003;35:245–50.
11. Brown CJ, Mackinnon SE, Dellon AL, et al. The sensory potential of free flap donor sites. Ann Plast Surg 1989;23:135–40.
12. Koshima I, Murashita T, Soeda S. Free vascularized deep peroneal neurocutaneous flap for repair of digital nerve defect involving severe finger damage. J Hand Surg Am 1991;16:227–9.
13. Rose EH, Buncke HJ. Free transfer of a large sensory flap from the first web space and dorsum of the foot including the second toe for reconstruction of a mutilated hand. J Hand Surg Am 1981;6:196–201.
14. Reddy H, Floyer A, Donaghy M, et al. Altered cortical activation with finger movement after peripheral denervation: comparison of active and passive tasks. Exp Brain Res 2001;138:484–91.
15. Schweizer R, Braun C, Fromm C, et al. The distribution of mislocalizations across fingers demonstrates training-induced neuroplastic changes in somatosensory cortex. Exp Brain Res 2001;139:435–42.
16. Blake DT, Byl NN, Merzenich MM. Representation of the hand in the cerebral cortex. Behav Brain Res 2002;135:179–84.
17. Imai H, Tajima T, Natsumi Y. Successful reeducation of functional sensibility after median nerve repair at the wrist. J Hand Surg Am 1991;16:60–5.
18. Kato H, Ogino T, Minami A, et al. Restoration of sensibility in fingers repaired with free sensory flaps from the toe. J Hand Surg Am 1989;14:49–54.
19. Winograd JM, Mackinnon SE. Peripheral nerve injuries: repair and reconstruction. In: Mathes SJ, Hentz VR, eds., Plastic Surgery. New York: W.B. Saunders. In press.
20. Jones NF, Lister GD. Free skin and composite flaps. In: Green DP, Hotchkiss RN, Pederson WC, eds., Green's Operative Hand Sugery. New York: Churchill-Livingstone, 1999:1159–200.
21. Chen HC, Tang YB, Mardini S, et al. Reconstruction of the hand and upper limb with free flaps based on musculocutaneous perforators. Microsurgery 2004;24:270–80.
22. Kim KS, Kim ES, Kim DY, et al. Resurfacing of a totally degloved hand using thin perforator-based cutaneous free flaps. Ann Plast Surg 2003;50:77–81.
23. Walker MA, Hurley CB, May JW Jr. Radial nerve cross-finger flap differential nerve contribution in thumb reconstruction. J Hand Surg Am 1986;11:881–7.

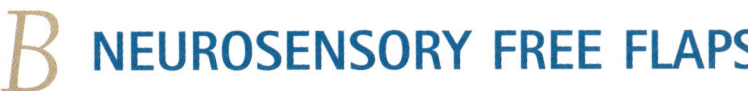

B NEUROSENSORY FREE FLAPS

Bradon J. Wilhelmi and W.P. Andrew Lee

INTRODUCTION

Over the years several advances have been established in the treatment of mutilating hand injuries through soft tissue, bone, tendon, and joint reconstruction. However, the ultimate is to not only provide durable coverage, but also restore protective sensation. An insensate hand is prone to further injury and less likely to be functional than a hand that is sensate and stiff. Therefore, reconstruction with sensate soft tissue can be extremely important in hand reconstruction.

With the development of microsurgery and free tissue transfer, neurosensory flaps became a useful technique for sensory restoration to the injured upper extremity.[1–4] The innervation of the free flap is reestablished by coapting the nerve in the flap to a nerve in the recipient site. Because free flap procedures require extensive surgery and risk entire flap embarrassment, criteria need to be met when this option is considered.[5,6]

1. The potential regenerating axons at the area of tissue loss are insufficient or at too great a distance for local spontaneous sensory neurotization to occur reliably.
2. Sensate tissue coverage cannot be achieved by local or regional tissue transfer.
3. Sensory restoration to the injured part is critical for hand function such as with volar thumb.

The palm of the hand, dorsum, or web spaces are less important as a fine tactile surface, although a large insensate area would be prone to further injury and could benefit from sensory restoration. The pulp of the index finger is less deserving of a free sensate flap if the middle finger is intact, as the index finger will be bypassed for the sensate middle finger.[7]

DONOR SELECTION FOR NEUROSENSORY FLAPS

Several neurosensory free flaps have been described. However, appropriate flap selection requires an understanding of the sensory receptors in the recipient site and donor skin. Cutaneous sensory receptors convert mechanical stimuli into impulses transmitted by peripheral nerve fibers to the central nervous system.[8] The majority of sensory receptors are unencapsulated free nerve endings. Unencapsulated free nerve endings are responsible for the sensation of pain and temperature. Additionally, there are four types of encapsulated mechanoreceptors, including Meissner and Pacinian corpuscles, Merkel cell neurite complexes, and Ruffini end organs. Meissner and Pacinian corpuscles are quickly adapting receptors that sense low and high frequency vibration, respectively. The Merkle cell neurite complexes and Ruffini end organs are slowly adapting receptors that sense constant touch and skin stretch, respectively.

The glabrous skin of the hand and feet has the highest density of peripheral nerves, which provides for fine tactile sensation. The ultimate sensibility of the flap depends on the number of cutaneous sensory receptors in the neurosensory flap. As the glabrous skin has a high density of sensory receptors, it provides the best discriminatory sensation.[9] Another desirable characteristic of a neurosensory flap is for the skin to be thin and malleable, similar to the skin of the hand.[6,10,11] A pedicle with large-caliber vessels and predictable anatomy are other appealing features of a neurososensory flap, as well as a consistent and axial nerve supply, which facilitates flap dissection and the microsurgical repairs. However, donor site functional and aesthetic morbidity must be considered against the benefit of the neurosensory flap reconstruction.

In selecting the most appropriate neurosensory flap, it is important to delineate between critical sensibility and protective sensibility in the hand.[12] Critical sensibility is needed for reconstruction of the digital pulp and distal amputation stump. Protective sensibility is required when reconstructing the dorsal or palmer aspect of the hand. The best tissue for discriminatory sensory reconstruction is glabrous skin from the hand and feet. Thus, the selection of a neurosensory flap

depends on the location and size of the defect versus the potential donor morbidity.

OPTIONS FOR CRITICAL SENSORY RESTORATION

First Web–Space Flap

The gold standard neurosensory flap is the first web-space flap. This flap is discussed in Chapter 11A.

Toe Pulp Transfers

Another option for critical sensory restoration is the toe pulp transfer, which is a modification of the first web-space flap. This flap is applicable to small defects of the digital volar pads. The toe pulp flap is based on the plantar digital artery and vein, which can be dissected into the plantar arch or the dorsal inflow if greater pedicle length is required. The corresponding plantar nerve is harvested with this flap. Clinical series have reported this flap to provide two point discrimination of 3 to 7 mm.[13,14] The advantage of this flap is the minimal donor disfigurement, as it allows for skin grafting or direct closure.

Wrap-Around Flap

When the defect requires near circumferential digital reconstruction including the nail, a wrap-around flap can be considered. A wrap-around flap includes the entire soft tissue envelope of the great or second toe, excluding a strip of medial skin around the toe tip.[15] The flap dimensions are 7 cm transversely and 6 cm longitudinally. This flap includes the nail, which provides for pulp stability and improved aesthetics. The wrap-around flap is based on the first dorsal metatarsal artery and plantar digital nerves. Like the first web-space flap, the pedicle can be lengthened with extension to include the dorsalis pedis artery and saphenous superficial vein to provide a pedicle length of 6 to 10 cm. Harvesting this lengthened pedicle requires the preservation of the distal communication of the dorsalis pedis artery to the plantar system digital arteries by the deep communicating artery to the first plantar metatarsal artery. Lengthening the pedicle of this flap allows for repair of the dorsalis pedis artery end to side to the larger caliber radial artery in the snuff box. Pulp sensibility is supplied by both the medial and lateral plantar digital nerves. The wrap-around flap is most suitable for reconstruction of combined digital volar pad and nail loss. When reconstructing the thumb the ipsilateral great toe is preferred to avoid an incision on the ulnar aspect of the thumb. This flap can also be used to reconstruct the whole thumb in conjunction with an iliac bone graft, thus preserving the great toe, even though a simpler technique of total thumb reconstruction is with an entire toe transfer.[16–19] The great toe can be preserved by covering the donor wound with a skin graft or alternatively the volar great toe pad can be reconstructed with a cross-toe flap from the dorsum of the second toe and the dorsum of the great toe and second toe covered with a skin graft. Skin graft take can be optimized by allowing the wound to granulate for 2 weeks before grafting. The wrap-around flap provides a return of two-point discrimination of 6 to 10 mm after transfer.[20] The advantage to the use of the wrap-around flap is that it provides like tissue in reconstructing circumferential digital defects with sensate glabrous tissue and a viable nail.

Plantar Flap

The medial planter flap is a glabrous fasciocutaneous flap that can be used for neurosensory restoration of hand defects. Plantar skin, with its concentration of mechanoreceptors can provide tactile discrimination. The plantar fasciocutaneous flap can be harvested based on the medial or lateral plantar artery or both. Use of the medial plantar artery flap allows for potential of primary closure of the donor site. Small fingertip wounds can be reconstructed with the medial plantar free flap.[21] The venous return from this flap is through the venae comitantes with the artery. The pedicle is 3 to 5 cm long with a vessel diameter of 1 to 2 mm.[21,22] The pedicle can be extended to include the posterior tibial artery to the bifurcation of the medial and lateral plantar artery. The innervation of this flap is by cutaneous branches from the medial plantar nerve. The two-point discrimination of this flap has been reported between 5 to 20 mm.[21,22] The disadvantage of this flap is that it can be bulky, and separation of the cutaneous branches of the medial plantar nerve may be difficult, often requiring sacrifice of the common digital nerve of the second web space. Another potential problem is donor morbidity with the risk of developing hyperkeratosis and unstable scar at the donor site. Therefore the medial plantar flap is considered a second choice option for glabrous defects.

Spare Parts—Index Finger

Special circumstances may allow for use of spare parts to restore sensation to glabrous hand and finger defects. An example of this includes a multiple digit injury such as a thumb and index finger, whereby a devascularized index finger can be used as a free neurosensory flap to reconstruct a volar thumb soft tissue defect, through microsurgical repair of vessels and nerves (Fig. 11B–1).

OPTIONS FOR PROTECTIVE SENSATION RESTORATION

Neurosensory flaps from thin, sometimes hair-bearing areas other than the glabrous skin, can be used to restore

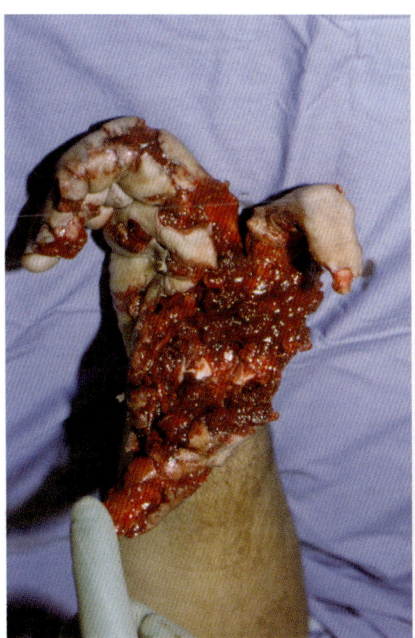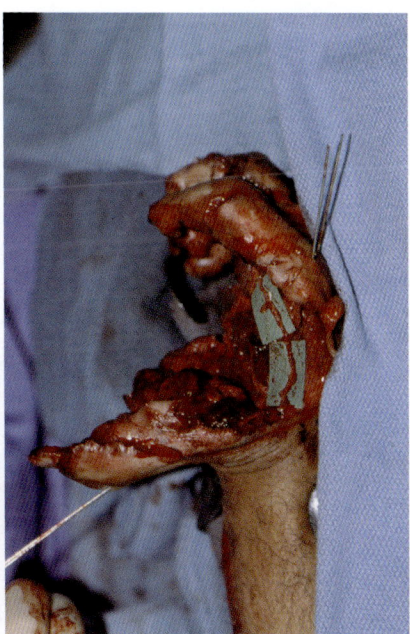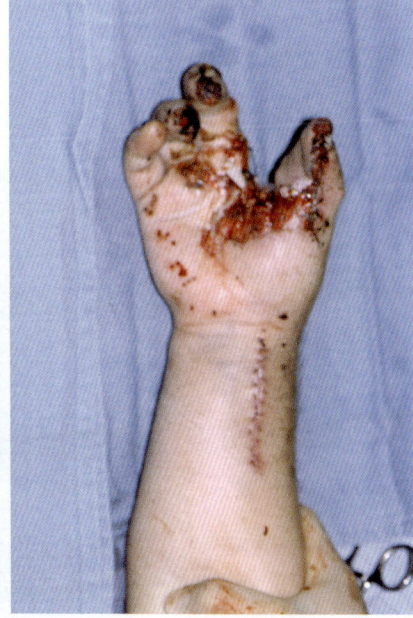

Figure 11B–1 A firework exploded in the hand of this patient, which resulted in a defect of volar thumb and mutilating devascularizating injury of the index finger. The index was used as a neurosensory flap to restore tactile discrimination to his thumb.

sensation to the denervated hand. Even though these neurosensory flaps do not contain the same concentration of cutaneous sensory receptors, these flaps are capable of providing protective sensibility.

Dorsalis Pedis Flap

The dorsalis pedis flap was first described in 1975, and this was a commonly used neurosensory flap.[3,4,23,24] The flap is based on small branches from the dorsalis pedis artery and the first dorsal metatarsal artery (Fig. 11B–2). A patent posterior tibial artery circulation to the foot is necessary to allow for the use of this flap. Therefore, an angiogram should be obtained preoperatively. During harvesting of this flap it is critical to avoid separation of the skin from the arterial pedicle.[25] If a longer pedicle is required, the artery can be extended proximally under the extensor retinaculum. The superficial saphenous veins or deep venae comitantes are used for venous drainage of the flap. This flap can also be harvested with the underlying extensor tendons and second metatarsal if needed[26,27] (Fig. 11B–3 A to F). The superficial peroneal nerve innervates the dorsum of the foot. Studies have demonstrated the in situ two-point discrimination of the dorsalis pedis flap averages between 32 and 34 mm.[28,29] Again, after transfer, flap two-point discrimination is usually half that of the donor. Thus, this flap inferior to the first web-space flap as it is unable to provide fine discriminatory sensation after transfer.

Therefore, this flap is most suitable to reconstruct areas requiring only protective sensation, especially an area such as the dorsum of the hand when tendon and bone is also needed. The flap dimension is 15 by 12 cm. However, due to the multifascicular nature of the super-

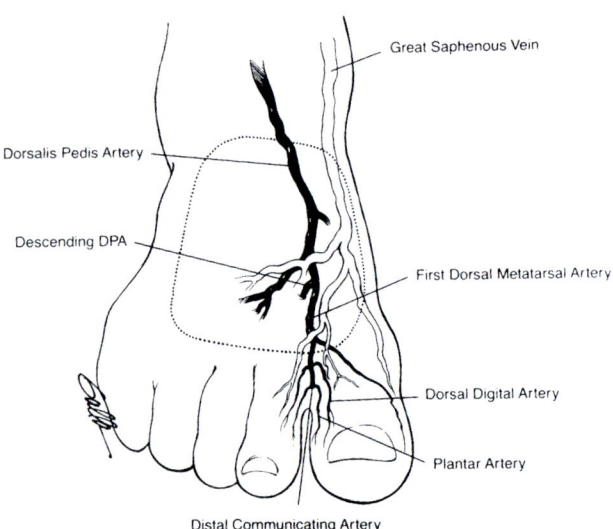

Figure 11B–2 The dorsalis pedis flap is based on the dorsalis pedis artery and either its venae comitantes or a superficial saphenous vein. (From Orgel MG. Innervated free flaps and free vascularized nerve grafts in the hand. In: McCarthy JG, May JW Jr, Littler JW, eds., Plastic Surgery, vol. 7. Philadelphia: W.B. Saunders, 1990:4859,[6] with permission.)

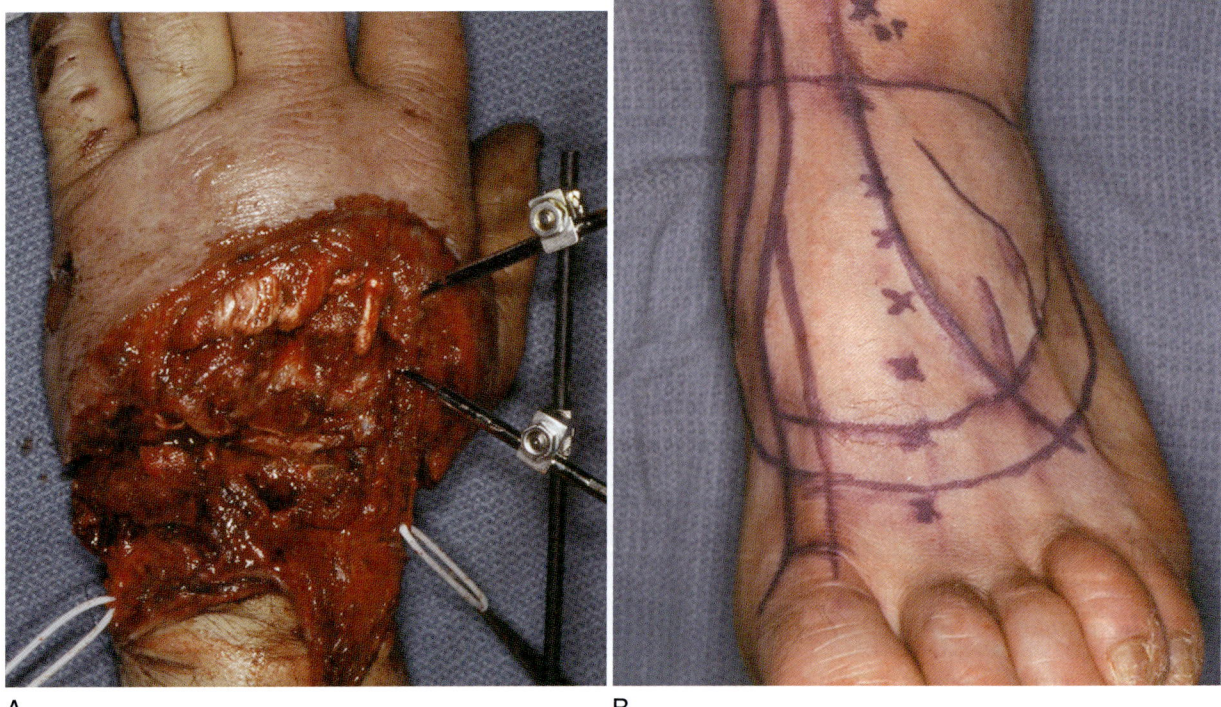

A   B

Figure 11B–3 **A** to **E:** This patient had a dorsal hand wound reconstructed with neurosensory dorsalis pedis flap.

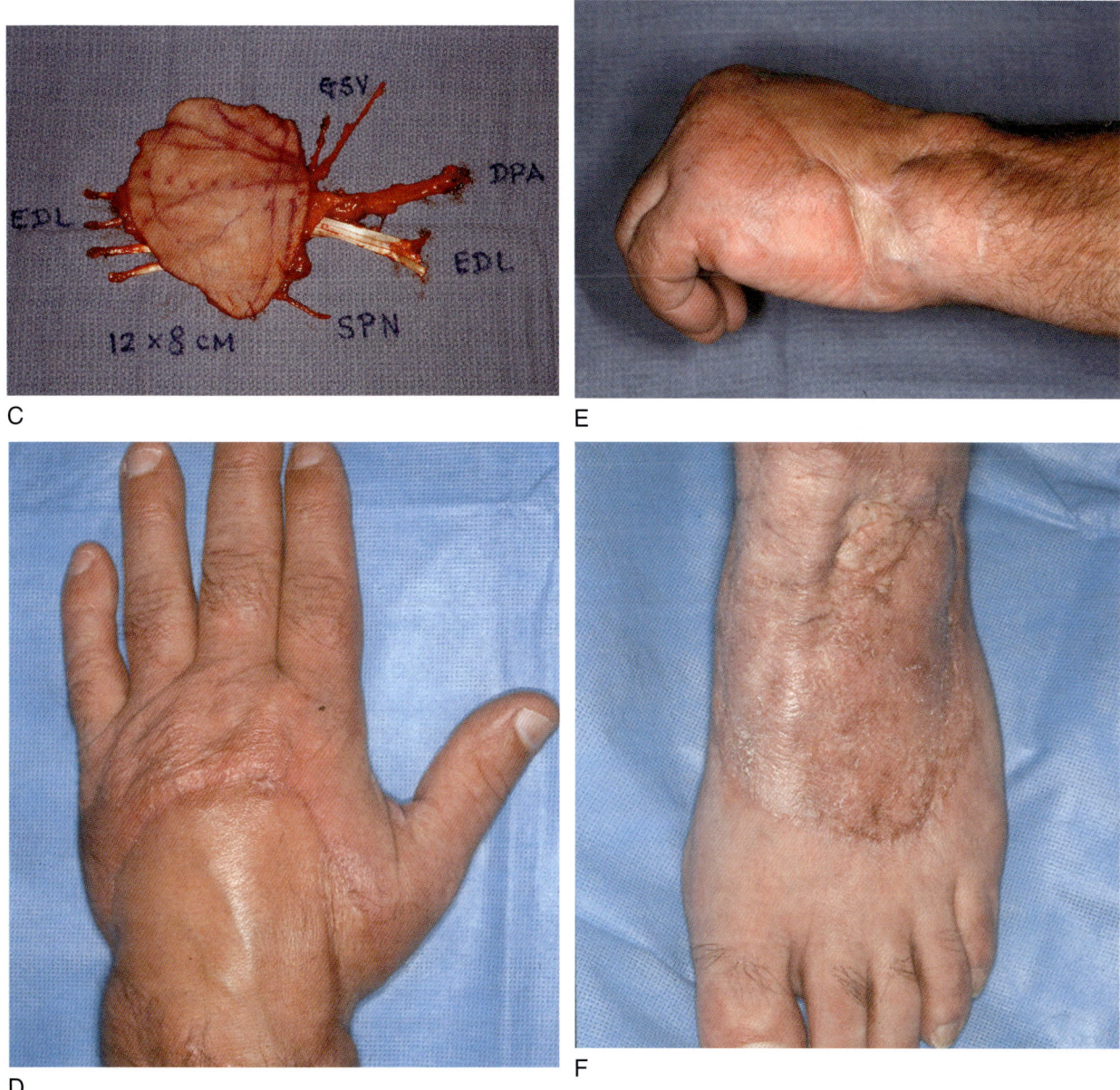

Figure 11B–3—Cont'd

ficial peroneal nerve that makes its innervation unpredictable, electrophysiologic sensory mapping is needed for precise determination of the flaps neural boundary.[23] An additional disadvantage for this flap is donor morbidity. It is critical with flap dissection to preserve the underlying paratenon to provide a bed for skin grafting of the donor site. However, even with paratenon preservation, prolonged healing and unstable scarring are common complications of this donor site.[3,23]

Radial Forearm Flap

The radial forearm flap is similar to the dorsalis pedis flap. This flap involves harvesting volar forearm skin based over septocutaneous branches of the radial artery (Fig. 11B–4). Venous drainage of this flap is through the basilic or cephalic or venae comitantes. The flap dimensions are 25 by 12 cm of skin innervated by the lateral and medial cutaneous nerves of the forearm. The two-point discrimination of this volar forearm skin has been measured in situ at 15 to 25 mm.[30] However two-point discrimination of this innervated flap after transfer has been reported at 22 to 32 mm.[31] Thus this flap does not provide fine discriminatory sensation. Provided the patient has a satisfactory Allen's test, a preoperative angiogram is usually not required to confirm adequate collateral flow to the hand through the ulnar artery before sacrificing the radial artery. Moreover, intraoper-

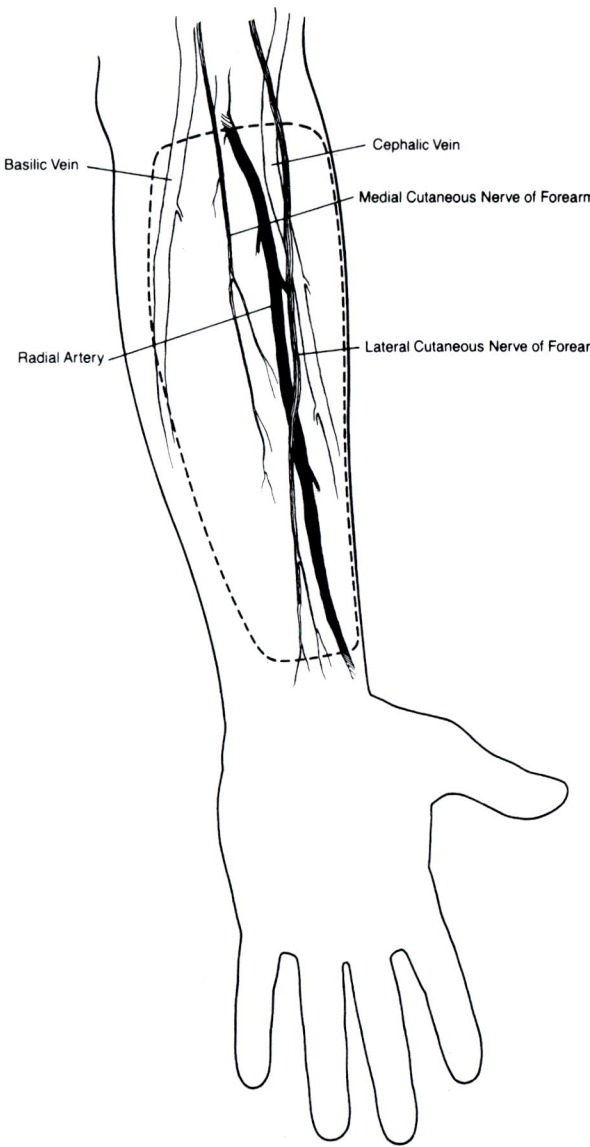

Figure 11B–4 The radial forearm flap is based on the radial artery, cephalic or basilic vein, and the lateral and medial cutaneous nerves of the forearm. (From Orgel MG. Innervated free flaps and free vascularized nerve grafts in the hand. In: McCarthy JG, May JW Jr, Littler JW, eds., Plastic Surgery, vol. 7. Philadelphia: W.B. Saunders, 1990:4859,[6] with permission.)

atively the radial artery can be temporarily clamped and tourniquet deflated to confirm that the hand is adequately perfused through the ulnar artery. The large caliber of the vessels to the radial forearm flap make this an attractive free flap to use. The skin paddle to the radial forearm flap can be proximal or distal. Placing the skin paddle distally allows for the advantage of a longer pedicle, but risks potential exposure of tendons and a less favorable donor site. A proximal skin territory design can sometimes allow for primary closure of the donor but results in a shorter pedicle (Fig. 11B–5 A

through E). With this proximal skin paddle the flap can be based on retrograde circulation, but this compromises venous return and mandates use of the less reliable venae comitante system. Therefore, the antegrade design is more practical when using the radial forearm flap for free tissue transfer. This flap can also be based distally as a pedicled flap through retrograde flow across the deep palmer arterial arch if it is patent. When used as a retrograde pedicle flap, the problem of nerve coaptation can be avoided by turning the flap over the dorsal web space, thus positioning the proximal portion of the flap for coaptation to appropriate recipient nerves in the hand.[12] Part of the radius can also be included in the radial forearm flap.[30] Another disadvantage to the use of this flap in addition to higher two-point discrimination and an unsightly donor is the sacrifice of a major artery to the hand, the radial artery. Arterial reconstruction of the radial artery can be considered, but some of this graft will be less protected under the skin graft within the donor site. Moreover, the side by side nerve supply to this flap makes sensory return unpredictable without the aid of neuromapping or preoperative nerve block study. Furthermore, caution must be exercised when a sensate radial arm flap innervated by the lateral antebrachial cutaneous nerve is raised, because sometimes this nerve innervates the radial side of the thumb. Again, this flap provides protective sensory restoration at best.

Lateral Upper Arm Flap

The cutaneous territory of the lateral arm septocutaneous flap includes the skin over the longitudinal axis from the deltoid insertion to the lateral epicondyle. The flap dimensions are 6 cm transversely and 12 cm longitudinally. The lateral arm flap is supplied by the posterior radial collateral artery, a branch of the profunda brachii artery (Fig. 11B–7). The posterior radial collateral artery can be found to arise along the lateral intramuscular septum, after coursing through the lateral intermuscular septum it terminates in a fascial and subdermal vascular network.[32] The arterial pedicle can be 4 to 8 cm long with a vessel diameter of 1.5 to 2 mm.[33] The venous return of this flap is from two systems—the superficial veins draining of the cephalic vein and the deep venae comitantes. The artery is accompanied by the posterior cutaneous nerve of the arm, which is a branch of the radial nerve and the innervation to the flap. This flap can provide thin sensate skin to reconstruct upper extremity defects. However, in obese patients this flap can be bulky. The two-point discrimination of this flap has been reported at 30 mm.[34] Therefore, this flap can provide protective sensation only, and not tactile discrimination. The lateral arm flap is a suitable option for reconstruction of palmer defects with

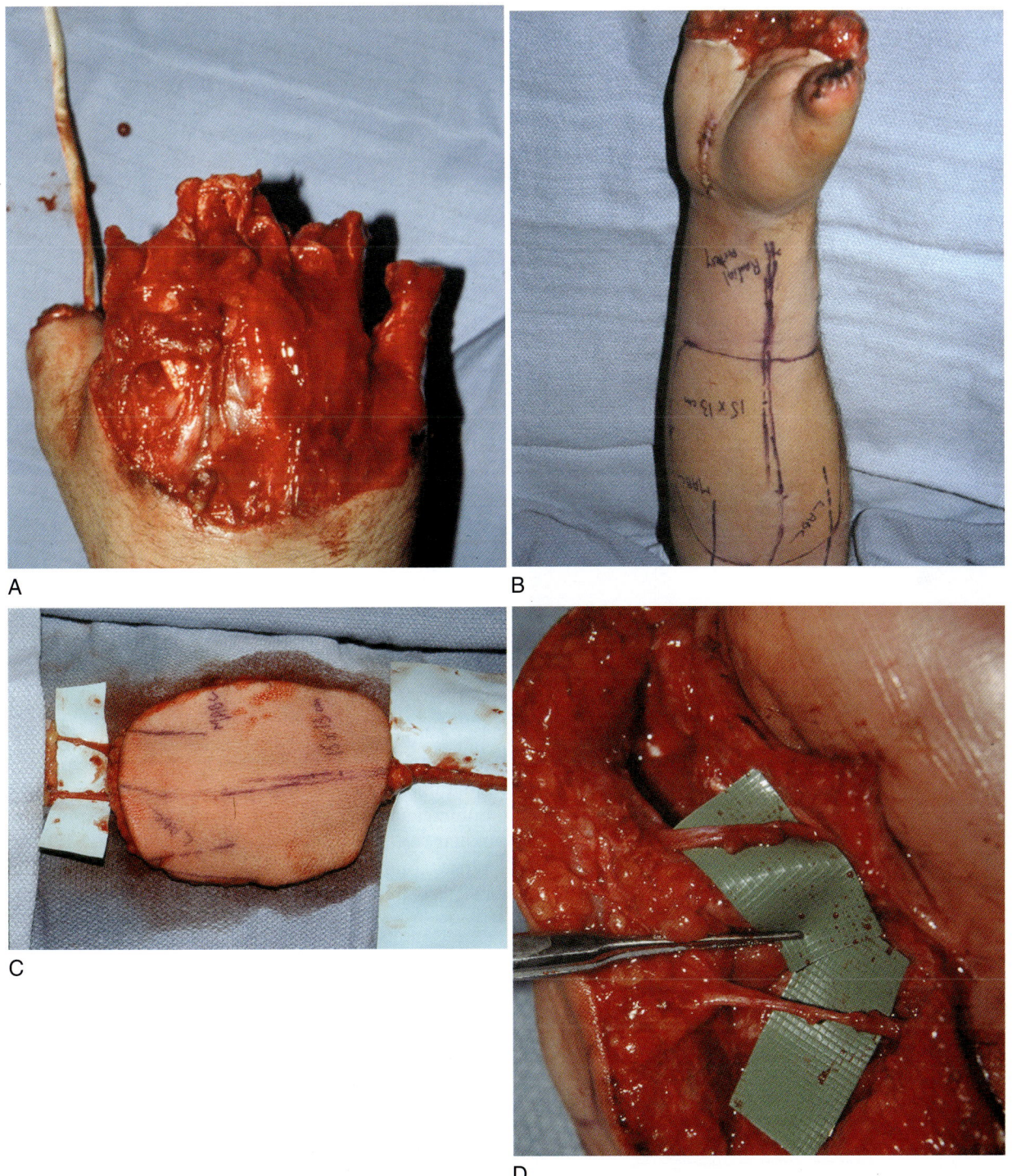

A

B

C

D

Figure 11B–5   This patient had a hand wound reconstructed with the neurosensory radial forearm flap.

soft tissue and requiring protective sensation. Another disadvantage of the lateral arm flap is the loss of sensation in the superolateral forearm provided by the posterior cutaneous nerve. Advantages with this flap are that it can be harvested under tourniquet control, with bone, and if the flap design is 6 cm in width, the donor site can be closed primarily.

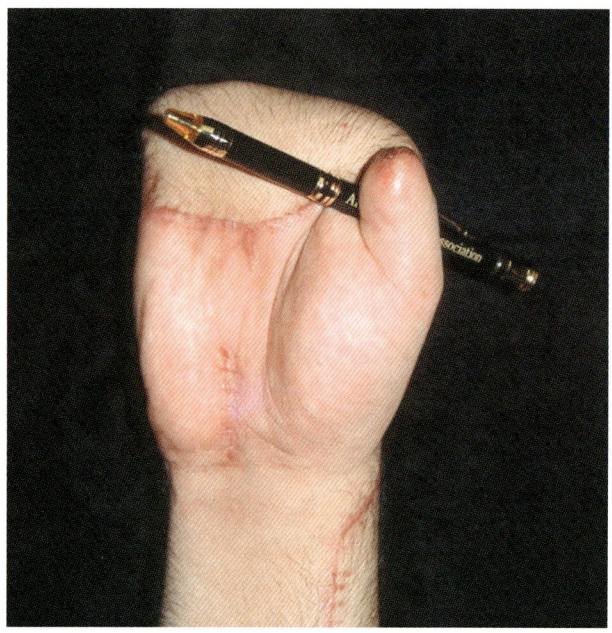

E

Figure 11B–5—Cont'd

Medial Upper Arm Flap

The medial arm flap is a 6-by-12-cm fasciocutaneous flap based on either the superior ulnar collateral artery or a direct fasciocutaneous branch from the brachia artery or both.[35] There are no direct fasciocutaneous branches from the superior ulnar collateral artery (SUCA) in 20%. If no direct fasciocutaneous branches from the SUCA are found, dissection in the proximal direction will facilitate a direct fasciocutaneous branch from the brachial or profunda brachii artery. The venous drainage of this flap is either the superficial basilic vein or the deep venae comitantes. The length of the vascular pedicle is 4 to 5 cm with vessel diameter of 1.0 to 2.0 cm. Because the pedicle enters the midportion of the flap, the functional length of the flap makes the microanastomosis awkward. The innervation of the medial arm flap is the medial brachial cutaneous nerve, which provides sensory feedback from the distal one third of the medial arm. One advantage of the medial arm flap is the inconspicuous donor site, which can be closed primarily if less than 6 cm in width. The variability of the blood supply to the medial arm flap and short pedicle make this a less reliable and a secondary option for neurosensory restoration.

Deltoid Flap

The deltoid flap is a fasciocutaneous flap harvested from the posterolateral deltoid muscle based on the posterior circumflex humeral artery. The posterior circumflex humeral artery is a branch from the third portion of the axillary artery. The venous drainage of this flap is by two venae comitantes with the artery. This flap's pedicle length is 6 to 8 cm with a vessel diameter of 2 to 4 mm.

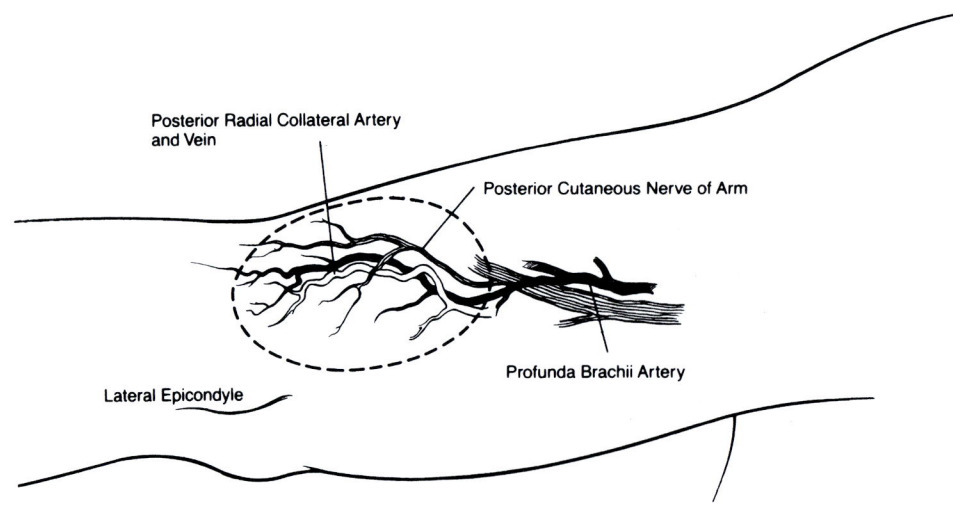

Posterior Radial Collateral Artery and Vein

Posterior Cutaneous Nerve of Arm

Lateral Epicondyle

Profunda Brachii Artery

Figure 11B–6 The lateral upper arm flap is supplied by the posterior radial collateral artery and vein and the posterior cutaneous nerve of the arm. (From Orgel MG. Innervated free flaps and free vascularized nerve grafts in the hand. In: McCarthy JG, May JW Jr, Littler JW, eds., Plastic Surgery, vol. 7. Philadelphia: W.B. Saunders, 1990:4859,[6] with permission.)

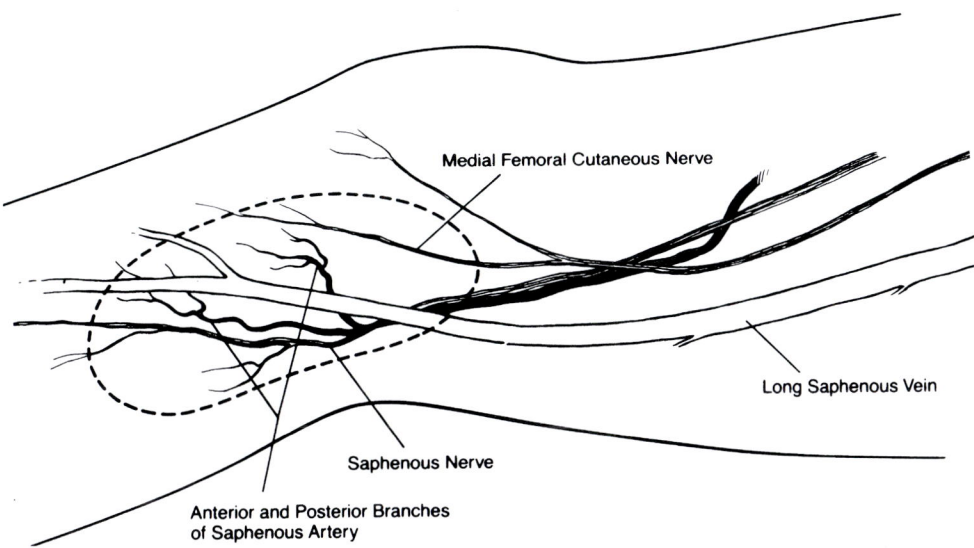

Figure 11B-7 Based on the saphenous branches of the descending genicular artery, the saphenous flap is innervated proximally by the medial femoral cutaneous nerve and distally by the saphenous nerve. (From Orgel MG. Innervated free flaps and free vascularized nerve grafts in the hand. In: McCarthy JG, May JW Jr, Littler JW, eds., Plastic Surgery, vol. 7. Philadelphia: W.B. Saunders, 1990:4859,[6] with permission.)

The innervation of the deltoid flap is the lateral brachial cutaneous nerve, the terminal sensory branch of the axillary nerve.[36] The neurovascular bundle exits the quadrangular space. The neurovascular pedicle can be located preoperatively with the patient in an upright position at the intersection of a line drawn from acromion to the medial epicondyle and the deltoid triceps groove.[37] This skin territory of the deltoid flap is large is 24 by 34 cm. The nerve innervates on average a 15-by-10-cm portion of the flap centered over the deltoid triceps groove. The two-point discrimination of this flap has been reported at 20 mm or more after flap transfer. Therefore, this flap does not provide tactile discrimination. This flap is thin and an occasional option for providing sensate skin to the glabrous palm. The disadvantage of this flap is that the arterial supply to the skin is inconsistent which can result in partial necrosis. Furthermore, the donor site can be unacceptable, especially in women. Sometimes the donor can be closed primarily if less than 7 cm in width.

Tensor Fascia Lata Flap

The tensor fascia lata flap (TFL) is a myocutaneous flap based on the small tensor fascia lata muscle. This flap can provide up to 40 by 15 cm of sensate skin for reconstruction.[38,39] The arterial supply to the TFL flap is the transverse branch of the lateral femoral circumflex artery. The venous drainage of this flap is venae comitante traveling with this artery. The cutaneous territory of the TFL flap is innervated by two distinct sensory nerves the lateral cutaneous branch of T12 proximally and the lateral cutaneous nerve of the thigh L2–L3 dis-

tally. The two-point discrimination of this flap after transfer has been reported to be poor at 40 to 50 mm.[11] In overweight patients, this flap is bulky, especially with the inclusion of the muscle. Accordingly, this flap is not commonly used to reconstruct the hand. The bulk of this flap makes it more appropriate for restoring protective sensibility to the forearm or upper limb amputation stump.

Anterolateral Thigh Flap

The anterolateral thigh flap is a fasciocutaneous flap based on cutaneous perforators of the descending branch of the lateral femoral circumflex vessels. The arterial pedicle if 8 to 12 cm in length with vessel diameter of 2 mm. This flap can provide a large skin quantity 12 by 38 cm. The anterolateral thigh flap is innervated by the lateral femoral cutaneous nerve.[40] The venous drainage of this flap is the venae comitante that travel with the artery. Like the TFL flap, the anterolateral thigh flap can be bulky, hair bearing and result in an unacceptable donor site scar, and therefore has a limited role in upper extremity reconstruction.

Saphenous Flap

The saphenous flap is a cutaneous flap over the medial aspect of the knee based on the saphenous artery (Fig. 11B–8). The saphenous artery is a terminal branch of the descending genicular artery that arises from the medial side of the femoral artery 15 cm above the knee just proximal to where the femoral artery passes through the adductor hiatus. This flap has two venous drainage

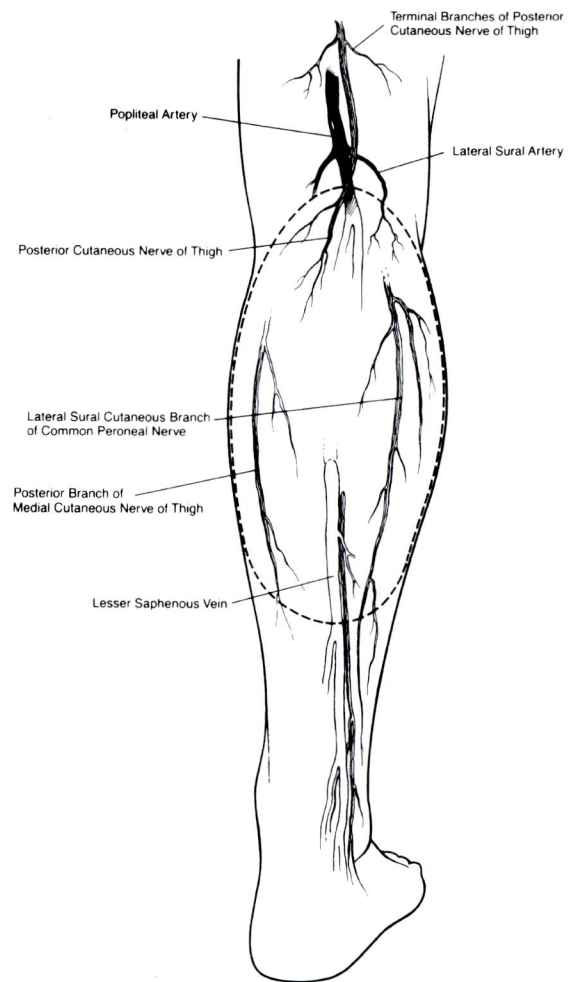

Popliteal Artery

Terminal Branches of Posterior
Cutaneous Nerve of Thigh

Lateral Sural Artery

Posterior Cutaneous Nerve of Thigh

Lateral Sural Cutaneous Branch
of Common Peroneal Nerve

Posterior Branch of
Medial Cutaneous Nerve of Thigh

Lesser Saphenous Vein

Figure 11B–8 The posterior calf flap is supplied by branches of the popliteal or lateral sural artery and their venae comitantes. Its sensory innervation comes form multiple cutaneous nerves. (From Orgel MG. Innervated free flaps and free vascularized nerve grafts in the hand. In: McCarthy JG, May JW Jr, Littler JW, eds., Plastic Surgery, vol. 7. Philadelphia: W.B. Saunders, 1990:4859,[6] with permission.)

systems superficial through the saphenous vein and deep by venae comitantes with the artery. The pedicle of this flap is 15 cm long and 1.5 to 2.0 mm in diameter.[1] The saphenous artery can be absent in 5% of patients.[1] The saphenous flap is innervated proximally by the medial femoral cutaneous nerve and distally by the saphenous nerve. The numbness of the donor site after skin grafting can be bothersome. The donor site can be closed primarily if less than 7 cm width, but is still unacceptable in women. The flap is thin and can provide a variable size skin paddle from 2 by 3 cm to 8 by 29 cm. A two-point discrimination of 9 to 14 mm after transfer has been reported in one case.[1] The advantage of this flap is that it is a thin flap with a long pedicle. However, the donor site appearance and numbness can be unacceptable, and there is little experience reported on the recovery of sensation with this flap. Furthermore,

the dissection is technically difficult, and sometimes necessitates division of the sartorius muscle.

Posterior Calf Flap

The posterior calf flap is a fasciocutaneous based on either a descending fasciocutaneous branch of the popliteal artery or the lateral sural artery. The dominant axial artery originates from either the popliteal (50%) or lateral sural artery (45%), and can be identified in the interval between the posterior midline of the calf and the fibular head.[41] Sometimes the dominant blood supply to the flap is via the medial sural artery (4%). The venous drainage of this fasciocutaneous flap is more reliable by the two venae comitantes that course deep with the artery into the fascia, than by the lesser saphenous vein that drains the subcutaneous tissue and not fascia. This flap is innervated by the lateral sural nerve or medial sural nerve, but there is much variability with the innervation of the posterior calf skin, which makes flap dissection tedious. When the flap is based on the medial sural artery the lateral sural nerve is preserved and the medial sural nerve can be preserved when the flap is based laterally. One series reported 6 to 12 mm of two-point discrimination with this flap. This flap can provide a large skin territory, but since the innervation is unpredictable, this flap is less useful for sensory restoration. Furthermore, significant donor morbidity, such as prolonged lower extremity edema, hematoma formation, graft loss, and loss of sural nerve sensation has been reported with this flap

Posterior Interosseus Flap

The posterior interosseous flap is a septocutaneous flap. The maximum flap dimensions are 10 by 6 cm.[42] The flap is based on the posterior interosseous artery, a branch of the common interosseous artery. The arterial pedicle is short and the vessel diameter is only 0.8 to 1.2 mm. The common interosseous artery arises from the ulnar artery at the level of the radial tuberosity and divides into posterior and anterior branches. The posterior interosseous artery courses with the posterior interosseous nerve under the superficial portion of the supinator. After exiting the supinator, the posterior interosseous artery enters the septum between the extensor digiti minimi and extensor carpi ulnaris. Along its course, the posterior interosseous artery gives off several cutaneous arteries (7 to 14 in number). The largest of these perforating branches is proximal. The posterior artery travels with the posterior interosseous nerve to the midwrist along a longitudinal vector from the lateral epicondyle to the dorsal midline of the wrist at the distal radioulnar joint. Since the posterior interosseous nerve has motor and sensory components it has to be preserved in harvesting this flap to avoid denervation of the wrist and finger extensors.

The posterior interosseous flap can be designed as an antegrade or retrograde flap. The retrograde arterial flow to the posterior interosseous artery is by anastomoses at the wrist with the perforating branch of the anterior interosseous artery, the dorsal carpal arch and the vascular plexus surrounding the ulnar head. The venous drainage of this flap is more reliable when an antegrade design is used. For the antegrade flap the venous drainage is best by local superficial veins and not venae comitante. However, when basing the flap on retrograde flow, the venae comitante have to be used. The retrograde design can be used as a pedicle flap for reconstructing hand defects. The antegrade flap can be used as a free flap or as pedicle to reconstruct distal elbow defects.

This flap can be used as a sensate flap. This flap is named after its arterial supply and not innervation. The sensory component of the posterior interosseous nerve is to the wrist. The innervation of this cutaneous territory is the medial antebrachial cutaneous nerve. The donor site can be closed primarily if the flap width is less than 3 cm; otherwise, a skin graft is used. The two-point discrimination achieved with free transfer of this flap was 15 mm in one report.[42] These authors discouraged its use to restore tactile discrimination. Other disadvantages of the free posterior interosseous flap are the tedious dissection, short pedicle, narrow vessels, somewhat bulky flap, and hair-bearing skin not suitable for palmar reconstruction.

Other Flaps

Other neurosensory flaps that have been described include the distal unlar artery flap, transverse cervical flap, sensate superior gluteal artery perforator flap, sensate deep inferior epigastric muscluocutaneous flap, sensate myocutaneous latissimus flap, sensate osteocutaneous fibula flap, and the lateral intercostal flap.[35,43–51] However, many of these flaps have been reported to provide protective sensation to other areas, such as the head and neck, breast, or other areas, and not enough clinical experience has been obtained to establish their usefulness in sensor reconstruction of the hand.

SUMMARY

Neurosensory free flaps can provide sensibility, vascularity, and soft tissue coverage to an injured hand. In determining the most suitable means of reconstructing a defect, the benefit of the reconstruction has to outweigh the risk of donor morbidity. Appropriate selection of a neurosensory flap is based primarily on the need for tactile discrimination or protective sensation. Because of its thin glabrous skin, constant vascular and neural anatomy, minimal donor morbidity and in situ two-point discrimination, the first web-space flap of the foot (or its variants) are considered to be the best choice for restoration of critical sensibility to the digital tips or first web space of the hand. Several other neurosensory flaps have been described that can be used to restore protective sensation for other areas on the hand. But the return of sensation with these other flap options is variable, and it is therefore critical to scrutinize individual reports on the use of these flaps to appropriately determine the chance for long-term sensory ability in selecting a donor neurosensory flap.

REFERENCES

1. Acland RD, Schusterman M, Godina M, et al. The saphenous neurovascular free flap. Plast Reconstr Surg 1981;67:763.
2. Daniel RK, Terzis J, Schwartz G. Neurovascular free flaps: a preliminary report. Plast Reconstr Surg 1975;56:13.
3. Ohmori K, Harii K. Free dorsalis pedis sensory flap to the hand with microneurovascular anastomoses. Plast Reconstr Surg 1976;58:546.
4. Robinson DW. Microsurgical transfer of the dorsalis pedis neurovascular island flap. Br J Plast Surg 1976;29:209.
5. Hing DN, Buncke HJ, Alpert BS, et al. Free flap coverage of the hand. Hand Clin 1985;1:741.
6. Orgel MG. Innervated free flaps and free vascularized nerve grafts in the hand. In: McCarthy JG, May JW Jr, Littler JW, eds., Plastic Surgery, vol. 7. Philadelphia: W.B. Saunders, 1990: 4859.
7. Littler JW. Neurovascular pedicle transfer of tissue in reconstructive surgery of the hand. J Bone Joint Surg Am 1956;38:917.
8. Terzis JK, Michelow BJ. Sensory receptors. In: Gelberman RH, ed., Operative Nerve Repair and Reconstruction, vol. 1. Philadelphia: J.B. Lippincott, 1991:85.
9. Dellon AL. Evaluation of Sensibility and Reeducation of Sensation in the Hand. Baltimore: Williams & Wilkins, 1981.
10. Gilbert A, Morrison WA, Tubiana R. Transfer sur la main d'un lambeau libre sensible. Chirurugie 1973;101:691.
11. Strauch B, Greenstein B. Neurovascular flaps to the hand. Hand Clin 1985;1:327.
12. Swartz WM. Restoration of sensibility in mutilating hand injuries. Clin Plast Surg 1979;16:170.
13. Buncke HJ, Rose EH. Free toe to fingertip neurovascular flaps. Plast Reconstr Surg 1979;63:607.
14. Foucher G, Merle M, Maneaud M, et al. Microsurgical free partial toe transfer in hand reconstruction: a report of 12 cases. Plast Reconstr Surg 1980;65;616.
15. Morrison WA, O'Brien BM, MacLeod AM. Thumb reconstruction with free neurovascular wraparound flap from the big toe. J Hand Surg 1980;5:575.
16. Leung P-C, Ma F-Y. Digital reconstruction using the toe flap report of 10 cases. J Hand Surg 1982;7:366.
17. May JW Jr. Microvascular great toe to hand transfer for reconstruction of the amputated thumb. In: McCarthy JG, May JW Jr,

Littler JW, eds., Plastic Surgery, vol. 8. Philadelphia: W.B. Saunders, 1990:5153.

18. May JW Jr, Daniel RK. Great toe to hand transfer. Clin Orthop 1978;133:140.

19. Tsai TM, Falconer D. Modified great toe wrap for thumb reconstruction. Microsurgery 1986;7:193.

20. Kato H, Ogino T, Minami A, et al. Restoration of sensibility in fingers repaired with free sensory flaps from the toe. J Hand Surg Am 1989;14:49.

21. Lee Hb, Tark KC, Rar DK, et al. Pulp reconstruction of fingers with very small sensate medial plantar free flap. Plast Reconstr Surg 1998;101:999.

22. Narsete TA. Anatomic design of a sensate plantar flap. Ann Plast Surg 1997;38:538.

23. Daniel RK, Terzis J, Midgley RD. Restoration of sensation to an anesthetic hand by a free neurovascular flap from the foot. Plast Reconstr Surg 1976;57:275.

24. McCraw JB, Furlow LT. The dorsalis pedis arterialized flap. A clinical study. Plast Reconstr Surg 1975;55:177.

25. Man D, Acland RD. The microarterial anatomy of the dorsalis pedis flap and its clinical applications. Plast Reconstr Surg 1980;65:419.

26. Taylor GI, Townsend PLG. Composite free flap and tendon transfer. An anatomical study and clinical technique. Br J Plast Surg 1979;32:170.

27. Zuker RM, Manktelow RT. The dorsalis pedis free flap technique of elevation, foot closure, and flap application. Plast Reconstr Surg 1986;77:93.

28. May JW Jr, Chait LA, Cohen BE, et al. Free neurosensory vascular flap from the first web of the foot in hand reconstruction. J Hand Surg 1977;2:387–93.

29. Morrison WA, O'Brien BM, MacLeod AM, et al. Neurovascular free flaps from the foot for innervation of the hand. J Hand Surg 1978;3:235.

30. Foucher G, van Genechten F, Merle N, et al. A compound radial artery forearm flap in hand surgery an original modification of the Chinese forearm flap. Br J Plast Surg 1984;37:139.

31. Muhlbauer W, Herndl E, Stock W. The forearm flap. Plast Reconstr Surg 1982;70:336.

32. Song R, Song Y, Yu U, et al. The upper arm free flap. Clin Plast Surg 1982;9:27.

33. Katsaros J, Schusterman M, Beppu M, et al. The lateral upper arm flap. Anatomy and clinical applications. Ann Plast Surg 1984;12:489.

34. Katsaros J, Tan E, Zoltie N, et al. Further experience with the lateral arm free flap. Plast Reconstr Surg 1991;87:902.

35. Newsom HT. Medial arm free flap. Plast Reconstr Surg 1981;67:63.

36. Franklin JD. The deltoid flap. Anatomy and clinical applications. In: Buncke HJ, Furnas DW, eds. Symposium on Clinical Frontiers in Reconstructive Microsurgery, vol. 24. St. Louis: C.V. Mosby, 1983:63.

37. Russell RC, Guy RJ, Zook EG, et al. Extremity reconstruction using the free deltoid flap. Plast Reconstr Surg 1985;76:586.

38. Hill HL, Nahai F, Vasconez LO. The tensor fascia lata myocutaneous free flap. Plast Reconstr Surg 1978;61:517.

39. Nahai F, Hill HL, Hester TR. Experiences with the tensor fascia lata flap. Plast Reconstr Surg 1978;63:788.

40. Pribaz JJ, Orgill DP, Epstein MD, et al. Anterolateral thigh free flap. Ann Plast Surg 1995;34:585.

41. Walton RL, Bunkis J. The posterior calf fasciocutaneous free flap. Plast Reconstr Surg 1984;74:76.

42. Chen HC, Tang YB, Chuang D, et al. Microvascular free posterior interosseous flap and a comparison with the pedicled posterior interosseous flap. Ann Plast Surg 1996;36:542.

43. Badran HA, El Helaly MS, Safe I. The lateral intercostals neurovascular free flap. Plast Reconstr Surg 1984;73:17.

44. Morris RL, Dillman D, McCabe JS, et al. The transverse cervical neurovascular free flap. Ann Plast Surg 1983;10:90.

45. Woerdeman LA, Chaplin BJ, Griffioen FM, et al. Sensate osteocutaneous fibula flap anatomic study of the innervation pattern of the skin flap. Head Neck 1998;20:310.

46. Wei FC, Chuang SS, Yim KK. The sensate fibula osteoseptocutaneous flap: a preliminary report. Br J Plast Surg 1994;47:544.

47. Mawera G, Kalangu KK, Muguti GI. The sensate deep inferior epigastric musculocutaneous flap and the twelfth thoracic nerve. Br J Plast Surg 1995;48:455.

48. Blondeel PN. The sensate free superior gluteal artery perforator (S-GAP) flap: a valuable alternative in autologous breast reconstruction. Br J Plast Surg 1999;52:185.

49. Schultes G, Karcher H, Gaggl A. Sensate myocutaneous latissimus dorsi flap. J Reconstr Microsurg 1998;14:541.

50. Muguti GI, Mawera G, Kalangu KK. The sensate deep inferior epigastric musculocutaneous flap: details of the operative technique. Cent Afr J Med 1997;43:340.

51. Mawera G, Kalanu KK, Muguti GI. The sensate deep inferior epigastric musculocutaneous flap and the twelfth thoracic nerve. Br J Plast Surg 1995;48:455.

12

Direct Muscular Neurotization

Giorgio A. Brunelli

INTRODUCTION

Reconstructive surgeons have to face more and more frequently cases in which, because of high velocity traumas, the wound has either avulsed the motor nerve from the muscle or destroyed its "neural part," that is, the part of the muscle in which the divisions of the nerve endings form the neuromuscular synapses, or the motor end plates. In these cases, traditional surgery such as end-to-end or end-to-side nerve sutures, nerve grafts, or nerve conduits, cannot be performed. The same is true for surgical "en bloc" removal of the "neural zone" of the muscle because of various pathologies. Classically, only tendon transfers could be done.

In 1970, I started to search for the possibility of reinnervating the denervated muscles. Upon reviewing the literature, I learned that experiments of implanting nerves into muscles had been done since the early 20th century (Heineke, 1914,[1] Erlacher, 1914,[2] Steindler, 1915,[3] Elsberg, 1917[4]). Experiments were followed by clinical applications, mainly for muscles affected by poliomyelitis. Results were inconstistent, and the technique was abandoned.

Later Aitken (1950)[5] and Guth and Zalewsky (1963)[6] tried experimental implantation of nerves into denervated muscles. In 1964, Katz and Miledi[7] showed that just by laying a motor nerve on a denervated muscle, acetylcholine (ACh) sensitivity could be induced. The receptors for ACh in denervated muscles spread all over the muscular fibers. The sparse receptors allow the branches of an implanted nerve to "take" in the muscle and to form new functioning motor end plates, even in heterotopic places.

RATIONALE

It is known that a normally innervated muscle cannot accept a new innervation because its sensitivity to ACh is restricted to the very point of motor end plates so that *no* new nerve fibers put inside the muscle can form new motor end plates. Motor end plates are not anatomic structures, but rather constitute physiologic alteration of the nerve ending and muscular membrane when in touch with each other. During denervation, the nerve ending disappears due to Wallerian degeneration. Only the Schwann cells that myelinated the axon remain, and the muscular membrane loses its characteristic folding and the concentration of ACh receptors.

Hence, the biological bases for direct muscular neurotization are as follows:

1. A normally innervated muscle does not accept a new innervation.
2. A denervated muscle can accept a new innervation because its sensitivity to ACh is spread all over the muscle.
3. New motor end plates form when nerve endings get in touch with denervated muscular fiber.

As mentioned above, this is possible because in denervated muscles the receptors for ACh are spread all over the muscular fiber. In fact, the transmembrane molecular channels for Na containing the receptors for ACh, normally grouped under the nerve ending, after nerve lesion and Wallerian degeneration scatter all over the muscle.

Due to the scattering of ACh receptors and of agrins, which normally gather at the ending of axons, new synapses (motor end plates) can be formed even if in heterotopic sites, because they can find ACh receptors and because other ACh receptors, scattered all over the muscle, group under the new nerve ending due to the action of agrins.

PERSONAL RESEARCH

To check if it were possible to effectively reinnervate a denervate muscle by direct implantation of a nerve, I began my research in 1970 first in rats and then in rabbits.[8,9]

Material and Methods

The first series of animals (1970) consisted of 21 rabbits. The distal portion of the tibial nerve with its intramuscular branches was removed to denervate the gastrocnemius muscle. The peroneal nerve was severed and implanted into the proximal portion of the lateral head of that muscle in an aneural zone. (This zone would not, under normal conditions, exhibit motor end plates.) Physiologic muscle responses were obtained, and formation of new motor end plates in aneural zones of muscle was noted (Fig. 12–1).

In 1973, the experimental model was modified: the nerve was divided in several fascicles to obtain a larger area of reinnervation (Fig. 12–2). Over the next few years of animal research, more technical modifications were made, consisting mainly of the meticulous microsurgical division of the nerve in more and more artificial fascicles, and in the wider distribution of these divisions both in width and depth. These technical improvements gave better results.

Electrical stimulation of the peroneal nerve demonstrated good functional reinnervation as early as 1 month after surgery. Muscle fibers in which new motor end plates had formed regained trophicity and showed normal morphology.

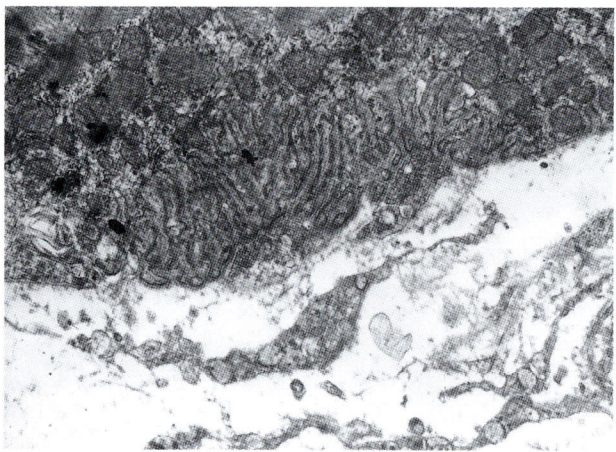

Figure 12–1   TEM photography of newly formed motor end plates after direct muscular neurotization in a previously aneural zone of the muscle. Nerve ending with synaptic vesicles; the synaptic cleft is enlarged by the folding of the muscular membrane.

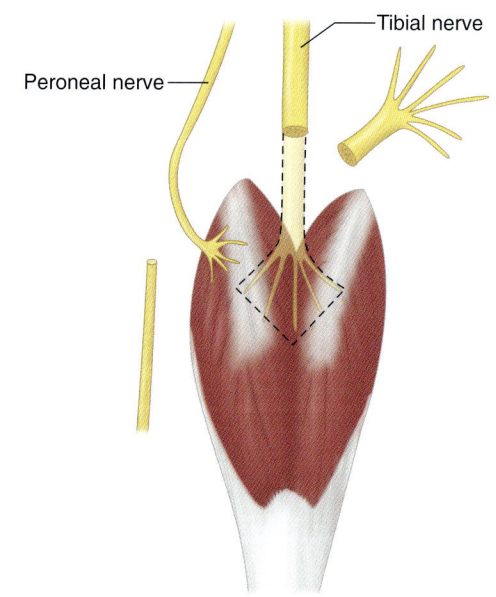

Figure 12–2   Scheme of the experimental surgery (late protocol): the tibial nerve is cut and its branches to the muscle removed from the so-called motor end plates. The peroneal nerve is then cut, divided into thin slips, and introduced into small slits in the proximal part of the muscle, the aneural zone where normally no motor end plate exists.

In contrast, the nonreinnervated fibers showed dystrophic appearance (Figs. 12–3 and 12–4). Transmission electron microscopy demonstrated normal motor end plates with bare axon branches rich in presynaptic vescicles in direct contact with the membranes of muscle fibers that had normal-appearing folds (Fig. 12–1).

Presynaptic vesicles and mytochondria were noted in the axon branches, while only a single layer of Schwann cytoplasm was present over the axon on the opposite

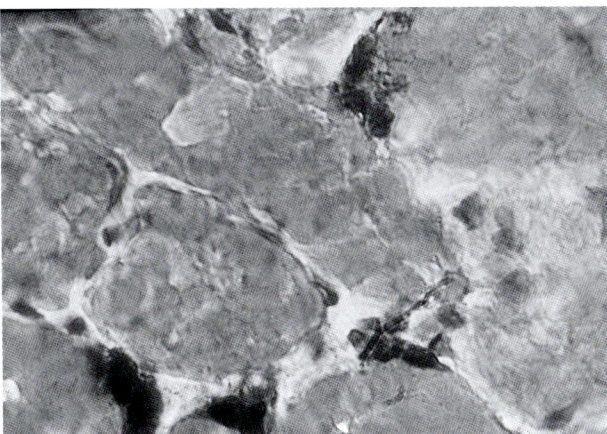

Figure 12–3 The muscular fibers are still degenerated. Motor end plates start to be evident after 1½ months of experimental surgery.

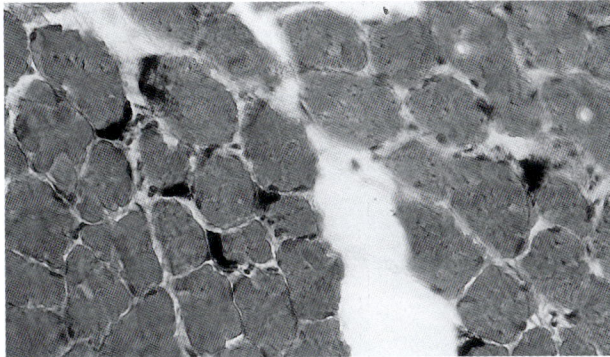

Figure 12–4 The muscular fibers are much more trophic where motor end plates formed; still distrophic where they have not yet appeared.

side of the muscle. There were no connective elements between the axon branches and the muscle.

In subsequent research, nerve specimens were stained for ACh, using the technique described by Koelle and Tsuge. The fact that some of the fibers in the newly implanted nerve did not take up the stain, is indirect evidence that both afferent and efferent fibers regenerated.

These encouraging results may also have been caused by the adoption phenomenon, which depends on the chemotactic appeal exerted by the denervated muscle fibers on the surrounding regenerated axons. The latter send out sprouts, which then become branches. They may issue from a node of Ranvier, or from the axon immediately above the motor end plate, or even from motor end plate itself. By reinnervation of orphan fibers, giant motor units are formed that are two or three times bigger than normal units, demonstrated by electromyography (EMG). These giant motor units constitute a large part of the newly functioning muscle. A sound or regenerated axon is probably able to adopt orphan muscle fibers belonging to three or four (and possibly more) nonregenerated axons.

In 1972, Sakellarides et al.[10] published similar results from experiments performed on dogs. Unfortunately, these authors did not continue the experiments nor clinical application.

Clinical Application

After obtaining encouraging experimental results, I began clinical direct muscular neurotization in 1975. Candidates were patients who had sustained injuries in which the proximal nerve stump was available, but the distal branches were missing because of the traumatic or surgical loss of the muscle portion in which the motor nerve branches and motor end plates are located. Contraindications included a long interval of denervation such that the reparative ability of anterior horn cells were exhausted. The procedure was also deemed inappropriate if too large a portion of muscle had been destroyed, if the remaining muscle was extremely fibrotic, or if there were other extramuscular limiting conditions, such as marked joint stiffness exist.

The ideal candidate was a *young,* intelligent and cooperative man/woman who underwent avulsion of the nerve endings from one muscle or from a group of muscles having similar function (e.g., extensor carpi radialis longus [ECRL], extensor carpi radialis brevis [ECRB], extensor digitorum longus [EDL], extensor pollicis longus [EPL], extensor indicis proprius [EIP], extensor digiti minimi [EDM], extensor pollicis brevis [EPB]). The time of denervation must not be too long, and the muscle to be innervated must be still trophic enough and show fibrillation at EMG examination. The surrounding tissue must be in good condition without severe scarring, and the blood supply of the muscle must still be adequate.

Anagraphic age is less important than biological age. As mentioned previously, young people are preferentially chosen, but adults up to middle age are eligible if the lacking function is paramount for their lifestyle or profession, especially if tendon transfers are not practicable.

Indications

Indications are listed below.

Avulsion of the nerve (with its terminal branches) from the muscle.
Surgical removal of the "neural" zone of the muscle for various pathologies.
Traumatic removal of the same part of the muscle.
Practically all conditions of muscle denervation.

Eligibility conditions are as follows:

Remaining muscular mass large enough for an efficient function.

Remaining trophism of the muscle demonstrated by EMG (fibrillation).

There are no fixed time periods: a denervated muscle may undergo atrophy in a short time interval; in contrast, it can remain trophic for a long time if massage and physiotherapy have been applied. Trophicity and EMG fibrillation are the parameters that allow surgery independently from the elapsed time.

Contraindications are the following:

1. Atrophy of the muscle, without fibrillation at EMG.
2. Necessity of more important surgery to the same limbs (or elsewhere).
3. Advanced old age (biological).
4. Bad general health condition.
5. Extensive local scar.
6. Devascularization.
7. Severe stiffness of the joint(s) to be mobilized.
8. Scarce patient cooperation.
9. Infections.
10. Too large muscular removal so that the remaining muscular mass is inadequate for an effective function.

Surgical Technique and Practical Tips

As the muscles to be operated are different, the patient position, skin incision, and dissection will vary also depending on the site and type of nerve avulsion from the muscle, and on the traumatic or surgical loss of the neural part of the muscle. The incision should be extended up to the donor nerve that can be the proximal stump of the proper nerve or another nerve selected by the surgeon with the agreement of the patient.

There is no particular preference for the type of anesthesia. It can be general, regional, or locoregional. If general anesthesia is used, muscle relaxants should be avoided in order to allow intraoperative electrical stimulation of the muscle, even if generally it is not necessary. In most cases, a simple surgical locator is enough.

All operations shall be done under tourniquet ischemia (if possible). Instrumentation is very simple: Adson forceps, knife 20 and 11, dissection scissors, retractors, two microsurgical forceps (no. 5). After the incision is done, the donor nerve is retrieved and transversally cut up to visualize good internal fascicles. Then the muscular belly or bellies are dissected. The best part of the muscle is identified. This part must be as proximal as possible according to the lesion, that is, more or less at the junction of the proximal quarter with the three distal quarter of the muscular belly. The reddest (most highly vascularized) part of the muscle is selected.

A sural nerve graft of adequate length is withdrawn from the leg following the usual technique. According

to the size of the donor nerve and the size and number of the muscle to be reinnervated, one or two grafts are used. The graft must be end to end sutured to the donor nerve and laid down in a soft and vascularized bed up to the muscle. At this point, a colored plastic sheet is passed under the distal ending of the graft that has to be trimmed at a convenient length.

Then, under operating microscope or loupe magnification, the epineurium of the graft has to be removed over 1.5 to 2 cm. The distal part of the nerve, freed from the epineurium, is artificially divided in as many as possible artificial fascicles (Figs. 12–5 and 12–6). At this point, the tourniquet is released and a very careful homeostasis has to be implemented. The epineurium of the graft is then sutured to the epimysium in order to prevent the recession of the graft.

Next, with a no. 11 blade, slits (corresponding to that of the artificial fascicles) are prepared in an area corresponding to the wider extension of the fascicles (Fig.

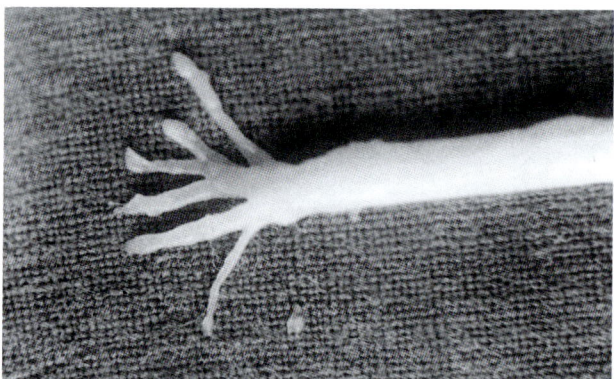

Figure 12–5 Artificial division of a graft in six artificial branches.

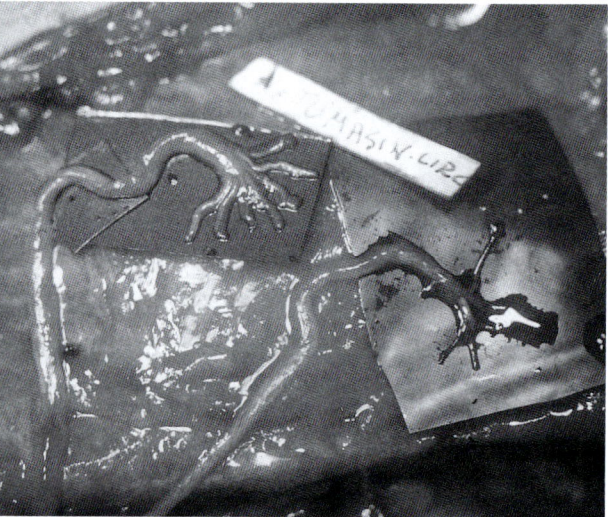

Figure 12–6 Two sural nerve grafts artificially divided in several slips, ready to be implanted into the muscle.

12–7). The slits must have different depths in order to reach the maximum possible number of muscular fibers, and must be implanted in as wide an area as possible.

The artificial fascicles of the nerve graft are then introduced into the slits, while checking that they can remain in place thanks to the autologous fibrin glue and to the anchorage of the epinerium (Figs. 12–8 and 12–9). Then the operated muscle must be gently and carefully covered with healthy skin. If necessary, a rotational skin flap can be used.

The operated limbs has to be immobilized for 10 days. Then careful and prudent re-education is started consisting in mobilization and electrotherapy. To avoid scar constriction at the level of the suture, x-ray therapy at antifibroblast dosage (800 r) must be done at the level of the suture, starting at the 10th day.

Surgical Series and Results

As seen in Table 12–1, results[11–16] are at least as good as those obtained by traditional nerve grafting (Figs.

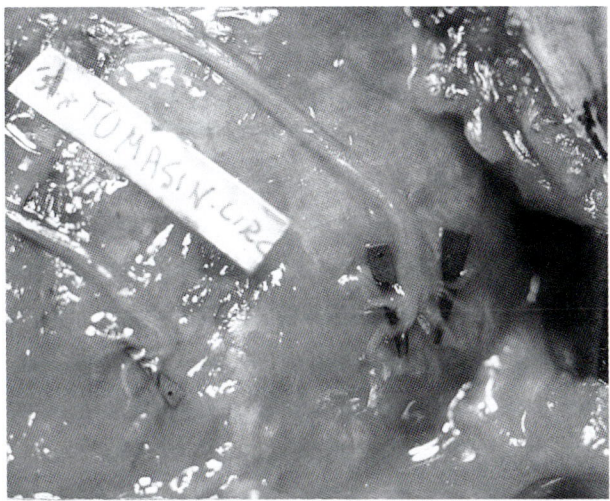

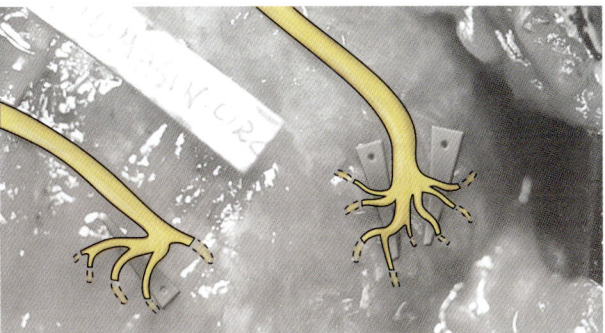

Figure 12–8 Shows how the artificial branches in which the graft has been divided must be implanted into the muscle.

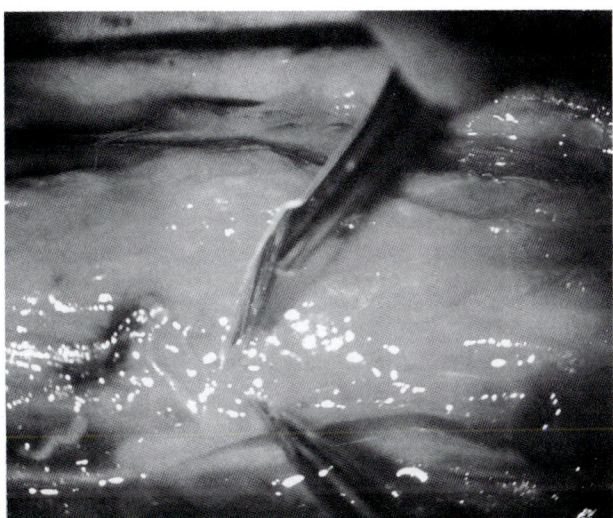

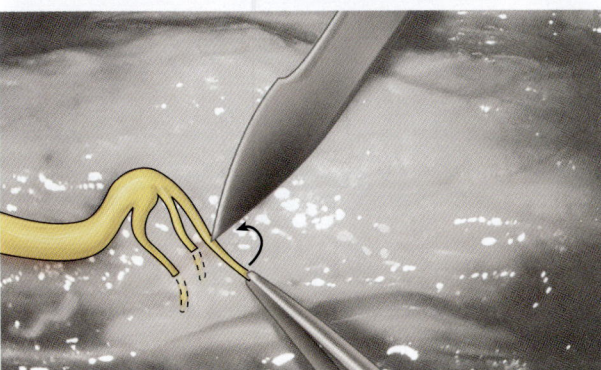

Figure 12–7 By means of a no. 11 blade some small slits are prepared in the muscle. The microsurgical forceps will then introduce the artificial slip into the slits.

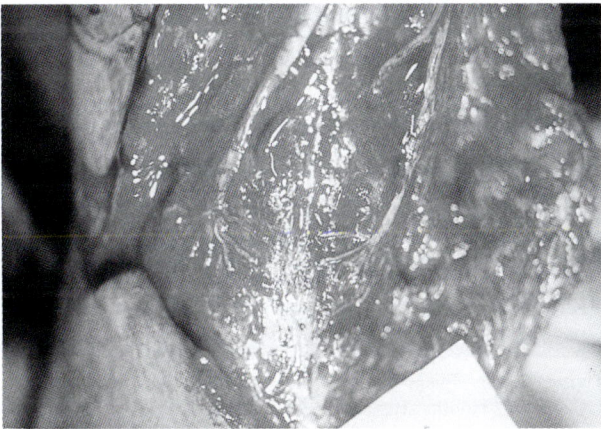

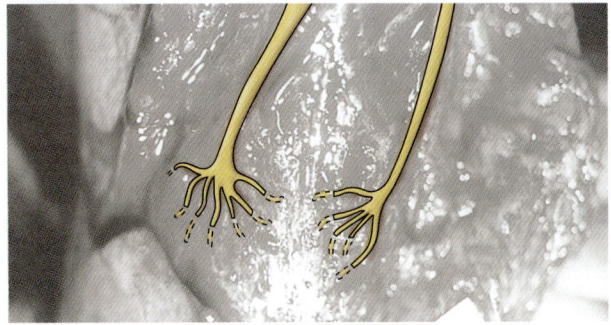

Figure 12–9 Another example of implantation.

TABLE 12–1

Results of Direct Muscular Neurotization: Personal Series

	Number of Cases	>M4	MN	M3	<M3
Extensor muscles at forearm	17	11	4	2	0
Extensor muscles at leg	18	13	4	1	0
Trapezium	7	4	2	1	0
Supraspinatus	1	0	1	0	0
Biceps	8	4	3	1	0
Thenarian muscles	4	3	1	0	0
EPL	1	0	1	0	0
Deltoid	7	1	4	1	1
Muscles of the tongue	2	1	1	0	0
Total	65	37	21	6	1
Various muscles studied by different authors; survey overview of communications	206	106	39	29	32

EPL, extensor pollicis longus; MN, median nerve.

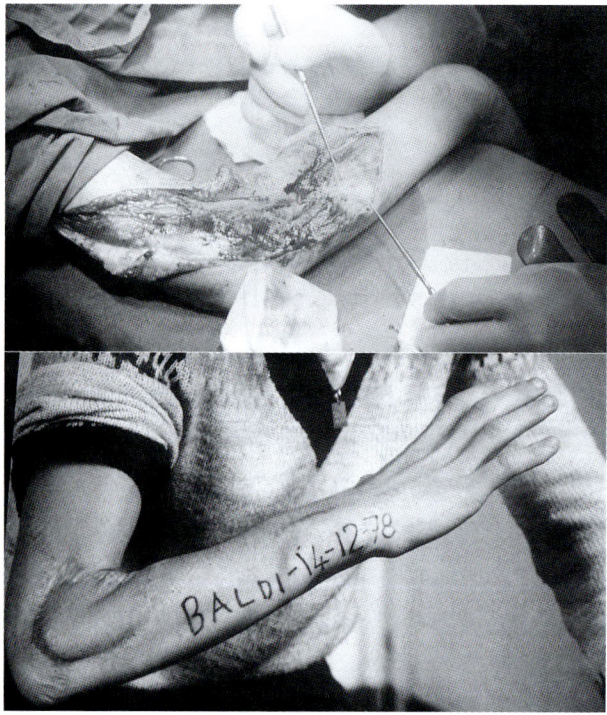

Figure 12–10 This was the first case, operated on in 1975. The patient presented 12 months after a propeller of a motor boat had avulsed the proximal (neural) third of the extensor muscles of the right forearm, with osteoarthritis at elbow. Four more months were necessary to cure the osteoarthritis, and to cover the large loss of soft tissue by means of a free scapular flap. Then a graft of two segments of sural nerve was sutured to the proximal stump of the radial nerve and implanted in the very short distal bellies of the extensor muscles after having divided them in several artificial branches. Result after 3 years.

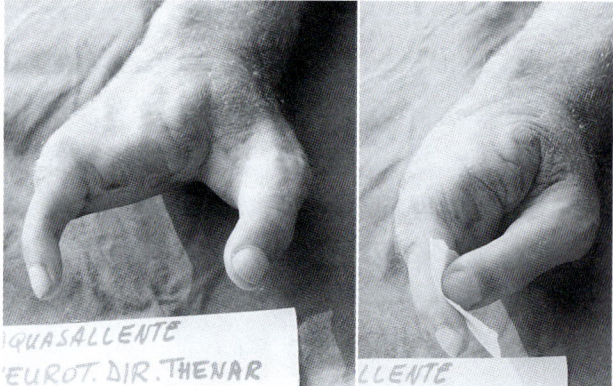

Figure 12–11 Result of direct muscular neurotization of thenarian muscles.

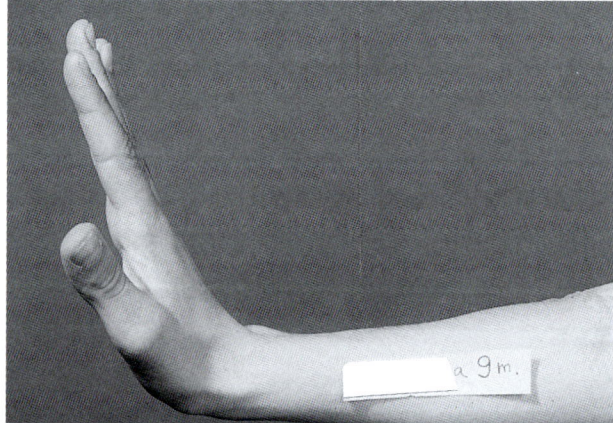

Figure 12–12 Result of direct muscular neurotization of extensor muscles of the wrist and digits after traumatic removal of the proximal (neural) part of the muscles.

12–10, 12–11, 12–12, 12–13, 12–14, and 12–15). Surprisingly (as generally the operations on the peroneal nerve give the poorest results), the best results were obtained in the direct neurotization of the extensors at the leg after avulsion of the neural part of the muscle

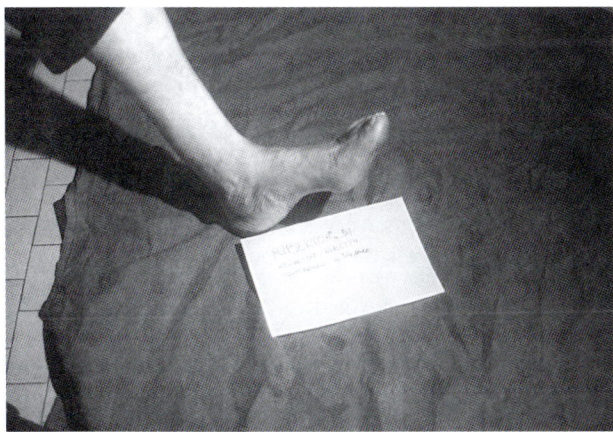

Figure 12–13 Result of direct muscular neurotization of the extensor muscles of the leg.

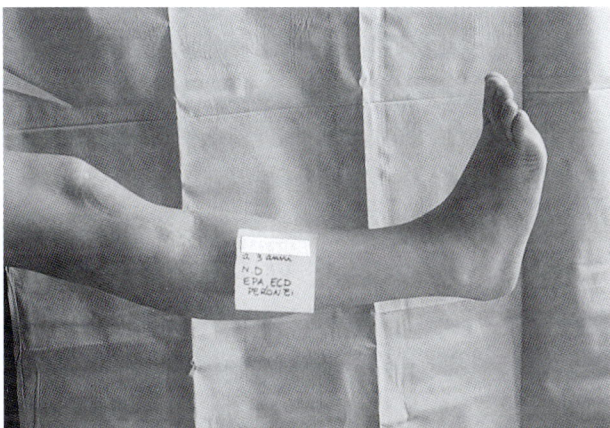

Figure 12–14 Very good results after direct muscular neurotization of the extensor muscles of the foot due to traumatic removal of the proximal part of the muscles. Note loss of muscles at the proximal leg.

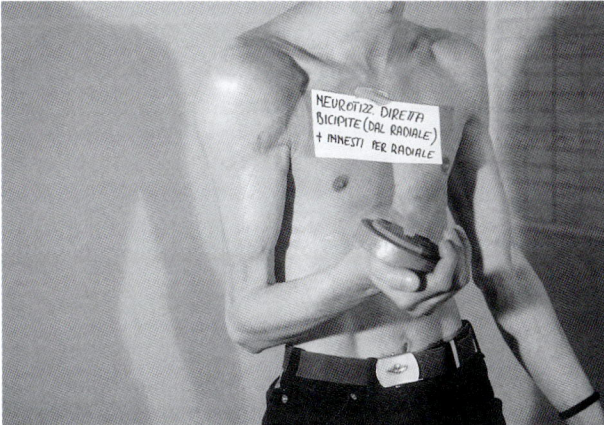

Figure 12–15 Good result of direct neurotization of the biceps muscle after traumatic removal of part of its proximal belly and avulsion of the musculocutaneous nerve. A branch to the triceps of the radial nerve was used for neurotization.

even when the left belly was short. A possible explanation is that the peroneal nerve is often in precarious conditions because of its compression at the head of the fibula due to leg crossing so that suture of such a fibrotic nerve gives lesser results that the substitution of that part of the nerve done by performing direct neurotization.

After surveying surgeons who adopted my technique all over the world (Table 12–1), I was able to ascertain that results were satisfying in their series as well: of more than 200 cases checked in 1995, 72% were very good or good.

Following a relatively short "learning curve" for the surgical technique, *if the indication was correct* and postoperative re-education was appropriate, results were very good or good. Of course, results depend also on the phenomenon of adoption and on the formation of giant motor units.

The time needed for reinnervation to occur depends on the distance from the proximal nerve stump to the point of implantation (nerve regenerates at an average speed of 1 mm/day). In three of the cases in which the proximal stump was unavailable for reinnervation (because of avulsion of the brachial plexus from the spinal cord), a foreign donor nerve was used. In one case, even an antagonist nerve (a radial nerve branch of the triceps to the biceps) was transferred (Fig. 12–15). In all of these cases, functional results were good. In the reported series, 61 of the 65 cases were operated on by connecting the proper nerve with the muscle by means of sural nerve graft.

CONCLUSION

There are no traditional techniques by means of which reinnervation can be obtained when the distal ending of a nerve has been avulsed from the muscle or the neural part of it has been removed. In these cases, traditional surgery can do either tendon transfers or arthrodesis. Both of them are partially crippling procedures. If the proximal nerve is available and the remaining part of the muscle is large enough, direct muscular neurotization can provide very satisfying results.

REFERENCES

1. Heineke D. Die directs Einflanzung des Nerfs in den Muskel. Zentralb Chir 1914;41:465.
2. Erlacher P. Ueber die motorischen nervendigungen. Z Orthop Chir 1914;34:561.
3. Steindler A. The method of direct neurotisation of paralysed muscles. Am J Orthop Surg 1915;13:33.
4. Elsberg CA. Experiments on motor nerve regeneration and the direct neurotisation of paralysed muscles by their own and by foreign nerves. Science 1917;45:318.
5. Aitken JT. Growth of nerve implants in voluntary muscle. J Anat 1950;84:38.

6. Guth L, Zalewski AA. Disposition of colinesterase following implantion of nerve into denervate muscle. Exp Neurol 1963;7:316.
7. Katz B, Miledi R. The development of acetylcholine sensitivity in nerve free segments of skeletal muscle. J Physiol 1964;170:389.
8. Brunelli G, Monini L, Antonucci A, et al. Neurotizzazione in zona aneurale di muscoli denervati. Il Policlinico 1976;83:611–6. (Presented at first meeting of the Society of Research in Surgery, Rome, 1975.)
9. Brunelli G. Direct neurotisation of severely damaged and denervated muscles. In: Freilinger GA, et al., eds., Muscle Transplantation. New York: Springer Verlag, 1981:283–6.
10. Sakellarides HT, Sorbie C, James L. Reinnervation of denervated muscles by nerve transplantation. Clin Orthop 1972;83:194–9.
11. Brunelli G, Monini L. Direct muscular neurotisation. J Hand Surg 1985;10:993–7.
12. Brunelli GA. Direct neurotisation of severely damaged muscles. J Hand Surg 1982;7:572.
13. Brunelli G, Monini L, Brunelli F. Direct muscular neurotisation. Ann Chir Main 1990;9:290.
14. Brunelli G. Direct muscular neurotisation. In: Gelbermann RH, ed., Operative Nerve Repair and Reconstruction. Philadelphia: Lippincott, 1991:783–91.
15. Brunelli GA, Brunelli GR. Direct muscle neurotisation. J Reconstr Microsurg 1993;9:81.
16. Brunelli GA, Brunelli GR. Direct muscular neurotisation. In: Hunter LH, Schneider EJ, Mackin E, eds., Tendon and Nerve Surgery in the Hand. Philadelphia: Mosby, 1997:221–5.

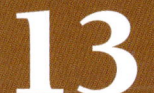

Nerve Repair in Upper Extremity Replantation and Toe-to-Hand Transfers

Sean M. Bidic and Neil F. Jones

INTRODUCTION

The purpose of this chapter is to provide a practical guide to nerve repairs in upper extremity replantation and toe-to-hand transfers. A review of the anatomy, physiology, techniques, and outcomes relevant to the nerve repairs in these related reconstructive procedures is presented. Although the anatomic, physiologic, and technical repair aspects of replants and toe transfers are similar, the outcomes reporting is understandably divergent in the literature.

Upper extremity replantation after a traumatic amputation can be done at any level from the fingertip to the glenohumeral joint. The nature of the injury may be sharp, crushing, or an avulsion. The patient's age and mechanism of injury (two surgeon-independent factors) are major determinants of sensory (and motor) recovery success. Other factors pertinent to successful nerve regeneration to the target organ include repair delays, employment of nerve grafts/conduits, and smoking history. Toe transfers are performed for two main indications: (1) for traumatic thumb and finger amputations that cannot be replanted due to the nature of the initial insult, prolonged ischemia time, or a failed replantation attempt; and (2) for congenital anomalies in which thumb or opposable fingers are absent.

With advances in nerve repair techniques, microscopic magnification, and the recognition of conditions unfavorable to nerve repair—functional recovery has become expected.[1,2] As reconstructive hand surgeons we must remember that a well-perfused replant or toe transfer alone is not a success since the ultimate goal includes a sensate, pain-free digit. For this reason, attention to nerve repair is critical.

ANATOMY AND PHYSIOLOGY

At the proximal stump, axons degenerate back to the most distal node of Ranvier *not involved with the injury*. Therefore, in a toe-to-hand transfer for a congenital malformation, minimal proximal nerve preparation is necessary, but for a replant following a Skilsaw accident, the degeneration begins at a site *just proximal to the zone of injury*, not at the site just proximal to the laceration.

Knowledge of finger/thumb and toe nerve anatomy is important for expectation of sensibility following toe transfers. Palmar digital nerves have three to four times as many axons as do plantar digital nerves.[3]

A physiologic concept central to toe transfers is that of central nervous system adaptation of the transferred toe. Transfers for traumatic losses require only that the neo-finger/thumb regain the previous cortical representation once held by the lost digit. Congenitally absent digits are unlikely to have cortical representation, but central reorganization may be stimulated by a toe transfer.[4] Older children, with more established functions, will unlikely incorporate the neo-digit into spontaneous use.[5]

TIMING OF NERVE REPAIR

Repairs that take place within 7 days of the injury when the proximal and distal stumps of a transected nerve are coapted are called primary nerve repairs. The two ends of the injured nerve should be reapproximated without tension in a well-vascularized bed of surrounding soft tissue. Primary nerve repairs are preferred for replantation after sharp amputations.

A secondary nerve repair is undertaken when the two ends of the injured nerve are repaired later than 7 days after the injury either with an end-to-end repair or with nerve grafting. Nerve repairs for replants and toe transfers fall into this category only when a large zone of injury exists or the tension of an end-to-end repair cannot be alleviated by bone shortening.

INDICATIONS

The patient and family should be told that complete sensory (or motor) recovery is not expected, and that the goal is a sensate, pain-free distal segment (with less than 100% motor recovery if a motor nerve is involved). The ideal candidate for nerve repair in either a replant or post-traumatic toe transfer scenario is a young non-smoker with a sharp transection and without a soft tissue crush/avulsion component. The likelihood of a successful nerve repair is also increased by performing the definitive (primary/graft/conduit) repair sooner rather than later, once the surrounding soft tissue bed has achieved a healing equilibrium. Protective sensory recovery (i.e., static two-point discrimination [S2PD] <15 mm) has been noted to occur years after a definitive repair,[4] but motor recovery decreases with each day of delay due to continuous decrease in motor end plate density. The regenerating axons advance approximately 1 mm per day or 1 inch per month. For motor nerve injuries, the surgeon should be aware that motor end-plate density decreases approximately 1% to 2% per week. Experimentally, this decrease can be limited by intramuscular electrical stimulation. The goal is to get the regenerating axon to the motor end plates before they have disappeared. This occurs between 1 and 2 years, and equates to a laceration to target distance of 12 to 24 inches (if repaired on the day of injury).

TECHNIQUES OF NERVE REPAIR

For nerve preparation and definitive repair—three instrumentation components are required: (1) a set of microsurgery instruments (needle driver, jeweler's forceps, straight adventitia scissors, and curved dissecting scissors); (2) an operative microscope or loupe magnification of greater than 4.5; and (3) nonabsorbable suture ranging from 8-0 to 10-0. A BV-100 needle is preferred for its acute needle arc.

Nerve repairs in replants and toe transfers involve two types of end-to-end repairs (epineurial and group fascicular), end-to-side repairs, interpositional nerve grafting, and nerve conduits (both vein and synthetic).

Epineurial Repair

The goal of this technique is to coapt the epineurium while not capturing any nerve substance. The nerve ends should meet without tension, herniation or misalignment of any nerve fascicles. For a digital nerve in digital replantation or toe transfers, three to four simple 10-0 nylon sutures are usually adequate.

Group Fascicular Repair

This technique is used when a distinct group of fascicles can be identified and where fascicular crossover is not known to occur (the median and ulnar nerves in the distal forearm or the radial nerve at the elbow). After identification and matching, the internal epineurium surrounding each group fascicle is coapted using 9-0 or 10-0 sutures. Group fascicular repair is used in replantation at the wrist and distal forearm level.

An intraoperative group fascicular matching technique can be performed using a nerve stimulator. After dissection of the group fascicles in the proximal and distal nerve stumps, the tourniquet should be let down for approximately 20 minutes to reverse any nerve ischemia and the patient awakened. Then the nerve stimulator producing a stimulus of 0.2 to 0.5 mA is delivered first to the proximal group fascicles. Stimulating a sensory group fascicle will produce the perception of a localized hand sensation, while stimulation of a motor group fascicle will produce no response or a vague pain. A stimulus delivered to a distal motor group fascicle will produce contraction of intrinsic hand muscles, but only in the first several days after injury.

Identification of motor and sensory group fascicles has also been reported using special staining techniques for carbonic anhydrase and acetyl cholinesterase, but this method is not usually amenable for traumatic amputations.

Individual Fascicular Repair

Multiple individual fascicles are identified and coapted using sutures in their perineurial sheaths. This technique is not used in replantation or toe transfers (Fig. 13–1).

Interpositional Nerve Grafts

For digital nerves, grafts can be harvested from the posterior interosseous nerve in the distal forearm.[6] For larger nerve grafts, the sural nerve is preferred. The graft length should be determined such that tension does not occur at the maximal extended position. A tension-free epineurial repair should be performed for digital nerves. More proximally, the nerve grafts should be interposed and coapted to corresponding group fascicles. Interpositional nerve grafts are typically used secondarily in replantation when primary end-to-end repair would produce too much tension on the nerve repair, or in toe transfers when the recipient nerve is too proximal to

allow end-to-end repair to the digital nerves in the toe transfer. Occasionally, nerve grafts can be performed primarily in replantation..

Cable grafts are no longer performed because revascularization of the internal portion of the graft is delayed and will likely result in a poorly functional graft secondary to prolonged ischemia.[6] Vascularized nerve grafts have been described, but they have not been shown to significantly improve motor or sensory function.[6] A possible indication for a vascularized nerve graft would be secondary reconstruction after forearm or wrist replantation with an extensively scarred bed or a previously failed conventional sural nerve graft.

End–to–Side Repairs

This technique should only be used clinically if the options of end-to-end nerve repair or nerve grafting are not available. End-to-side nerve repairs are useful in toe transfers when the number or size of the toe donor nerves is greater than the recipient hand nerves. Neurotropic factors from Schwann cells, denervated muscle, or nerve stumps stimulate intact axons to sprout collateral branches that advance distally to reinnervate a target organ.[7] Performing an epineurial window at the site of an end-to-side repair will increase axonal counts traversing the repair[8] (Fig. 13–2).

Autologous Venous Nerve Conduits or Synthetic Nerve Conduits

Vein grafts or synthetic bioabsorbable polyglycolic tubes have been described to bridge sensory nerve gaps of up to 3 cm in length in an end-to-end fashion. They may be considered in replantation and toe transfers to obviate the harvest of a sural nerve graft.[9]

NERVE REPAIR IN REPLANTATION

Shortening the bone cannot be overstressed. For finger replants, 0.5- to 1-cm bone shortening with an oscillating saw usually from the distal segment (to permit as much length as possible in case of replant failure) should be considered. This degree of shortening will often permit nerve (and blood vessel) overlap, thereby allowing a tension-free repair. Shortening may entail the sacrifice of an interphalangeal or metacarpophalangeal joint, especially in the thumb. Loss of a joint will be better tolerated than an insensate, cold intolerant, or painful digit. For more proximal replants, shortening the radius, ulna, or humerus up to 5 cm is well tolerated. Inherent anatomical features on the nerve stumps will aid in proper alignment for epineurial repairs. Occasionally a vasa nervorum can be identified on each nerve stump to allow the proper alignment.

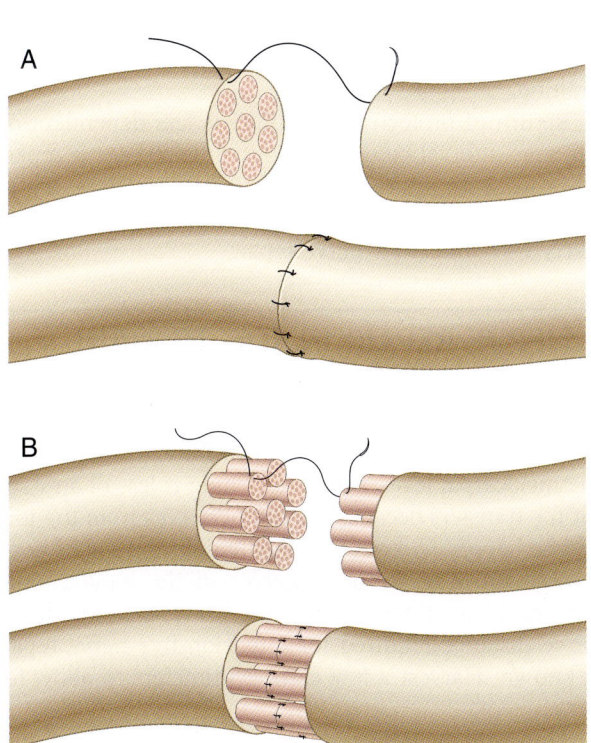

Figure 13–1   Various techniques of primary nerve repair. **A:** Epineurial repair. **B:** Group fascicular repair.

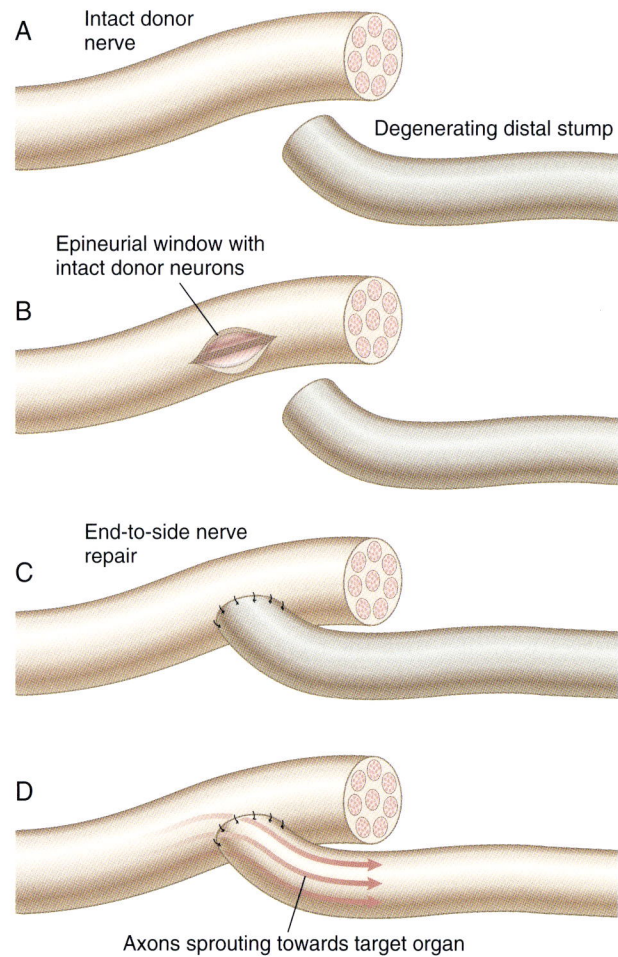

A   Intact donor nerve

                       Degenerating distal stump

B   Epineurial window with intact donor neurons

C   End-to-side nerve repair

D

Axons sprouting towards target organ

Figure 13–2 Axonal regeneration following end-to-side nerve repair.

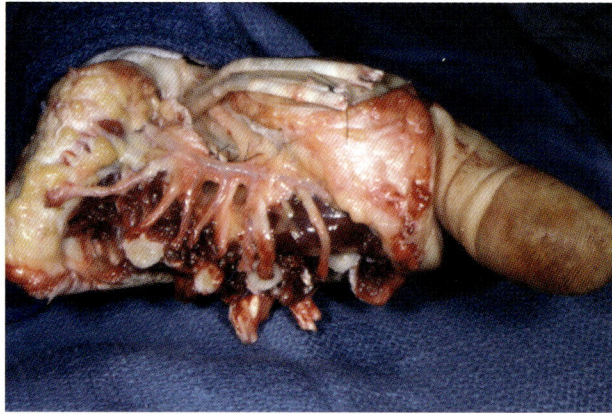

Figure 13–3 Dissection of the common digital nerves during trans-metacarpal amputation of the left hand.

Replantation at the mid-carpal level and in the fingers usually involves a tension-free epineurial repair (Fig. 13–3). A sensory nerve gap of less than 3 cm can be bridged by a vein or synthetic conduit.[9] For nerve repairs in replants distal to the thumb interphalangeal joint or distal interphalangeal joint in the fingers, direct neurotization can be considered.[10]

For major limb replants at the level of the wrist or distal forearm, a group fascicular repair of the median and ulnar nerves is often feasible (Fig. 13–4). The topography of the median nerve is such that with the hand supine, the motor fascicles are situated at the 6 o'clock position, while in the ulnar nerve, the motor fascicles are situated at the 12 o'clock position. Motor recovery is more likely when the delay in nerve repair is less than 6 months due to a progressive loss of the motor end plates over time. A chance of some motor recovery exists for up to 2 years.

Digital nerve repair and median and ulnar nerve repair at the wrist must be tension free, otherwise conduits or secondary nerve grafting should be considered.

For sensory nerves, if a gap of up to 3 cm exists between the nerve ends, the immediate use of a vein or synthetic conduit should be considered.[11] If a gap of greater than 3 cm exists, the nerve ends should be tagged with a non-absorbable suture and a secondary nerve graft should be employed once the soft tissues have healed. A 3-month interval is often sufficient. Motor nerves should be repaired with nerve grafts and not conduits if a tension-free primary repair cannot be achieved, but motor function may be restored by more guaranteed techniques such as tendon transfers.

If the patient has not regained the expected sensory recovery by 6 months after repair, and no advancing Tinel sign exists, the patient should be considered for re-exploration, resection of the neuroma, and nerve grafting.

Return of protective sensibility is less dependent on the time interval between amputation and nerve repair, and can occur with a nerve repair years after the initial injury. However, a more favorable sensory recovery is likely with an earlier nerve repair.

NERVE REPAIR IN TOE–TO–HAND TRANSFERS

The bone of a toe transfer is often fixed to the hand at the metacarpal level. Bone shortening is less of an issue for toe transfers because the donor nerves from the foot can be harvested more proximally than the site of bony transection. The recipient nerves in the hand should have been identified prior to toe harvest, so the donor nerve distance required for a tension-free nerve repair is known. Harvest a few extra centimeters to allow for nerve recoil.

The distal digital nerves, and the distal median, ulnar, and superficial radial nerves provide the recipient nerves in the hand. The nerves in the donor toe are

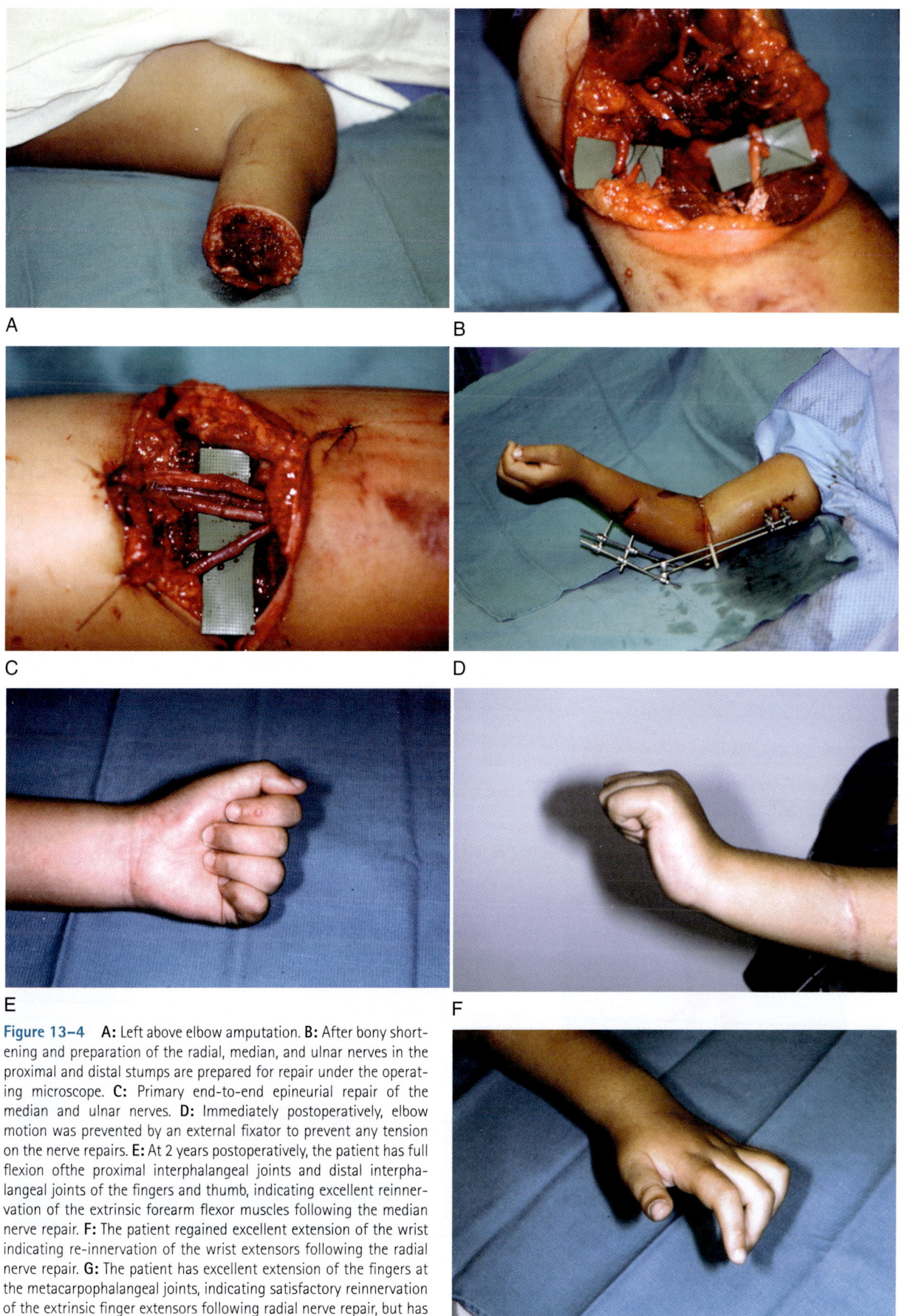

Figure 13–4 **A:** Left above elbow amputation. **B:** After bony short-ening and preparation of the radial, median, and ulnar nerves in the proximal and distal stumps are prepared for repair under the operat-ing microscope. **C:** Primary end-to-end epineurial repair of the median and ulnar nerves. **D:** Immediately postoperatively, elbow motion was prevented by an external fixator to prevent any tension on the nerve repairs. **E:** At 2 years postoperatively, the patient has full flexion of the proximal interphalangeal joints and distal interpha-langeal joints of the fingers and thumb, indicating excellent reinner-vation of the extrinsic forearm flexor muscles following the median nerve repair. **F:** The patient regained excellent extension of the wrist indicating re-innervation of the wrist extensors following the radial nerve repair. **G:** The patient has excellent extension of the fingers at the metacarpophalangeal joints, indicating satisfactory reinnervation of the extrinsic finger extensors following radial nerve repair, but has slight clawing of the fingers at the pip joints due to less than optimal reinnervation of the extrinsic.

always the medial and lateral digital nerves (Fig. 13–5), and occasionally the deep peroneal nerve. The medial and lateral digital nerves of the donor toe should be dissected as far proximally as possible, if necessary, dissecting the common digital nerve to the great toe–second toe web space using microscissors to achieve as long a length as possible for the two donor nerves. In optimal circumstances, especially in post-traumatic toe transfers, the medial and lateral digital nerves of the toe are repaired end to end to the radial and ulnar digital nerves in the thumb or finger stump. Occasionally, in post-traumatic toe transfers and especially in congenital toe transfers, the recipient nerves are the more proximal segments of the common digital nerves originating from the median and ulnar nerves, and the intervening distance has to be reconstructed with an interpositional nerve graft. Sural nerve grafts may be harvested from the ipsilateral leg, but more frequently we utilize segments of the deep or superficial peroneal nerves from the toe dissection as interpositional nerve grafts (Fig. 13–6). Occasionally in congenital toe transfers, the superficial radial nerve may be more developed than the median or ulnar nerve, and one of the medial or lateral digital nerves of the toe transfer can be coapted to the superficial branch of the radial nerve. Finally, the medial and lateral digital nerves of the toe transfer may be much larger than any of the recipient nerves in a congenital hand anomaly; in these circumstances, one toe digital nerve is repaired end-to-end to a common digital nerve or the median or ulnar nerve. Subsequently, the other toe digital nerve is sutured end-to-side to the previously repaired toe digital nerve. Vein or synthetic conduits can be used in post-traumatic or congenital toe transfers, but nerve grafts are preferred.

RESULTS OF NERVE REPAIR AFTER REPLANTATION AND TOE TRANSFERS

A universally accepted standard for reporting the return of sensibility or motor function following nerve repairs does not exist in the literature. The British Medical Research Council classification, Mackinnon and Dellon's modifications for sensibility grades,[12,13] and Highet and Sanders' modifications for motor grades[9] provide criteria in which some interobserver variability exists (Table 13–1).

SENSORY RECOVERY AFTER REPLANTATION

Tamai[16] reviewed his large series of 293 upper extremity replantations over a 22-year period. An epineuroperineurial suture was utilized for nerve repair. An

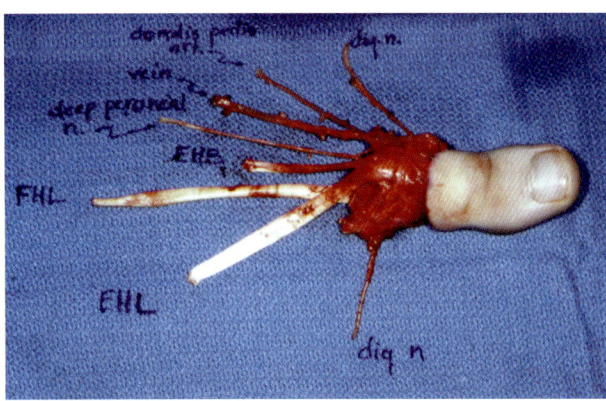

A

B

Figure 13–5   Dissection of a great toe transfer **(A)** and a trimmed toe transfer **(B),** illustrating the medial and lateral digital nerves.

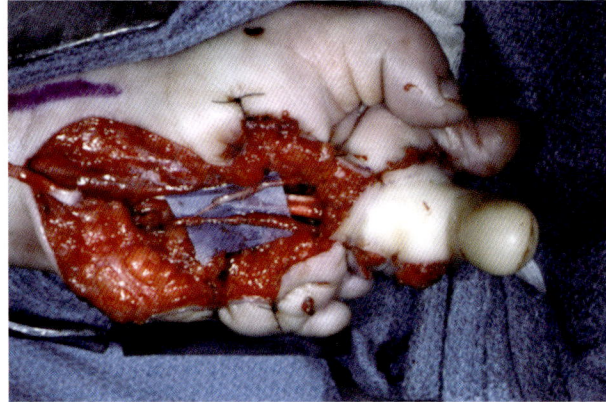

Figure 13–6   Second toe transfer for a congenital failure of formation of the digits. The medial and lateral digital nerves of the second toe transfer were extended with interposition nerve grafts from the superficial peroneal nerve at the level of the wrist.

TABLE 13–1

Sensibility Grading

S0	No sensory recovery
S1	Recovery of deep cutaneous pain sensibility
S2	Recovery of superficial cutaneous pain sensibility
S2+	As in S2, but with over-response
S3	Recovery of pain and touch sensibility with disappearance of over-response Two-point discrimination >15 mm
S3+	As in S3, but localization of the stimulus is good Two-point discrimination 7–15 mm
S4	Complete recovery Two-point discrimination 2–6 mm

Note: British Medical Research Council classification with MacKinnon and Dellon's modification delineating correlation with static two-point discrimination.

elaborate grading system, incorporating the BMRC criteria, to evaluate functional recovery was described. An S2PD of less than 15 mm was documented in 70% of digital replants, but sensory recovery of major (forearm and upper arm) replants was poor. The best motor functional recovery occurred after replantation of the distal half of the forearm. The worst results were seen in the proximal third of the forearm where the motor nerves entered the extrinsic muscles of the hand (Fig. 13–2).

Lister et al.[15] reviewed the functional recovery of 347 upper and lower extremity replants in 245 patients. In this inclusive study, the only comment regarding recovery of sensibility was that "60% of all patients had 2PD of 15 mm."

Chiu et al.[5] performed a multivariate analysis on their series of 169 digital replants (including some revascularization procedures) at the middle and proximal phalangeal level. Using Tamai's functional recovery scale,[16] age, mechanism of injury, level of injury, and rehabilitation protocols were evaluated to determine whether these factors had any significant influence on sensory recovery. Younger patients with more distal amputations had significantly better sensory recovery. Whether a patient followed a rehabilitation protocol and the type of amputation (sharp vs. crush) did not significantly affect the sensory recovery. Sensory reeducation was not part of the rehabilitation protocol and the authors commented that this might have a beneficial effect on sensory recovery.

Cheng et al.[7] performed a long-term follow-up study of 43 pediatric digital replants. The vast majority were sharp amputations. Eight-eight percent recovered S4, 9% recovered S3+, and one patient recovered S3 sensation.

May et al.[18] evaluated 35 replanted digits to investigate which factors most contributed to full sensory return. They found a significant correlation between return of sensation and digital vascularity. A

pulse pressure (a function of both arterial inflow and venous outflow) of greater than 85% of normal correlated with a return of S2PD of less than 8 mm, whereas a pulse pressure of less than 70% of normal correlated with a S2PD of greater than 15 mm. Sharp distal amputations in younger patients all contributed to improved return of sensation. Cold intolerance was experienced by all patients and was directly related to the restoration of normal vascularity.

Glickman and Mackinnon[8] performed a meta-analysis of 12 series, incorporating 367 finger replants and 87 thumb replants over a 12-year period. The mean S2PD in sharp thumb replants was 9.3 mm versus 12.1 mm in crush/avulsion thumb replants. The mean S2PD in sharp finger replants was 8 mm versus 15 mm in crush/avulsion finger replants. Sixty-one percent of thumb replants and 54% of finger replants regained a useful S2PD of less than 15 mm or S3+ or more. Factors that improved return of sensibility included a younger age, distal level of amputation, sharp mechanism of amputation, and postoperative sensory re-education protocol. Cold intolerance was a significant problem, with 80% of replanted digits experiencing moderate to severe cold intolerance. Although none of the series in this meta-analysis utilized a distinct sensory re-education program, the authors stressed the importance of this modality to enhance and hasten sensory recovery after digital replantation.[20] At the time of this report, there were no publications in the literature proving the beneficial effects of sensory reeducation after replantation.

Shieh et al.[6] evaluated the effectiveness of sensory reeducation following digital replantation. Patients in the group receiving sensory re-education achieved significantly improved moving two-point discrimination and Semmes-Weinstein thresholds when compared to controls.

Chu[22] analyzed 14 adult patients after digital replantation by clinical sensory testing and somatosensory evoked potential (SSEP). Patients showed a hypersensitivity to cold, with near-complete recovery of pinprick, touch, and heat sensations. Vibration and two-point discrimination were impaired, with an average S2PD of 8.6 mm for replanted digits compared with 3.0 mm for a normal finger. The SSEP conduction times were normal in 50% of patients. More severe and proximal injuries correlated with a worse sensory recovery and prolonged SSEP latency.

SENSORY RECOVERY IN TOE-TO-HAND TRANSFERS

Yu-dong et al.[14] evaluated the functional recovery of 300 toe transfers. A total of 296 transfers were for traumatic reconstructions, 4 for congenital anomalies, and 248 for thumb reconstruction. This report does not mention a standard technique for nerve repair, but stressed the importance of utilizing the median and ulnar nerves as recipient nerves in the hand. After 5 years, 236 of 240 toe transfers had S3 or better sensation and 216 had S2PD of less than 10mm. An important finding from this study was that sensory recovery improved progressively and substantially over a 2-year period.

Lister et al.[15] reviewed 54 toe transfers, including 51 for traumatic reconstruction and 3 for congenital reconstruction. They stressed the importance of performing the nerve repair as far distal on the recipient hand nerve as possible so that the regeneration distance to the transferred sensory end organs was as short as possible. Static touch was not appreciated in any patient until 9 months, but only 38 patients in this cohort were followed for 9 months or longer. Of those followed for over 2 years, 9 of 12 had S2PD of less than 10mm, and of those followed between 9 and 24 months, only 6 of 16 had S2PD of less than 10 mm.

Wei and Ma[24] demonstrated a significant improvement in static and moving two-point discrimination in 13 patients with 22 toe-to-hand transfers when a delayed, at-home sensory re-education protocol was employed. The protocol was initiated at a mean of 38 months after the toe transfer and lasted approximately 3.3 months. Each of the 22 toe transfers improved sensibility by an average of 7mm in static, and 6mm in moving, two-point discrimination.

Rowan[25] examined the effect of sensory re-education in 30 toe transfers after traumatic amputations. This study divided the cohort into those with sharp, distal amputations, and those with severe scarring. The re-education process included an early phase starting at 3 to 6 weeks postoperatively, which incorporated light touch and vibratory stimuli. Once sensation to the transplanted tip was definite, the second stage—training for tactile gnosis—began. For sharp injuries, utilizing the re-education protocol hastened and improved the final good results for both study patients and controls. For severely scarred injuries, sensory recovery did not proceed as fast as that in the sharp injury group, but those patients utilizing the re-education protocol had a much faster and much improved sensory recovery. This study therefore argues that a better-than-normal toe sensory recovery can be achieved with a formal sensory re-education protocol.

Chu[22] evaluated the recovery of sensation and SSEPs after toe transfers in adults following traumatic amputations. The average delay between amputation and toe transfer was 7 months. The order of return of sensibility was temperature, pinprick, touch, vibration, and S2PD. The overall sensory recovery of the transferred toes was more like normal toes than normal fingers. This should be expected because of the decreased axonal density and sensory end organs in the toe when compared to the finger or thumb. The S2PD of a normal finger was 2.9mm, 6.2mm for a normal toe, and 9.1 for a transferred toe. The SSEP data suggested that performing toe transfers within 1 month after the injury was critical in preventing proximal (median) nerve amplitude reduction and digital nerve latency prolongation.

There is a paucity of studies reviewing the return of sensation following toe transfers for reconstruction of congenital anomalies in the current literature.

COMPARISON OF SENSORY RECOVERY AFTER REPLANTATION AND AFTER TOE-TO-HAND TRANSFERS

Dellon[26] reviewed the sensory recovery in replants and toe transfers in a mixed adult and pediatric population. Five factors affected sensory recovery: (1) age of the patient at the time of repair; (2) the level of injury (proximal versus distal); (3) the mechanism of injury (sharp versus crush/avulsion); (4) sensory re-education; and (5) digital anesthetic block at the time of final evaluation. Younger patients with sharp distal nerve repairs who had sensory re-education postoperatively[13] and a digital nerve block of the adjacent uninjured digital nerves during testing, had an improved reported sensory outcome. The ischemia time of the amputated segment or the transferred toe did not seem to alter sensibility recovery.

Ahean et al.[17] compared the sensory recovery between 13 adult patients with 22 replanted digits, and 12 adults and adolescents with 14 post-traumatic toe transfers. Electrophysiologic, ninhydrin, and clinical testing 2 years or longer after nerve repair revealed that replanted digits had a better overall sensory recovery when compared to toe transfers. The authors noted that the traumatic finger or thumb injuries preceding the toe transfers were devastating and included electrical, thermal and explosive injuries. Toe transfers for congenital anomalies were not included in this study.

Chu et al.[9] performed a conduction study of digital nerve functional recovery comparing toe transfers for traumatic injuries and digital replants. Nerve action potentials (NAPs) of replanted digits measured between 2 and 3 years postoperatively were similar to normal digits, but NAPs of the toe transfers showed reduced amplitude, prolonged latency, and slowed conduction velocity. This suggests that digital nerve functional recovery is worse after toe transfers and better after replantation. The authors speculated that the more severe injuries sustained in the toe transfer group, delays in nerve repair, retrograde injury to the median nerve (sustained after 1 month without repair), mismatch in size between donor and recipient nerves, and discrepancies in receptor density between recipient fingers and donor toes all contributed to the poorer recovery of NAPs in the toe transfer group. In a later study, Chu[27] compared the recovery of sympathetic skin responses in digital replants and toe transfers after traumatic injury. After digital replantation, comparison of the sympathetic skin responses between the replanted and contralateral normal digit were almost identical. In contrast, the sympathetic responses of the toe transfers showed prolonged latency and reduced amplitude.

CONCLUSIONS

For digital replants and transmetacarpal replantation, bone shortening should allow primary end-to-end epineurial repair of the proper digital nerves and common digital nerves without tension. For nerve gaps between 0.5 and 3 cm, vein conduits or synthetic conduits may occasionally be used in an acute replantation. Interposition nerve grafts performed either acutely or secondarily are more appropriate for sensory nerve grafts greater than 3 cm. For replants at the level of the wrist or distal forearm, primary repair of the median and ulnar nerves is performed using a group fascicular technique without tension. If a nerve gap still exists after bony shortening, the proximal and distal nerve stumps should probably be tagged, and group fascicular nerve grafting performed secondarily. For replants proximal to the distal forearm, bony shortening of the humerus and radius and ulna should allow primary nerve repair using an epineurial technique. Sensory recovery after replantation is better after a sharp transection compared with a crush or avulsion injury, in younger patients and in nonsmokers.

In toe-to-hand transfers, the medial and lateral digital nerves of the donor toe should be harvested as far proximally as possible to obviate the need for nerve grafting. If there is still an intervening defect between the recipient nerve and the digital nerves of the toe transfer, then the nerve gap can be reconstructed either using a vein conduit, a synthetic conduit, an immediate interpositional nerve graft harvested from the superficial or deep peroneal nerves, or occasionally, by end-to-side repair of one of the toe digital nerves to the other toe digital nerve. The axonal density and sensory end organs in a donor toe are less than in a finger or a thumb; therefore, the sensory recovery in a toe-to-hand transfer is closer to that of an uninjured toe rather than an uninjured digit. Return of sensation after toe-to-hand transfers for congenital anomalies should be expected to be better than toe-to-hand transfers for traumatic amputations due to the younger age of the patients and the wider zone of injury and the delay between amputation

and secondary nerve reconstruction, but such a comparison study has not been published.

All patients undergoing replantation or toe-to-hand transfers should be enrolled in a postoperative protocol of sensory re-education. Patients should be informed that cold intolerance is common following replantation and toe transfers. If return of sensation and muscle re-innervation is not seen or is less than optimal after the usual calculated interval for nerve regeneration has elapsed (1 mm per day or 1 inch per month), or if the patient complains of a painful neuroma at the site of the nerve repair, then re-exploration of the previous nerve repair, excision of the neuroma, and nerve grafting should be considered.

REFERENCES

1. Allan CH. Functional results of primary nerve repair. Hand Clin 2000;16:67–72.
2. Bunke RF, Bunke HJ, Kind GM, et al. The harvest and clinical application of the superficial peroneal sensory nerve for grafting motor and sensory nerve defects. Plast Reconstr Surg 2002; 109:145–51.
3. Millesi H. Techniques of nerve grafting. Hand Clin 2000;16:73–91.
4. Wei FC, El-Gammal TA, Chen HC, et al. Toe-to-hand transfer for traumatic digital amputations in children and adolescents. 1997;100:605–9.
5. Chiu HY, Shieh SJ, Hsu HY. Multivariate analysis of factors influencing the functional recovery after finger replantation or revascularization. Microsurgery 1995;16:713–7.
6. Shieh SJ, Chiu HY, Lee JW, et al. Evaluation of the effectiveness of sensory reeducation following digital replantation and revascularization. Microsurgery 1995;16:578–82.
7. Cheng GL, Pan DD, Zhang NP, et al. Digital replantation in children: a long-term follow-up study. J Hand Surg Am 1998; 23:635–46.
8. Glickman LT, Mackinnon SE. Sensory recovery following digital replantation. Microsurgery 1990;11:236–42.
9. Chu NS, Chuy EC, Yu JM. Conduction study of digital nerve function recovery following toe-to-digit transplantation and a comparison with digit-to-digit replantation. Muscle Nerve 1995; 18:1257–64.
10. MacKinnon SE, Dellon AL. Surgery of the Peripheral Nerve. New York: Thieme Medical Publishers, 1988.
11. Stephane F, Aymetic L, Dautel G, et al. Adjacent and spontaneous neurotization after distal digital replantation in children. 2003; 111:159–65.
12. MacKinnon SE, Dellon AL. Clinical nerve reconstruction with a bioabsorbable polyglycolic acid tube. Plast Reconstr Surg 1990: 85;419–24.
13. Dellon AL. Evaluation of Sensation and Re-education of Sensation in the Hand. Baltimore: Williams & Wilkins, 1981.
14. Yu-dong G, Gao-meng Z, De-shong C, et al. Great toe transfer for the thumb and finger reconstruction in 300 cases. Plast Reconstr Surg 1993;91:693–700.
15. Lister G, Kalisman M, Tsai TM. Reconstruction of the hand with free microneurovascular toe-to-hand transfers: experience within 54 toe transfers. Plast Reconst Surg 1983:372–84.
16. Tamai S. Twenty years' experience of limb replantation—review of 293 upper extremity replants. J Hand Surg Am 1982;549–56.
17. Ahean U, Arnez ZM, Janko M, et al. Regeneration of sudomotor and sensory nerve fibers after digital replantation and microneurovascular toe to hand transfer. Br J Plast Surg 1997:50;227–35.

18. May JW, Smith RJ, Peimer CA. Toe-to-hand free tissue transfer for thumb reconstruction with multiple digit aplasia. Plast Reconstr Surg 1981;67:205–13.

19. Chu N. Current perception thresholds in toe to digit transplantation and digit to digit replantation. Muscle Nerve 1996;19:183–6.

20. Romero-Zarate JL, Pastrana-Figueroa JM, Granados-Martinez R. Upper extremity replantation: three-year experience. Microsurgery 2000;20:202–6.

21. Gilbert A. Toe transfers for congenital hand defects. J Hand Surg Am 1982;7:118–24.

22. Chu NS. Recovery of finger sensibility and somatosensory evoked potentials following digit-to-digit replantation in man. Scand J Rehab Med 1996;28:125–31.

23. Stephane F, Aymetic L, Dautel G, et al. Adjacent and spontaneous neurotization after distal digital replantation in children. 2003;111:159–65.

24. Wei FC, Ma HS. Delayed sensory reeducation after toe-to-hand transfer. Microsurgery 1995;16:583–5.

25. Rowan PR, Long-En C, Urbaniak JR. End-to-side nerve repair. Hand Clin 2000;16:151–9.

26. Dellon AL. Sensory recovery in replanted digits and transplanted toes: a review. J Reconstr Microsurg 1986;2:123–9.

27. Chu NS. Recovery of sympathetic skin responses after digit to digit replantation and toe to digit replantation in human. Ann Neurol 1996;40:67–74.

14 Muscle–Tendon Transfers for Traumatic Nerve Injuries

George E. Omer, Jr.

INTRODUCTION

Reconstructive procedures after peripheral nerve injuries include skeletal stabilization, muscle–tendon transfers, and redistribution of sensibility. Motor reconstruction should be done before sensory reconstruction because precise sensibility depends on precise muscle control as well as appropriate sensory end organs. The result should be a limited, but balanced, functional performance done by redistributing assets rather than creating new ones, except in circumstances where it is possible to perform a free functional muscle transfer by microvascular means.

PATIENT EVALUATION

Tissue equilibrium, or homeostasis, should be regained before tendon transfers are performed. Chronic wounds are contraindications to elective surgery. Soft tissues should be free of scar contractures. There should be stable skeletal alignment. Tendon transfers across a bony nonunion fail because the telescoping skeleton prevents adequate tension for functional muscle power. Joints should have normal motion and the functional motion expected after surgery should be demonstrated passively before surgery. However, it is rare for return of good muscle strength two joints distal to the nerve injury.[1,2]

Muscle imbalance is usually static after traumatic injuries, and unusual functional loss may indicate additional progressive neuromuscular impairment. Following deep muscle laceration, intact nerves must regenerate across the site of injury, and distal tissue separated from the intramuscular nerve must be reinnervated in order to recover functional tension and shorten appropriately.[3] Even with reinnervation, the increased fibrotic tension from scar and shorter residual fiber length results in decreased total tension and diminished function of the involved muscle. One should not transfer muscles that have had even temporary total denervation, even if they later regain function.[4]

PREOPERATIVE REHABILITATION

Maintaining a mobile extremity without deforming contracture demands a planned and persistent rehabilitation program. The extremity is immobilized in a position to maintain the desired result. The functional performance expected after tendon transfer should be possible to effect by passive movement before surgery.

The timing of tendon transfers varies with the level and severity of the nerve injury. When a patient with a distal nerve laceration has had a precise nerve repair, the prognosis for reinnervation of the paralyzed muscles has improved over the past decade.[5–7] In these patients, selected tendon transfers may be performed early as internal splints to support partial function and prevent deformity while awaiting the potential nerve recovery.

More severe wounds are less predictable. A prospective study[1] was done of 648 nerve lesions of the upper extremity with the involved nerve demonstrated to be in continuity at the time the wound was debrided. Spontaneous recovery took 1 to 4 months for 85% of fracture-dislocations or crush injuries, and 3 to 9 months for 70% of gunshot wounds.

MOTOR MUSCLE SELECTION

In the normal forearm and hand, there are 50 muscles to activate movement. Normal amplitude approximates 33 mm for wrist movers, 70 mm for finger flexors, and 50 mm for finger extensors and the thumb extrinsic muscle tendons.[8] Although the excursion of a specific tendon cannot be increased, a muscle can be converted from monoarticular to multiarticular by effectively using the natural dynamic tenodesis effect. For example, when the flexor carpi ulnaris or the flexor carpi radialis is transferred to the extensor digitorum communis, it is converted to a multiarticular muscle, and the effective amplitude of the tendon transfer is significantly increased over the absolute amplitude of the muscle fibers by active volar flexion of the wrist, thereby allowing the transferred wrist flexor to fully extend the fingers.[9] A second technique to increase excursion is dissection of the muscle from its surrounding fascial attachments,[10] but this may bring unwelcome hemorrhage or denervation.

The motor muscle selected for transfer should be 4+ to 5 on the Highet scale, because it will have to pull itself free of the healing process after surgery and usually loses one grade of strength on Highet's clinical scale.[11] After reconstruction, the muscle selected for transfer should have work capacity equal to that of the antagonist muscle.[12] The present action of the selected motor muscle should be synergistic with the anticipated action, or be trainable by conscious control.[13] Paralyzed muscles that have regained function after nerve suture usually lack the individualized control and strength desirable for successful transfer.[14]

The amplitude of a muscle is the distance that it can be stretched from its resting position, plus the distance that it contracts from its resting position.[15,16] Stimulating the muscle after tendon transfer is an effective technique to evaluate the functional outcome of synergistic muscles.[17] If tissue homeostasis is good, tendon tension can be evaluated and determined at operation.[18] Tension is judged best while the extremity is placed in the position it will assume when the transferred tendon contracts. The motion expected after tendon transfer cannot exceed the passive motion that is present preoperatively. For extensor tendons, the resting tension should be strong enough to hold the extremity passively against gravity. However, one must be sure that the wrist has the potential for a normal arc of flexion. Flexor tendons often cross more than one joint and should be fixed at somewhat greater than normal tension against gravity.

Goldner (Goldner JL, personal communication, May 26, August 28, September 29, 2003) uses a practical technique to determine tension for the muscle–tendon unit. The extremity and the recipient tendon are positioned in functional position, and the tendon to be transferred is positioned in resting length. Traction is then applied to the tendon to be transferred, and the distance marked in the wound. Sixty percent of the distance between the resting and traction length is marked as the position of the transferred muscle when the final insertion is initiated. Cooney[19] also has reported an intraoperative technique to determine position for the tendon to be transferred. The distance that the muscle to be transferred contracts after release from its normal insertion is measured. The lost length is restored at the time of transfer, plus slightly more tension to "pick up" the connective tissue elasticity within the muscle. The tourniquet is deflated when final tension is set for the transfer so that muscle ischemia does not contract the muscle to such a degree that the tension is too loose.

OPERATIVE TECHNIQUES

Incisions should be transverse to the subcutaneous path of the transferred tendon. The transferred tendon should not cross bare bone. Muscle–tendon units that must move through fascial planes, such as interosseous membrane, should have as large an opening in the fascia as practicable. The muscle should be drawn into the fascia window, because the exterior muscle fibers will "freeze," but the interior muscle fibers will retain motion. If the tendon is placed in the fascial window, it will bind fast and motion will be lost.[14]

An appropriate moment arm should be selected for the direction of muscle–tendon action.[15] Most muscles are parallel to bone, and the angle of approach between the transferred tendon and its new insertion should be small. The more distal to the axis of motion of a joint that the transfer is anchored, the more force the muscle can exert on the joint, but also the more excursion required of the tendon to provide a normal range of motion in the joint. If the insertion of a transferred tendon is split, the motor will act primarily on the slip under greater tension. A tendon transfer is more effective when it crosses only one joint. If a tendon "bowstrings" across a proximal joint, its mechanical advantage at that joint will be so great that it may force that joint into unwanted movement or use up all its amplitude so that it cannot move the distal joint. An example is the transfer of the brachioradialis muscle to the flexor pollicis longus: when the elbow and wrist are extended, the patient can hold an object tightly, but when the elbow is fully flexed the muscle power is dissipated at the elbow, and the patient drops the object.

Tendon fixation should result in minimal tissue reaction.[20] Suture material can be relatively large, such as 2-0 for forearm transfers. Some potential ischemia is prevented when the suture is inserted through the center of the tendon and then circles only one-half of the tendon; sutures along the length of the tendon should alternate the circle to be tied from side to side to further protect circulation. "Lacing" a transferred tendon into a group of paralyzed muscle–tendon units should be avoided because it creates bulk, twist, and scar, and increases friction; a precise insertion point should be selected. A second technique is leaving the recipient tendon in its bed, and passing the transferred tendon over it. This is an oblique transfer, and there should be a double line of nonabsorbable sutures to prevent shifting in the tension. A third technique would excise the paralyzed and fibrous muscle from the recipient tendon. However, excision of the muscle may result in hemorrhage and should not be done unless the fibrous muscle mass is causing deformity.

COMPLETE LESIONS OF INDIVIDUAL NERVES

Isolated Radial Palsy

The functional needs after radial palsy are (1) wrist extension (2) finger and thumb extension, and (3) thumb proximal stability.[21–23] (See Table 14–1 for abbreviations used in tendon transfer discussed in this chapter.) Preoperative management should maintain a full passive range of motion in all joints of the hand and wrist while preventing contractures such as the thumb–index web (Table 14–2).

TABLE 14–1

Abbreviations Used in Tendon Transfers

ADQ	Abductor digiti quinti
AP	Adductor pollicis
APB	Abductor pollicis brevis
APL	Abductor pollicis longus
BR	Brachioradialis
ECRB	Extensor carpi radialis brevis
ECRL	Extensor carpi radialis longus
ECU	Extensor carpi ulnaris
EDC	Extensor digitorum communis
EDM	Extensor digitorum minimi (quinti)
EIP	Extensor indicis proprius
EPB	Extensor pollicis brevis
EPL	Extensor pollicis longus
FCR	Flexor carpi radialis
FCU	Flexor carpi ulnaris
FDP	Flexor digitorum profundus
FDS	Flexor digitorum superficialis (sublimis)
FPL	Flexor pollicis longus
IP	Interphalangeal (PIP, proximal; DIP, distal)
MP	Metacarpophalangeal
PL	Palmaris longus
PT	Pronator teres

TABLE 14–2

Early Tendon Transfers as Internal Splints

Palsy	Functional Need	Available Motors
Low median	Thumb abduction (APB)	EIP to APB (and EPL) or EDM or PL or FDS (ring)
Radial	Wrist extension	PT to ECRB
Low ulnar	Thumb adduction, improve clawed fingers, improve metacarpal arch	FDS (long) with one-half tendon to AP, pulley of flexor sheath for flexion, or dorsal apparatus for extension

For wrist extension, a longitudinal incision is made over the radial aspect of the forearm, the PT is freed with a tongue of periosteum from the radius. The PT is bluntly freed and is passed subcutaneously over the BR and ECRL muscles to be attached only to the ECRB muscle–tendon junction. After surgery, the wrist should rest in 45 degrees of extension for 4 to 6 weeks (Fig. 14–1 A and B).

For digital extension, the oldest procedure uses the FCU[8] (Fig. 14–2 A to C). Through a longitudinal incision over the muscle, the FCU is freed from its fascial attachments. The limiting factor is the innervation that enters the proximal 5 cm of the muscle. A longitudinal incision is made over the dorsal surface of the forearm, and the FCU is directed subcutaneously around the

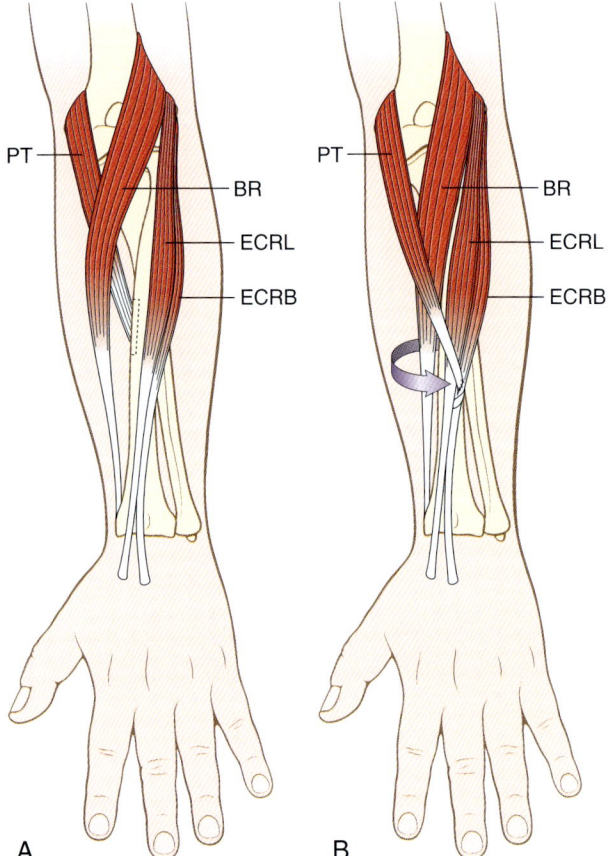

Figure 14–1   PT to ECRB transfer. **A:** The PT is freed with a tongue of periosteum from the radius *(dotted line)*. **B:** The PT is passed subcutaneously over the BR and ECRL muscles to be attached only to the ECRB muscle–tendon junction.

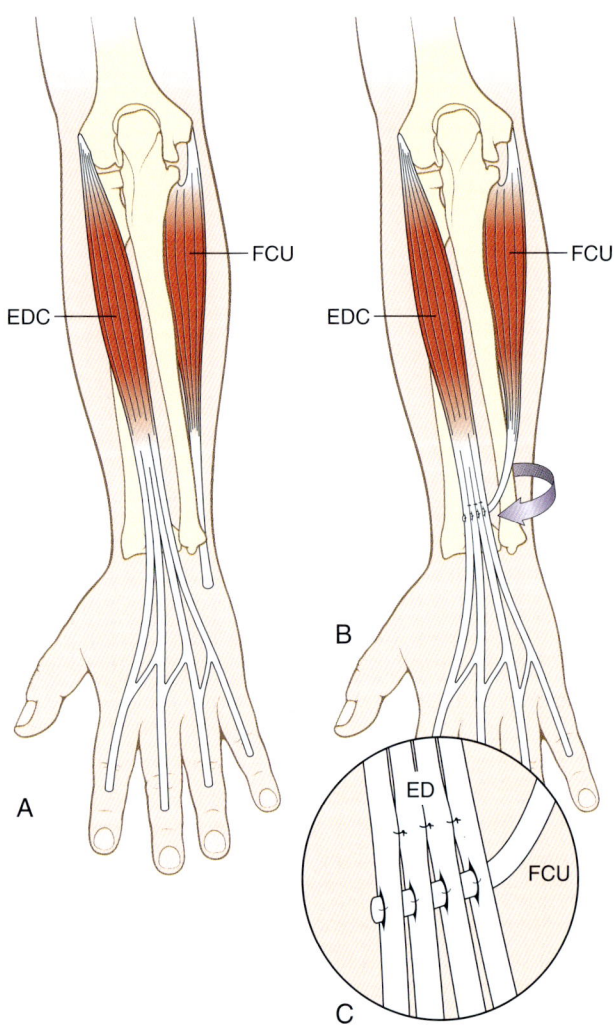

Figure 14–2   FCU to EDC transfer. **A:** The FCU is freed from its fascial attachments. **B:** The FCU is directed subcutaneously around the forearm, and superficial to the EDC tendons in their compartment. **C:** The transferred tendon is attached in an oblique line of sutures proximal to the dorsal retinaculum to each EDC tendon.

forearm and superficial to the EDC tendons in their compartment. The transferred tendon is attached in an oblique line of sutures proximal to the dorsal retinaculum, and is attached proximally and distally to each EDC tendon. The EDM is not included unless the EDC slip to the little finger is absent.

Tension on individual EDC tendons should be adjusted to demonstrate the appropriate finger position in extension. The EPL is then included to fit the digital pattern in extension. This full FCU transfer often results in a slight radial deviation of the hand at the wrist. If the patient has significant radial deviation at the wrist, the insertion of the ECRL should be transferred to the ECU or the FCU transfer should not be done. The PL, if present, may be used to activate the EPL (Fig. 14–3 A to C).

The fingers and thumb also can be extended by the FDS tendons to the long and ring fingers.[8] The FDS tendons are exposed through a transverse incision in the distal palm and a longitudinal incision in the volar forearm. The tendons are divided proximal to the chiasma, separated from the profundi tendons, and delivered into the forearm. Proximal to the pronator

quadratus, two windows are incised in the interosseous membrane, one on each side of the anterior interosseous artery. The two windows should be as large as practical.[18] The two tendons are passed to the dorsum of the forearm through the interosseous windows with the long FDS to the radial side of the FDP and the ring FDS to the ulnar side of the FDP. If there has been potential injury to either the anterior or posterior interosseous vessels, the tourniquet should be deflated and hemostasis obtained. If it is not possible to pull the FDS muscle units through the interosseous windows, then the FDS units are routed around both sides of the forearm. A passive fist is formed with the wrist held in 45 degrees of extension, and the transferred tendons are sutured at "normal" tension. The ring FDS is attached to the EDC similar to the FCU transfer, and the long FDS is attached to the EPL and the EIP. The anastomoses should be well proximal to the dorsal retinaculum.

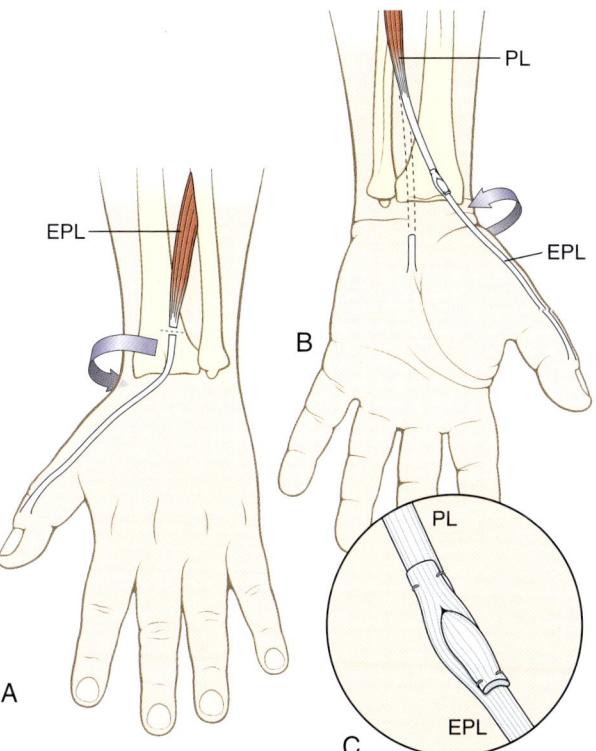

Figure 14–3 PL to EPL transfer. **A:** The EPL is released at Lister's tubercle. **B:** The distal EPL tendon is routed volarly and sutured to the proximal PL tendon. **C:** Pulvertaft juncture.

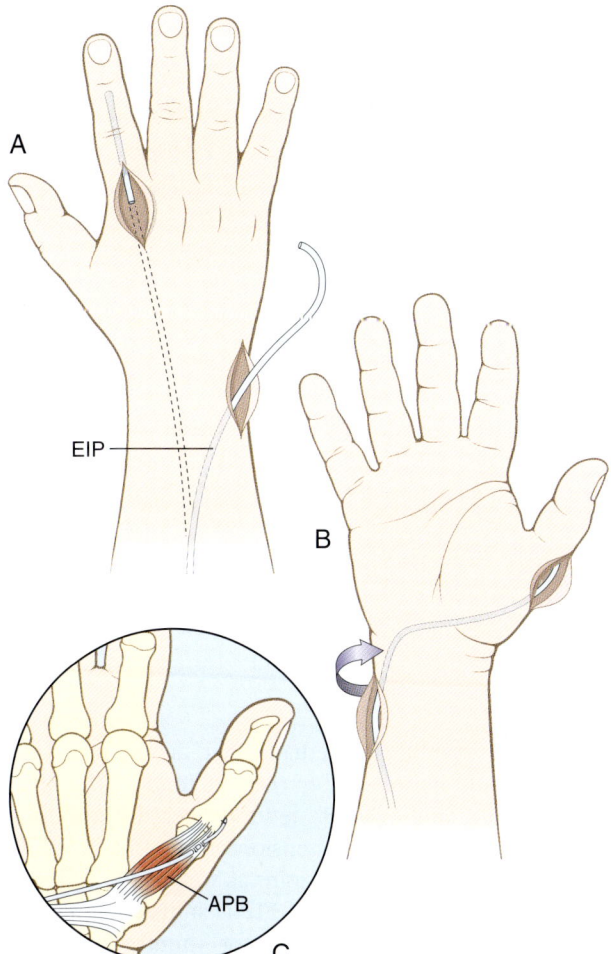

Figure 14–4 EIP to APB transfer. **A:** the EIP is freed at the index MCP joint and rerouted to the ulnar wrist incision just distal to the pisiform. **B:** The EIP tendon is passed around the ulnar border of the forearm, using the pisiform and its ligaments as the pulley. **C:** The EIP tendon is advanced to the thumb MP joint and sutured to either the APB tendon and/or the capsule and EPL tendon.

When the passive fist is released, the digits should posture in functional extension against gravity. Full flexion of the wrist is uncommon after reconstruction.

For proximal stability of the thumb, the EPB is mobilized from the first dorsal compartment and tenodesed to the PL. The PL tendon is absent in about 20% of the population.[24] An alternative is using the FCR to both the APL and EPL tendons.

Following surgery, the elbow is held at 90 degrees, the forearm at neutral 0 degrees, the wrist at 45 degrees, the MP joints near full extension, and the thumb in full extension and radial abduction. The DIP and PIP joints begin active motion. The position is maintained for four to six weeks in a long arm cast, then a removable short arm splint is used. and all joints begin active motion. Functional recovery is anticipated by 6 months.

Isolated Median Palsy

The functional need after low median palsy is thumb abduction.[24] Preoperative management should maintain a full passive range of abduction and pronation for the thumb. At surgery,[25] the EIP is identified through a longitudinal minimal zigzag incision over the index MCP joint (Fig. 14–4 A to C). It is appropriate to make a short transverse incision distal to the dorsal retinaculum to free the tendon of the EIP from the index tendon of the EDC. A second short transverse incision is made

proximal to the dorsal retinaculum in line with the EIP tendon. A third transverse incision will allow the EIP tendon to be freed up to the muscle tendon junction. An ulnarward short transverse incision is made just distal to the pisiform. A tendon passer is used to pass the EIP tendon around the ulnar border of the forearm, using the pisiform and its ligaments as the pulley. A longitudinal incision is made along the radial border of the thumb, and the tendon of the APB is identified. A tendon passer is used to develop a subcutaneous tunnel across the palm from the pisiform to the index MP joint. The EIP tendon is advanced to the thumb MP joint. A short incision can be made over the thenar muscle area and an intramuscular tunnel created for the EIP tendon, which results in less "bowline" effect across the base of the palm. The distal attachment of the EIP tendon vary with the clinical problem. In isolated low median palsy, the tendon can be attached only to the tendon of the

TABLE 14–3

Isolated Radial Palsy

Needed Function	Available Motor	Motor Retained for Balance
Wrist extension Finger and thumb extension	PT to ECRB FCU to EDC and EPLFDS (long and ring) to EDC, EIP and EPL	Pronator quadratus FCR and PL FDP
	FCR to EDC and PL to FPL	FCU
Proximal thumb stability	FCR split insertion to APL and FCR	PL and FCU
	Tenodesis of PL and EPB, (mobilized from first dorsal compartment)	FCU

TABLE 14–4

Isolated Median Palsy

Needed Function	Preferred Motor	Alternate Transfer
Low Palsy: Thumb abduction	EIP to APB (and EPL)	EDM, PL, FDS (ring)
High Palsy: Thumb flexion Finger flexion (index and long)	BR to FPL Tenodesis of FDP (ring and little) to FDP (index and long)	ECRL to FPL ECRL to FDP (index) and tenodesis of FDP (long) to FDP (ring and little)
Sensibility of thumb-index volar pinch	Ulnar digital nerve translocation	Neurovascular cutaneous island pedicle, free nerve grafts, superficial radial neurocutaneous flap

APB. In a combined median-ulnar nerve loss, the tendon should be attached to the APB tendon, the MCP joint capsule, and the EPL tendon over the proximal phalanx. By increasing the tension on the EPL, the FPL becomes a flexor of the MP joint as well as the IP joint. The tension of the transferred EIP is adjusted while the wrist is flexed 30 degrees and the thumb is held in maximum opposition (Table 14–3).

The functional needs after high (proximal) median palsy include (1) thumb abduction, (2) index and long finger flexion, and (3) thumb flexion. A midline longitudinal slightly zigzag incision is made from approximately 2.5 cm above the wrist crease to the proximal third of the forearm. For index- and long-finger flexion, the tendons of the FDP are pulled proximally until all finger pulps are in transverse alignment instead of oblique alignment. The tendons of the index and long FDP are tenodesed to the tendons of the ulnar innervated ring and little FDP. A double line of sutures is important to prevent shifting of the tendons during power grasp. Index finger flexion can be individualized by transferring the tendon of the ECRL to the tendon of the index FDP, leaving the middle FDP to be powered by the ring and little FDP.

After finger flexion, the FPL and BR tendons are identified. The BR should be freed from its tissue attachments so that it has approximately 5 cm of passive mobility.[26] The FPL must glide freely, especially distal to the wrist. The BR tendon is interwoven into the tendon of the FPL and held with nonabsorbable sutures. Tension is adjusted so that there is full extension of the thumb when the wrist is in 30 degrees of flexion.

The forearm and hand should be immobilized for 3 to 4 weeks after surgery. The elbow is supported in 90 degrees of flexion, the wrist in 15 to 20 degrees of flexion, the thumb in full opposition, and the fingers supported in a flexion position of 30 degrees at the PIP and DIP joints. By the 6th or 7th week, soft-tissue healing is strong enough to withstand resistance.

Isolated Ulnar Palsy

Paralysis of seven interossei muscles and the abductor digiti quinti prevents active abduction and adduction of the fingers, and with instability of the transverse metacarpal arch, results in significant loss of hand strength. There is no universally "accepted" program for reconstruction (Table 14–4).

Functional needs after low ulnar palsy are (1) thumb adduction, (2) thumb–index tip pinch, (3) power for gross grip, and (4) adduction of the little finger, plus (5) ring and little finger flexion in high ulnar palsy.[27] Biomechanical studies demonstrate 75% to 80% loss of power pinch in patients with ulnar palsy.[28] For thumb adduction, the ECRB or BR is released from its insertion and attached to a free tendon graft (Fig. 14–5). The graft is passed into the palm through the third intermetacarpal space and tunneled superficial (volar) to the AP and deep (dorsal) to the flexor tendons and neurovascular structures.[29] The graft is attached to the tendon of the APB, which improves thumb pronation for pinch.

For thumb–index tip pinch, an accessory slip of the APL can be elongated with a free tendon graft and transferred to the tendon of the first dorsal interosseous

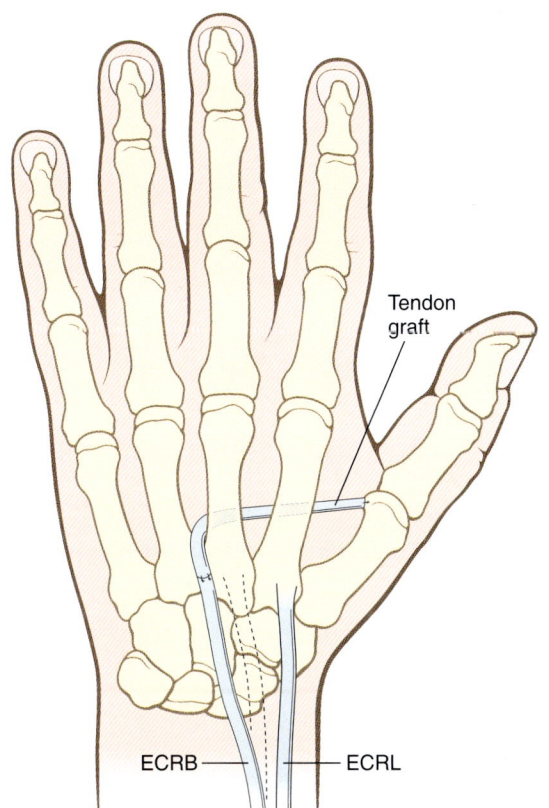

Figure 14–5   For thumb adduction, the ECRB is attached to a free tendon graft, passed through the third intermetacarpal space, and attached to the APB tendon.

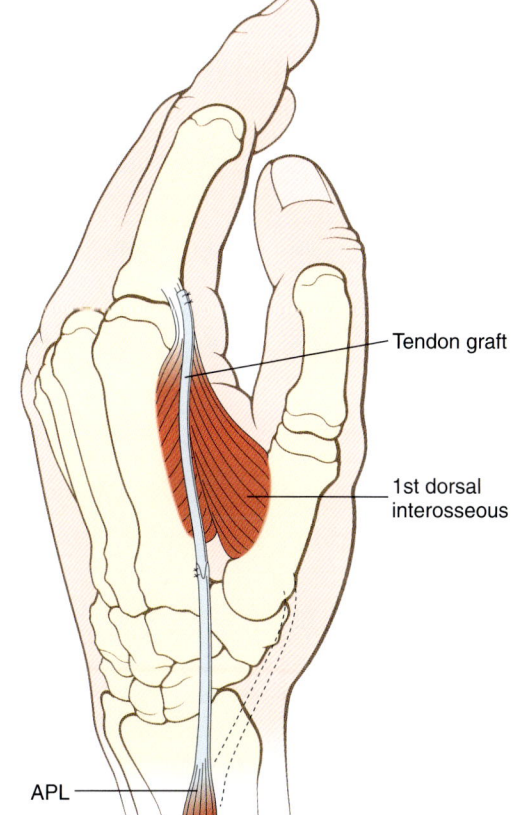

Figure 14–6   For thumb-index tip pinch, an accessory slip of the APL can be elongated with a free tendon graft, and transferred to the tendon of the first dorsal interosseous.

(Fig. 14–6). This transfer does not appreciably increase the force of tip pinch, but stabilizes the index finger. An alternate is arthrodesis of the MP joint of the thumb.

A reliable procedure to increase power for gross grip is to add a muscle–tendon unit to the power train for flexion of the proximal phalanx. Burkhalter and Strait[30] prolonged the ECRL with a free graft, usually PL or plantaris (Fig. 14–7 A to C). The free graft is split into two slips and passed through the intermetacarpal spaces between the long–ring fingers and the ring–little fingers. A four-tailed graft can be used. The tendon slips pass volar to the deep transverse metacarpal ligament, and are sutured either into the A2 pulley of the flexor sheath or into the lateral band of the extensor apparatus. The flexor pulley insertion does not assist in finger extension, and the extensor apparatus insertion is a potential "swan neck" deformity. Postoperative immobilization is for 4 weeks, with the wrist at 45 degrees dorsiflexion and the MP joints in 60 degrees flexion. The ECRL contracts during finger flexion.

Instability (flattening) of the transverse arch may contribute to recurrent clawing after lumbrical replacement procedures. Blacker et al.[31] found that the EDM had the potential to abduct the little finger through its indirect insertion into the abductor tubercle on the proximal phalanx. This action is normally balanced by the third palmar interosseous, which is inactive in ulnar palsy. The ulnar half of the EDM is passed between the fourth and fifth metacarpals into the palm (Fig. 14–8). If the little finger is clawed as well as abducted, the tendon slip is inserted through the A2 pulley of the flexor sheath. If the little finger is not clawed, the tendon slip is passed beneath the deep transverse metacarpal ligament and sutured into the radial collateral ligament of the MP joint of the little finger.

If there is marked weakness of the ring and little fingers in high ulnar palsy, one can tenodese the FDP of the ring and little fingers to the FDP of the long finger in the forearm. The index FDP is left free. One should consider tenodesis of the FDP across the distal IP joints of the ring and little fingers.

Ulnar deviation is as important for wrist flexion as radial deviation is for wrist extension. It is useful to transfer the FCR tendon to the insertion of the FCU in the patient with high ulnar palsy who performs activities requiring strong wrist flexion.

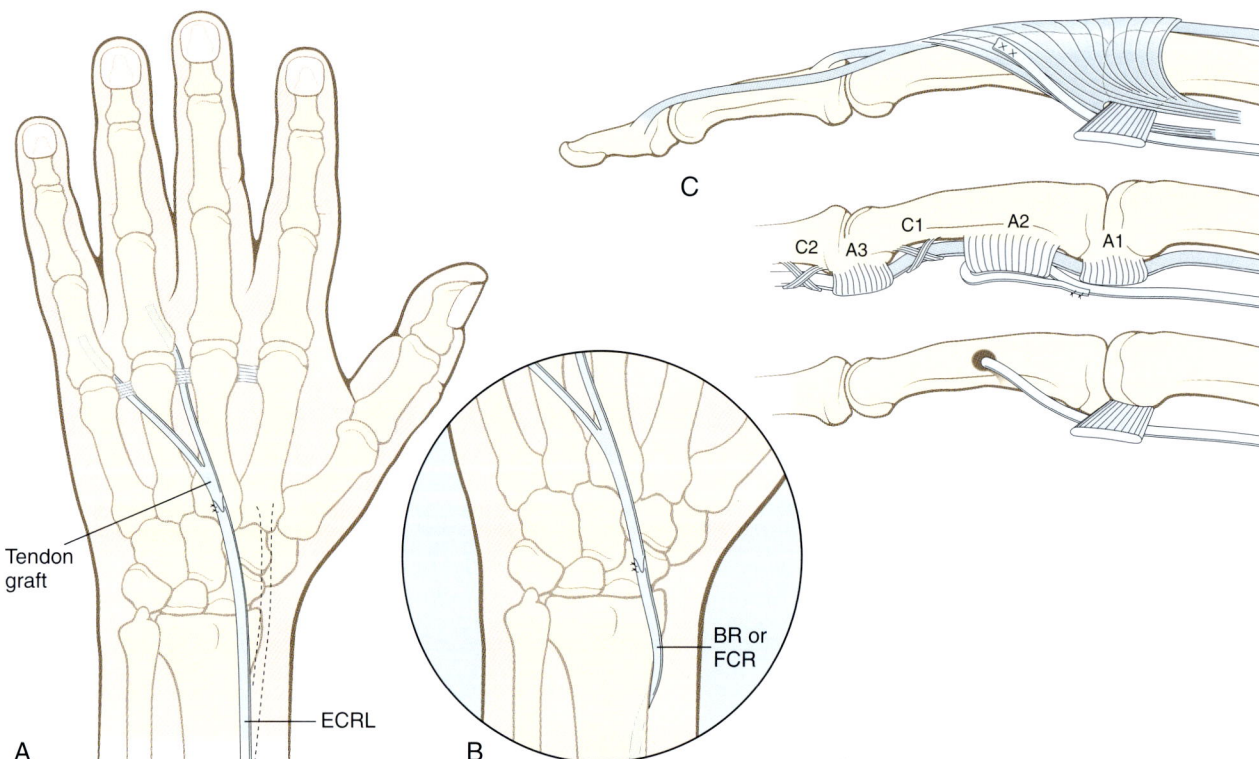

Figure 14–7 **A:** The ECRL is prolonged with a free graft split into two slips and volar to the deep transverse metacarpal ligament. **B:** The BR or FCR may be substituted. **C:** The graft is sutured either into the A2 pulley of the flexor sheath, or into the lateral band of the extensor apparatus.

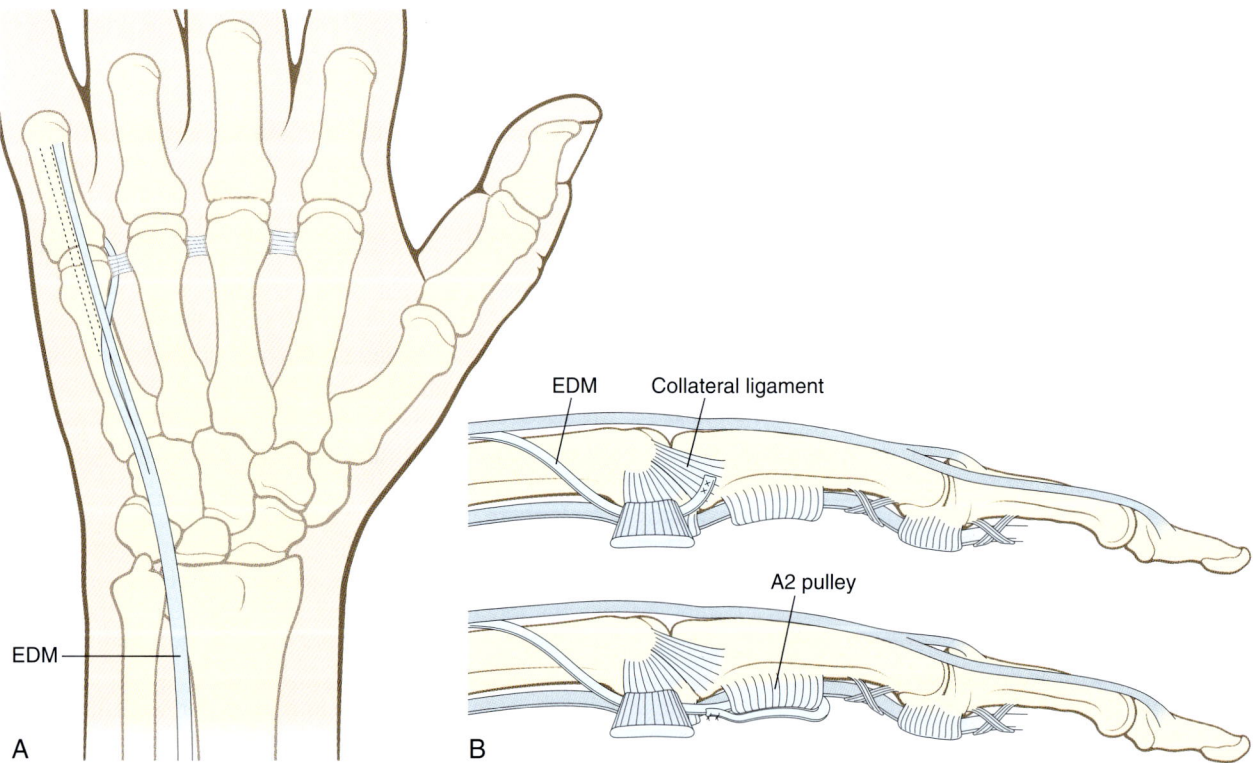

Figure 14–8 **A:** The ulnar half of the EDM is passed between the fourth and fifth metacarpals into the palm. **B:** If clawing is present, insert the tendon slip through the A2 pulley. If clawing is not present, the tendon slip is passed beneath the deep transverse metacarpal ligament, and sutured into the radial collateral ligament of the MP joint of the little finger.

EARLY TENDON TRANSFERS AS INTERNAL SPLINTS

Appropriate early tendon transfers enhance function while awaiting the return of nerve control and total muscle function. The objectives are to stimulate sensibility re-education and to improve the coordination of residual muscle–tendon units. The combined results of early muscle transfer plus the reinnervation from nerve repair often are better than those of either procedure separately.[32–35]

Radial Palsy: Extension of the Wrist

The PT transferred to the ECRB will produce active wrist extension. Increasing dorsal extension power of the wrist by an increment of one may increase power grip three to five times.[34] Postoperatively, the wrist should rest for 5 weeks in 20 degrees of extension.

Low Median Palsy: Abduction of the Thumb

The EIP transferred to the APB[35] is appropriate, except in patient with very mobile MP joints. In these patients, the transfer also should include an EPL tendon insertion. Postoperatively, the thumb is held in full abduction for 5 weeks. If there is continued instability in the longitudinal arch of the thumb, the MP joint should be arthrodesed.

Low Ulnar Palsy: Adduction of the Thumb

The long FDS tendon can improve thumb adduction, the clawed position of the ring and little fingers, and the flattened metacarpal arch. The FDS is detached at the PIP joint level with tenodesis of the radial half across the joint. The tendon is further split, and the radial half of the tendon passes volar to the AP and dorsal to the FDP tendons into the insertion of the APB. The ulnar half of the tendon is again split into two slips that are directed distally and volar to the deep transverse metacarpal ligament and looped through the A2 pulley of the flexor sheath for the ring and little fingers. The pulley for this transfer is the distal edge of the palmar fascia inserted into the third metacarpal. Postoperatively, the wrist is in slight dorsiflexion, the thumb is adducted and pronated, the MP joints of the fingers are flexed, and the IP joints of the fingers are extended (the "hoe-hand" position). This intrinsic-plus position is maintained for 4 weeks before active extension is permitted.

TABLE 14–5

Isolated Ulnar Palsy

Needed Function	Preferred Motor	Alternate Transfer
Low Palsy:		
Thumb adduction for key pinch	ECRB, with free tendon graft between 3rd and 4th metacarpals, to tendon of APB	FDS (long) to abductor tubercle of thumb, with palmar fascia as pulley
Thumb–index tip pinch	Slip of APL to 1st dorsal interosseous tendon, and arthrodesis MP joint of thumb	EPB to 1st dorsal interosseous tendon, if MP joint of thumb arthrodesed
Proximal phalanx power flexion and integration of MP and IP motion (clawed fingers)	ECRL with 2 or 4 tailed graft passed volar to deep transverse metacarpal ligament to either A2 pulley of flexor sheath or radial band of the dorsal apparatus	If wrist flexion contracture, FCR with 4 tailed graft to either flexor sheath (A2 pulley) or lateral bands of dorsal apparatus
Metacarpal (palmar) transverse arch and adduction for little finger	EDM tendon is split and ulnar half transferred volar to deep transverse metacarpal ligament to radial collateral ligament of proximal phalanx or A2 pulley of the flexor sheath (EDC little finger must be effective)	If little finger is clawed as well as abducted, insert ulnar half of EDM only into A2 pulley
Volar sensibility for ring and little fingers	Proximal median digital nerve translocated to distal ulnar digital nerve	Free or vascularized nerve graft
High Palsy:		
Distal finger flexion, for ring and little finger	FDP (long) tenodesed to FDP (ring and little), with possible tenodesis of distal IP joints in the ring and little fingers	
Wrist flexion, ulnar side	FCR to insertion of FCU	PL to insertion of FCU

Combined Nerve Palsies of the Forearm and Hand

Tendon transfers in combined nerve palsies may be more complicated than isolated nerve palsies secondary to complex extremity injuries. Muscle–tendon units are often lacerated and sometimes avulsed, resulting in poor proprioception and distorted sensibility. Circulation is usually impaired, with pain and increased fibrosis. The need for multiple operations complicates rehabilitation[36-40] (Table 14–6).

With appropriate splinting, all tendon transfers can be done at one time. Adduction contracture of the thumb–index web must be prevented. Following transfers, the residual loss of sensibility is likely to be the greater functional problem than motor patterns for grasp and pinch (Table 14–7).

The major clinical problem is the total loss of volar sensibility, while atrophy of the finger pulps will discourage both precision and power grip. If the other hand is normal, focus on improving key pinch and simple grasp (Table 14–8).

Surgical rehabilitation is difficult because surgical procedures need to be performed both for finger extension and flexion and for thumb adduction and abduction. Surgery should be staged, perhaps at 3-month intervals. Tlhe first phase might include wrist and digit extension with thumb abduction. The second phase might include digit flexion and thumb abduction.

Splints need modification for each phase. Sensibility procedures are the final stage of surgical reconstruction, and should be delayed until all tendon transfers have healed (Table 14–9).

These transfers will result in a extremity that functions only slightly more effectively than a prosthesis. Many adult patients do not regain precise cortical orientation, and it is difficult to determine the advantages and disadvantages of digital nerve translocation to restore sensation.

LONG-TERM FOLLOW-UP

There have been only a few reports of long-term evaluation of tendon transfers after trauma. Dunnet et al.[41] reported on radial palsy. Transfers were done an average of 32 months after injury, and followed an average of 66 months before reporting. All patients demonstrated functional improvement after surgery, but 66 months later, 55% had difficulty grasping or releasing large objects, 64% had impaired coordination and dexterity, and 82% had premature fatigue with wrist extension. In the patient with traumatic radial palsy, what is the usual $5\frac{1}{2}$ year outcome? In radial palsy, what are the usual functional changes for median and ulnar innervated muscles-with or without tendon transfers? We need more long-term studies to measure function before and after tendon transfers.

TABLE 14–6

Combined Low (Distal) Median and Ulnar Palsy

Needed Function	Preferred Motor	Alternate Transfer
Thumb adduction, key pinch	ECRB with free tendon graft between 3rd and 4th metacarpals, to APB tendon	FDS (long) to abductor tubercle of thumb, with palmar fascia and flexor tendons as pulleys
Thumb abduction, opposition	EIP around pisiform pulley and through thenar muscle tunnel to APB tendon insertion and EPL tendon	PL to APB tendon insertion, (or) FDS (ring) to APB tendon
Thumb–index tip pinch	APL slip with free tendon graft to first dorsal interosseous tendon and arthrodesis thumb MP joint	EPB or PL to first dorsal interosseous tendon, with arthrodesis thumb MP joint
Metacarpal (palmar) transverse arch and adduction for little finger	EDM tendon split and ulnar half passed volar to deep transverse metacarpal ligament to radial collateral ligament of MP joint of the little finger or the A2 pulley of the flexor sheath	FDS (little) to deep transverse metacarpal ligament between 4th and 5th metacarpals, or FDS (long or ring) combined as single transfer for thumb adduction and metacarpal arch
Power flexion for proximal phalanges and integration of MP and interphalangeal motion (clawed fingers)	ECRL or BR to all four fingers using four-tailed free tendon graft and insertion in flexor sheath (A2 pulley) or lateral bands of dorsal apparatus	FCR (if wrist flexion contracture) with four-tailed free tendon graft to either flexor sheath (A2 pulley) or dorsal apparatus
Median and ulnar volar sensibility	Superficial radial nerve translocation or cutaneous neurovascular island	Cross-finger index-to-thumb fillet flap (superficial radial nerve)

TABLE 14–7

Combined High (Proximal) Median and Ulnar Palsy

Needed Function	Preferred Motor	Alternate Transfer
Thumb adduction (AP), key pinch	ECRB with free tendon graft between 3rd and 4th metacarpals to APB tendon	BR or EIP with free tendon graft between 3rd and 4th metacarpals to abductor tubercle of thumb (APB tendon)
Thumb flexion (IP joint)	BR to FPL in forearm	Tenodesis of FPL distal to MP joint of thumb
Thumb abduction (APB)	EIP with pisiform pulley to insertion APB tendon (plus) EPL tendon	EPL or ECU with free graft around pisiform pulley to APB tendon (thumb MP is arthrodesed and no active motion at thumb IP joint)
Thumb, index tip pinch	Thumb MP joint arthrodesis; and APL slip with free tendon graft to 1st dorsal interosseous tendon	EPB or PL to 1st dorsal interosseous, and fusion of thumb MP joint
Finger flexion (FDP)	FCRL to all four tendons of FDP with possible tenodesis of DIP of ulnar three fingers	Biceps brachii extended with FCR tendon to tendons of FDP
Power for flexion of proximal phalanx with integration of MP and IP motion (clawed fingers)	Tenodesis of all four digits with free tendon graft from dorsal carpal ligament volar to deep transverse metacarpal ligament to lateral bands of extensor apparatus or from deep transverse metacarpal ligament to extensor apparatus	Capsulodesis of MP volar capsule, arthrodesis of PIP joints, or arthrodesis of MP joints
Metacarpal (palmar) arch and adduction for little finger	EDM to deep transverse metacarpal ligament (EDC of little finger must be active)	EDM to radial lateral bands (extensor hood) of the ring and little finger
Wrist flexion		ECU to insertion of FCU
Median and ulnar volar sensibility	Superficial radial innervated index fillet flap to palm	Superficial radial nerve translocation
	First dorsal metacarpal artery neurovascular island pedicle flap	Free vascularized nerve graft

TABLE 14–8

Combined High (Proximal) Ulnar and Radial Palsy

Needed Function	Preferred Motor	Alternate Transfer
Wrist extension	PT to ECRB	
Thumb adduction, key pinch, and clawed fingers: metacarpal (palmar transverse arch) and power flexion of proximal phalanx and integration of MP and IP motion	One-half of FDS (long) as split transfer to abductor tubercle of thumb, and one-half of FDS (long) in two slips to A2 pulley of flexor sheath for ring and little fingers, and later, if unable to fully extend	Tenodesis with free tendon graft from radial lateral band of dorsal apparatus to deep transverse metacarpal ligament, or capsulodesis of MP volar capsule
Thumb–index tip pinch	Arthrodesis of thumb MP joint	
Proximal thumb stability for abduction and wrist flexion (radial side)	Tenodeis of APL to radius	FCR (yoke insertion) to APL and EPB
Wrist flexion (ulnar aspect)		PL to insertion of FCU
Finger and thumb extension	FDS (index and ring) through interosseous membrane to EDC and EPL	PL to EDC and EPL
Finger flexion (ring and little)	Tenodesis of FDP (long) as active motor to ring and little FDP, and tenodesis of DIP joint of ring and little fingers, using FDP tendons	
Volar sensibility, ring and little fingers	Median digital nerve translocation	Free vascularized nerve grafts, or neurovascular cutaneous island pedicle

TABLE 14–9

Combined High (Proximal) Median and Radial Palsy

Needed Function	Preferred Motor	Alternate Transfer
Forearm pronation	Biceps brachii tendon rerouting around the radius	
Wrist extension and flexion	Radiocarpal arthrodesis	
Finger flexion	Tenodesis of FDP ring and little fingers (active motors) to FDP index and long fingers	
Finger and thumb extension	FCU to tendons of EDC and EPL	
Proximal thumb stability	Arthodesis of thumb MP joint, and tenodesis of APL tendon to radius	
Thumb abduction (opposition)		ADQ to the insertion of the APB, or AP tendon insertion from adductor tubercle to abductor tubercle
Thumb flexion	Tenodesis of FPL across thumb IP joint	
Radiovolar sensibility	Ulnar digital nerve translocation	Neurovascular cutaneous island pedicle from ring finger, or free vascularized nerve graft

REFERENCES

1. Omer GE Jr. Injuries to nerves of the upper extremity. J Bone Joint Surg Am 1974;56:1615–24.
2. Omer GE Jr. Peripheral nerve testing and suture techniques. Instr Course Lect 1975;24:122–143.
3. Garrett WE Jr, Seaber AV, Boswick J, et al. Recovery of skeletal muscle after laceration and repair. J Hand Surg Am 1984;9:683–92.
4. Moneim MS, Omer GE Jr. Latissimus dorsal muscle transfer for restoration of elbow flexion after brachial plexus disruption. J Hand Surg Am 1986;11:135–9.
5. Birch R, Raji ARM. Repair of median and ulnar nerves: primary suture is best. J Bone Joint Surg Br 1991;73:281–7.
6. Mailander P, Berger A, Schaler E, et al. Results of primary nerve repair in the upper extremity. Microsurgery 1989;10:147–50.
7. Millesi H. Peripheral nerve repair today: turning point or continuous development? J Hand Surg Br 1990;15:281–7.
8. Boyes JW. Tendon transfers for radial palsy. Bull Hosp Joint Dis 1960;21:97–103.
9. Green DL. Radial nerve palsy. In: Green DL, Hotchkiss R, Pederson WC, eds., Operative Hand Surgery, 4th ed. New York: Churchill-Livingstone 1999:1481–96.
10. Freehafer AA, Mast WA. Transfer of the brachioradialis to improve wrist extension in high spinal cord injuries. J Bone Joint Surg Am 1967;49:648–52.
11. Omer GE Jr. Evaluation and reconstruction of the forearm and hand after traumatic peripheral nerve injuries. J Bone Joint Surg Am 1968;50:1454–78.
12. Brand PW, Beach RB, Thompson DE. Relative tension and potential excursion of muscles in the forearm and hand. J Hand Surg Am 1981;6:209–19.
13. Littler JW. Principles of tendon transfers. In: Converse JM, ed., Reconstructive Plastic Surgery, vol. 4. Philadelphia: W.B. Saunders, 1964:1678–80.
14. Omer GE Jr. The technique and timing of tendon transfers. Orthop Clin North Am 1974;5:243–52.
15. Freehafer AA, Peckman PH, Keith MW. Determination of muscle–tendon unit properties during tendon transfer. J Hand Surg Am 1979;4:331–9.
16. Floyd WE III. Tendon transfers. Hand Surg Update, Am Soc Surg Hand 1999;159–67.
17. Omer GE Jr, Vogel JA. Determination of physiological length of a reconstructed muscle–tendon unit through muscle stimulation. J Bone Joint Surg Am 1965;47:304–12.
18. Brand PW. Clinical Mechanics of the Hand. St. Louis: C.V. Mosby, 1985.
19. Cooney WP. Tendon transfers for median nerve palsy. Hand Clin 1988;4:155–65.
20. Omer GE Jr. Reconstruction of the forearm and hand after peripheral nerve injuries. In: Omer GE Jr, Spinner M, Van Beek AL, eds., Management of Peripheral Nerve Problems, 2nd ed. Philadelphia: W.B. Saunders, 1998:675–705.
21. Schneider LH. Tenon transfers for radial nerve palsy. In: Gelberman RH ed., Operative Nerve Repair and Reconstruction. Philadelphia: J.B. Lippincott, 1991:697–709.
22. Omer GE Jr. Tendon transfers in radial nerve palsy. In: Hunter JM, Schneider LH, Mackin EJ, eds., Tendon Surgery in the Hand. St. Louis: C.V. Mosby, 1987:425–31.
23. Omer GE Jr. Reconstructive procedures for extremities with peripheral nerve defects. Clin Orthop 1985;163:80–91.
24. Burkhalter WE. Median nerve palsy. In: Green DP, ed., Operative Hand Surgery, 3rd ed. New York: Churchill-Livingstone, 1993:1419–48.
25. Burkhalter WE, Christensen RC, Brown P. Extensor indicis proprius opponens plasty. J Bone Joint Surg Am 1973;53:725–32.
26. Eversmann WW. Median nerve palsy. In: Gelberman RH, ed., Operative Nerve Repair and Reconstruction. Philadelphia: J.B. Lippincott, 1991:711–28.
27. Omer GE Jr. Ulnar nerve palsy. In: Green DP, Hotchkiss RN, Pederson WC, eds., Green's Operative Hand Surgery, 4th ed. New York: Churchill-Livingstone, 1999:1521–41.
28. Omer GE Jr. Restoring power grip in ulnar palsy. Proceedings of the American Society for Surgery of the Hand. J Bone Joint Surg Am 1971;53:814.
29. Omer GR Jr. The palsied hand. In: Evarts CMC, ed., Surgery of the Musculoskeletal System, 2nd ed. New York: Churchill-Livingstone, 1990:849–78.
30. Burkhalter WE, Strait JL. Metacarpophalangeal flexor replacement for intrinsic muscle paralysis. J Bone Joint Surg Am 1973;55:1656–76.
31. Blacker GJ, Lister GD, Kleinert HE. The abducted little finger in low ulnar palsy. J Hand Surg Am 1976;1:190–6.
32. Omer GE Jr. Early tendon transfers in the rehabilitation of the median, radial, and ulnar palsies. Ann Chir Main 1982;1:187–90.
33. Burkhalter WE. Early tendon transfers in upper extremity peripheral nerve injury. Clin Orthop 1974;104:68–79.

34. Omer GE Jr. Tendon transfers as early internal splints following peripheral nerve injury in the upper extremity. In: Hunter JM, Schneider LH, Mackin EJ, et al., eds., Rehabilitation of the Hand. St. Louis: C.V. Mosby, 1978:292–303.

35. Omer GE Jr. Early tendon transfers as internal splints after nerve injury. In: Hunter JM, Schneider LH, Mackin EJ, eds., Tendon Surgery in the Hand. St. Louis: C.V. Mosby, 1987:413–8.

36. Littler JW. Tendon transfers and arthrodeses in combined median and ulnar nerve paralysis. J Bone Joint Surg Am 1949;31:225–34.

37. Riordan DC. Tendon transplantation in median nerve and ulnar nerve paralysis. J Bone Joint Surg Am 1953;35:312–20.

38. Omer GE Jr, Blair WF. Tendon transfers in combined nerve palsies of the forearm and hand. In: Chapman MW, ed., Orthopaedic Surgery, 3rd ed. Philadelphia: Lippincott Williams & Wilkins, 2001:1669–86.

39. Omer GE Jr. Tendon transfers for combined traumatic nerve lesions of the forearm and hand. J Hand Surg Br 1992;17:603–10.

40. Omer GE Jr. Combined nerve palsies. In: Green DP, Hotchkiss RN, Pederson WC, eds., Green's Operative Hand Surgery, 4th ed. New York: Churchill-Livingstone, 1999:1542–56.

41. Dunnet WJ, Housden PL, Birch R. Flexor to extensor tendon transfers in the hand. J Hand Surg Br 1995;20B:26–8.

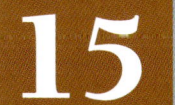

Compression Neuropathies of the Median Nerve

Robert M. Szabo and Jason T. Koo

The greatest obstacle to discovery is not ignorance—it is the illusion of knowledge.

DANIEL J. BOORSTIN

Life is short and the art is long; the occasion fleeting; experience fallacious, and judgment difficult.

HIPPOCRATES

INTRODUCTION

Historically, median nerve compression neuropathies have presented as either post-traumatic sequelae or as manifestations of idiopathic progressive paresthesias and/or pain in predominantly middle-aged patients. Recently, however, the medical community and popular press have increasingly focused on a category of disorders known as cumulative trauma disorders or repetitive stress injuries, and have erroneously grouped compressive neuropathies together with them.[1] The weak association between repetitive stress and compression neuropathies has been described.[2] Nevertheless, this has had a tremendous impact on the medicolegal and workers' compensation arenas, especially with regard to carpal tunnel syndrome. Although it is accepted that certain activities or prolonged positioning of the extremities can induce symptoms of compression neuropathy,[2] it is still controversial whether an a priori relationship exists between compression neuropathy and certain occupations. The shift to the workplace requires a concomitant change in the physician's approach to managing the condition. This approach is best realized by discussing different risk factors for the neuropathy with the patient rather than immediately attributing the "cause" to the workplace. A successful outcome is more likely if the patient plays an active role in the treatment process.[3]

PATHOPHYSIOLOGY

The term "compression neuropathy" implies compression of the nerve by an adjacent anatomic structure. The cervical spine and the wrist are common sites of compression, and give rise to various well-known nerve compression syndromes. This concept of nerve compression, however, is simplistic; there are a myriad of other factors that may confound the clinical picture.

Systemic conditions such as diabetes,[4] myxedema from hypothyroidism,[5] hyperthyroidism,[6] sarcoidosis,[7] metabolic disorders such as mucopolysaccharidosis,[8–11] alcoholism, or exposure to industrial solvents including toxic metal or chemical poisoning[12] may contribute to the increased susceptibility of peripheral nerves to injury secondary to compression. In some people, aging has a similar effect.[13] Patients on long-term hemodialysis have high incidences of carpal tunnel syndrome.[14–16]

The dramatic relief of symptoms that sometimes occurs following surgical decompression suggests an ischemic etiology to many compression neuropathies.[17–23] According to this theory, the mechanical cause of nerve compression obstructs venous return. This results in segmental anoxia, capillary vasodilatation, and edema.[24] The edema compounds the compressive effects, and leads to abnormal axonal and cellular exchange. Surgical release at this early stage generally yields good results. Prolonged compression, however, results in intraneural fibrosis, after which nerve recovery is less likely to occur after decompression.[25] Experimentally, the first manifestations of injury appear at 20 to 30 mm Hg of compression, and include reduced epineurial blood flow and impairment of axonal transport.[26] With prolonged compression, an increase in endoneurial fluid pressure, which may interfere with intrafascicular capillary flow, is seen.[21] Neurophysiologic changes and symptoms of paresthesias have been induced in human volunteers with 30 to 40 mm Hg compression on the median nerve.[19]

By necessity, nerves of the upper extremity have considerable mobility throughout their length. Compression may tether the nerve and restrict its mobility, thereby causing traction of the nerve in response to joint motion. Traction alone can cause conduction block. It is likely, although not yet demonstrated, that many upper extremity compression neuropathies include traction on the nerve as a component of the pathophysiology.[27,28]

The double-crush phenomenon, as postulated by Upton and McComas,[29] suggests that the presence of a proximal lesion renders the distal nerve trunk more vulnerable to the effects of compression. This is likely due to disturbances in axonal flow kinetics and the disruption of the neurofilament architecture. The nerve cell body synthesizes enzymes, polypeptides, polysaccharides, free amino acids, neurosecretory granules, mitochondria, and tubulin subunits which are necessary for the survival and normal function of the axon. These substances travel anterograde down the axon, while metabolic breakdown products return retrograde by a combination of fast and slow axoplasmic transport mechanisms. Any disruption of the synthesis or blockage of the transport of these materials will increase the susceptibility of axons to the effects of compression.[30,31]

Because of this phenomenon, the outcome of surgical decompression may be disappointing unless both entrapments are treated. For instance, a lower degree of compression (as measured by distal sensory latency) of the median nerve at the carpal tunnel is needed to produce symptoms when a proximal forearm lesion is present. Concurrent proximal forearm compression is one of the reasons for persistent residual symptoms following carpal tunnel release.

CLINICAL PRESENTATION

The median nerve may be compressed as it travels from the C5–T1 nerve roots down towards the hand, causing specific compression syndromes. Carpal tunnel syndrome is the best known and most common, but pronator teres syndrome and anterior interosseous nerve syndrome are also clinically significant.[32]

PRONATOR SYNDROME

Seyffarth first coined the term pronator syndrome, in his report on the nonoperative management of 17 patients in 1951, to describe a compression neuropathy of the median nerve as it passes through the pronator teres.[33] Johnson and Spinner characterized this syndrome based on observations in 103 operative decompressions.[34,35] Pronator syndrome now is a term used to describe a pain syndrome resulting from compression of the median nerve by any structure in the proximal forearm and elbow.

Clinical symptoms of pronator syndrome include forearm pain as well as paresthesias and hypoesthesia in the cutaneous distribution of the median nerve, that is, the thumb, index, long, and radial half of the ring finger. These symptoms may be attributed to carpal tunnel syndrome. However, while the symptoms from carpal tunnel syndrome are frequent at night, those of pronator syndrome occur primarily from use during the daytime. These sensory symptoms may also be present over the thenar eminence in the distribution of the palmar cutaneous branch of the median nerve, which, having branched from the median nerve proximal to the wrist, does not travel through the carpal tunnel. Patients may also complain of perceived weakness in the extremity secondary to pain.

ANTERIOR INTEROSSEOUS SYNDROME

In 1948, Parsonage and Turner reported six patients with paralysis of the flexor pollicis longus (FPL) and the flexor digitorum profundus (FDP) to the index finger, and attributed the condition to an anterior horn cell lesion.[36] Kiloh and Nevin, in 1952, reported an "isolated neuritis" of the anterior interosseous nerve (AIN) in two patients with these findings.[37] In 1965, Fearn and Goodfellow were the first to propose mechanical compression as the cause of the syndrome; they suggested that it be treated surgically.[38] Isolated anterior interosseous nerve palsy is a rare occurrence; it accounts for less than 1% of all upper extremity peripheral neuropathies.[39] The debate continues as to whether AIN is a neuritis, compression neuropathy, or both.

CARPAL TUNNEL SYNDROME

Sir James Paget first described carpal tunnel syndrome in 1854, when he published his *Lectures on Surgical Pathology*.[40,41] In 1880, Putnam reported a series of 37 patients with pain and paresthesia in the median nerve distribution, and concluded that the sensory changes were caused by changes in blood supply to the nerve endings supplying the areas of the hand, similar to the vasomotor disorder described by Raynaud.[42,43] The first carpal tunnel release was probably performed in 1924 by Herbert Galloway.[44] Although the term, "carpal tunnel syndrome" was termed by Moersch in 1938,[40] the condition was not widely recognized until a series of articles by Phalen, the first in 1950.[45–48] It is now estimated that 1 million adults in the United States are diagnosed with carpal tunnel syndrome each year.[49] Medical costs resulting from carpal tunnel syndrome exceed $1 billion per year, and over 200,000 surgical procedures are performed annually.[50]

In recent times, some members of the medicolegal community, popular media, and insurance industry have incorporated certain compressive neuropathies into a group of disorders known as cumulative trauma disorders or repetitive stress injuries. Carpal tunnel syndrome accounts for approximately 40% of lost workdays because of repetitive motion problems.[51] An association between repetitive stress and compression neuropathies has been explored.[52] Common task-related factors attributed to occupational carpal tunnel syndrome are repetition, force, mechanical stress, posture, vibration, and temperature. However, the mechanisms by which they produce neuropathy are not well known. Job-related factors do not necessarily predict the development of carpal tunnel syndrome.[53] Attempts by companies to reduce workers' compensation expenses related to carpal tunnel syndrome by screening workers with pre-employment median nerve tests was found not to be cost-effective in a retrospective dynamic cohort study based on 2150 workers.[54]

There is little scientific evidence supporting the concept that carpal tunnel syndrome is primarily caused by work. One problem is that cases of occupational carpal tunnel syndrome believed to be caused by work activities are almost always accompanied by other upper extremity symptoms that are poorly characterized and difficult to diagnose.[55] It has been shown that 81% of the electrophysiologic slowing in the median nerve was due to body mass index, age, and the wrist depth/width ratio, whereas only 8% was due to job-related factors.[56] Gerr and Letz finally concluded that "carpal tunnel syndrome is closely correlated with health habits and life-style but is only peripherally related to workplace activities."[53]

Carpal tunnel syndrome is the most common and best known of the compression neuropathies of the upper extremity. The clinical picture of pain and paresthesias in the palmar radial aspect of the hand, often worse at night and/or exacerbated by repetitive forceful use of the hand, is readily recognized. Carpal tunnel syndrome represents a constellation of signs and symptoms in which no one test absolutely confirms its diagnosis. The validity and reliability of many of the diagnostic tests used for carpal tunnel syndrome are described.[57,58]

ANATOMY

Median Nerve

The median nerve arises from the medial and lateral cords of the brachial plexus. It accompanies the brachial artery as it passes between the biceps tendon and the brachialis muscle. At the distal humerus, nerve and artery pass through the antecubital fossa underneath a fibrous sheath, the bicipital aponeurosis (lacertus fibrosis), which originates from the biceps tendon and the fascia of the flexor-pronator mass. Although the median nerve can take different paths in relation to the pronator teres (PT),[59] it most commonly passes between the deep (ulnar) and superficial (humeral) heads of the PT, which originate from the proximal ulna and medial epicondyle, respectively. The PT receives one to four branches from the median nerve. Despite separating from the bulk of the nerve proximal to the elbow joint, these branches share its perineurial sheath. Branches that originate from the median nerve before it passes through the PT include branches to the palmaris longus (PL), flexor carpi radialis (FCR), and flexor digitorum superficialis (FDS), and rarely the flexor digitorum profundus (FDP).[60]

The fibrous arch of the PT (the pronator arch) lies 3 to 7.5 cm below the humeral epicondylar line. The fibrous arch of the FDS (the superficialis arch), which is always distal to the pronator arch, lies 6.5 cm below the humeral epicondylar line in its most proximal position.[60] The median nerve enters the forearm deep to the fibrous arch of the FDS, and emerges beneath the radial side of the muscle belly of the middle finger superficialis where it is quite superficial and near the PL tendon.[61] The anterior interosseous nerve (AIN) arises from the median nerve in the distal part of the cubital fossa. The fascicles of the AIN are grouped separately from the remaining median nerve before the nerve divides into its main and anterior interosseous branches.[62]

In 1848 and 1854, John Struthers wrote about sites of compression of the median nerve in the upper extremity. He is best known for describing entrapment of the median nerve by a ligament (the ligament of Struthers) from a supracondylar process to the medial epicondyle of the humerus.[63] A series of nine abnormal arcades were described; all but one is a potential site of median nerve/brachial artery compression. Only two of these have been associated with clinical symptoms, Arcades VII and VIII.[64–66]

Arcade VII is characterized by an aberrant origin of the superficial head of the PT from the supracondylar ridge rather than the medial epicondyle. This may be associated with the presence of a supracondylar process.[65,67] Lateral displacement and compression of the neurovascular bundle may result.[61]

Arcade VIII consists of a supracondylar process and ligament of Struthers that spans the supracondylar process and medial epicondyle, thus creating an arcade that contains the median nerve and brachial artery.[67] With an incidence of 1%, the supracondylar process is a projection of bone from the anteromedial aspect of the distal humerus, which arises 3 to 5 cm proximal to the medial epicondyle and is 2 to 20 mm in length.[68] It may be identified only on oblique x-rays of the elbow,[69] and is a rare cause of compression of the underlying median nerve and brachial artery.[67,68] The ligament of Struthers has also been described in the absence of an associated supracondylar process, and may alone cause median nerve compression.[64,65]

In the forearm, the median nerve can be compressed by the pronator teres, the flexor superficialis arch, or the bicipital aponeurosis (lacertus fibrosus), in descending order of frequency[35,70] (Fig. 15–1). In dissecting 31 cadaver arms, Dellon and Mackinnon found that the PT always had a superficial head and usually a deep head, that the FDS varied greatly in its site of origin, and that the median nerve might be crossed by two, one, or no fibroaponeurotic arches.[71] Dissections revealed either a fibrous band on the dorsum of the superficial head of the pronator overlying the median nerve, or a fibrous band as a component of the deep head of the pronator. When the deep ulnar head was absent, a separate fibrous band was found attached to the coronoid process of the ulna proximally.[61,71] In some instances, fibrous bands were noted on both heads, which formed a definite fibrous arcade.[35] A fibrous arcade was also observed in approximately one-third of the dissections at the proximal margin of the FDS to the middle finger.[35] Finally, entrapment of the median nerve at the bicipital aponeurosis was the least common cause of median nerve entrapment in the proximal forearm, and may have been secondary to hypertrophy or enlargement of the bicipital aponeurosis.[35]

The median artery has been associated with both carpal tunnel and pronator syndromes.[70,72,73] In pronator syndrome, the median artery has been noted to penetrate the median nerve, and also to form vascular leashes that constricted the nerve.[72,73] The median artery is normally a transitory vessel that develops from the axial artery of the upper extremity during early embryonic life. When the radial and ulnar arteries develop, the median artery usually involutes.[73] A persistent median artery in adults occurs with an incidence of 1% to 17%,[73] and is usually a long, thin vessel that arises from the anterior interosseous artery and passes distally between the FDP and FPL to the median nerve. It supplies the median nerve throughout its course in the forearm,[68] and in approximately 8% of individuals, is a large vessel that continues into the palm to help form the superficial palmar arterial arch[74] (Fig. 15–2).

Several accessory and variant muscles have been noted as compressing structures, including Gantzer's muscle, an accessory head of the FPL, the palmaris profundus, and the flexor carpi radialis brevis.[65] Gantzer's muscle was present in 45%[71] to 52%[75] of cadavers studied. It is innervated by the AIN, arises from the medial epicondyle 85% of the time, and has a dual origin from the epicondyle and coronoid process of the ulna in the remainder.[61] There is some controversy regarding the association of Gantzer's muscle and pronator syndrome. Dellon and Mackinnon stated that Gantzer's muscle always lay posterior to both the median nerve and the anterior interosseous nerve,[71] a finding confirmed by al-Qattan.[75] However, two instances of compression by Gantzer's muscle have been reported. In the first, a slip of Gantzer's muscle inserted to the underside of the FDS in the vicinity of the superficialis arch,[76] while in the second, the median nerve was perforated by Gantzer's muscle itself in the forearm.

Pure sensory disturbances have also been reported at the level of the bicipital aponeurosis by a snapping brachialis tendon.[77] Cubital bursitis has also been reported as a cause of median nerve irritation by causing swelling in the cubital fossa.[78]

Anterior Interosseous Nerve

The anterior interosseous nerve is the largest muscular branch that emerges from the median nerve.[61] It innervates the FDP to the index and middle fingers, the FPL, and the pronator quadratus (PQ). The terminal portion also provides sensory innervation to the carpal joints.[61] The AIN arises from the median nerve on the dorsoradial surface about 5 to 8 cm distal to the medial epicondyle. According to Sunderland, the AIN becomes a separate group of fascicles 2.5 cm proximal to the branch point.[79] The AIN travels between the FDS and FDP, and then passes dorsally in the interval between

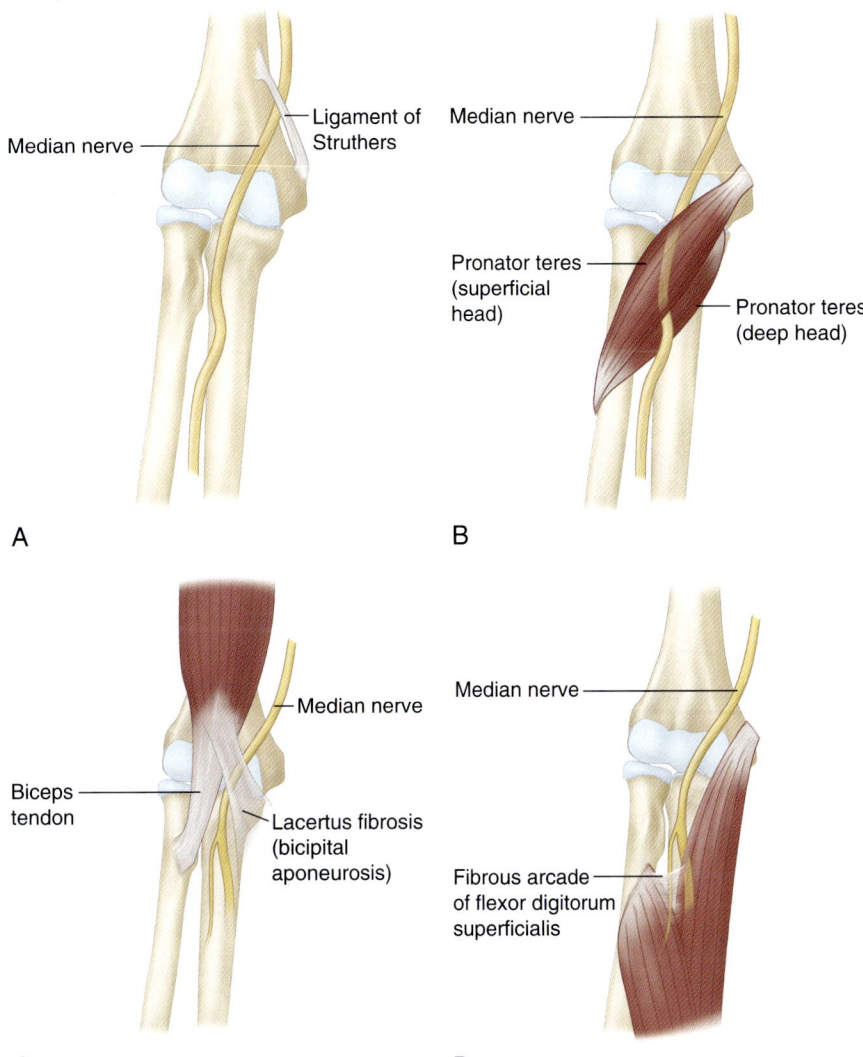

Median nerve

Ligament of Struthers

Median nerve

Pronator teres (superficial head)

Pronator teres (deep head)

Median nerve

Biceps tendon

Lacertus fibrosis (bicipital aponeurosis)

Median nerve

Fibrous arcade of flexor digitorum superficialis

A   B

C   D

Figure 15–1 Possible sites of compression in pronator syndrome. **A:** Ligament of Struthers (Arcade VIII). **B:** Pronator teres. **C:** Bicipital aponeurosis. **D:** Fibrous arcade at the proximal margin of the FDS to the middle finger. (From Koo J, Szabo RM. Compression neuropathies of the median nerve. J Am Soc Surg Hand 2004;4:156–75,[32] with permission. Data from Doyle J, Botte MJ. Surgical Anatomy of the Hand and Upper Extremity. Philadelphia: Lippincott Williams & Wilkins, 2003,[61] with permission.)

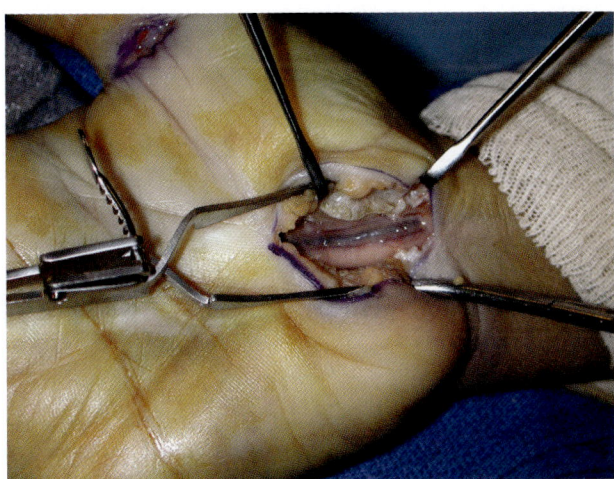

Figure 15–2 Persistent median artery seen during a carpal tunnel release.

the FPL and FDP, giving off two to six branches to each of these muscles. The nerve reaches the anterior surface of the interosseous membrane and travels with the anterior interosseous artery to the PQ where it penetrates the muscle proximally and passes deep to the belly to innervate the muscle.[61] It ends by sending sensory afferent branches to the intercarpal, radiocarpal, and distal radioulnar joints.[80]

The AIN may be compressed by fibrous bands from the deep (most common) or superficial head of the PT to the brachialis fascia.[81] Other possible sites of compression include the fibrous tissue arcade of the FDS under which the AIN passes,[70] enlarged bursae or tumors, aberrant or thrombosed vessels,[82] an accessory bicipital aponeurosis overlying the nerve,[83] compression of the nerve as it runs deep to both heads of the PT, and fractures of the forearm and distal humerus.[70,81] Aberrant muscles have been associated with AIN syndrome, including Gantzer's muscle, the palmaris profundus, and the flexor carpi radialis brevis[70,84,85] (Fig. 15–3).

Lister[86] and Spinner[87] have both implicated Gantzer's muscle as a possible cause of AIN syndrome. Al-Qattan showed that the median nerve is closely related to Gantzer's muscle when it passed deep to the deep head of the PT, or when the deep head of the pronator was absent.[75] Doyle and Botte demonstrated the possibility of a "pincer-like effect" when they dissected a forearm with a Gantzer's muscle present, and found that the median

nerve and AIN passed through the interval between the muscle and the adjacent anterior FDS, which shared a common origin on the medial epicondyle.[61]

Carpal Tunnel

The carpal tunnel is open ended proximally and distally, but behaves like a closed compartment physiologically and maintains its own distinct tissue fluid pressure levels.[88] It is a fibro-osseous canal that is dorsally bounded by the concave arch of the carpal bones, and

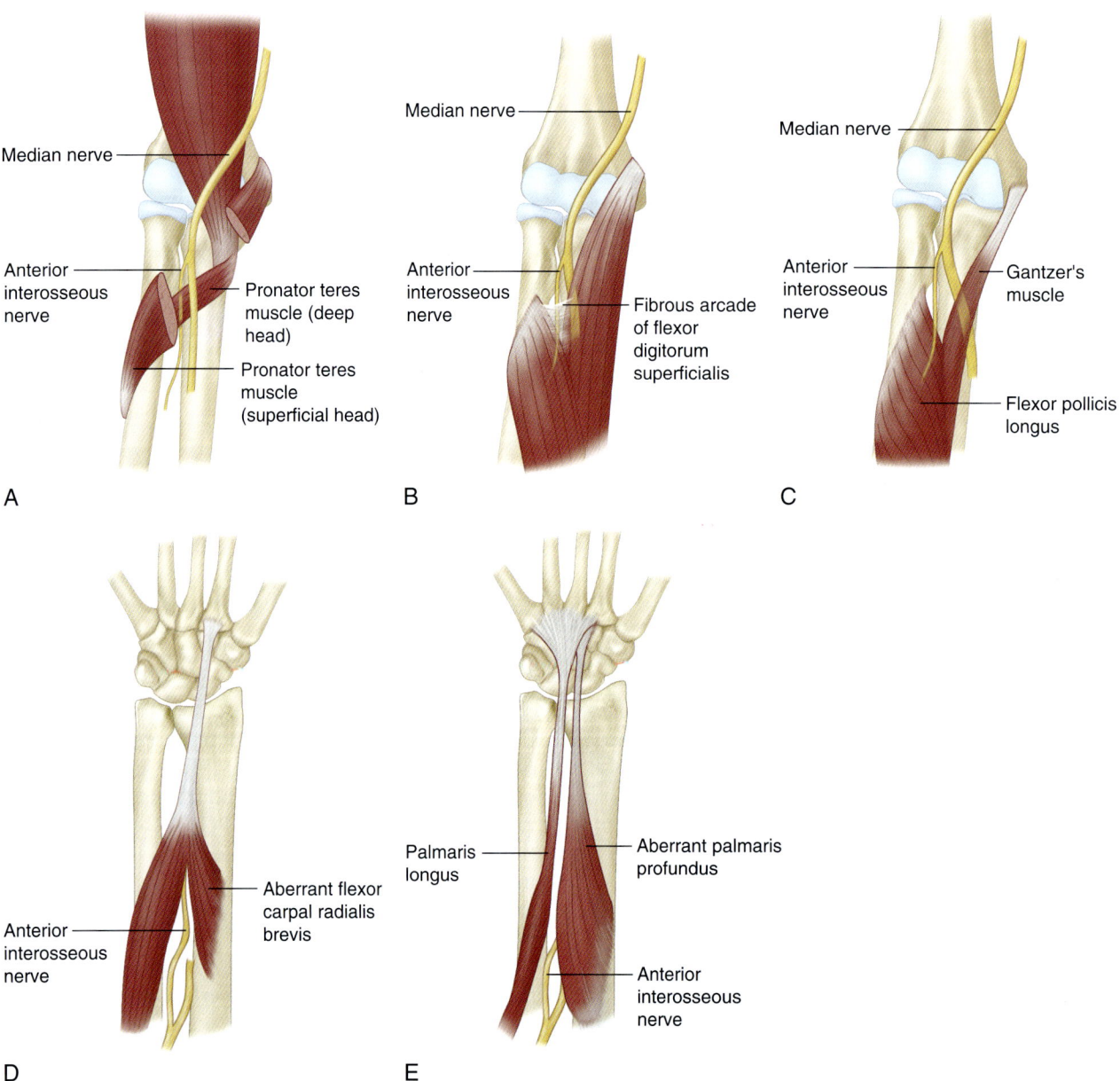

Figure 15–3 Possible sites of compression in anterior interosseous nerve syndrome. **A:** Deep head of the pronator. **B:** Fibrous arcade at the proximal margin of the FDS to the middle finger. Aberrant muscles have been associated with AINS, including **(C)** Gantzer's muscle, **(D)** the flexor carpi radialis brevis, and **(E)** the palmaris profundus. (From Koo J, Szabo RM. Compression neuropathies of the median nerve. J Am Soc Surg Hand 2004;4:156–75,[32] with permission. Data from Doyle J, Botte MJ. Surgical Anatomy of the Hand and Upper Extremity. Philadelphia: Lippincott Williams & Wilkins, 2003,[61] with permission.)

the flexor retinaculum (FR) volarly. There are actually two separate layers of fascia over the volar carpal canal. The more superficial is the thickened antebrachial fascia proximally and the palmar fascia distally, while the deep layer is the FR. The hook of the hamate, triquetrum, and pisiform form the ulnar border, while the radial border consists of the scaphoid, trapezium, and the fascial septum overlying the FCR.

Cobb et al. observed that the FR consists of three distinct and continuous segments that extend from the distal radius to the base of the long finger metacarpal[89] (Fig. 15–4). The proximal segment is continuous with the deep forearm fascia and is inseparable from the thickened antebrachial fascia, while the transverse carpal ligament (TCL) makes up the second part of the FR. The TCL arises from the scaphoid tuberosity and trapezial beak radially and from the pisiform and hook of the hamate ulnarly. The distal segment of the FR consists of the aponeurosis between the thenar and hypothenar muscles.

The median nerve becomes superficial in the forearm approximately 5 cm proximal to the wrist, lies between the tendons of the FDS and FCR, and is dorsal or dorsoradial to the palmaris longus. It passes under the FR in the radiopalmar portion of the carpal tunnel at a level that corresponds to the volar flexion crease of the wrist. At the distal edge of the retinaculum, the nerve normally divides into six branches: the recurrent motor branch, three proper digital nerves, and two common digital nerves. In 78% of cases, the motor fascicles occupy a radiopalmar position in the nerve; in the remainder, they are located in the central palmar portion of the nerve.[90]

The motor branch passes through a separate fascial tunnel immediately before entering the thenar muscles in 56% of specimens.[55] The first lumbrical muscle is innervated by motor branches that originate from the radial digital nerve to the index finger. The second lumbrical is innervated by motor branches that originate from the common digital nerve to the index and long fingers.[91] The palmar cutaneous branch (PCN) originates from the radiopalmar aspect of the median nerve, about 5 cm proximal to the wrist crease. After traveling with the main nerve for 1.6 to 2.5 cm, it courses separately under the antebrachial fascia between the PL and FCR tendons.[92,93] It emerges through the fascia 0.8 cm proximal to the wrist crease, and then divides into a radial and one or more ulnar branches. Within the subcutaneous tissue overlying the flexor retinaculum, the terminal portions of the ulnar PCN branch may be encountered as transverse sensory nerves during routine carpal tunnel decompression.

Variations of median nerve anatomy in the carpal tunnel have been well characterized by Lanz.[47] He described eight patterns. High divisions of the median nerve (Group III) may arise in the proximal or middle third of the forearm and travel a parallel course, separated by a persistent median artery or an aberrant muscle, and may rejoin distal to the TCL. Amadio reported a unilateral variation of the high-division/closed-loop anomaly that included a separate compartment within the carpal tunnel through which passed the radial half of a bifid median nerve.[44] Szabo and Pettey reported a bilateral Group III variation in which the radial-most branch of each median nerve occupied an accessory ligamentous compartment beneath its transverse carpal ligament[94] (Fig. 15–5).

The recurrent motor branch passes through or around the distal edge of the TCL in one of three pat-

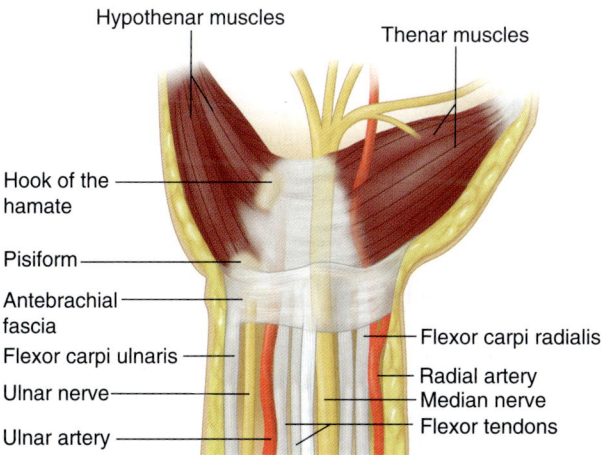

Figure 15–4 Flexor retinaculum (transverse carpal ligament). The proximal segment (1) is continuous with the deep forearm fascia and is inseparable from the thickened antebrachial fascia, whereas the TCL makes up the second portion (2). The distal segment of the FCR (3) consists of the aponeurosis between the thenar and hypothenar muscles. (From Koo J, Szabo RM. Compression neuropathies of the median nerve. J Am Soc Surg Hand 2004;4:156–75,[32] with permission. Data from Doyle J, Botte MJ. Surgical Anatomy of the Hand and Upper Extremity. Philadelphia: Lippincott Williams & Wilkins, 2003,[61] with permission.)

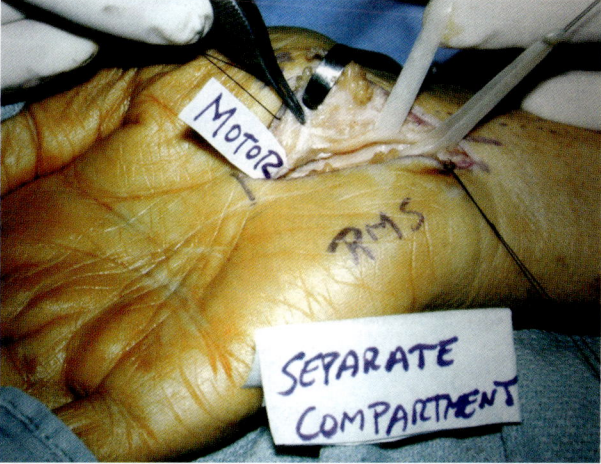

Figure 15–5 During a routine carpal tunnel release, the radial-most branch of this patient's median nerve occupied an accessory ligamentous compartment beneath its transverse carpal ligament.

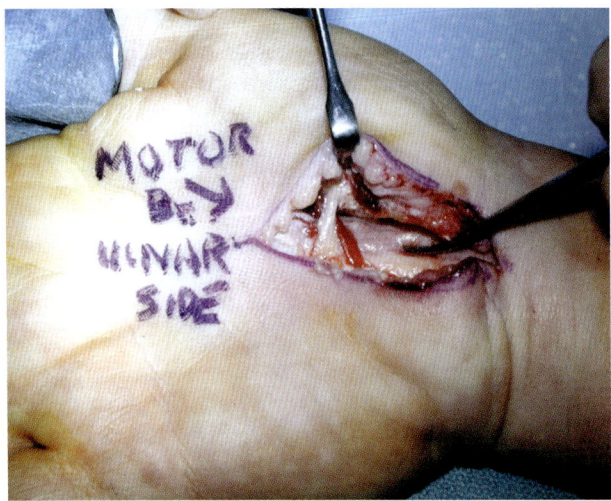

Figure 15–6 This patient's motor branch originated from the ulnar side of the median nerve in the distal carpal tunnel.

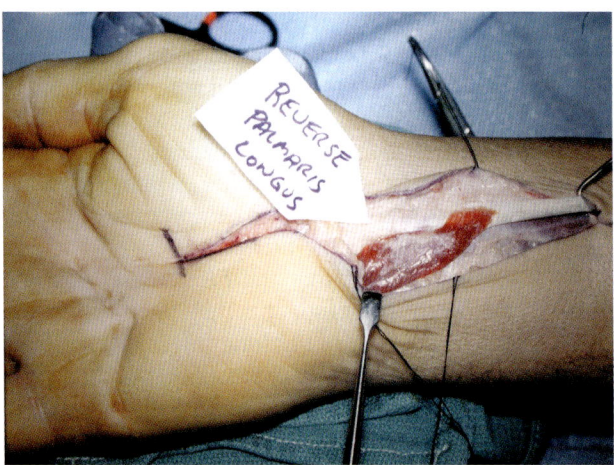

Figure 15–7 This patient had a reverse palmaris longus muscle where the muscle itself inserted distally on the transverse carpal ligament.

terns: extraligamentous (46% to 90%), subligamentous (31%), and transligamentous (23%).[95] Rarely, it may take off from the ulnar aspect of the median nerve[47,96] (Fig. 15–6). In 4% of cases, Amadio found that there may be multiple recurrent branches.[97] When multiple recurrent branches were present, about 50% of them passed through the FR.

The median and ulnar nerves can be connected in the forearm by Martin-Gruber connections 15% of the time.[98] In 50% of cases, this communication originates from the AIN. Some of the intrinsic hand muscles in 7.5% of limbs are thus supplied by the median nerve.[61]

The palmar cutaneous branch (PCN) originates 5 cm proximal to the proximal wrist crease. It travels with the median nerve for 1.6 to 2.5 cm before it separates, enters a short tunnel immediately medial to the FCR tendon, and innervates the skin of the thenar eminence.[93] This area of sensibility is important in differentiating proximal median nerve compression from carpal tunnel syndrome.[61] It varies in its exact branching pattern.[99–101] In one study the PCN was noted to pierce the PL tendon 1 to 1.5 cm proximal to its insertion into the palmar fascia,[102] but it can emerge through the antebrachial fascia as far as 2.6 cm proximal to the wrist crease.[99]

Anatomically, two areas of the carpal tunnel may cause median nerve compression. The first is at the proximal edge of the TCL, where compression may be produced by acute flexion of the wrist, which explains the positive Phalen's test (wrist flexion test) in carpal tunnel syndrome. The second is adjacent to the hook of the hamate, where Doyle most commonly observed the location of the hourglass deformity in the median nerve seen at carpal tunnel release.[61]

Compression within the carpal tunnel may also result from any space-occupying lesion.[103–105] Common causes

include flexor tenosynovitis, fractures and dislocations of the floor of the canal and distal radius, tumors, and ganglia. These space-occupying lesions increase the pressure within the noncompliant carpal tunnel compartment thus compressing the median nerve. Some cases are attributed to "nonspecific synovitis" (nonrheumatoid), although the synovium from the carpal canal in these cases usually fails to reveal signs of inflammation. Biopsies of tenosynovium from 177 wrists undergoing carpal tunnel release revealed inflammatory cells in only 10%; however, edema and vascular sclerosis were consistently present 98% of the time,[106,107] which themselves may be secondary to compression rather than the primary cause of the entrapment neuropathy.[108,109] Nakamichi and Tachibana have also reported a case of median nerve compression after release of the antebrachial fascia during a carpal tunnel release. The nerve was compressed by a palmaris longus tendon that was inserted radially into the thenar fascia.[110] Other muscle variations are found to contribute to median nerve compression in the carpal canal (Figs. 15–7 and 15–8).

INVESTIGATION

Prontator Syndrome

Physical examination reveals tenderness on palpation of the median nerve in the proximal forearm. The PT muscle can be tender and firm, or appear to be enlarged.[35] There is no weakness of the median-innervated intrinsic or extrinsic muscles. Palpation of the medial humeral condyle and distal diaphysis may reveal a bony prominence, the supracondylar process. AP, lateral, and oblique x-rays of the elbow should be obtained to rule out its presence. The absence of a supracondylar process does not rule out the existence

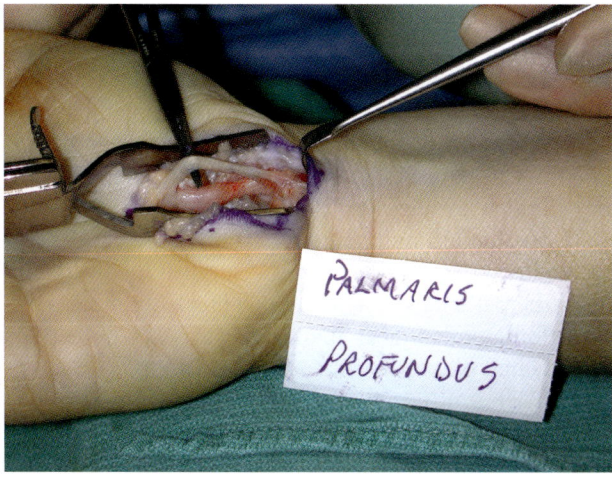

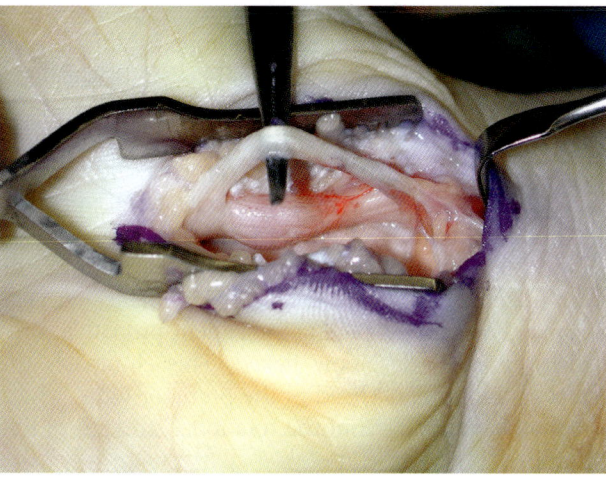

Figure 15–8   Example of a palmaris profundus. **A:** The muscle belly can be seen just under the proximal retractor. The tendon inserts underneath the transverse carpal ligament. **B:** Closer view demonstrates the tendon coursing from ulnar to radial crossing the median nerve contributing to compression.

of a ligament of Struthers and entrapment at this site,[65] nor does its presence ensure that the ligament of Struthers is indeed the site of compression. This is a very rare site of entrapment.[25] Threshold testing with Semmes-Weinstein monofilaments may reveal decreased sensibility over the distribution of the median nerve, including the thenar eminence.[111]

Phalen's wrist flexion test should be negative, but may be positive.[112,113] Tinel's nerve percussion test, in which the median nerve in the proximal forearm is percussed, elicits tingling and paresthesias proximal to the wrist in contrast to carpal tunnel syndrome, where this test is positive distally at the wrist. The pronator compression test has been found to be an accurate and dependable physical sign in the diagnosis of pronator syndrome. Manual compression of the median nerve at or near the pronator muscle usually reproduced pares-

thesias in the median-innervated distribution within 30 seconds.[112,114]

Several provocative manuevers can be utilized to try to localize the site of median nerve compression. Complaints resulting from flexion of the elbow against resistance when the elbow is at 120 to 135 degrees of flexion may suggest compression by a ligament of Struthers. Pain or paresthesias produced by resisted forearm supination in combination with resisted elbow flexion beyond 120 degrees implicates compression at the bicipital aponeurosis.[33,34,115,116] Paresthesias resulting from resisted forearm pronation while the elbow is slowly extended from full flexion suggests compression between the two heads of the PT.[34,80,115] Resisted proximal interphalangeal joint flexion of the middle finger producing paresthesias in the radial three digits suggests entrapment under the fibrous origin of the FDS.[35,115]

Even in patients with a clinical history and physical findings compatible with pronator syndrome, fewer than 50% can be confirmed by electrodiagnostic testing.[113] Mysiew and Colachis were unable to improve this yield by the use of three test maneuvers (elbow flexion, forearm pronation, and finger flexion against resistance) in conjunction with conventional nerve conduction studies.[117]

Median nerve compression neuropathies in the distal arm and forearm are extremely uncommon when compared to carpal tunnel syndrome.[55] In a review of 4838 electromyographic (EMG) studies, Gross and Jones found that 0.2% of the patients tested had findings of proximal median nerve compression as compared with 23% with median neuropathy at the wrist.[118] However, the value in obtaining these studies is to evaluate for possible carpal tunnel syndrome. A normal conduction velocity at the wrist in conjunction with the signs and symptoms of pronator syndrome supports a diagnosis of proximal compression of the median nerve. A study consistent with carpal tunnel syndrome necessitates treatment directed at the wrist, but does not rule out a more proximal lesion, the double-crush phenomenon.[25] Failed carpal tunnel releases that respond to subsequent operative release in the proximal forearm support the occurrence of simultaneous lesions.[112]

Nerve conduction velocity measurement of the median nerve in the proximal forearm is misleading because reduced velocity of conduction in the forearm has been noted in 20% to 32% of patients with carpal tunnel syndrome.[55] This slowing had been attributed to artifact in the electrodiagnostic method rather than pathology in the forearm. Pease et al. confirmed that forearm median nerve conduction velocities in patients with carpal tunnel syndrome are significantly slower than those in normal subjects by using direct evaluation of the forearm median nerve by the stimulation and recording of the forearm nerve action potential (FNAP) proximal to the wrist. This suggested that retrograde degeneration of the nerve axons may result from entrapment in the carpal tunnel.[119] Using the same technique, Chang et al. confirmed that retrograde degeneration of the median nerve does exist in carpal tunnel syndrome. However, retrograde degeneration contributed little to the reduced forearm median motor conduction velocity (MMCV), which resulted from the block of faster conduction fibers at the wrist. They concluded that technique artifact did, in fact, play a role in the proximal slowing found in standard electrodiagnosis.[120] Moreover, Anastasopoulos compared motor velocities calculated by F-waves obtained from muscles with the same root and nerve supply but different median branches, one emerging before the carpal tunnel (pronator quadratus muscle) and one passing through the tunnel (abductor pollicis brevis), and showed that slowing of median nerve proximal conduction velocity in patients with carpal tunnel syndrome is restricted to the fibers that distally pass through the carpal tunnel and does not necessarily imply an additional proximal lesion.[121] Finally, Olehnik found that electrodiagnostic studies were a poor predictor of outcome after surgical decompression in a series of 36 patients.[112]

Anterior Interosseous Syndrome

AIN syndrome must be differentiated from Parsonage-Turner syndrome, also known as brachial plexus neuritis or neuralgic amyotrophy. In a brachial neuritis, pain in the arm, elbow, and/or forearm often precedes the motor symptoms, and there is no history of trauma. The pain symptoms may be unrelated to the motor findings, and can appear spontaneously,[122] following a viral illness[123-125] or vaccination,[126,127] or be expressed as part of a hereditary syndrome.[128] There have also been cases of brachial neuritis associated with acute Q fever,[129] infective endocarditis,[130] and HIV seroconversion.[131] In Parsonage and Turner's original description, 10% of the patients had antecedent surgery. Malamut et al. reported six patients with postsurgical neuralgic amyotrophy.[132] There have also been reports of epidemiologic clustering in geographic locations.[133]

By contrast, the patient with a localized compression neuropathy will usually have a history of trauma or repetitive injury, may have associated sensory findings in the distribution of the median nerve, will not have preceding pain except that associated with trauma, and will not have proximal brachial plexus abnormalities.[134] Bilateral involvement should alert one to the possibility of Parsonage-Turner syndrome, however, Braun and Spinner reported a patient with bilateral AINS secondary to compression by enlarged communicating veins.[135] Szwejbka et al. reported a patient who developed bilateral anterior interosseous neuropathy following an abdominal surgical procedure most likely representing a neuritis.[24]

Electrodiagnostic findings can be identical in these two conditions.[55] Shoulder girdle EMG studies should be obtained in all AIN syndrome patients to exclude neuralgic amyotrophy, with possible supplementation by magnetic resonance images (MRI).[136,137] It is important to make this diagnosis because treatment recommendations are highly specialty oriented. Good results were obtained in both the surgical and medical specialties, with 90% of patients in the surgical literature and all of the patients in the neurology literature recovering. Therefore, nonsurgical management is recommended for brachial plexus neuritis–induced AIN palsy.[134]

In AIN syndrome, patients typically present with complaints of vague, aching pain in the proximal forearm that occurs at rest and is exacerbated by activity. The patient may have difficulty with writing and activities that require tip pinch. The thumb and index finger assume a classic position during pinch in this syndrome (Fig. 15–9). The index finger extends at the distal interphalangeal joint with compensatory increased flexion at the proximal interphalangeal joint. The thumb hyperextends at the interphalangeal joint and displays increased flexion of the metacarpophalangeal joint.

AIN syndrome is characterized by loss of function of the FPL and FDP to the index, and sometimes the long finger and the PQ. Sensibility is unaffected. The PQ may be tested by having the patient pronate against resistance with the elbow flexed. This eliminates the effect of the humeral head of the pronator teres, which is responsible for 75% of the rotational strength of this muscle.[138]

AIN syndrome can be present with varying levels of severity. An incomplete syndrome can occur with either weakness or absence of the FPL or FDP of the index

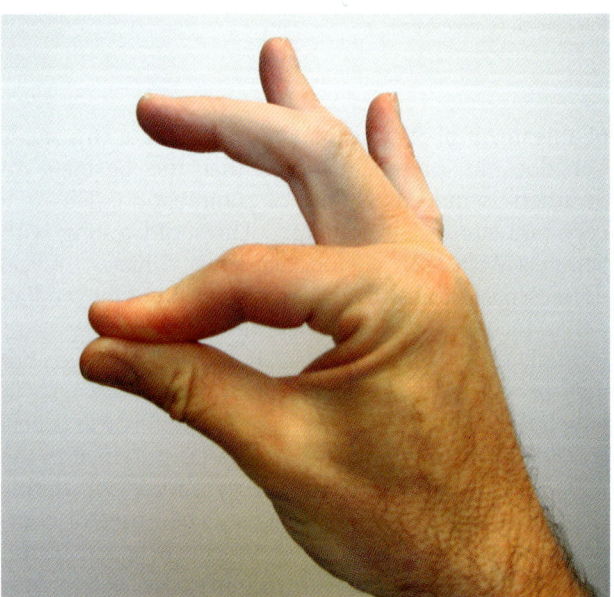

Figure 15–9   Pinch disturbance seen with anterior interosseous nerve palsy.

finger alone with normal PQ function.[81] All of the profundus tendons may be AIN innervated, with subsequent weakness of all the fingers.[79,139,141]

Martin-Gruber connections (variant connection from the median nerve or AIN to the ulnar nerve in the forearm) occur in about 15% of individuals[61,142]; 50% of Martin-Gruber connections arise from the AIN. Therefore, hand intrinsic muscles may be affected resulting from weakness of the first dorsal interosseous, adductor pollicis, and/or abductor digiti minimi.[82] In 30% of specimens studied, the FDS was innervated from the AIN,[79,140] so patients may present with weakness in this muscle as well.[80]

One must differentiate between AIN syndrome and rupture of the FDP or FPL, which may occur from rheumatoid arthritis, Keinböck's disease, and scaphoid nonunion. In Hill's series of 33 patients, 10 patients had an initial diagnosis of tendon rupture.[81] This is assessed by looking for the tenodesis effect of the FPL and the index FDP while flexing and extending the wrist.[143]

Carpal Tunnel Syndrome

Threshold sensory tests, such as the Semmes-Weinstein monofilaments and vibrometry, and direct compression and Durkan pressure tests are the most sensitive.[144–149] Electromyographic studies of the thenar muscles can help quantitate the severity of median nerve compression by looking for signs of denervation.

Although MRI and ultrasound have been used to evaluate carpal tunnel syndrome,[150–153] electrodiagnosis is considered the "gold standard," and all predictors of carpal tunnel syndrome are judged against it.[154] Some authors, observing that neurophysiologic exams afford the only objective test of median nerve function, have concluded that carpal tunnel syndrome should be diagnosed solely on the basis of electrodiagnostic exams.[155,156] Nerve conduction studies can provide objective evidence of impaired conduction, but standards vary widely.[157,158] In general, distal motor latencies of more than 4.5 ms and distal sensory latencies of more than 3.5 milliseconds (ms) are considered abnormal. Asymmetry of conduction between both hands of more than 1 ms for motor conduction or 0.5 ms for sensory conduction time is also considered abnormal. Nevertheless, a group of 12 medical researchers agreed by consensus that a positive electrodiagnostic test with absent symptoms cannot lead to a diagnosis of carpal tunnel syndrome.[159] They were also unable to come to agree on the diagnosis of subjects with classic symptoms of carpal tunnel syndrome and negative electrodiagnostic findings.[159]

Phalen's wrist flexion test, direct compression of the median nerve, Tinel's nerve percussion test,[45] and a hand diagram in which the patient marks on an outline of the dorsal and palmar aspects of the hand the location of pain, numbness, or tingling[160] are easily performed clinical tests. Clinical history and physical exam including provocative tests are more easily performed than electrodiagnostic studies, and they are the most appropriate diagnostic tools in the ambulatory setting.[58]

Szabo et al. found that Durkan's compression test (89%), Semmes-Weinstein testing after Phalen's maneuver (83%), and hand diagram scores (76%) were the most sensitive tests for the diagnosis of carpal tunnel syndrome. Night pain was a sensitive symptom predictor (96%). The most specific tests were the hand diagram (76%) and Tinel's sign (71%). If a patient had an abnormal hand diagram, abnormal sensibility by Semmes-Weinstein testing in wrist-neutral position, a positive Durkan's test, and night pain, the probability of having carpal tunnel syndrome was 0.86. If all four of these conditions were normal, the probability of having carpal tunnel syndrome was 0.0068. They concluded that the addition of electrodiagnostic tests did not increase the diagnostic power of the combination of four clinical tests.[58]

TREATMENT

Prontator Syndrome

Nonoperative Management

In patients with symptoms of short duration, relief may be achieved by modification or cessation of the provocative activities. Steroid injections have little to offer in the nonoperative management of proximal median nerve compression. Anti-inflammatory medications in combination with immobilization in a removable long-arm splint (with the elbow in 90 degrees flexion, forearm in slight pronation, and wrist in slight flexion) for 4 to 6 weeks may relieve pressure and traction on the median nerve because symptoms in pronator syndrome are often caused by repetitive elbow flexion/extension and forearm pronation/supination. In pronator syndrome, 50% of patients will respond to nonoperative therapy,[34] but failure to improve is an indication for exploration and release of the entire course of the proximal median nerve.

Operative Technique

A tourniquet is inflated, and the incision is usually started medially, 5 cm proximal to the elbow flexion crease (Fig. 15–10). However, if either a supracondylar process or accessory bicipital aponeurosis has been identified, the incision should begin at least 10 cm proximal to the elbow crease. The incision is curved distally just medial to the biceps tendon, crosses the antecubital crease in a lazy-S, and gently curves radially for 5 cm in the proximal forearm.[161] The medial antebrachial

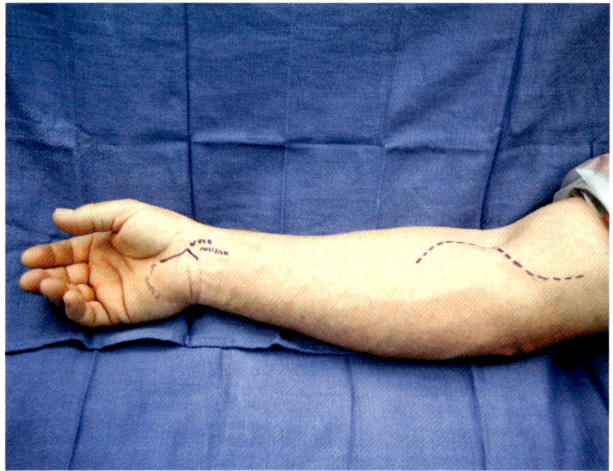

Figure 15–10   Incision in proximal forearm/elbow for exploration of median nerve. This patient had recurrent median nerve symptoms after previous carpal tunnel release. He was referred with the diagnosis of recurrent carpal tunnel syndrome, but had symptoms of pronator syndrome (positive provocative signs and decreased sensation in the palmar cutaneous nerve). He also had a positive Tinel sign distal to his previous carpal tunnel incision. Both areas were explored.

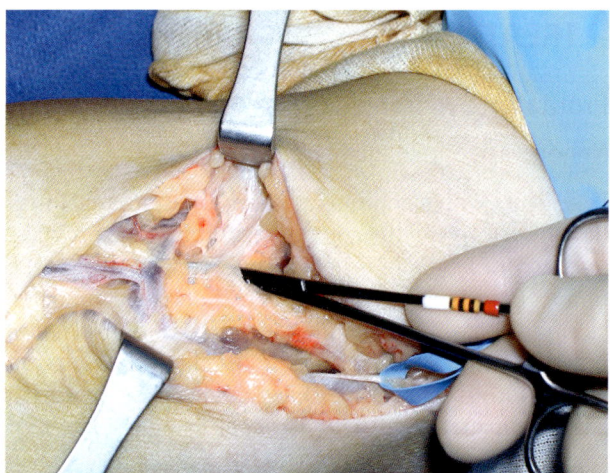

Figure 15–11   Identification of the bicipital aponeurosis under the hemostat. The medial antebrachial cutaneous nerve is tagged with a rubber dam.

cutaneous nerve is identified and gently retracted as it courses next to the basilic vein.[162] The median nerve is identified proximal to the elbow and tagged. The bicipital aponeurosis is incised (Fig. 15–11). If a supracondylar process or accessory bicipital aponeurosis has been diagnosed preoperatively, the median nerve must be located at the most proximal extent of the incision and traced distally. The ligament of Struthers and the supracondylar process are excised, and if present, the accessory bicipital aponeurosis is divided (Fig. 15–12).

Because other sites of compression may be present, the median nerve must be explored distally. The nerve is traced to the proximal border of the superficial head of the PT. Retraction of the superficial head will assist in recognizing any variation of the nerve's course in relation to the two heads of the pronator. Tendinous or fibrous bands within the pronator are identified and incised. If a persistent median artery is found to penetrate the median nerve, passage of the artery can be enlarged by interfascicular dissection. Ligation of this artery is avoided because it provides the dominant blood supply to the proximal median nerve in 30% of cases, and significantly contributes to the blood supply of the index and long fingers in the presence of an incomplete superficial palmar arterial arch.[73] However, if muscular branches from the persistent median artery are found crossing the nerve, they should be ligated.

Most of the time, the median nerve passes between the two heads of the pronator teres. If visualization of the anterior interosseous nerve is inadequate, the insertion of the superficial head can be divided and tagged for later reattachment. If a variant is encountered (i.e., the median and anterior interosseous nerves passing deep to both heads of the pronator teres), the deep head can be detached at its tendinous insertion on the radius and reflected proximally and ulnarly to fully expose the distal course of the nerves. If further exposure is needed, the radial origin of the superficialis can be released.

Attention is next directed to the superficialis arcade. The anterior interosseous and median nerves pass deep to the superficialis arch distal to the pronator teres. This arch is incised because it may be a source of compression, particularly if it is thickened (Fig. 15–13). Careful dissection just distal to the arch is continued, with attention directed at finding anatomic variants such as accessory muscles. Any site of compression is relieved.

The tourniquet is deflated and careful hemostasis is obtained with bipolar cautery. The PT is reattached if detachment was necessary. The muscle should not be shortened or tightened lest a new compressive lesion be created. Epineurotomy or internal neurolysis is not necessary and may, in fact, be harmful.[55] Subcutaneous transposition of the median nerve is also not recommended. The subcutaneous layer is closed with 4-0 interrupted absorbable sutures, and skin is approximated with 5-0 nylon simple sutures (or alternatively with a running subcuticular 4-0 nylon suture).

Postoperative Management

Postoperatively, the arm is placed for comfort in a bulky, above elbow plaster splint that maintains the elbow at 90 degrees of flexion, the forearm in 45 degrees of pronation, and the wrist in slight flexion. Sutures are removed at 7 to 10 days and Steri-Strips are applied. This incision tends to spread, and careful attention to detail will improve final cosmesis. Gentle elbow range-

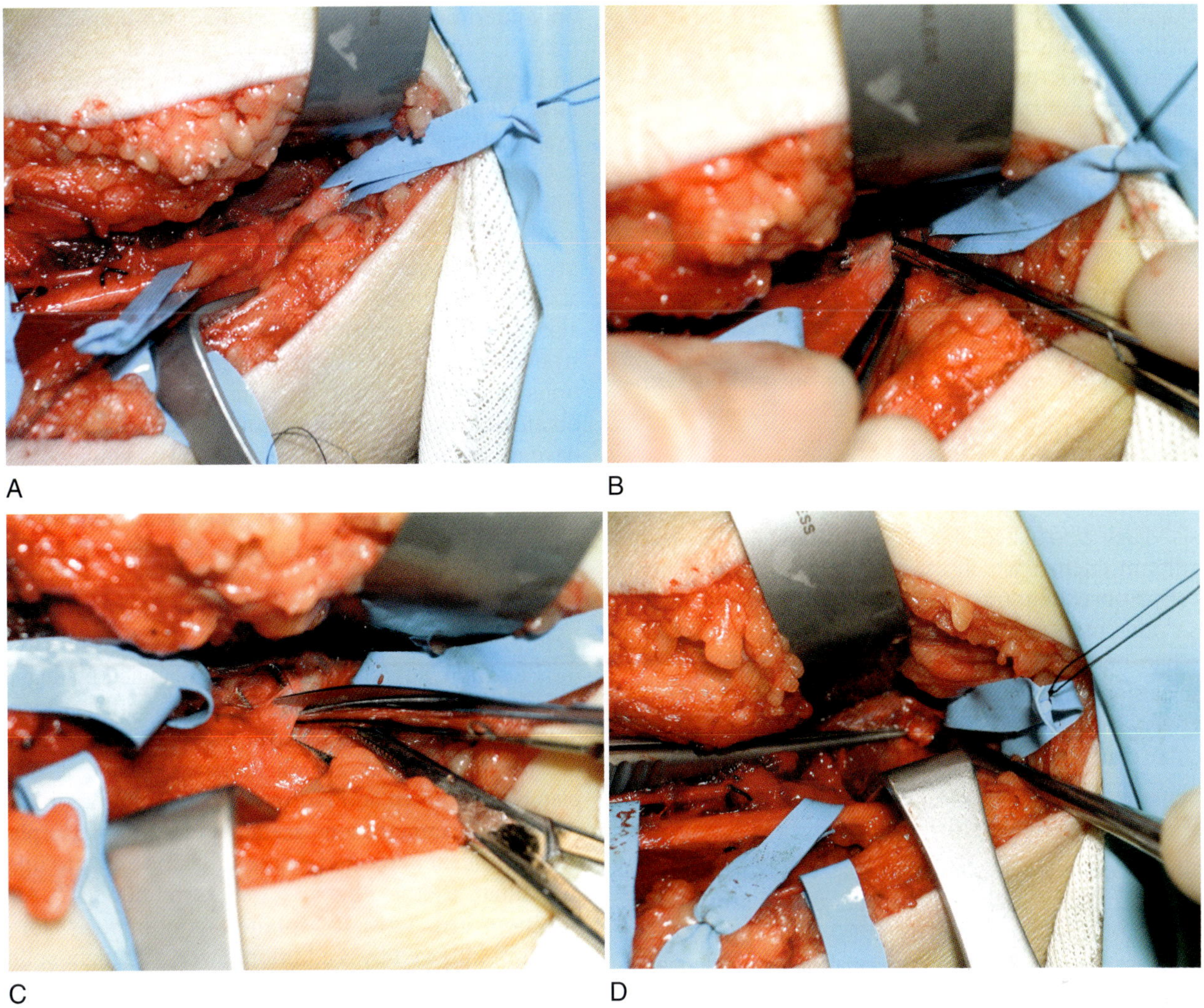

Figure 15–12   The median nerve was compressed by a ligament of Struthers. **A:** Rubber dams surround the nerve proximally and distally to the site of compression. **B:** Extent of ligament identified. **C:** Ligament incised. **D:** The supracondylar process (from which the ligament of Struthers originated) at the end of forceps was then excised.

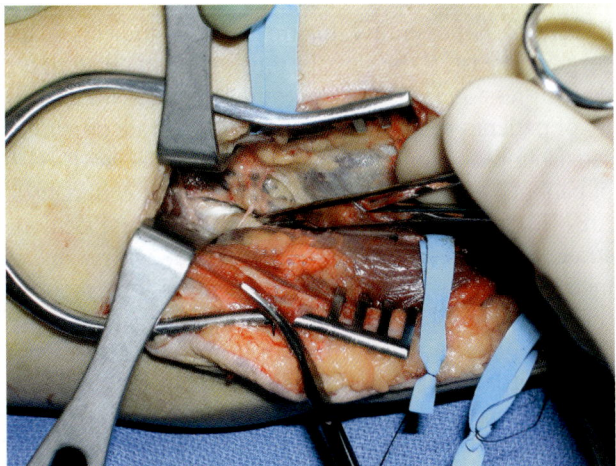

Figure 15–13   The median nerve is coursing under the superficialis arcade, which was very tight in this patient.

of-motion exercises are begun. Resistive activities are avoided until 6 to 8 weeks after surgery.

Surgical decompression generally yields good results. Olehnik et al. reported improvement in 77% of their patients,[112] while Johnson et al.[34] and Hartz et al.[113] reported improvement in 92% of patients. In the series by Olehnik et al., 33 of 36 patients returned to work, 25 to their original jobs.

Anterior Interosseous Syndrome

Nonoperative Management

Three weeks should be allowed to elapse before baseline electrodiagnostic studies are obtained. This is to allow Wallerian degeneration to be detected electromyographically. If there is no improvement either clinically or by EMG studies by 4 to 6 months after diagnosis, surgical exploration is indicated. Even though return of function has been reported up to 18 months after onset of symptoms, expectant treatment is less predictable than surgical intervention, and recovery is often incomplete.[37,71,163]

Operative Technique

The surgical approach and postoperative management for AIN palsy is essentially the same as for pronator syndrome, with one caveat. Microscope-assisted interfascicular neurolysis of the AIN within the substance of the median nerve (2 to 7.5 cm above the elbow) should be considered in any patient in whom an obvious compression site cannot be localized.[164,165] Nagano et al. explored the AIN in nine patients with spontaneous palsy, and found hourglass-like fascicular constrictions in eight of them only after performing internal neurolysis. They postulated that inflammation in the nerve results in edema, which causes the fascicles to adhere locally. Subsequent traction by elbow flexion and extension pulls more strongly on the shorter segment of the median nerve forming the anterior interosseous nerve fascicles and causes them to become constricted. Good recovery was obtained in their series following interfascicular neurolysis.

Postoperative Management

Postoperative care is similar to that for pronator syndrome. The arm is placed in a bulky, long arm plaster splint that maintains the elbow at 90 degrees of flexion, the forearm in 45 degrees of pronation, and the wrist in slight flexion. This immobilization is primarily for patient comfort. Full return of function can take longer than 6 months.

Carpal Tunnel Syndrome

Nonoperative Management

Nonoperative therapy may include splinting the wrist in neutral position, oral anti-inflammatory drugs, diuretics, and management of underlying systemic diseases.[166–168] In a small study, Gerritsen suggested that wrist splinting alone had a low chance of success, and that only the subset of patients with a brief history of carpal tunnel syndrome complaints (1 year or less) and mild to moderate severity of paresthesias at night (a score of 6 or less out of 10) had a 62% chance of success.[169] The great interest in pyridoxine (vitamin B6) for the treatment of carpal tunnel syndrome has faded because it does not appear to modify the natural history of this disease.[170]

Steroid injection offers transient relief to 80% of patients, but only 22% will be symptom-free 12 months later. Those most likely to benefit from conservative management have had symptoms for less than 1 year,

only intermittent numbness, normal two-point discrimination, only 1- to 2-ms prolongation of distal motor and sensory latencies, and no motor findings (no weakness, thenar atrophy, or denervation potentials on EMG examination).[166] Forty percent of this group will remain symptom free for longer than 12 months. Complications from intraneural injections can mostly be avoided when a soluble preparation of dexamethasone is injected and proper technique is used by physicians knowledgeable about carpal tunnel surgery.[171,172] Steroid injection may also serve a diagnostic purpose. Green has demonstrated a strong correlation between the results of injections and subsequent operations in that a patient who obtained a good response from steroid injection will have a high probability of responding to surgical management.[173] This was confirmed recently by Edgell et al.[174] However, poor relief from injection did not necessarily mean that the patient was a poor candidate for surgery.[173]

A 22- or 25-gauge needle may be used. At a point 1 cm proximal to the distal wrist flexion crease between the PL and FCR tendons, the needle is angled 45 degrees distally and dorsally, and is advanced until it touches the floor of the canal. It is then withdrawn 0.5 cm. If median paresthesias are elicited, the needle is completely withdrawn and redirected.[175] A solution of 1 mL (4 mg) of dexamethasone acetate and 2 mL of 1% plain lidocaine is then injected. Some surgeons prefer to inject just ulnar to the palmaris longus tendon.[17,168] After injection, the wrist is splinted continuously for 3 weeks[166] followed by 3 additional weeks of night splinting.[176] While ergonomic interventions may create a more comfortable work environment, there is no compelling evidence to suggest efficacy in the treatment of documented carpal tunnel syndrome.

Surgical Management

Failure of nonoperative treatment is an indication for surgical release of the carpal tunnel. Open median nerve decompression leads to symptomatic relief in the majority of patients. Osterman reported a 96% rate of patient satisfaction and improvement of symptoms, with 84% of patients returning to their original jobs after surgery.[30] An MRI study of 15 hands after open release demonstrated consistent increases in volume, with a mean increase of 24%, and a change in morphology of the tunnel from oval to circular.[177,178]

Influenced by the arthroscopic revolution that has redefined joint surgery, several endoscopic methods to release the carpal tunnel have been introduced in an effort to decrease postoperative morbidity. Proponents of these techniques cite the smaller scar and an earlier rehabilitation as advantages. Although many variations have been introduced,[179,180] there are fundamentally two competing endoscopic techniques: the two-portal

Chow technique,[181–183] and the single proximal incision Agee technique.[184–186] "Minimally invasive" or minimal scar techniques have also been described.[187–190]

Safety, efficacy, and cost issues are still under scrutiny.[191] Cadaver studies have demonstrated incomplete release in as high as 50% of specimens.[192–194] Pillar pain has not been reduced and palmar tenderness has not been eliminated. After open carpal tunnel release, patients typically regain their preoperative baseline grip strength within 3 months, and pinch strength within 6 weeks.[195] Endoscopic carpal tunnel release shortens this period only minimally. These small benefits must be weighed against the significant disadvantage of poor or absent visualization, the attendant risk of iatrogenic injury to the neurovascular structures,[196–203] and the inability to identify anatomic variants involved with the pathology. In one series, Lindley and Kleinert documented 31 anomalies during the course of 526 elective carpal tunnel releases.[204]

Concannon et al. performed open releases on 103 patient hands and 88 endoscopic releases. Average follow-up time was 29 months for the open group and 22 months for the endoscopic group. They found no recurrences in the open group and six recurrences in the endoscopic group (7%, p = 0.008). However, long-term data on recurrence rates in patients after endoscopic release are still not available.[205]

In an effort to come to a happy medium between open and endoscopic releases, several surgeons have described minimally invasive approaches.[205–209] However, there have been no studies demonstrating that minimal incision carpal tunnel release is superior to traditional open release.

In advanced cases of nerve compression, longstanding endoneurial edema induces fibroblast invasion and fibrosis. Patients in this stage of carpal tunnel syndrome have profound sensory loss and thenar atrophy, and carpal tunnel release alone may not eliminate all symptoms. Several adjunctive procedures have been used in an effort to improve the results of surgical release of the carpal tunnel. These include internal neurolysis and epineurotomy. Internal neurolysis, described by Curtis and Eversmann in 1973, involves splitting the epineurium and gently teasing apart the fascicles of the nerve by using sharp pointed scissors and small forceps.[210] Clinical studies, however, have failed to demonstrate any benefit from neurolysis, and it has fallen out of favor.[211–216]

Epineurotomy, on the other hand, releases the epineurium of a peripheral nerve, and was a frequently used as an adjunct to carpal tunnel release at around the same time.[217] However, its efficacy is not supported by two prospective clinical studies.[218,219] Borisch and Haussmann, in a randomized prospective clinical trial on 273 patients, found no statistically significant difference between simple decompression and decompression combined with epineurotomy.[220] Additionally, Blair et al. found that epineurotomy based on intraoperative observations even in selected patients had no benefit.[218]

Routine reconstruction of the TCL has been proposed as insurance against bowstringing of the flexor tendons when the wrist is flexed.[221] However, postoperative bowstringing of the tendons is not usually a problem, and a short period of immobilization allows sufficient healing of the TCL to prevent bowstringing when mobilization is finally initiated. As described, the operation requires considerably more dissection, with release of Guyon's canal and mobilization of the ulnar nerve and artery. Until prospective randomized studies confirm any benefits, this procedure should be reserved for when it is necessary to immobilize the wrist in some flexion after releasing the carpal tunnel, such as with a concomitant flexor tendon repair.[55]

Sometimes patients with carpal tunnel symptoms have sensory symptoms in the little finger. Some surgeons have advocated release of Guyon's canal. However, magnetic resonance imaging demonstrates that the dimensions of Guyon's canal enlarge with carpal tunnel release alone. Clinically, symptoms resulting from compression in Guyon's canal improve after carpal tunnel release alone,[222] and therefore release of Guyon's canal is not indicated.

Finally, routine tenosynovectomy does not provide better results than carpal tunnel release alone. In a prospective randomized study of 87 patients, Shum et al. observed no benefit with the performance of a flexor tenosynovectomy at the time of carpal tunnel release.[223] Although no added morbidity was observed, the theoretical increased risk of postoperative hematoma may worsen symptoms and cause adhesions between the nerve and tendons. Synovectomy is recommended only in cases of proliferative or invasive tenosynovitis (i.e., gout, inflammatory arthritis, or tuberculosis).

Despite the advanced state of medical knowledge and technology today, many of the treatment modalities utilized still depend on anecdotal reports. Standardization of results, resolution of so-called controversies, and advancement in practice can only come through the broadened use of evidence-based medicine. There are but scattered studies that guide our current treatment recommendations. Thoma et al.[224] identified seven reviews that compared endoscopic to open carpal tunnel release, and assessed them for methodologic quality using the 18-point scale by Hoving et al.,[225] a modified version of the validated scale of Oxman and Guyatt.[226,227] They deemed three to be of high methodologic quality.

Feuerstein et al.[228] concluded that the outcomes for endoscopic carpal tunnel release and open release were similar, but based on three nonrandomized, prospective, multiple group studies,[191,229,230] endoscopic release resulted in a more rapid return to work and less weakness and tenderness postoperatively.

Boeckstyns and Sorensen[231] compared rates of complications between endoscopic and open release, and found that while there was no difference in the rate of irreversible nerve damage (0.3% and 0.2% respectively), there was a higher risk for reversible nerve damage during endoscopic procedures (4.3% versus 0.9%).

Gerritsen et al.[232] reviewed 14 randomized clinical trials for surgical treatments of carpal tunnel syndrome and concluded that none of the alternatives to standard open release provided better relief of symptoms. They concluded that standard open carpal tunnel release is still the preferred method of treatment for carpal tunnel syndrome since it is just as effective as the alternatives, but is technically less demanding and therefore subjects the patient to a lower risk of complications and lower costs.

Recently, Chapell et al. performed a meta-analysis on the results of eight studies that compared the global outcomes of patients who underwent carpal tunnel release with and without adjunctive neurolysis or epineurotomy. They found that patients who underwent such procedures tended to have poorer global outcomes than those who did not, and suggested that neural surgery is potentially harmful for most patients with carpal tunnel syndrome.[233]

Preferred Operative Technique

Although any form of anesthesia may be used, axillary block or local anesthesia is preferred for most cases. General anesthesia is rarely indicated, and intravenous regional block can obscure normal tissue planes and thus make the operation more difficult.

A number of landmarks should be identified to avoid injuries to the palmar cutaneous branch (PCN), recurrent motor branch, superficial arch, and the ulnar nerve and artery. Kaplan's cardinal line is drawn from the apex of the thumb–index web toward the hook of the hamate, parallel with the proximal palmar crease (Fig. 15–14). The intersection of the cardinal line with the long finger flexed onto the thenar eminence localizes the recurrent motor branch. The deep palmar arch lies under the cardinal line, whereas the superficial palmar arch is located between the cardinal line and the proximal palmar crease. Palpation of the ulnar artery and hook of the hamate will prevent an excessively ulnar incision and usually protect the ulnar neurovascular bundle, although the surgeon should be aware of and look for possible positional variations of these structures. These landmarks are used to make the incision in the palm just ulnar to the median nerve. At the wrist, the incision stays ulnar to the palmaris longus to protect the PCN and its distal branches. The skin incision is marked, and local anesthetic is infiltrated

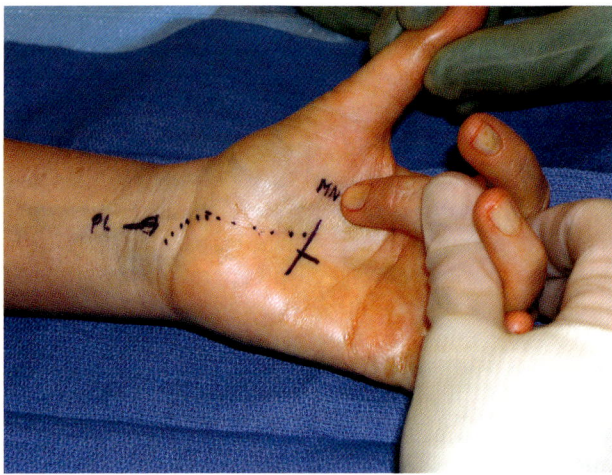

Figure 15–14 Incision planning for open carpal tunnel release. Kaplan's lines are also drawn. MN, motor nerve (the recurrent motor branch lies at the tip of the flexed long finger); PL, palmaris longus (the incision at the wrist crease curves proximally just ulnar to the palmaris longus).

into the subcutaneous tissue plane along the proposed incision.

The limb is exsanguinated, a tourniquet is inflated, and a curvilinear incision is made beginning just proximal to Kaplan's line, 2 to 3 mm ulnar to and parallel with the thenar crease. Remaining ulnar to the palmaris longus or the flexed ring finger at the distal wrist crease, the incision can be brought 5 mm into the distal forearm in an oblique direction ulnarly if needed, to provide additional proximal exposure. Blunt dissection is used to spread the subcutaneous tissue transversely to permit identification of the antebrachial and palmar fascia. The TCL is visualized after gentle spreading of the palmar fascia while remaining ulnar to the palmaris longus. Since the palm is heavily and variably innervated by the palmar cutaneous branches of the median and ulnar nerves, the nerve of Henle, and multiple transverse ulnar cutaneous branches, care must be taken to preserve these branches to avoid persistent incisional tenderness.[99,234] A fine hemostat is used to penetrate the antebrachial fascia in the proximal wound and the underlying median nerve identified. Under direct vision, the antebrachial fascia is then divided. It has been cited as a possible cause of compression in certain patients.[235] The nerve is then traced distally, and the underside of the TCL is freed from adherent tenosynovium.

The TCL is sharply divided along its ulnar border. Distally, it is divided in layers to protect the superficial arch. The surgeon should be aware of the deep motor branch of the ulnar nerve coursing around the hook of the hamate, inasmuch as three cases of injury at this level have been reported.[236] The distal median nerve and recurrent motor branch are then inspected. Residual fibers of the FR at the level of the arch as well as those fibers compressing a transligamentous motor branch are carefully divided. The flexor tendons may be retracted radially to inspect the floor of the canal for ganglia, calcifications, or osteophytes. The tourniquet is deflated, the wound irrigated, meticulous hemostasis achieved, and skin closed with 5-0 nylon horizontal mattress sutures.

Postoperative Management

The FR at the wrist serves as a pulley to restrain the digital flexor tendons when the wrist is flexed. The theoretical concern that division of this structure in the course of carpal tunnel release would permit bowstringing of the tendons or entrapment of the median nerve is the rationale for postoperative splinting of the wrist. A survey of American hand surgeons found that 81% splinted patients' wrists for 2 to 4 weeks following carpal tunnel surgery.[237] However, in studies by Das and Brown, Nathan et al., and Cook et al., no incidents of tendon bowstringing or median nerve entrapment were observed as a result of foregoing postoperative splinting.[238–240]

We believe that 2 weeks of splinting after carpal tunnel surgery is excessive and should not be routine. If used, splinting should be limited to 7 to 10 days. Some patients complain of weakness in their thumb postoperatively because release of the carpal tunnel has the same effect as a muscle slide procedure particularly if the thumb is splinted in radial abduction. For this reason, we splint the thumb in palmar abduction. Finger motion is encouraged immediately. Afterwards, the patient is instructed to exercise the wrist and fingers separately while avoiding simultaneous finger and wrist flexion (which may cause bowstringing).

RECURRENCE

Recurrent entrapment neuropathies present a challenging problem. Recurrent carpal tunnel syndrome occurs in 0% to 19% of patients following carpal tunnel release, with up to 12% requiring re-exploration.[241] Common causes include incomplete release of the TCL, fibrous proliferation, or recurrent tenosynovitis.[241–244] There are higher recurrence rates and poorer outcomes in patients with occupation-related carpal tunnel syndrome.[241]

Adequate exposure of the median nerve and carpal tunnel is required. The preferred surgical approach is through a second, more ulnar incision.[245] External lysis of the nerve should then be performed by gently but completely mobilizing it from surrounding adherent scar tissue. Although there is no published data that conclusively determines that internal neurolysis yields superior results,[246] many advocate its use.[245,247,248] Interposition of a biologic barrier between the nerve and sur-

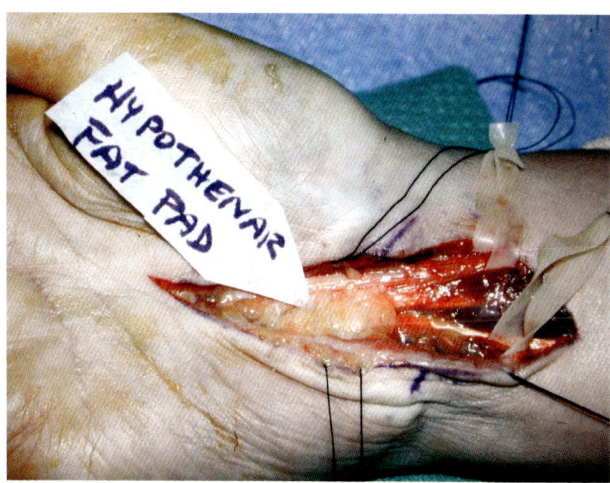

Figure 15–15 Hypothenar fat flap. This patient had failed endoscopic carpal tunnel release and a very sensitive median nerve following a subsequent open release. The hypothenar fat was mobilized to cover the scarred median nerve.

rounding tissues may discourage scarring and provide a nutrient bed for axonal regeneration.[247] The advantage of local muscle or fat flaps like the ADQ, pronator quadratus, and hypothenar fat flap,[249] palmaris brevis muscle flap,[247,250] and circumferential vein wrapping[251,252] is the ease with which they can be used, but length limitations may restrict their utility. After simpler techniques have been ruled out as options, it may be necessary to employ technically complex free tissue transfers.[252] Early postoperative mobilization of the wrist and fingers is mandatory to encourage tendon and nerve gliding. Our preference is to use a hypothenar fat flap when possible (Fig. 15–15).

Dedication

To Mary, my best friend and wife. To the memory of my father, Gustav Szabo, for his love and inspiration.—Bob Szabo

REFERENCES

1. Szabo R, King K. Repetitive stress injury: diagnosis or self-fulfilling prophecy? J Bone Joint Surg Am 2000;82: 1314–22.
2. Szabo R. Occupational carpal tunnel syndrome. In: Kasdan M, ed., Occupational Hand and Upper Extremity Injuries and Diseases. Philadelphia: Hanley and Belfus, 1998:113.
3. Szabo R, Madison M. Carpal tunnel syndrome as a work-related disorder, in repetitive motion disorders of the upper extremity. In: Gordon SL, Blair SJ, Fine LJ, eds. Rosemont IL: American Academy of Orthopaedic Surgery, 1995:421–34.
4. Phalen G. The carpal tunnel syndrome—clinical evaluation of 598 hands. Clin Orthop 1972;83:29–40.
5. Purnell DC, Daly DD, Lipscomb PR. Carpal tunnel syndrome associated with myxedema. Arch Intern Med 1961;108: 751–6.
6. Roquer J, Cano JF. Carpal tunnel syndrome and hyperthyroidism. A prospective study. Acta Neurol Scand 1993;88: 149–52.

7. Yanardag H, et al. An increased frequency of carpal tunnel syndrome in sarcoidosis. Results of a study based on nerve conduction study. Acta Med (Hradec Kralove) 2003;46:201–4.

8. Gschwind C, Tonkin MA. Carpal tunnel syndrome in children with mucopolysaccaridosis and related disorders. J Hand Surg Am 1992;17:44–7.

9. Bona I, et al. Carpal tunnel syndrome in Mucopolysaccharidoses. A report of four cases in child. Electromyogr Clin Neurophysiol 1994;34:471–5.

10. Norman-Taylor F, Fixsen JA, Sharrard WJ. Hunter's syndrome as a cause of childhood carpal tunnel syndrome: a report of three cases. J Pediatr Orthop B 1995;4:106–9.

11. Wraith JE, Alani SM. Carpal tunnel syndrome in the mucopolysaccharidoses and related disorders. Arch Dis Child 1990;65:962–3.

12. Dobyns J. Carpal tunnel release in patients with peripheral neuropathy. In: Gelberman R, ed., Operative Nerve Repair and Reconstruction. Philadelphia: J.B. Lippincott, 1991:963–5.

13. Nakasato YR. Carpal tunnel syndrome in the elderly. J Okla State Med Assoc 2003;96:113–5.

14. Schwarz A, et al. Carpal tunnel syndrome: a major complication in long-term hemodialysis patients. Clin Nephrol 1983;22:133–7.

15. McClure J, Bartley CJ, Ackrill P. Carpal tunnel syndrome caused by amyloid containing beta 2 microglobulin: a new amyloid and a complication of long term haemodialysis. Ann Rheum Dis 1986;45:1007–11.

16. Gilbert M, et al. Carpal tunnel syndrome in patients who are receiving long-term hemodialysis. J Bone Joint Surg Am 1988;70:1145–53.

17. Gelberman R, et al. Carpal tunnel syndrome: a scientific basis for clinical care. Orthop Clin North Am 1988;19:115–24.

18. Gelberman RH, Szabo RM. Pressure effects on human peripheral nerve function. In: Hargens AR, ed., Tissue Nutrition and Viability. New York: Springer-Verlag, 161–83.

19. Gelberman RH, et al. Tissue pressure threshold for peripheral nerve viability. Clin Orthop 1983;285–91.

20. Lundborg G, Dahlin LB. [Carpal tunnel syndrome—easy to treat but the etiology is unclear]. Lakartidningen 1990;87:2485–7.

21. Lundborg G, Myers R, Powell H. Nerve compression injury and increased endoneurial fluid pressure: a "miniature compartment syndrome." J Neurol Neurosurg Psych 1983;46:1119–24.

22. Szabo RM, Gelberman RH. Peripheral nerve compression. Etiology, critical pressure threshold, and clinical assessment. Orthopaedics 1984;7:1461–6.

23. Szabo RM, et al. Effects of increased systemic blood pressure on the tissue fluid pressure threshold of peripheral nerve. J Orthop Res 1983;1:172–8.

24. Szwejbka PE, et al. Bilateral anterior interosseous neuropathy following surgery: a case report. Electromyogr Clin Neurophysiol 2004;44:183–6.

25. Halikis M, Taleisnik J, Szabo RM. Compression neuropathies of the upper extremity. In: Chapman M., ed., Chapman's Orthopaedic Surgery. Philadelphia: Lippincott Williams & Wilkins, 2000.

26. Dahlin LB, et al. Mechanical effects of compression of peripheral nerves. Trans ASME 1986;108:120–2.

27. Rath T, Millesi H. [The gliding tissue of the median nerve in the carpal tunnel]. Handchir Mikrochir Plast Chir 1990;22:203–5.

28. Szabo RM, et al. Median nerve displacement through the carpal canal. J Hand Surg Am 1994;19:901–6.

29. Upton ARM, McComas AJ. The double crush in nerve-entrapment syndromes. Lancet 1973;2:359–62.

30. Osterman A. The double crush syndrome. Orthop Clin North Am 1988;19:147–55.

31. Osterman AL. Double crush and multiple compression neuropathy. In Gelberman RH, ed., Operative Nerve Repair and Reconstruction Philadelphia: J.B. Lippincott, 1991:1211–29.

32. Koo J, Szabo RM. Compression neuropathies of the median nerve. J Am Soc Surg Hand 2004;4:156–75.

33. Seyffarth H. Primary myoses in the m. pronator teres as cause of the n. medianus (the pronator syndrome). Acta Psychiatr Scand 1951;74(Suppl):251–4.

34. Johnson RK, Spinner M. Median nerve compression in the forearm: the pronator tunnel syndrome. In: Szabo RM, ed., Nerve Compression Syndromes—Diagnosis and Treatment. Thorofare, NJ: Slack Inc., 1989:137–51.

35. Johnson RK, Spinner M, Shrewsbury MM. Median nerve entrapment syndrome in the proximal forearm. J Hand Surg Am 1979;4.48–51.

36. Parsonage MJ, Turner JW. Neuralgic amyotrophy: the shoulder-girdle syndrome. Lancet 1948:974–8.

37. Kiloh LG, Nevin S. Isolated neuritis of the anterior interosseous nerve. BMJ 1952;1:850–1.

38. Fearn CBDA, Goodfellow JW. Anterior interosseous nerve palsy. J Bone Joint Surg Br 1965;47:91–3.

39. Nigst H, Dick W. Syndromes of compression of the median nerve in the proximal forearm (pronator teres syndrome: anterior interosseous nerve syndrome). Arch Orthop Trauma Surg 1979;93:307–12.

40. Moersch F. Median thenar neuritis. Proc Staff Meet Mayo Clin 1938:220–2.

41. Paget J. Lectures on Surgical Pathology, 3rd ed. Philadelphia: Lindsey & Blakiston, 1854.

42. Putnam J. A series of cases of paresthesias, mainly of the hand, or periodic recurrence, and possibly of vaso-motor origin. Arch Med 1880;4:147–62.

43. Pfeffer GB, et al. The history of carpal tunnel syndrome. J Hand Surg Br 1988;13:28–34.

44. Amadio PC. The first carpal tunnel release? J Hand Surg Br 1995;20:40–1.

45. Gellman H, et al. Carpal tunnel syndrome: an evaluation of the provocative diagnostic tests. J Bone Joint Surg Am 1986;68:735–7.

46. Katz JN, et al. The carpal tunnel syndrome: diagnostic utility of the history and physical examination findings. Ann Intern Med 1990;112:321–7.

47. Lanz U. Anatomical variations of the median nerve in the carpal tunnel. J Hand Surg Am 1977;2:44–53.

48. Phalen G. Spontaneous compression of the median nerve at the wrist. JAMA 1951;145:1128–33.

49. Michelsen H, Posner M. Medical history of carpal tunnel syndrome. Hand Clin 2002;18:257–68.

50. Patterson JD, Simmons BP. Outcomes assessment in carpal tunnel syndrome. Hand Clin 2002;18:359–63, viii.

51. Tanaka S, Petersen M, Cameron L. Prevalence and risk factors of tendinitis and related disorders of the distal upper extremity among U.S. workers: comparison to carpal tunnel syndrome. Am J Ind Med 2002;39:328–35.

52. Gelberman R, Hergenroeder PT, Hargens AR, et al. The carpal tunnel syndrome: a study of carpal canal pressures. J Bone Joint Surg Am 1981;63:380.

53. Gerr F, Letz R. Risk factors for carpal tunnel syndrome in industry: blaming the victim? J Occup Med 1992;34:1117–9.

54. Franzblau A, Werner RA, Yihan J. Preplacement nerve testing for carpal tunnel syndrome: is it cost effective? J Occup Environ Med 2004;46:714–9.

55. Szabo R. Entrapment and compression neuropathies. In: Green D, ed., Green's Operative Hand Surgery. Philadelphia: Churchill-Livingstone, 1999:1404–47.

56. Nathan PA, et al. Obesity as a risk factor for slowing of sensory conduction of the median nerve in industry. A cross-sectional and longitudinal study involving 429 workers. J Occup Med 1992;34:379–83.
57. Palumbo CF, Szabo SM. Examination of patients for carpal tunnel syndrome sensibility, provocative, and motor testing. Hand Clin 2002;18:269–77, vi.
58. Szabo RM, et al. The value of diagnostic testing in carpal tunnel syndrome. J Hand Surg Am 1999;24:704–14.
59. Megele R. Anterior interosseous nerve syndrome with atypical nerve course in relation to the pronator teres. Acta Neurochir (Wien) 1988;91:144–6.
60. Fuss FK, Wurzl GH. Median nerve entrapment. Pronator teres syndrome: surgical anatomy and correlation with symptom patterns. Surg Radiol Anat 1990;12:267–71.
61. Doyle J, Botte MJ. Surgical Anatomy of the Hand and Upper Extremity. Philadelphia: Lippincott Williams & Wilkins, 2003.
62. Sunderland S. The median nerve. Anatomical and physiological features. Nerves and Nerve Injuries, 2nd ed. Edinburgh: Churchill-Livingstone, 1978:655–90.
63. De Jesus R, Dellon AL. Historic origin of the "arcade of Struthers." J Hand Surg Am 2003;28:528–31.
64. Struthers J. On some points in the abnormal anatomy of the arm. Br Foreign Med Chir Rev 1854:14:170–9.
65. Smith RV, Fisher RG. Struthers ligament: a source of median nerve compression above the elbow. J Neurosurg 1973;38:778–9.
66. Vesley DG, Killian JT. Arcades of Struthers. J Med Assoc State Ala 1983;52:33–4, 36–7.
67. al-Qattan MM, Husband JB. Median nerve compression by the supracondylar process: a case report. J Hand Surg Br 1991;16:101–3.
68. Williams P. Gray's anatomy, 38th ed. New York: Churchill-Livingstone, 1995.
69. Ivins GK. Supracondylar process syndrome: a case report. J Hand Surg Am 1996;21:279–81.
70. Eversmann W. Entrapment and compression neuropathies. In: Green D, ed., Operative Hand Surgery, 3rd ed. New York: Churchill-Livingstone, 1993:1423–78.
71. Dellon AL, Mackinnon SE. Musculoaponeurotic variations along the course of the median nerve in the proximal forearm. J Hand Surg Br 1987;12:359–63.
72. Gainor BJ, Jeffries JT. Pronator syndrome associated with a persistent median artery. A case report. J Bone Joint Surg Am 1987;69:303–4.
73. Jones NF, Ming NL. Persistent median artery as a cause of pronator syndrome. J Hand Surg Am 1988;13:728–32.
74. Tountas C, Bergman RA. Anatomic Variations of the Upper Extremity. New York: Churchill-Livingstone, 1993.
75. al-Qattan MM. Gantzer's muscle. An anatomical study of the accessory head of the flexor pollicis longus muscle. J Hand Surg Br 1996;21:269–70.
76. Kaplan E, Spinner M. Important muscular variations of the hand and forearm. In: Spinner M, ed., Kaplan's Functional and Surgical Anatomy of the Hand. Philadelphia: J.B. Lippincott, 1984:335–49.
77. Coonrad RW, Spinner RJ. Snapping brachialis tendon associated with median neuropathy. J Bone Joint Surg Am 1995; 77:1891–3.
78. Karanjia ND, Stiles PJ. Cubital bursitis. J Bone Joint Surg Br 1988;70:832–3.
79. Sunderland S. The intraneural topography of the radial, median, and ulnar nerves. Brain 1945;68:243–99.
80. Spinner M. Injuries to the Major Branches of Peripheral Nerves of the Forearm, 2nd ed., vol. 1. Philadelphia: W.B. Saunders, 1978.
81. Hill NA, Howard FM, Huffer BR. The incomplete anterior interosseous nerve syndrome. J Hand Surg Am 1985;10:4–16.
82. Spinner M. The Median Nerve. Injuries to the Major Branches of Peripheral Nerves of the Forearm, 2nd ed. Philadelphia: W.B. Saunders, 1972:262–92.
83. Spinner RJ, Carmichael SW, Spinner M. Partial median nerve entrapment in the distal arm because of an accessory bicipital aponeurosis. J Hand Surg Am 1991;16:236–44.
84. Carstam N. A rare anomalous muscle, palmaris profundus, found when operating at the wrist for neurological symptoms. A report of two cases. Bull Hosp Jt Dis Orthop Inst 1984; 44:163–7.
85. Mangani U. Flexor pollicis longus muscle: its morphology and clinical significance. J Bone Joint Surg Am 1960;42:467–70.
86. Lister G. The Hand: Diagnosis and Indications, 2nd ed. Edinburgh: Churchill-Livingstone, 1984.
87. Spinner M. Nerve compression lesions in the forearm, elbow and arm. In: Tubiana R., ed., The Hand. Philadelphia: W.B. Saunders, 1993:400–32.
88. Cobb TK, et al. The carpal tunnel as a compartment. An anatomic perspective. Orthop Rev 1992;21:451–3.
89. Cobb TK, et al. Anatomy of flexor retinaculum. J Hand Surg Am 1993;18:91–9.
90. Mackinnon SE, Dellon AE. Anatomic investigations of nerves at the wrist. I. Orientation of the motor fascicle of the median nerve in the carpal tunnel. Ann Plast Surg 1988;21:32–5.
91. Lauritzen RS, Szabo RM, Lauritzen DB. Innervation of lumbrical muscles. J Hand Surg Br 1996;21:57–8.
92. Bezerra AJ, Carvalho VC, Nucci A. An anatomical study of the palmar cutaneous branch of the median nerve. Surg Radiol Anat 1986;8:183–8.
93. Taleisnik J. The palmar cutaneous branch of the median nerve and the approach to the carpal tunnel: an anatomical study. J Bone Joint Surg Am 1973;55:1212–7.
94. Szabo RM, Pettey J. Bilateral median nerve bifurcation with an accessory compartment within the carpal tunnel. J Hand Surg Br 1994;19:22–3.
95. Tountas CP, et al. Variations of the median nerve in the carpal canal. J Hand Surg Am 1987;12:708–12.
96. Caffee HH. Anomalous thenar muscle and median nerve: a case report. J Hand Surg Am 1979;4:446–7.
97. Amadio P. Anatomic variation of the median nerve within the carpal tunnel. Clin Anat 1988;1:23–31.
98. Thomson A. Third annual report on the Committee of Collective Investigation of the Anatomical Society of Great Britain and Ireland for the year 1891–1892. J Anat Physiol 1893;27:183.
99. DaSilva MF, et al. Anatomy of the palmar cutaneous branch of the median nerve: clinical significance. J Hand Surg Am 1996; 21:639–43.
100. Martin CH, Seiler JG, Lesesne JS. The cutaneous innervation of the palm: an anatomic study of the ulnar and median nerves. J Hand Surg Am 1996;21:634–8.
101. Watchmaker GP, Weber D, Mackinnon SE. Avoidance of transection of the palmar cutaneous branch of the median nerve in carpal tunnel release. J Hand Surg Am 1996;21: 644–50.
102. Dowdy PA, Richards RS, McFarlane RM. The palmar cutaneous branch of the median nerve and the palmaris longus tendon: a cadaveric study. J Hand Surg Am 1994;19:199–202.
103. Chidgey LK, Szabo RM, Wiese DA. Acute carpal tunnel syndrome caused by pigmented villonodular synovitis of the wrist. Clin Orthop 1988:254–7.
104. Lee KE. Tuberculosis presenting as carpal tunnel syndrome. J Hand Surg Am 1985;10:242–5.
105. Weiss AP, Steichen JB. Synovial sarcoma causing carpal tunnel syndrome. J Hand Surg Am 1992;17:1024–5.
106. Fuchs PC, Nathan PA, Myers LD. Synovial histology in carpal tunnel syndrome. J Hand Surg Am 1991;16:753–8.

107. Schuind F, Ventura M, Pasteels JL. Idiopathic carpal tunnel syndrome: histologic study of flexor tendon synovium. J Hand Surg Am 1990;15:497–503.

108. Kerr CD, Sybert DR, Albarracin NS. An analysis of the flexor synovium in idiopathic carpal tunnel syndrome: report of 625 cases. J Hand Surg Am 1992;17:1028–30.

109. Nakamichi K, Tachibana S. Histology of the transverse carpal ligament and flexor tenosynovium in idiopathic carpal tunnel syndrome. J Hand Surg Am 1998;23:1015–24.

110. Nakamichi K, Tachibana S. Median nerve compression by a radially inserted palmaris longus tendon after release of the antebrachial fascia: a complication of carpal tunnel release. J Hand Surg Am 2000;25:955–8.

111. Szabo R, Gelberman RH. Peripheral nerve compression. Etiology, critical pressure threshold, and clinical assessment. Orthopedics 1984;7:1461–6.

112. Olehnik WK, Manske PR, Szerzinski J. Median nerve compression in the proximal forearm. J Hand Surg Am 1994; 19:121–6.

113. Hartz CR, et al. The pronator teres syndrome: compressive neuropathy of the median nerve. J Bone Joint Surg Am 1981; 63:885–91.

114. Gainor BJ. The pronator compression test revisited. A forgotten physical sign. Orthop Rev 1990;19:888–92.

115. Spinner M. Management of nerve compression lesions of the upper extremity. In: Omer G, Spinner M, eds., Management of Peripheral Nerve Problems. Philadelphia: W.B. Saunders, 1980:569–92.

116. Barnard L, McCoy SM. The supracondyloid process of the humerus. J Bone Joint Surg Am 1946;28:845.

117. Mysiew WJ, Colachis S. The pronator syndrome. An evaluation of dynamic maneuvers for improving electrodiagnostic sensitivity. Am J Phys Med Rehabil 1991;70:274–7.

118. Gross PT, Jones HJ. Proximal median neuropathies: electromyographic and clinical correlation. Muscle Nerve 1992; 15:390–5.

119. Pease WS, Lee HH, Johnson EW. Forearm median nerve conduction velocity in carpal tunnel syndrome. Electromyogr Clin Neurophysiol 1990;30:299–302.

120. Chang MH, et al. Proximal slowing in carpal tunnel syndrome resulting from either conduction block or retrograde degeneration. J Neurol 1993;240:287–90.

121. Anastasopoulos D, Chroni E. Effect of carpal tunnel syndrome on median nerve proximal conduction estimated by F-waves. J Clin Neurophysiol 1997;14:63–7.

122. Gonzalez-Alegre P, Recober A, Kelkar P. Idiopathic brachial neuritis. Iowa Orthop J 2002;22:81–5.

123. Puechal X, et al. Neuralgic amyotrophy and polyarthritis caused by parvovirus B19 infection. Ann Rheum Dis 1998; 57:262.

124. Brown JL. Brachial neuritis following infection with Epstein-Barr virus. J Infect 1987;15:173–6.

125. Janes SE, Whitehouse WP. Brachial neuritis following infection with Epstein-Barr virus. Eur J Paediatr Neurol 2003;7: 413–5.

126. Stratton KR, Howe CJ, Johnston RB Jr. Adverse events associated with childhood vaccines other than pertussis and rubella. Summary of a report from the Institute of Medicine. JAMA 1994;271:1602–5.

127. Hamati-Haddad A, Fenichel GM. Brachial neuritis following routine childhood immunization for diphtheria, tetanus, and pertussis (DTP): report of two cases and review of the literature. Pediatrics 1997;99:602–3.

128. van Alfen N, et al. The natural history of hereditary neuralgic amyotrophy in the Dutch population: two distinct types? Brain 2000;123:718–23.

129. Post JJ, et al. Acute Q fever and brachial neuritis: case report and literature review. Infection 2002;30:400–2.

130. English P, Maciver D. Neuralgic amyotrophy as a presenting feature of infective endocarditis. Postgrad Med J 2000; 76:710–1.

131. Louis E, et al. [Bilateral amyotrophic neuralgia (Parsonage Turner syndrome) with HIV seroconversion]. Rev Neurol (Paris) 2003;159:685–7.

132. Malamut RI, et al. Postsurgical idiopathic brachial neuritis. Muscle Nerve 1994;17:320–4.

133. Auge WK 2nd, Velazquez PA. Parsonage-Turner syndrome in the Native American Indian. J Shoulder Elbow Surg 2000; 9:99–103.

134. Wong L, Dellon A. Brachial neuritis presenting as anterior interosseous nerve compression—implications for diagnosis and treatment: a case report. J Hand Surg Am 1997;22: 536–9.

135. Braun RM, Spinner RJ. Spontaneous bilateral median nerve compressions in the distal arm. J Hand Surg Am 1991; 16:244–7.

136. Bredella MA, et al. Denervation syndromes of the shoulder girdle: MR imaging with electrophysiologic correlation. Skeletal Radiol 1999;28:567–72.

137. Helms CA, Martinez S, Speer KP. Acute brachial neuritis (Parsonage-Turner syndrome): MR imaging appearance—report of three cases. Radiology 1998;207:255–9.

138. Geissler WB, Fernandez DL, Graca R. Anterior interosseous nerve palsy complicating a forearm fracture in a child. J Hand Surg Am 1990;15:44–7.

139. Sunderland S, Ray LJ. Metrical and non-metrical features of the muscular branches of the median nerve. J Comp Neur 1946; 85:191–201.

140. Sunderland S. The innervation of the flexor digitorum profundus and lumbrical muscles. Anat Rec 1945;93:317–21.

141. Siegel D, Gelberman RH. Ulnar nerve: applied anatomy and operative exposure. In: Gelberman R, ed., Operative Nerve Repair and Reconstruction. Philadelphia: J.B. Lippincott, 1991: 413–24.

142. Mannerfelt L. Studies of anastamoses between the median and ulnar nerves in the forearm. Acta Univ Lund 1964;6:1–7.

143. Mody B. A simple clinical test to differentiate rupture of flexor pollicis longus and incomplete anterior interosseous paralysis. J Hand Surg Br 1992;17:510.

144. Bell-Krotoski J. Advances in sensibility evaluation. Hand Clin 1991;7:527–46.

145. Dellon AL. The vibrometer. Plast Reconstr Surg 1983;71: 427–31.

146. Durkan JA. A new diagnostic test for carpal tunnel syndrome. J Bone Joint Surg Am 1991;73:535–8.

147. Durkan JA. The carpal-compression test. An instrumented device for diagnosing carpal tunnel syndrome. Orthop Rev 1994;23:522–5.

148. Szabo RM, Gelberman RH, Dimick MP. Sensibility testing in patients with carpal tunnel syndrome. J Bone Joint Surg Am 1984;66:60–4.

149. White KM, et al. Vibrometry testing for carpal tunnel syndrome: a longitudinal study of daily variations. Arch Phys Med Rehabil 1994;75:25–8.

150. Buchberger W. Radiologic imaging of the carpal tunnel. Eur J Radiol 1997;25:112–7.

151. Kele H, et al. The potential value of ultrasonography in the evaluation of carpal tunnel syndrome. Neurology 2003;61: 389–91.

152. Jarvik JG, Yuen E, Kliot M. Diagnosis of carpal tunnel syndrome: electrodiagnostic and MR imaging evaluation. Neuroimaging Clin N Am 2004;14:93–102, viii.

153. Horch RE, et al. Median nerve compression can be detected by magnetic resonance imaging of the carpal tunnel. Neurosurgery 1997;41:76–82, discussion 82–3.
154. Johnson EW. Diagnosis of carpal tunnel syndrome. The gold standard [editorial]. Am J Phys Med Rehabil 1993;72:1.
155. Buch-Jaeger N, Foucher G. Correlation of clinical signs with nerve conduction tests in the diagnosis of carpal tunnel syndrome. J Hand Surg Br 1994;19:720–4.
156. deKrom MC, Knipschild PG, Kester AD, et al. Efficacy of provocative tests for diagnosis of carpal tunnel syndrome. Lancet 1990;335:393–5.
157. Practice parameter for electrodiagnostic studies in carpal tunnel syndrome. Neurology 1993;43:2404–5.
158. Jablecki CK, et al. Literature review of the usefulness of nerve conduction studies and electromyography for the evaluation of patients with carpal tunnel syndrome. AAEM Quality Assurance Committee. Muscle Nerve 1993;16:1392–414.
159. Rempel D, et al. Consensus criteria for the classification of carpal tunnel syndrome in epidemiologic studies. Am J Public Health 1998;88:1447–51.
160. Katz JN, et al. A self-administered hand symptom diagram for the diagnosis and epidemiologic study of carpal tunnel syndrome. J Rheumatol 1990;17:1495–8.
161. Szabo RM. Median nerve release: proximal forearm. In: Blair WF, ed., Techniques in Hand Surgery. Baltimore: Williams & Wilkins, 1996:754–64.
162. Masear VR, Meyer RD, Pichora DR. Surgical anatomy of the medial antebrachial cutaneous nerve. J Hand Surg Am 1989;14:267–71.
163. Spinner M. The anterior interosseous-nerve syndrome. With special attention to its variations. J Bone Joint Surg Am 1970;52:84–94.
164. Haussmann P, Patel MR. Intraepineural constriction of nerve fascicles in pronator syndrome and anterior interosseous nerve syndrome. In: George V., ed., Peripheral Nerve Compressions of the Upper Extremity. Philadelphia: W.B. Saunders, 1996:339–44.
165. Nagano A, et al. Spontaneous anterior interosseous nerve palsy with hourglass-like fascicular constriction within the main trunk of the median nerve. J Hand Surg Am 1996;21:266–70.
166. Gelberman R, Aronson D, Weisman M. Carpal tunnel syndrome: results of a prospective trial of steroid injection and splinting. J Bone Joint Surg Am 1980;62:1181–4.
167. Goodman H, Foster J. Effect of local corticosteroid injection on median nerve conduction in carpal tunnel syndrome. Ann Phys Med 1962;6:287–94.
168. Weiss AP, Sachar K, Gendreau M. Conservative management of carpal tunnel syndrome: a reexamination of steroid injection and splinting. J Hand Surg Am 1994;19:410–5.
169. Gerritsen AA, et al. Splinting for carpal tunnel syndrome: prognostic indicators of success. J Neurol Neurosurg Psychiatry 2003;74:1342–4.
170. Amadio PC. Bifid median nerve with a double compartment within the transverse carpal canal. J Hand Surg Am 1987;12:366–8.
171. Linskey ME, Segal R. Median nerve injury from local steroid injection in carpal tunnel syndrome. Neurosurgery 1990;26:512–5.
172. McConnell JR, Bush DC. Intraneural steroid injection as a complication in the management of carpal tunnel syndrome. A report of three cases. Clin Orthop 1990;250:181–4.
173. Green DP. Diagnostic and therapeutic value of carpal tunnel injection. J Hand Surg Am 1984;9:850–4.
174. Edgell SE, et al. Predicting the outcome of carpal tunnel release. J Hand Surg Am 2003;28:255–61.
175. Szabo RM. Carpal tunnel syndrome. In: Szabo RM, ed., Nerve Compression Syndromes—Diagnosis and Treatment. Thorofare, NJ: Slack Inc., 1989:101–20.
176. Szabo RM. Carpal tunnel syndrome—general. In: Gelberman RH, ed., Operative Nerve Repair and Reconstruction. Philadelphia: J.B. Lippincott, 1991:869–88.
177. Richman J, et al. Carpal tunnel syndrome: morphologic changes after release of the transverse carpal ligament. J Hand Surg Am 1989;14:852–7.
178. Richman J, et al. Carpal tunnel volume determination by magnetic resonance imaging three dimension reconstruction. J Hand Surg Am 1987;12:712–7.
179. Cobb TK, Knudson GA, Cooney WP. The use of topographical landmarks to improve the outcome of Agee endoscopic carpal tunnel release. Arthroscopy 1995;11:165–72.
180. Seiler JG III, et al. Endoscopic carpal tunnel release: an anatomic study of the two-incision method in human cadavers. J Hand Surg Am 1993;17:996–1002.
181. Chow JC. Endoscopic release of the carpal ligament: a new technique for carpal tunnel syndrome. Arthroscopy 1989;5:19–24.
182. Chow JC. Endoscopic release of the carpal ligament for carpal tunnel syndrome: 22-month clinical result. Arthroscopy 1990;6:288–96.
183. Chow JC. Endoscopic carpal tunnel release. Two-portal technique. Hand Clin 1994;10:637–46.
184. Agee JM, McCarroll HR, North ER. Endoscopic carpal tunnel release using the single proximal incision technique. Hand Clin 1994;10:647–59.
185. Agee JM, et al. Endoscopic release of the carpal tunnel: a randomized prospective multicenter study. J Hand Surg Am 1993;17:987–95.
186. Agee JM, et al. Endoscopic carpal tunnel release: a prospective study of complications and surgical experience. J Hand Surg Am 1995;20:165–71, discussion 172.
187. Bromley GS. Minimal-incision open carpal tunnel decompression. J Hand Surg Am 1994;19:119–20.
188. Nathan PA, Meadows KD, Keniston RC. Rehabilitation of carpal tunnel surgery patients using a short surgical incision and an early program of physical therapy. J Hand Surg Am 1993;18:1044–50.
189. Wilson KM. Double incision open technique for carpal tunnel release: an alternative to endoscopic release. J Hand Surg Am 1994;19:907–12.
190. Huang JH, Zager EL. Mini-open carpal tunnel decompression. Neurosurgery 2004;54:397–9, discussion 399–400.
191. Palmer DH, Hanrahan LP. Social and economic costs of carpal tunnel surgery. Instr Course Lect 1995;44:167–72.
192. Lee DH, et al. Endoscopic carpal tunnel release: a cadaveric study. J Hand Surg Am 1993;17:1003–8.
193. Rowland EB, Kleinert JM. Endoscopic carpal-tunnel release in cadavers. An investigation of the results of twelve surgeons with this training model. J Bone Joint Surg Am 1994;76:266–8.
194. Van Heest A, et al. A cadaveric study of the single-portal endoscopic carpal tunnel release. J Hand Surg Am 1995;20:363–6.
195. Gellman H, et al. Analysis of pinch and grip strength after carpal tunnel release. J Hand Surg Am 1989;14:863–4.
196. Arner M, Hagberg L, Rosen B. Sensory disturbances after two-portal endoscopic carpal tunnel release: a preliminary report. J Hand Surg Am 1994;19:548–51.
197. Bande S, De Smet L, Fabry G. The results of carpal tunnel release: open versus endoscopic technique. J Hand Surg Br 1994;19:14–7.
198. Bozentka DJ, Osterman AL. Complications of endoscopic carpal tunnel release. Hand Clin 1995;11:91–5.

199. De Smet L, Fabry G. Transection of the motor branch of the ulnar nerve as a complication of two-portal endoscopic carpal tunnel release: a case report. J Hand Surg Am 1995;20:18–9.
200. Erdmann MW. Endoscopic carpal tunnel decompression. J Hand Surg Br 1994;19:5–13.
201. Kelly CP, Pulisetti D, Jamieson AM. Early experience with endoscopic carpal tunnel release. J Hand Surg Br 1994;19:18–21.
202. Murphy RX Jr, Jennings JR, Wukich DK. Major neurovascular complications of endoscopic carpal tunnel release. J Hand Surg Am 1994;19:114–8.
203. Stark RH. Ulnar nerve transection as a complication of two-portal endoscopic carpal tunnel release [letter, comment]. J Hand Surg Am 1994;19:522–3.
204. Lindley SG, Kleinert JM. Prevalence of anatomic variations encountered in elective carpal tunnel release. J Hand Surg Am 2003;28:849–55.
205. Concannon MJ, Brownfield ML, Puckett CL. The incidence of recurrence after endoscopic carpal tunnel release. Plast Reconstr Surg 2000;105:1662–5.
206. Klein RD, Kotsis SV, Chung KC. Open carpal tunnel release using a 1-centimeter incision: technique and outcomes for 104 patients. Plast Reconstr Surg 2003;111:1616–22.
207. Luchetti R, et al. Short palmar incision: a new surgical approach for carpal tunnel syndrome. Chir Organi Mov 1996;81:197–206.
208. Serra JM, Benito JR, Monner J. Carpal tunnel release with short incision. Plast Reconstr Surg 1997;99:129–35.
209. Frank CE. "Two stitch" carpal tunnel surgery. A mini-incision technique. Am J Orthop 1996;25:650.
210. Curtis RM, Eversmann WJ. Internal neurolysis as an adjunct to the treatment of the carpal-tunnel syndrome. J Bone Joint Surg Am 1973;55:733–40.
211. Gelberman RH, et al. Results of treatment of severe carpal tunnel syndrome without internal neurolysis of the median nerve. J Bone Joint Surg Am 1987;69:896–903.
212. Kendall WW. Results of treatment of severe carpal tunnel syndrome without internal neurolysis of the median nerve [letter]. J Bone Joint Surg Am 1988;70:151.
213. Lowry WEJ. Treatment of severe compression of the median nerve. In: Gelberman RH, ed., Operative Nerve Repair and Reconstruction. Philadelphia: J.B. Lippincott, 1991:921–6.
214. Lowry WEJ, Follender AB. Interfascicular neurolysis in the severe carpal tunnel syndrome: a prospective, randomized, double-blind, controlled study. Clin Orthop 1988;227:251–4.
215. Mackinnon S, McCabe S, Murray J. Internal neurolysis fails to improve the results of primary carpal tunnel decompression. J Hand Surg Am 1991;16:211–8.
216. Ting J, Weiland AJ. Role of ancillary procedures in surgical management of carpal tunnel syndrome: epineurotomy, internal neurolysis, tenosynovectomy, and tendon transfers. Hand Clin 2002;18:315–23.
217. Ariyan S, Watson HK. The palmar approach for the visualization and release of the carpal tunnel. An analysis of 429 cases. Plast Reconstr Surg 1977;60:539–47.
218. Blair WF, et al. Carpal tunnel release with and without epineurotomy: a comparative prospective trial. J Hand Surg Am 1996;21:655–61.
219. Foulkes GD, et al. Outcome following epineurotomy in carpal tunnel syndrome: a prospective, randomized clinical trial. J Hand Surg Am 1994;19:539–45.
220. Borisch N, Haussmann P. Neurophysiological recovery after open carpal tunnel decompression: comparison of simple decompression and decompression with epineurotomy. J Hand Surg Br 2003;28:450–4.
221. Jakab E, Ganos D, Cook F. Transverse carpal ligament reconstruction in surgery for carpal tunnel syndrome: a new technique. J Hand Surg Am 1991;16:202–6.
222. Silver MA, et al. Carpal tunnel syndrome: associated abnormalities in ulnar nerve function and the effect of carpal tunnel release on these abnormalities. J Hand Surg Am 1985;10:710–3.
223. Shum C, et al. The role of flexor tenosynovectomy in the operative treatment of carpal tunnel syndrome. J Bone Joint Surg Am 2002;84:221–5.
224. Thoma A, et al. A systematic review of reviews comparing the effectiveness of endoscopic and open carpal tunnel decompression. Plast Reconstr Surg 2004;113:1184–91.
225. Hoving JL, et al. A critical appraisal of review articles on the effectiveness of conservative treatment for neck pain. Spine 2002;26:196–205.
226. Oxman AD, Guyatt GH. Validation of an index of the quality of review articles. J Clin Epidemiol 1991;44:1271–8.
227. Oxman AD, et al. Agreement among reviewers of review articles. J Clin Epidemiol 1991;44:91–8.
228. Feuerstein M, et al. Clinical management of carpal tunnel syndrome: a 12-year review of outcomes. Am J Ind Med 1999;35:232–45.
229. Erdmann MW. Endoscopic carpal tunnel decompression. J Hand Surg Br 1994;19:5–13.
230. Kerr CD, Gittins ME, Sybert DR. Endoscopic versus open carpal tunnel release: clinical results. Arthroscopy 1994;10:266–9.
231. Boeckstyns ME, Sorensen AI. Does endoscopic carpal tunnel release have a higher rate of complications than open carpal tunnel release? An analysis of published series. J Hand Surg Br 1999;24:9–15.
232. Gerritsen A, et al. Systemic review of randomized clinical trials of surgical treatment for carpal tunnel syndrome. Br J Surg 2002;88:1285–95.
233. Chapell R, Coates V, Turkelson C. Poor outcome for neural surgery (epineurotomy or neurolysis) for carpal tunnel syndrome compared with carpal tunnel release alone: a meta-analysis of global outcomes. Plast Reconstr Surg 2003;112:983–90, discussion 991–2.
234. Lindsey JT, Watumull D. Anatomic study of the ulnar nerve and related vascular anatomy at Guyon's canal: a practical classification system. J Hand Surg Am 1996;21:626–33.
235. Ko CY, Jones NJ, Steen VD. Compression of the median nerve proximal to the carpal tunnel in scleroderma. J Hand Surg Am 1996;21:363–5.
236. Terrono A, et al. Injury to the deep motor branch of the ulnar nerve during carpal tunnel release. J Hand Surg Am 1993;18:1038–40.
237. Duncan KH, et al. Treatment of carpal tunnel syndrome by members of the American Society for Surgery of the Hand: results of a questionnaire. J Hand Surg Am 1987;12:384–91.
238. Cook AC, et al. Early mobilization following carpal tunnel release. A prospective randomized study. J Hand Surg Br 1995;20:228–30.
239. Nathan PA, Meadows KD, Keniston RC. Rehabilitation of carpal tunnel surgery patients using a short surgical incision and an early program of physical therapy. J Hand Surg Am 1993;18:1044–50.
240. Das SK, Brown HG. In search of complications in carpal tunnel decompression. Hand 1976;8:243–9.
241. Botte MJ, et al. Recurrent carpal tunnel syndrome. Hand Clin 1996;12:731–43.
242. Baranowski D, Klein W, Grunert J. [Revision operations in carpal tunnel syndrome]. Handchir Mikrochir Plast Chir 1993;25:127–32.

243. Kern BC, et al. The recurrent carpal tunnel syndrome. Zentralbl Neurochir 1993;54:80–3.

244. Kretschmer T, et al. [Pitfalls of endoscopic carpal tunnel release. Part 2: Conclusions from findings of open surgery]. Chirurg 2004.

245. Chang B, Dellon AL. Surgical management of recurrent carpal tunnel syndrome. J Hand Surg Br 1993;18:467–70.

246. Steyers CM. Recurrent carpal tunnel syndrome. Hand Clin 2002;18:339–45.

247. Rose EH. The use of the palmaris brevis flap in recurrent carpal tunnel syndrome. Hand Clin 1996;12:389–95.

248. Tung TH, Mackinnon SE. Secondary carpal tunnel surgery. Plast Reconstr Surg 2002;107:1830–43; quiz 1844, 1933.

249. Mathoulin C, Bahm J, Roukoz S. Pedicled hypothenar fat flap for median nerve coverage in recalcitrant carpal tunnel syndrome. Hand Surg 2000;5:33–40.

250. Rose EH, et al. Palmaris brevis turnover flap as an adjunct to internal neurolysis of the chronically scarred median nerve in recurrent carpal tunnel syndrome. J Hand Surg Am 1991;16: 191–201.

251. Varitimidis SE, et al. Treatment of recurrent compressive neuropathy of peripheral nerves in the upper extremity with an autologous vein insulator. J Hand Surg Am 2002;26:296–302.

252. Pizzillo MF, Sotereanos DG, Tomaino MM. Recurrent carpal tunnel syndrome: treatment options. J South Orthop Assoc 1999;8:28–36.

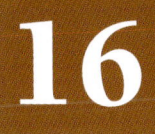

16

A DISTAL ULNAR NERVE ENTRAPMENT

Michael J. Botte, Lorenzo L. Pacelli, and Richard H. Gelberman

If I were asked what is the best thing once can expect in life,
I would say—the privilege of being useful.

ELEANOR ROOSEVELT

INTRODUCTION

In 1861, Jean Casimi Felix Guyon described an anatomic canal in the palmar-ulnar aspect of the wrist where the ulnar nerve is predisposed to compression.[1] Several anatomic studies have now more clearly delineated this space,[2-21] referred to as the ulnar tunnel or Guyon's canal (Fig. 16A–1 through Fig. 16A–4). These studies have allowed the clinician to predict specific sites and causes of compression by correlating presenting symptoms and signs with the unique anatomic features of the ulnar nerve in this area.[2] In addition, several studies and case reports have identified causes for the compression, which usually involve space-occupying lesions or are the result of acute or repetitive trauma.[22-159]

PHYSIOLOGY/CAUSES OF NERVE COMPRESSION

Neuropathy or compression of the ulnar nerve at the wrist occurs much less often than at the cubital tunnel. When it does occur, compression is often associated with an identifiable cause. These include tumors, anatomic anomalies, fractures or dislocations, edema following burns, repetitive occupational trauma, prolonged hyperextension stress of the wrist, and other miscellaneous causes. These causes are listed in Table 16A–1, based on the cumulative data of 243 reports in the literature.[22-159]

Benign Tumors

Benign tumors are the most common cause of ulnar tunnel syndrome, accounting for about 31% of identifiable causes. Tumors include ganglion cysts, lipomas, giant cell tumors, desmoid tumors, and foreign body granulomata (Table 16A–1). The ganglion is the most common, accounting for 29% to 45% of reported cases.[25,26,50,62,83,87,92,94,95,114,126,128,131,138,158] Most ganglia arise from the palmar aspect of the carpus in the proximal portions of the ulnar tunnel (Zones I and II, described below).

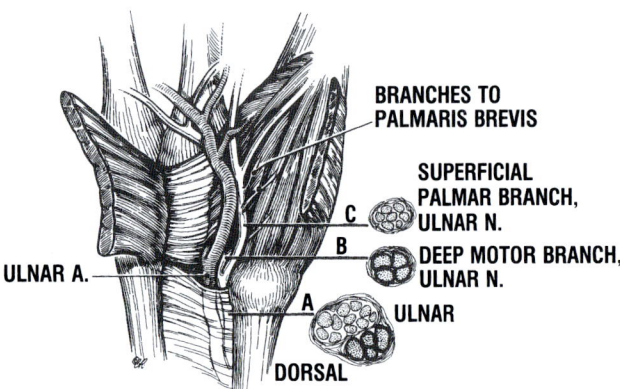

Figure 16A–1 Anatomical landmarks of the distal ulnar tunnel. **A:** Cross-section of the ulnar nerve in the region proximal to the bifurcation (Zone I). **B:** Cross-section of the ulnar nerve in the motor segment, following bifurcation (Zone II). **C:** Cross-section of the ulnar nerve in the sensory branch, distal to the bifurcation (Zone III). (From Gelberman RH. Ulnar tunnel syndrome. In: Gelberman RH, ed., Operative Nerve Repair and Reconstruction. Philadelphia: J.B. Lippincott, 1991:1131–43,[9] with permission.)

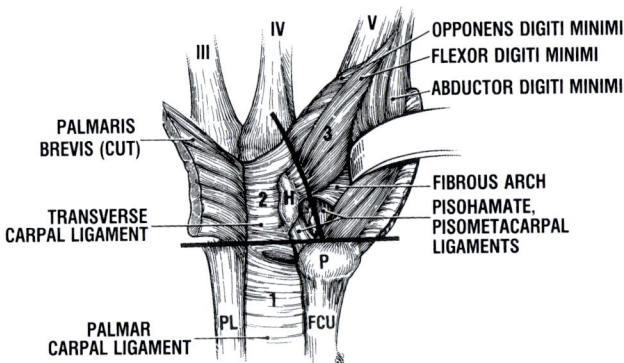

Figure 16A–2 Location of the three zones of the ulnar tunnel. Zone I is proximal to the bifurcation, Zone II encompasses the motor branch, and Zone III is the region surrounding the sensory branch. (From Gelberman RH. Ulnar tunnel syndrome. In: Gelberman RH, ed., Operative Nerve Repair and Reconstruction. Philadelphia: J.B. Lippincott, 1991:1131–43,[9] with permission.)

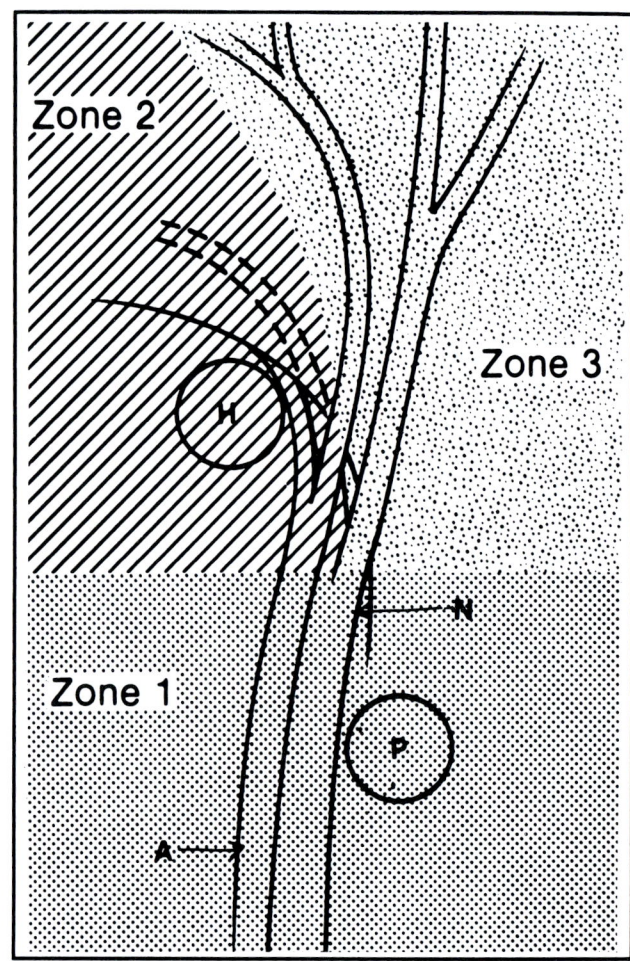

Figure 16A–3 Schematic drawing of the distal ulnar tunnel showing the location of the three zones. Zone I *(coarse stippling)*, Zone II *(lines)*, Zone III *(fine stippling)*. P, pisiform; H, hamulus; A, ulnar artery; N, ulnar nerve. (From Gross MS, Gelberman RH. The anatomy of the distal ulnar tunnel. Clin Orthop 1985;196:238,[2] with permission.)

Clinical symptoms may be insidious, and advanced neuropathy may develop before the patient seeks medical evaluation. A cystic mass may not be palpable, but is usually visualized by magnetic resonance imaging (MRI), computed tomography (CT), or diagnostic ultrasound.

Lipomas and benign giant cell tumors account for 3% and 2%, respectively, of reported cases of ulnar tunnel syndrome[34,60,96,98,106,112,113,152,157] (Table 16A–1). The tumors present as solitary masses in the proximal ulnar palm. The giant cell tumor may be palpable, firm, and may cause erosions of the hook of the hamate. A rare case of extra-abdominal desmoid tumor of the hand that produces ulnar tunnel syndrome has been reported.[116]

Isolated case reports have also noted an associated foreign body granuloma[37] and a schwannoma.[82]

Trauma

Trauma accounts for about 26% of cases of ulnar tunnel syndrome, and includes both acute and repetitive injury. Fractures and dislocations of the distal radius, ulna, or carpus have been associated with ulnar tunnel syndrome in about 12%.[23,31,47,72,105,119,147,149,159] Acute neuropathy can be caused by direct compression or by traction due to fracture fragment displacement. Secondary hematoma or edema contribute to compression. These injuries are usually associated with high-energy trauma and are often related to severe dorsally displaced fragments.[147] Fractures of the hook of the hamate may cause direct injury to the ulnar nerve, or secondary injury by displacement of fracture fragments, hematoma, or subsequent adhesions during healing.[23,47,105,119,147,149]

Ulnar tunnel syndrome can be caused from cyclic occupational trauma that involves repetitive blows or prolonged vibratory trauma. Those occurring from jackhammers or pneumatic drills[24,44,67,73,136] are often referred to as hypothenar hammer syndrome. Neuropathy is usually produced by or associated with injury when the wrist maintained in a dorsiflexed position while stabilizing a pneumatic tool.[24,39,67,71,73,155] Secondary ulnar artery dilation or thrombosis can occur, contributing to nerve compression. Ulnar neuropathy at the wrist has also been associated with chronic wrist motion sustained by meat packers,[136] and from chronic compression in professional parquet floor installers.[44]

Bicycling can precipitate ulnar tunnel syndrome from prolonged wrist dorsiflexion and maintained compression. This entity was originally noted in competitive bicyclists, and is now a well-recognized association with prolonged bike riding.[31,40,49,79,81,84] Eckman et al. originally noted three bicyclists who developed Zone I nerve compression following extended bike rides.[49] Two had combined motor and sensory symptoms and one had motor findings alone. It is unclear whether neuropathy

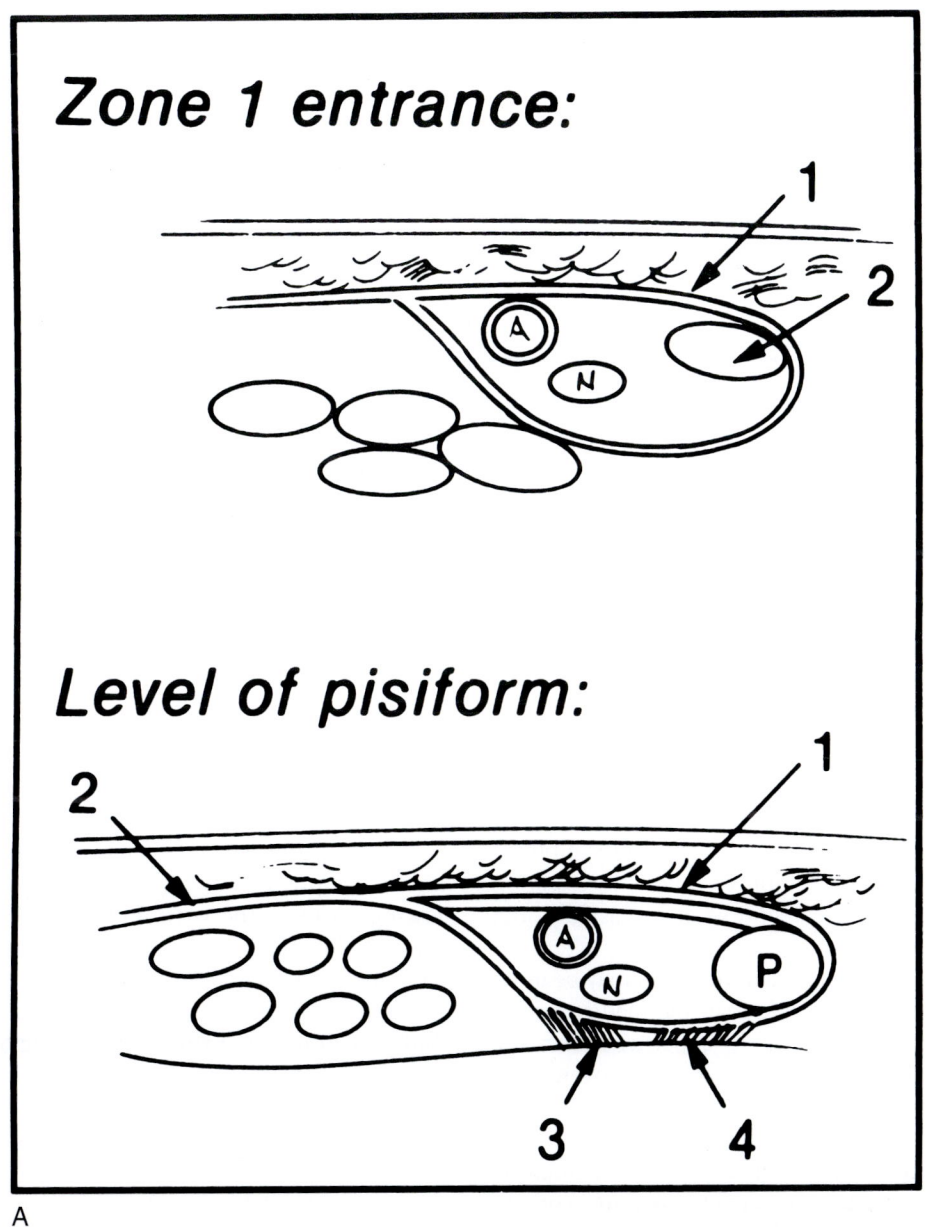

A

Figure 16A–4 **A:** Schematic cross-sections for the distal ulnar tunnel in Zone I. Entrance to Zone I: A, ulnar artery; N, ulnar nerve; 1, palmar carpal ligament; 2, tendon of the flexor carpi ulnaris. Level of the pisiform: A, ulnar artery; N, ulnar nerve; P, pisiform; 1, palmaris brevis; 2, transverse carpal ligament; 3, pisohamate ligament; 4, pisometacarpal ligament. (From Gross MS, Gelberman RH. The anatomy of the distal ulnar tunnel. Clin Orthop 1985;196:238,[2] with permission.)

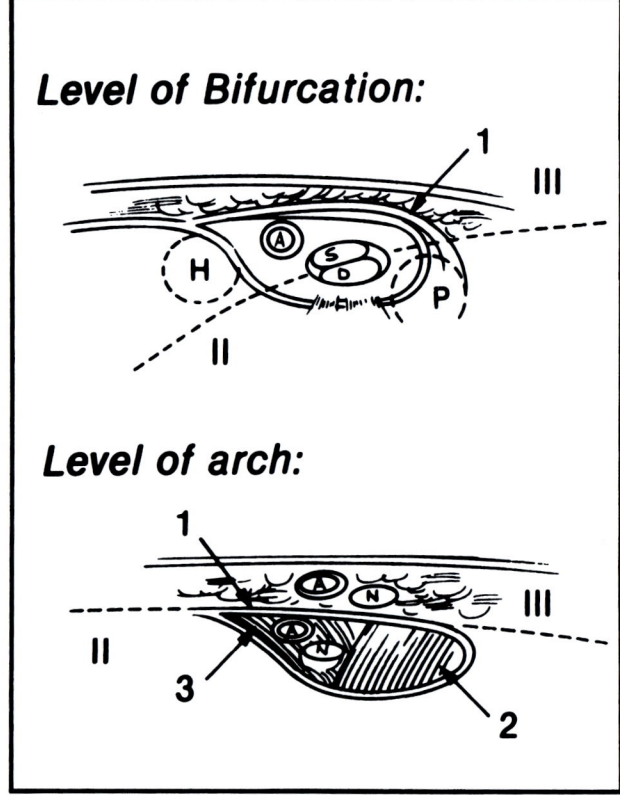

Level of Bifurcation:

Level of arch:

B

Figure 16A–4—Cont'd **B:** Schematic cross-sections of the distal ulnar tunnel at the proximal and distal ulnar boundaries of Zones II and III. Level of the bifurcation of the ulnar nerve: A, ulnar artery; S, superficial branch of the ulnar nerve; D, deep branch of the ulnar nerve; P, pisiform; H, hamulus; 1, palmaris brevis; II, Zone II; III, Zone III. Level of the fibrous arch of the hypothenar muscles: 1, fibrous arch of the hypothenar muscles; 2, abductor digiti minimi; 3, flexor digiti minimi. In Zone II: A, deep branch of the ulnar artery; N, deep branch of the ulnar nerve. In Zone III: A, superficial branch of the ulnar artery forming the superficial arch; N, superficial branch of the ulnar nerve. (From Gross MS, Gelberman RH. The anatomy of the distal ulnar tunnel. Clin Orthop 1985;196:238,[2] with permission.)

TABLE 16A–1		
Common Causes of Ulnar Nerve Compression at the Wrist Based on 243 Reported Cases 22–159		
Cause	Number	Percent
Tumors		31%
Ganglion	60	
Lipoma	6	
Giant cell tumor	5	
Schwannoma	1	
Hemangioma	1	
Desmoid tumor	1	
Hematic cyst	1	
Foreign body granuloma	1	
Trauma		26%
Fractures	29	
Repetitive trauma	21	
Edema following burns	10	
Other trauma	3	
Anatomic abnormalities		19%
Anomalous muscles	35	
Thickened ligaments	6	
Anomalous hamulus	5	
Anomalous pisiform	1	
Vascular pathology	23	9%
Idiopathic	14	6%
Inflammatory		4%
Rheumatoid arthritis	6	
Nodular synovitis 1	2	
Myositis ossificans	1	
Metabolic 3		1%
Calcinosis	3	
Degenerative arthritis	1	<1%
Iatrogenic		2%
Tendon transfers	4	
Injection injury	1	
Postoperative edema	1	
Other		
Dupuytren's contracture	1	<1%
	243 total	

is primarily caused by direct nerve compression or by maintained wrist hyperextension. Signs and symptoms are usually transient and improve following cessation of riding. Operative decompression is usually not required.

External compressive forces in the palm may be more likely to afflict the ulnar nerve than the median nerve, since the Guyon's canal is more superficial than the carpal tunnel. The ulnar nerve is also covered by the thinner palmar carpal ligament, and may be more vulnerable.

Wheelchair athletes are at risk for ulnar neuropathy at the wrist secondary to direct pressure and to repetitive wrist dorsiflexion required for wheelchair propulsion.[35] Similarly, race car driving has been noted to provoke ulnar nerve symptoms, probably related from both wrist positioning and from the associated vibration.[93]

Thermal injuries are a relatively rare cause of ulnar nerve compression, which develops from edema following burns in the wrist and hand.[55,57] The diagnosis may be difficult since the burn patient is usually in considerable pain, and muscle weakness may result from the primary thermal injury. Diagnosis can be established with a high index of suspicion leading to correlation of physical findings and electromyographic results.

Anatomic/Congenital Anomalies

Anatomic anomalies causing ulnar tunnel syndrome consist of anomalous muscle bellies or tendons, anomalous or thickened ligaments, and congenital or developmental carpal bone abnormalities (Table 16A–1). Anomalous muscles are the most frequent of these abnormalities, accounting for about 14% of reported cases of ulnar tunnel syndrome.[38,45,52,63,66,69,76,85,89,90,91,103,107,110,111,117,118,125,130,133,134,137,141,145] These muscles usually consist of those normally present with abnormal variations in size, shape, location, or with accessory muscles not normally present. Both intrinsic and extrinsic anomalous muscles have been noted. Extrinsic muscles often have an abnormal extension of tendon or muscle into the ulnar tunnel, and have included the palmaris longus, flexor carpi ulnaris, and flexor digitorum superficialis. Anomalous intrinsic muscles have included an accessory flexor digiti minimi, and an accessory abductor digiti minimi.[38,45,52,63,66,69,76,85,89,90,91,103,107,110,111,117,118,125,130,133,134,137,141,145]

A thickened pisohamate ligament has been reported to compress the ulnar nerve as the ligamentous band extends from the pisiform to the hook of the hamate anterior to the deep branch of the ulnar nerve in Zone II.[2]

Abnormalities of the pisiform or hook of the hamate have been associated with ulnar tunnel syndrome. Anomalies include variations in osseous size, shape or the presence of a bipartite hamulus.[22,28,64]

Vascular Pathology

Vascular lesions involving the ulnar artery are well-recognized associated conditions of ulnar tunnel syndrome, encompassing approximately 9% of reported cases of distal ulnar nerve compression (Table 16A–1).[41,42,51,65,75,81,84,99,124,127,132,140,144,150] Lesions include vascular thrombosis, true aneurysms, and false aneurysms. Dilation with an aneurysm or thrombosis can occur with repetitive trauma, as note above in the hypothenar hammer syndrome. Acute ulnar tunnel syndrome has been caused by rupture of an ulnar artery pseudoaneurysm.[51]

Inflammatory or Degenerative Conditions

Rheumatoid arthritis can precipitate ulnar tunnel syndrome from associated edema, tenosynovitis, synovial cysts, and osseous deformities of the carpus.[33,43,139] Approximately 4% of reported cases of ulnar tunnel syndrome have been associated with these inflammatory conditions, usually involving tenosynovitis of the flexor carpi ulnaris or the flexor digitorum superficialis. Rheumatoid synovial cysts can arise from the proximal edge of Guyon's canal.[3,139] Osteoarthritis can also contribute to distal ulnar neuropathy, from involvement of the pisotriquetral joint.[78]

Iatrogenic Causes

Iatrogenic causes of distal ulnar nerve compression have included compression following opponensplasty from tendon transfers that encroach on the ulnar nerve.[32,154]

Local steroid injection has also been reported to cause ulnar tunnel syndrome.[58]

Miscellaneous Conditions

Additional reported conditions associated with ulnar tunnel syndrome include insect bites with severe swelling in the region of Guyon's canal.[88] Calcinosis in patients with scleroderma[36,142] or uremic tumoral calcinosis associated with chronic renal failure[61] have been associated with compression of the ulnar nerve due to calcium deposition. Psuedomalignant myositis ossificans of the wrist can also cause ulnar nerve compression.[80]

Recently Murata et al. have brought attention to the occurrence of idiopathic distal ulnar nerve compression.[26] In 14 of 31 patients reviewed, there was no obvious anatomic or traumatic cause. The authors did note that most had concomitant carpal tunnel syndrome, and 6 of the 31 patients had diabetes mellitus.

CLINICAL PRESENTATION

Ulnar nerve compression at the wrist results in paresthesias or numbness in the palmar aspect of the little finger and palmoulnar aspect of the ring finger, along with paresis and atrophy of the ulnar innervated intrinsic muscles of the hand.[4,9,11,160–163] Sensibility is preserved on the dorsum of the ring and little fingers since the dorsal sensory branch leaves the ulnar nerve trunk in the forearm about 7 cm proximal to the ulnar tunnel. Muscles involved include the abductor digiti minimi, flexor digiti minimi, opponens digiti minimi, palmar and dorsal interossei, lumbricals to the ring and little fingers, and the adductor pollicis. Atrophy is usually most apparent in the first dorsal interosseous and abductor digiti minimi. Long-standing neuropathy will result in the intrinsic minus hand (claw hand deformity), characterized by hyperextension of the metacarpophalangeal joints, and flexion of the proximal and distal interphalangeal joints. Deformity is usually less severe in the index and long fingers due to remaining function of their lumbricals, which are innervated by the median nerve.

PERTINENT ANATOMY

The ulnar tunnel begins at the proximal edge of the palmar carpal ligament, and extends to the fibrous arch of the hypothenar muscles, spanning a length of about 4 to 4.5 cm.[2] Although this space varies in configuration from its proximal to distal extents, it functions pathophysiologically as a consistent tunnel with discrete anatomical landmarks (Figs. 16A–1 through 16A–4). The tunnel is divided into three zones that help correlate clinical symptoms with anatomical features of this region. The zones are based on a relationship between the internal topography of the nerve and the structures surrounding it. Zone I consists of the portion of the ulnar tunnel proximal to the bifurcation of the nerve, Zone II includes the areas surrounding the deep motor branch, and zone III includes the space through which the superficial branch of the nerve extends (Figs. 16A–2 through 16A–4) (Tables 16A–2 to 16A–4).[2,9]

Zone I is about 3 cm in length. It extends from the proximal edge of the palmar carpal ligament to the point at which the nerve bifurcates into the deep motor branch and the sensory branches. The palmar roof is formed by the palmar carpal ligament, a thickening of the antebrachial fascia that becomes distinct about 2 cm proximal to the pisiform. The ligament arises ulnarly from the flexor carpi ulnaris and inserts radially into the sheath of the palmaris longus tendon and the transverse carpal ligament. The dorsal surface is comprised of the flexor digitorum profundus tendons the ulnar portion of the transverse carpal ligament. The lateral boundary is composed of the distal fibers of the palmar carpal ligament, which extend radially and posteriorly to wrap around the neurovascular bundle, eventually merging with

fibers of the transverse carpal ligament. The medial wall is formed by the flexor carpi ulnaris tendon and the pisiform[2] (Figs. 16A–2 through 16A–4) (Table 16A–2).

Zones II and III lie adjacent to each other, and extend from the point of bifurcation of the nerve to the region just beyond the fibrous arch of the hypothenar muscles (Tables 16A–3 and 16A–4). Zone II encompasses the deep (motor) branch, and lies radial to Zone III. The palmar roof of Zone II is formed by the palmaris brevis muscle. The palmaris brevis is usually about 2.5 cm in length, and originates from the distal palmar aspect of the pisiform and hypothenar muscle fascia. It inserts into the ulnar margin of the palmar aponeurosis and transverse carpal ligament. The dorsal floor of Zone II is comprised of the pisohamate and pisometacarpal ligaments proximally and the opponens digiti minimi muscle distally. The pisohamate ligament arises from the distal radial aspect of the pisiform and inserts into the palmar-ulnar aspect of the hook of the hamate. Medial to the pisohamate ligament, the pisometacarpal ligament arises from the distal aspect of the pisiform and inserts into the palmar-radial aspect of the base of the small finger metacarpal[2] (Table 16A–3).

There is a divergence between the pisohamate and pisometacarpal ligaments that creates an opening in the floor of the tunnel. This opening is filled with fibro-fatty tissue, and lies over the capsule of the triquetrohamate joint. Laterally, the transverse carpal ligament forma a sloping wall that blends with the floor of the tunnel. At the distal extent of Zone II, the fibrous arch of the hypothenar muscles lies palmar to the nerve, the opponens digiti minimi muscle is dorsal, the hooks of the hamate and flexor digiti minimi muscle are lateral, and the abductor digiti minimi muscle is medial. Distally, as the deep branch of the nerve leaves the tunnel, it passes deep to the fibrous arch of the hypothenar muscles and penetrates the interval between the abductor digiti minimi and flexor digiti minimi muscles. The abductor digiti minimi receives a nerve branch that is given off just proximal to the intermuscular interval. The deep motor branch then pierces the opponens digiti minimi as it courses radially and dorsally around the hook of the hamate. It leaves the tunnel and continues trans-

TABLE 16A–2	
Boundaries of Zone I: Motor and Sensory Trunk	
Palmar	Palmar carpal ligament
Dorsal	Flexor digitorum profundus
	Transverse carpal ligament
Lateral	Palmar carpal ligament
Medial	Pisiform
	Flexor carpi ulnaris

Source: Gelberman RH. Ulnar tunnel syndrome. In: Gelberman RH, ed., Operative Nerve Repair and Reconstruction. Philadelphia: J.B. Lippincott, 1991:1131–43,[9] with permission.

TABLE 16A–3	
Boundaries of Zone II: Motor Branch	
Palmar	Palmaris brevis muscle
	Fibrous arch, hypothenar muscles
Dorsal	Pisohamate ligament
	Pisometacarpal ligament
	Triquetrohamate joint
	Opponens digiti minimi muscle
Lateral	Transverse carpal ligament
	Flexor digiti minimi muscle
	Hook of the hamate
Medial	Ulnar nerve, superficial branch
	Abductor digiti minimi muscle

Source: Gelberman RH. Ulnar tunnel syndrome. In: Gelberman RH, ed., Operative Nerve Repair and Reconstruction. Philadelphia: J.B. Lippincott, 1991:1131–43,[9] with permission.

TABLE 16A–4	
Boundaries of Zone III: Sensory Branch	
Palmar	Palmaris brevis muscle
	Ulnar artery, fibrofatty tissue
Dorsal	Hypothenar fascia
Lateral	Ulnar nerve, motor branch (Zone II)
Medial	Abductor digiti minimi muscle

Source: Gelberman RH. Ulnar tunnel syndrome. In: Gelberman RH, ed., Operative Nerve Repair and Reconstruction. Philadelphia: J.B. Lippincott, 1991:1131–43,[9] with permission.

versely across the deep palm, deep to the extrinsic flexors tendons and palmar to the to the interossei.[2]

The ulnar nerve bifurcates just distal to the boundary of Zone I. The sensory fibers angulate in a palmar-ulnar direction to enter Zone III. Zone III boundaries consist of the palmaris brevis muscle located palmary, the hypothenar fascia dorsally, the abductor digiti minimi muscle medially, and the border of Zone II dorsolaterally (Table 16A–4). The superficial branch continues distally to provide two small motor branches to the palmaris brevis muscle. The nerve is purely sensory distal to this point. The nerve then passes palmar to the fibrous arch of the hypothenar muscles, and continues deep and ulnar to the ulnar artery. At the distal end of Zone III, the nerve lies between the hypothenar fascia dorsally, and the ulnar artery and fibrofatty subcutaneous tissue palmarly.[2]

In Zone I, the ulnar nerve has both motor and sensory fibers contained within a common epineurial sheath. Cross-sections of the nerve in this zone show these two distinct groups of fascicles (Figs. 16A–1 and 16A–4 B). The palmar-radial fibers are destined to become the superficial branch of the nerve, and contain sensory fibers. The dorsal-ulnar fibers are destined to become motor and comprise the deep motor branch. The two groups of fascicles can be separated for a distance of 7.5 cm proximal to the bifurcation. Proximal to that region, there is significant plexus formation within the nerve. Throughout the proximal region of the ulnar tunnel (Zone I), the ulnar nerve is thus actually two nerves contained within a common sheath.

The deep motor branch of the nerve consists of an average of six fascicles. The nerve to the abductor digiti minimi muscle can be separated 15 mm proximal to the hypothenar fascia before significant intercommunications are noted. Nerves to the flexor digiti minimi and opponens digiti minimi muscles are separable for approximately 12 mm.[2]

The ulnar artery accompanies the ulnar nerve through Guyon's canal (Fig. 16A–1). The artery divides into two branches three to seven millimeters beyond the bifurcation of the nerve. The larger arterial branch travels with the superficial branch of the nerve, and eventually forms the superficial palmar arch along with the contribution from the superficial palmar branch of the radial artery. The smaller arterial branch accompanies the motor branch of the nerve into the adductor interosseous space, contributing to the deep palmar arch. Both arteries are located superficial and radial to the nerve that they accompany.

Correlation of Clinical Presentation to Anatomical Site of Compression

Clinically oriented anatomical studies of the ulnar tunnel have facilitated accurate localization of neural compression lesions, and can often allow correct preoperative identification of the cause.[2] Compression of the ulnar nerve in the ulnar tunnel can cause isolated motor loss, sensory loss, or combined motor and sensory loss.[4,9,11,160–163] These differences in clinical presentation can be attributed to specific sites of compression. When there is numbness that includes the dorsum of the ring and little fingers, along with weakness of the ulnar nerve–innervated intrinsic muscles, the site of compression occurs proximal to the branching of the dorsal sensory branch. The dorsal sensory branch exits the ulnar nerve trunk about seven centimeters proximal to the wrist crease, therefore compression occurs proximal to this area. These clinical findings usually indicate compression at the cubital tunnel. If there is associated numbness along the medial forearm, more proximal compression should be considered, such as at the level of the cervical spine, thoracic outlet, or lower brachial plexus.

Patients with numbness or paresthesias on the palmar aspects of the little finger and palmo-ulnar ring finger, along with weakness of the ulnar nerve-innervated intrinsic muscles usually have compression in Zone I.[2] Thirty-nine previously described patients with these combined sensory and motor deficits had compression in the proximal region of the ulnar tunnel where the nerve contains both sensory and motor fibers (Table 16A–5). Common causes of compression in this region were ganglia and fractures of the hook of the hamate or distal. In the absence of trauma, 86% of patients presenting with combined sensory and motor findings had ganglia encroaching on the nerve in the ulnar tunnel. Fractures of the hook of the hamate cause characteristic point tenderness in the palm 1 cm distal and lateral to the pisiform. Conformation is made with carpal tunnel view radiographs, CT, or MRI.

TABLE 16A–5

Distribution of Cases of Nerve Compression by Zone and Deficit 2

Zone	Motor/Sensory	Motor	Sensory	Total
I	39	1	7	47
II		36		36
III			10	10
Total (complete data)	39	37	17	93
Incomplete data				49
Total				142

Source: Gross MS, Gelberman RH. The anatomy of the distal ulnar tunnel. Clin Orthop 1985;196:238,[2] with permission.

Although most lesions in Zone I cause combined motor and sensory deficits, it is possible, with mild compression, to involve only the motor or only sensory fibers.[2] The motor fibers are located in the dorsal aspect of the nerve, and masses arising from the dorsal surface of the tunnel may compress only the motor fibers. The sensory fibers are located along the palmar aspect, and superficial palmar masses may compress initially sensory fibers only.

Patients presenting with impairment of the ulnar nerve-innervated intrinsic muscles only most often have compression within Zone II, which is distal to the bifurcation of the ulnar nerve[2] (Table 16A–5). The most common non-trauma cause of compression in this zone is a ganglion, usually arising from the triquetrohamate joint. Anomalous muscles and thickening of the fibrous proximal arch of the hypothenar muscles are additional causes of compression. Similar to Zone I lesions, if there is a history of trauma, fracture of the hamate hook is a probable cause.

Patients presenting with sensory impairment only usually have compression in Zone III (or possibly early in the course of Zone I compression). Zone III is distal to the bifurcation, and contains predominately sensory fibers. Common causes of compression in this zone are thrombosis of the ulnar artery and anomalous muscles.

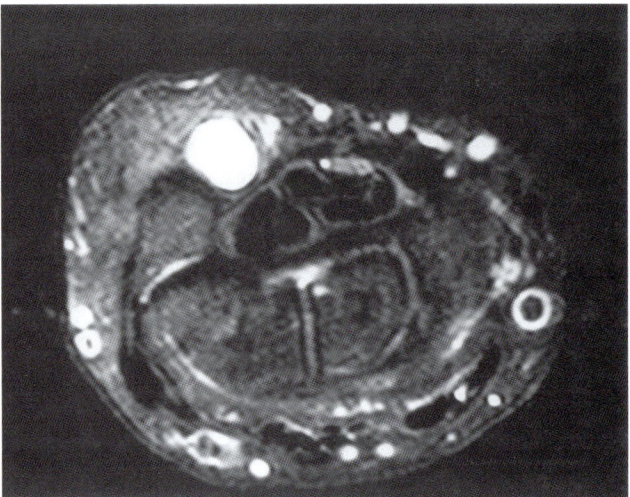

Figure 16A–5   Magnetic resonance imaging of the wrist showing ganglion in the ulnar tunnel.

INVESTIGATION

In the evaluation of the patient with suspected ulnar nerve entrapment in the ulnar tunnel, a history of trauma, including repetitive or occupational vibratory trauma, should be sought. Inflammatory afflictions such as rheumatoid arthritis and osteoarthritis, as well as systemic conditions that can contribute to peripheral neuropathy, should be considered. Associated signs or symptoms of compression of the median nerve in the carpal tunnel are also evaluated. The history should also include aspects concerning more proximal nerve lesions, such as in the cervical spine, thoracic outlet, or cubital tunnel.

Physical examination includes several areas of evaluations: elicitation of point tenderness, peripheral vascular examination, provocative testing, sensibility testing, and motor examination.[4,9,11,160] Point tenderness in the region of the hook of the hamate is indicative of possible fracture of the hook of the hamate. Peripheral vascular evaluation includes assessment of the pulses, timed Allen test (revascularization of the long finger by the ulnar artery within 5 seconds is normal), and an examination for bruits, pulsatile lesions, or evidence of a previous open injury. Provocative testing includes nerve percussion and the Phalen's test. Sensibility evaluation includes static two-point evaluation and the Semmes-Weinstein monofilament testing. Motor examination includes manual muscle testing of the extrinsic

and intrinsic median and ulnar-innervated muscles of the hand. The patient should be examined for more proximal areas of compression, including tenderness of the ulnar nerve in the cubital tunnel, strength testing of the flexor digitorum profundus to the ring and little fingers and the flexor carpi ulnaris, sensibility testing the dorsoulnar aspect of the hand, and provocative testing with the elbow held in flexion.

Initial imaging studies include standard radiographs. Additional studies include can include MRI, CT, electrodiagnostic studies, or vascular studies.[42,62,69,71,82,164–174] Radiographs include posteroanterior, lateral, oblique, and carpal tunnel views. CT is helpful for identification of fractures not visualized by standard radiographs, and will often visualize tumors, anomalous muscles, or vascular lesions.[42,62] MRI[82,121,164,165,167,168] or diagnostic ultrasound[37,69,121,171,172] of the wrist is generally more helpful in the evaluation of soft tissue afflictions such as tumors, muscle anomalies, aneurysm, or thrombosis (Fig. 16A–5). Arteriography also assists with evaluation of associated vascular lesions.[42,71,170]

Electromyography and nerve conductions studies are used to establish or confirm the diagnosis.[62,108,112,128,173] These electrodiagnositic studies are useful when multiple sites of compression are suspected, such as concomitant compression in the cervical spine, thoracic outlet, or cubital tunnel. Sparing of sensory of motor fibers in helpful in localizing the site of compression within the ulnar tunnel.

TREATMENT

Nonoperative treatment is usually initially indicated for neuropathies caused by repetitive trauma or in cases where a distinct space-occupying lesion or fracture is not identified.[4,9,11,160,161] Conservative management includes activity modification with avoidance of provocative activities, immobilization of the wrist in a neutral position with a splint or cast, nonsteroidal anti-inflammatory medication, and possible steroid injection.

When neuropathy occurs immediately following displaced fracture of the distal radius or ulna, fracture reduction should be carried out emergently. If nerve function does not improve in 24 to 36 hours following satisfactory closed reduction, nerve exploration and decompression should be performed.

In the patient who develops progressive ulnar neuropathy after fracture or following closed reduction, immediate exploration and decompression should be carried out.

Several anatomic differences help explain why ulnar neuropathy following fracture of the distal end of the radius is less common than neuropathy of the median nerve. Whereas both nerves have some protection by soft tissue at the level of the fracture, the median nerve is more firmly bound for a longer distance within the carpal canal. The ulnar tunnel, however, is short and farther from the fracture site, and greater excursion of the ulnar nerve is possible at the level of the injury.

In neuropathies where a space-occupying lesion can be identified (such as tumor, anomalous muscle, or vascular lesion), or in refractory cases in the absence of an identifiable cause, operative exploration and nerve decompression are usually indicated.[4,9,11,160,161,174–177]

Operative Decompression

Localization of the area of compression to one of the three zones is helpful in guiding preoperative evaluation and predicting causes of compression. However, operative treatment is aimed at exploring the nerve from the distal forearm into the palm throughout all three zones.

Preferred Surgical Approach

The patient is positioned supine, general or regional anesthesia administered, and the upper extremity is prepared and draped in the usually fashion. The skin incision is placed to lie in the interval between the palmar cutaneous branches of the median and ulnar nerves. The pisiform is palpated and marked with a skin marker. The hook of the hamate, located 1 cm distal and lateral to the pisiform, is palpated and marked. The extremity is exsanguinated and tourniquet inflated to 200 to 250 mm Hg. A curvilinear 7-cm incision is placed starting distally, bisecting the interval between the pisiform and hamate and crossing the transverse wrist creases obliquely (Figs. 16A–6 and 16A–7). The wrist creases are not crossed at right angles. The incision extends about 4 cm into the ulnar aspect of the palm and 3 cm into the distal forearm. Dissection is carried out from a proximal to distal direction. The flexor carpi ulnaris

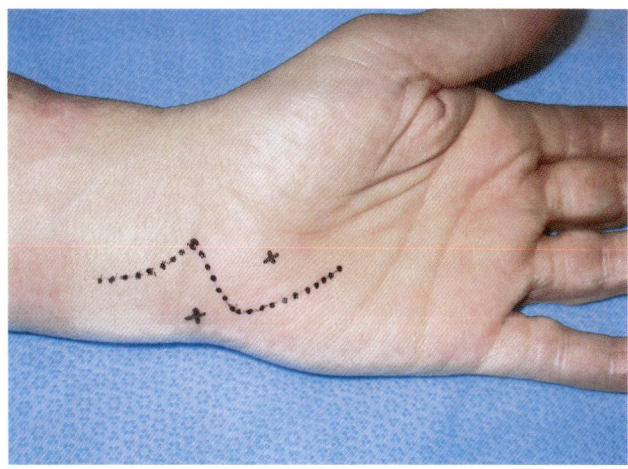

Figure 16A–6 Incision used for exploring the ulnar tunnel. The pisiform and hook of the hamate are marked. The incision avoids crossing the wrist crease at a right angle.

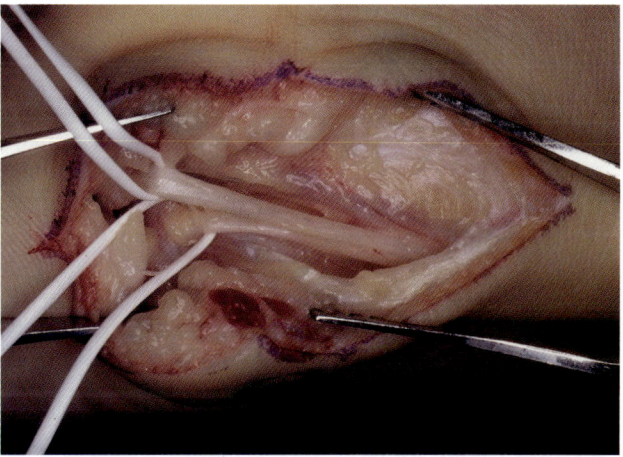

Figure 16A–7 Operative exploration and decompression of the ulnar nerve in the Guyon's canal. The vessel loops mark the branches distal to the bifurcation.

tendon is retracted ulnarly, exposing the ulnar nerve and artery. The artery is located palmar and radial to the nerve. The ulnar nerve is tagged with a rubber dam and the artery with a vessel loop. In the distal forearm, the neurovascular bundle is traced distally where it enters Guyon's canal deep top the palmar carpal ligament. The ligament, palmaris brevis, and hypothenar fat and fibrous tissue are incised, decompressing the nerve along its entire course through the canal.

Following nerve decompression, the floor of the canal is then explored, specifically examining the interval between the pisohamate and pisometacarpal ligaments. Masses such as ganglions, anomalous muscles, fibrous bands, osteophytes, and fracture fragments are identified and excised (Fig. 16A–8). The fibrous origin of the hypothenar muscles is located by palpating the hamate and identifying the fibrous proximal edge of the arch. A thickened fibrous origin of the hypothenar muscles is noted in about 40% of cases, and when

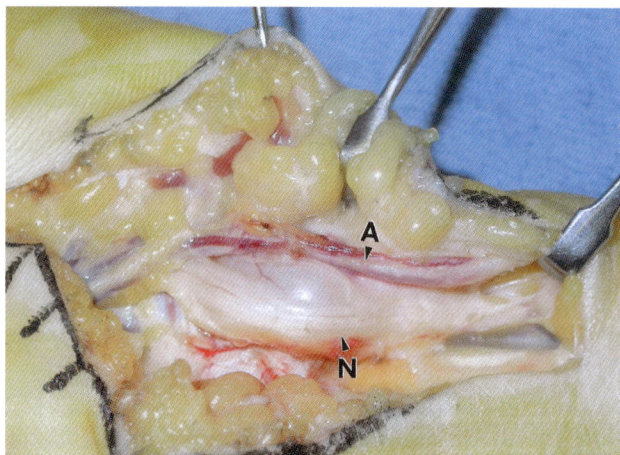

Figure 16A–8 Ganglion cyst found in the ulnar tunnel, emerging between the ulnar artery (A) and the ulnar nerve (N). Note the encroachment of the nerve by the ganglion.

present, the origin is divided.[20] The motor nerve is followed into the interval between the abductor digiti minimi and flexor digiti minimi muscles and through the origin of the opponens digiti minimi. The ulnar artery is explored throughout its course in the canal. The tourniquet is released, hemostasis obtained, and skin closed with 5-0 nylon sutures. The palmar carpal ligament is allowed to retract, and is not repaired. A bulky hand dressing with plaster splints is applied with the wrist in 20 degrees of dorsiflexion.

Postoperative Care

The hand dressing and sutures are removed in 7 to 10 days. A palmar splint is placed to maintain the wrist in 20 degrees of dorsiflexion for an additional 2 weeks. Splinting is discontinued in about 3 weeks.

In patients with concomitant carpal tunnel syndrome and ulnar tunnel syndrome, anatomic and clinical studies indicate that incision of the flexor retinaculum performed for carpal tunnel release may also relieve symptoms of ulnar tunnel syndrome by relaxing Guyon's canal and decreasing pressure on the ulnar nerve.[4,175,176]

Pain usually decreases or resolves immediately or in the early postoperative period. Sensibility and motor function improve gradually, depending on the length and magnitude of nerve compression.[20,43,48,102,122,177–179] Most studies lack details on time and completeness of motor recovery; however, tendon transfers are rarely needed, indicating a favorable prognosis for intrinsic muscle recovery.[180–188]

Dedication

To J. Leonard Goldner.—Dr. Gelberman

REFERENCES

1. Guyon F. Note sur une disposition anatomique propre a la face anterieure de la region du poignet et non encore decrite par le docteur. Bull Soc Anat Paris 1961;6:184.
2. Gross MS, Gelberman RH. The anatomy of the distal ulnar tunnel. Clin Orthop 1985;196:238.
3. McFarland RM, Mayer JR, Hugill JV. Further observations on the anatomy of the ulnar nerve at the wrist. Hand 1976;8:115.
4. Kuschner S, Gelberman RH. Ulnar nerve compression at the wrist. J Hand Surg Am 1988;13:577–80.
5. Kaplan EB. Variation of the ulnar nerve at the wrist. Bull Hosp Joint Dis 1963;24:85–8.
6. Kleinert HE, Hayes JW. Ulnar tunnel syndrome. Plast Reconstr Surg 1971;47:21.
7. Konig PS, Hage JJ, Bloem JJ, et al. Variations of the ulnar nerve and ulnar artery in Guyon's canal. A cadaveric study. J Hand Surg Am 1994;19:617–22.
8. Bergfield TG, Aulicino PL. Variation of the deep motor branch of the ulnar nerve at the wrist. J Hand Surg Am 1982;3:368–9.
9. Gelberman RH. Ulnar tunnel syndrome. In: Gelberman RH, ed., Operative Nerve Repair and Reconstruction. Philadelphia: J.B. Lippincott, 1991:1131–43.
10. Gonzalez MH, Brown A, Goodman D, et al. The deep branch of the ulnar nerve in Guyon's canal: branching and innervation of the hypothenar muscles. Orthopedics 1996;19:55–8.
11. Botte MJ, Gelberman RH. Ulnar nerve compression at the wrist. In: Szabo RM, ed., Nerve Compression Syndromes: Diagnosis and Treatment. Thorofare, NJ: Slack Inc., 1989:121–36.
12. Cobb TK, Carmichael SW, Cooney WOP. Guyon's canal revisited: an anatomic study of the carpal ulnar neurovascular space. J Hand Surg Am 1996;21:861–9.
13. Dodds GA, Hale D, Jackson WT. Incidence of anatomic variants in Guyon's canal. J Hand Surg Am 1990;5:352–5.
14. Fahrer M. The proximal end of the palmar aponeurosis. Hand 1980;12:33.
15. Lassa, R, Shrewsbury MM. A variation of the path of the deep branch of the ulnar nerve at the wrist. J Bone Joint Surg Am 1975;57:990.
16. Lindsey JT, Watumull D. Anatomic study of the ulnar nerve and related vascular anatomy at Guyon's canal: a practical classification system. J Hand Surg Am 1996;21:626–33.
17. Martin CH, Seiler JG 3rd, Lesesne JS. The cutaneous innervation of the palm: an anatomic study of the ulnar and median nerves. J Hand Surg Am 1996;21:634–8.
18. Jabaley ME, Wallace WH, Heckler FR. Internal topography of major nerves of the forearm and hand: a current view. J Hand Surg Am 1980;5:1.
19. Denman EE. The anatomy of the space of Guyon. Hand 1978;10:69.
20. Dellon AL, Mackinnon SE. Anatomic investigations of nerves at the wrist. II. Incidence of fibrous arch overlying motor branch of ulnar nerve. Ann Plast Surg 1988;21:36–7.
21. Harvie P, Patel N, Ostlere SJ. Prevalence and epidemiological variation of anomalous muscles at Guyon's canal. J Hand Surg Br 2004;29:26–9.
22. Antuna SA, Guitierrez CR, Paz Jimenez J. Ulnar nerve compression in Guyon's canal caused by a pseudotumor of the pisiform. Acta Orthop Belg 1995;61:245–8.
23. Baird DB, Predenberg ZB. Delayed ulnar nerve palsy following a fracture of the hamate. J Bone Joint Surg Am 1968;50:570.
24. Bakke JL, Wolff HG. Occupational pressure neuritis of the deep palmar branch of the ulnar nerve. Arch Neurol Psychiatry 1948;60:549.
25. Brooks DM. Nerve compression by simple ganglia. J Bone Joint Surg Br 1952;34:391.

26. Murata K, Shih JT, Tsai TM. Causes of ulnar tunnel syndrome: a retrospective study of 31 subjects. J Hand Surg Am 2003; 28:647–51.

27. Bayer WL, Shea JD, Curiel DC, et al. Excision of a pseudocyst of the hand in a hemophiliac (PTC-deficiency). Use of a plasma thromboplastin component concentrate. J Bone Joint Surg Am 1969;51:1423.

28. Berkowitz AR, Melone CP Jr, Belsky MR. Pisiform-hamate coalition with ulnar neuropathy. J Hand Surg Am 1992;17:657–62.

29. Bhatty MA, Thomas SS, Nancarrow JD. Delayed ulnar tunnel syndrome following a minor closed wrist injury. Injury 1995;26:341–2.

30. Bourrel P, Ferro RM. Nerve complication in closed fractures of the lower end of the radius. Ann Chir Main 1982;1: 119–26.

31. Bovim G, Andersen K. Nerve compression symptoms after a long bicycle ride—the Great Test of Strength. Tidsskr Nor Laegeforen 1992;112:2199–201.

32. Brutus JP, Mattoli JA, Palmer AK. Unusual complication of an opposition tendon transfer at the wrist: ulnar nerve compression syndrome. J Hand Surg Am 2004;29:625–7.

33. Budny PG, Regan PJ, Roberts AH. Localized nodular synovitis: a rare cause of ulnar nerve compression in Guyon's canal. J Hand Surg Am 1992;17:663–4.

34. Bui-Mansfield LT, Williamson M, Wheeler DT, Johnstone F. Guyon's canal lipoma causing ulnar neuropathy. AJR Am J Roentgenol 2002;178:1458.

35. Burnham RS, Steadward RD. Upper extremity peripheral nerve entrapments among wheelchair athletes: prevalence, location and risk factors. Arch Phys Med Rehabil 1994;75:519–24.

36. Chammas M, Meyer zu Reckendorf G, Allieu Y. Compression of the ulnar nerve in Guyon's canal by pseudotumoral calcinosis in systemic scleroderma. J Hand Surg Br 1995;20:794–6.

37. Choudhari KA, Muthu T, Tan MH. Progressive ulnar neuropathy caused by delayed migration of a foreign body. Br J Neurosurg 2001;15:263–5.

38. Comtet JJ, Quicot L, Moyen B. Compression of the deep palmar branch of the ulnar nerve by the arch of the adductor pollicis. Hand 1978;10:176.

39. Cantero J. Hypothenar hammer syndrome. Apropos of 2 cases. Ann Chir Main 1987;6:303–6.

40. Capitani D, Beer S. Handlebar palsy—a compression syndrome of the deep terminal (motor) branch of the ulnar nerve in biking. J Neurol 2002;249:1441–5.

41. Costigan DG, Riley JM, Coyh FE. Thrombofibrosis of the ulnar artery in the palm. J Bone Joint Surg Am 1959;41:702.

42. Coulier B, Goffin D, Malbecq S, et al. Colour duplex sonographic and multislice spiral CT angiographic diagnosis of ulnar artery aneurysm in hypothenar hammer syndrome. J Belg Radiol BTR 2003;86:211–14.

43. Dell PC. Compression of the ulnar nerve at the wrist secondary to a rheumatoid synovial cyst: case report and review of the literature. J Hand Surg Am 1979;4:468.

44. Dell'Omo M, Muzi G, Cantisani TA, et al. Bilateral median and ulnar neuropathy at the wrist in a parquet floorer. Occup Environ Med 1995;52:211–13.

45. De Smet L. Median and ulnar nerve compression at the wrist caused by anomalous muscles. Acta Orthop Belg 2002;68: 431–8.

46. Dumontier C, Apoil A, Meininger T, et al. Compression of the deep branch of the ulnar nerve as it exits the pisiform-unciform hiatus: report of an anomaly not yet described. Ann Chir Main Memb Super 1991;10:337–41.

47. Dunn WA. Fractures and dislocations of the carpus. Surg Clin North Am 1972;52:1513.

48. Dupont C, Cloutier GE, Prevost Y, et al. Ulnar-tunnel syndrome at the wrist. J Bone Joint Surg Am 1965;42:757.

49. Eckman PB, Perstein G, Altrocchi PH. Ulnar neuropathy in bicycle riders. Arch Neurol 1975;32:130.

50. Elias DA, Laz MJ, Anastakis DJ. Musculoskeletal images. Ganglion cyst of Guyon's canal cuasing ulnar nerve compression. Can J Hand Surg 2001;44:331–2.

51. Erdoes LS, Brown WC. Ruptured ulnar artery pseudoaneurysm. Ann Vasc Surg 1995;9:394–6.

52. Fahrer M, Millroy PJ. Ulnar compression neuropathy due to an anomalous abductor digiti minimi: Clinical and anatomic study. J Hand Surg Am 1981;6:266.

53. Fragiadakis EG, Lamb DW. An unusual cause of ulnar nerve compression. Hand 1970;2:14–15.

54. Fennay JB. Deep ulnar nerve paralysis resulting from an anatomical abnormality. J Bone Joint Surg Am 1965;47:1381.

55. Fissette J, Onkelinx A, Fandi N. Carpal and Guyon tunnel syndrome in burns at the wrist. J Hand Surg Am 1981;6:13–15.

56. Foucher G, Berard V, Snider G, et al. Distal ulnar nerve entrapment due to tumors of Guyon's canal. A series of ten cases. Handchir Mikrochir Plast Chir 1993;25:61–5.

57. Frank DH, Robson MD. Unusual occurrence of chronic nerve compression syndromes at the wrists of thermally injured patients. Orthop Rev 1979;8:180.

58. Frederick HA, Carter PR, Littler JW. Injection injuries to the median and ulnar nerves at the wrist. J Hand Surg Am 1992;17:645–7.

59. Fong EP, Mahaffey PJ. Ulnar tunnel syndrome-an unusual case. Hand Surg 2000;5:77–9.

60. Galeano M, Colonna M, Risitano G. Ulnar tunnel syndrome secondary to lipoma of the hypothenar region. Ann Plast Surg 2001;46:83–4.

61. Garcia S, Cofan F, Combalia A, et al. Compression of the ulnar nerve in Guyon's canal by uremic tumoral calcinosis. Arch Orthop Trauma Surg 2000;120–:228–30.

62. Giuliani G, Poppi M, Pozzati E, et al. Ulnar neuropathy due to a carpal ganglion: the diagnostic contribution of CT. Neurology 1990;40:1001–2.

63. Gloobe H, Pecket P. An anomalous muscle in the canal of Guyon. Anat 1973;133:477.

64. Greene MH, Hadied AM. Bipartite hamulus with ulnar tunnel syndrome-case report and literature review. J Hand Surg Am 1981;6:605.

65. Grossman, JA, Becker GA. Ulnar neuropathy caused by a thrombosed ulnar vein. Case report and literature review. Ann Chir Main Memb Super 1996;15:244–7.

66. Harrelson JM, Newman M. Hypertrophy of the flexor carpi ulnaris as a cause of ulnar-nerve compression in the distal part of the forearm: case report. J Bone Joint Surg Am 1975; 57:554–5.

67. Harris W. Occupational pressure neuritis of the deep palmar branch of the ulnar nerve. BMJ 1921;1:98.

68. Hart VL. Two unusual injuries of the wrist. J Bone Joint Surg Am 1941;23:948.

69. Harvie P, Patel N, Ostlere SJ. Ulnar nerve compression at Guyon's canal by an anomalous abductor digiti minimi muscle: the role of ultrasound in clinical diagnosis. Hand Surg 2003;8:271–5.

70. Hayes JR, Mulholland RC, O'Connor BT. Compression of the deep palmar branch of the ulnar nerve. J Bone Joint Surg Br 1969;51:469.

71. Heitmann C, Pelzer M, Trankle M, et al. The hypothenar hammer syndrome. Unfallchirurg 2002;105:833–6.

72. Howard FM. Ulnar nerve palsy in wrist fractures. J Bone Joint Surg Am 1961;43:1197.

73. Hunt JR. Occupational neuritis of the deep palmar branch of the ulnar nerve. J Nerv Ment Dis 1908;35:676.

74. Hunt JR. Thenar and hypothenar types of neural atrophy of the hand. BMJ 1930;2:642.

75. Jackson JP. Traumatic thrombosis of the ulnar artery in the palm. J Bone Joint Surg Br 1954;36:438.

76. Jeffrey AK. Compression of the deep palmar branch of the ulnar nerve by an anomalous muscle. J Bone Joint Surg Br 1971;53:718.

77. Jenkins SA. Solitary tumors of peripheral nerve trunks. J Bone Joint Surg Br 1952;34:401.

78. Jenkins SA. Osteoarthritis of the pisiform-triquetral joint. J Bone Joint Surg Br 1957;33:532.

79. Kalainov DM, Hartigan BJ. Bicycling-induced ulnar tunnel syndrome. Am J Orthop 2003;32:210–11.

80. Kaleli T, Temiz A, Ozturk H. Pseudomalignancy myositis ossificans of the wrist causing compression of the ulnar nerve and artery. A case report. Acta Orthop Belg 2003;69:289–91.

81. Kalisman M, Laborde K, Woldff TW. Ulnar nerve compression secondary to ulnar artery false aneurysm at the Guyon's canal. J Hand Surg Am 1982;7:137.

82. Kang HJ, Shin SJ, Kang ES. Schwannomas of the upper extremity. J Hand Surg Br 2000;25:604–7.

83. Kabayashi N, Koshino T, Nakazawa A, et al. Neuropathy of motor branch of median or ulnar nerve induced by midpalm ganglion. J Hand Surg Am 2001;26:474–7.

84. Koch H, Haas F, Pierer G. Ulnar nerve compression Guyon's canal due to a haemangioma of the ulnar artery. J Hand Surg Br 1998;23:242–4.

85. Lahey MD, Aulicino PL. Anomalous muscles associated with compression neuropathies. Orthop Rev 1986;15:199–208.

86. Lane CS, Kuschner SH. Causes of ulnar tunnel syndrome. J Hand Surg Am 2004;29:160.

87. Lavalle F, Pistre V, Alfandari B, et al. Compression of the deep motor branch of the ulnar nerve by a synovial cyst. A case report. Chir Main 2002;21:269–71.

88. Leslie IJ. Compression of the deep branch of the ulnar nerve due to edema of the hand. Hand 1980;12:271.

89. Lipscomb PR. Duplication of hypothenar muscles simulating soft tissue tumor of the hand. Report of a case. J Bone Joint Surg Am 1960;42:1058.

90. Lisanti M, Rosati M, Maltinti M. Ulnar nerve entrapment in Guyon's tunnel by an anomalous palmaris longus muscle with a persisting median artery. Acta Orthop Belg 2001;67:399–402.

91. Madhavi C, Holla SJ. Anomalous flexor digiti minimi brevis in Guyon's canal. Clin Anat 2003;16:340–3.

92. Mallet BL, Zilkha KJ. Compression of the ulnar nerve at the wrist by a ganglion. Lancet 1955;268:8901.

93. Masmejean EH, Chavane H, Chantegret A, et al. The wrist of the formula 1 driver. Br J Sports Med 1990;33:270–3.

94. Maynou C, Mestdagh H, Butruille Y, et al. Compression of the ulnar nerve at the wrist due to an arthrosynovial cyst. Apropos of 2 cases. Ann Chir Main Memb Super 1997;16:146–51.

95. Mc Dowell CL, Henceroth WD. Compression of the ulnar nerve in the hand by a ganglion. J Bone Joint Surg Am 1970;59:980.

96. McFarland GB, Hoffer MM. Paralysis of the intrinsic muscles of the hand secondary to lipoma in Guyon's tunnel. J Bone Joint Surg Am 1971;53:375.

97. Mellion MB. Common cycling injuries. Management and prevention. Sport Med 1991;11:52–70.

98. Milberg P, Lkeinert HE. Giant cell tumor compression of the deep branch of the ulnar nerve. Ann Plast Surg 1980;4:426.

99. Millender LH, Nalebuff E, Kasdon E. Aneurysms and thromboses of the ulnar artery in the hand. Arch Surg 1972;105:686.

100. Moneim MS. Ulnar nerve compression at the wrist: ulnar tunnel syndrome. Hand Clin 1992;8:337–44.

102. Muller LH. Anatomical abnormalities at the wrist joint causing neurological symptoms in the hand. J Bone Joint Surg Br 1963;45:431.

102. Nakano KK. The entrapment neuropathies. Muscle Nerve 1978;1:264.

103. Netscher D, Cohen V. Ulnar nerve compression at the wrist secondary to anomalous muscles: a patient with a variant of abductor digiti minimi. Ann Plast Surg 1997;39:647–51.

104. Nicolle FV, Woolhouse FM. Nerve compression syndromes of the upper limb. J Trauma 1965;5:313–18.

105. Nisenfield FG, Neviaser RJ. Fracture of the hook of the hamate: a diagnosis easily missed. J Trauma 1974;14:612.

106. Nucci F, Artico M, Antonini G, et al. Compression of the ulnar nerve in Guyon's canal by a giant cell tumor. Zentralbl Neurochir 1898;50:196–8.

107. O'Hara JJ, Stone JH. Ulnar neuropathy at the wrist associated with aberrant flexor carpi ulnaris insertion. J Hand Surg Am 1988;13:370–2.

108. Olney RK, Nanson M. AAEE case report 315: ulnar neuropathy at or distal to the wrist. Muscle Nerve 1988;11:828–32.

109. Pagliughi G, Vespasiani A. Unusual compression of the ulnar nerve caused by a hematic cyst. Chir Ital 1979;31:428–30.

110. Papierski P. Ulnar neuropathy at the wrist associated with a recurrent branch through the flexor carpi ulnaris tendon. J Hand Surg Br 1996;21:347–8.

111. Pribyl CR, Moneim MS. Anomalous hand muscle found in the Guyon's canal at exploration for ulnar artery thrombosis. A case report. Clin Orthop 1994;306:120–3.

112. Rafecas JC, Daube JR, Ehman RL. Deep branch ulnar neuropathy due to giant cell tumor: report of a case. Neurology 1988;38:327–9.

113. Rengachary SS, Arjunan K. Compression of the ulnar nerve in Guyon's canal by a soft tissue giant cell tumor. Neurosurgery 1981;8:400–5.

114. Richmond DA. Carpal ganglion with ulnar nerve compression. J Bone Joint Surg Am 1963;45:513.

115. Richmmond DR. Handlebar problems in bicycling. Clin Sports Med 1994;13:165–73.

116. Ritter MA, Marshall J, Straub LR. Extra-abdominal desmoid of the hand. A case report. J Bone Joint Surg Am 1969;51:1641.

117. Robinson SC. An anomalous flexor digitorum superficialis muscle-tendon unit associated with ulnar neuropathy. A case report. Clin Orthop 1985;194:169–71.

118. Robinson D, Aghasi MK, Halperin N. Ulnar tunnel syndrome caused by an accessory palmaris muscle. Orthop Rev 1989;18:345–7.

119. Rouhart F, Fourquet I, Tea SH, et al. Lesion of the deep branch of the ulnar nerve caused by fracture of the hook of the hamate. Neurophysiol Clin 1990;20.253–8.

120. Ruder JR, Wood VE. Ulnar nerve compression at the arch of the origin of the adductor pollicis muscle. J Hand Surg Am 1993;18:893–5.

121. Sakai K, Tsutsui T, Aoi M, et al. Ulnar neuropathy caused by a lipoma in Guyon's canal—case report. Neurol Med Chir (Tokyo) 2000;40:335–8.

122. Salgeback S. Ulnar tunnel syndrome caused by anomalous muscles. A case report. Scand J Plast Reconstr Surg 1977;11:255.

123. Santoro TD, Matloub HS, Gosain AK. Ulnar nerve compression by an anomalous muscle following carpal tunnel release: a case report. J Hand Surg Am 2000;25:740–4.

124. Sauerbier M, Krimmer H, Muller L, et al. Compression of the ulnar nerve in Guyon's canal by a traumatic aneurysm. A case report. Handchir Mikrochir Plast Chir 1998;30:303–5.

125. Schjelderup H. Aberrant muscle in the hand causing ulnar nerve compression. J Bone Joint Surg Br 1964;46:361.

126. Seddon HJ. Carpal ganglion as a cause of paralysis of the deep branch of the ulnar nerve. J Bone Joint Surg Br 1952;34:386.

127. Segal R, Machiraju U, Larkins M. Tortuous peripheral arteries: a cause of focal neuropathy. Case report. J Neurosurg 1992;76:701–4.

128. Seror P, Lestrade M, Vacher H. Ulnar nerve compression at the wrist by s synovial cyst successfully treated with percutaneous puncture and corticosteroid injection. Joint Bone Spine 2000;67:127–8.

129. Shea JD, McClain EJ. Ulnar nerve compression syndromes at and below the wrist. J Bone Joint Surg Am 1969;51:1095.

130. Sheppard JE, Prebble TB, Rahn K. Ulnar neuropathy caused by an accessory abductor digiti minimi muscle. Wis Med J 1991;90:628–31.

131. Shu N, Uchio Y, Ryoke K, et al. Atypical compression of the deep branch of the ulnar nerve in Guyon's canal by a ganlion. Case report. Scand J Plast Reconstr Surg Hand Surg 2000; 34:181–3.

132. Smith RJ. Ulnar nerve compression secondary to ulnar artery false aneurysm at the Guyon's canal. J Hand Surg Am 1982;7:631–2.

133. Soldado-Cerrera F, Vilar-Coromina N, Rodriguez-Baeza A. An accessory belly of the abductor digiti minimi muscle: a case report and embryologic aspects. Surg Radiol Anat 2000; 22:51–4.

134. Spinner M, Freundlich BD. An important variation of the palmaris longus. Bull Hosp Joint Dis 1967;28:126–30.

135. Stern PJ, Vice M. Compression of the deep branch of the ulnar nerve—case report. J Hand Surg Am 1983;8:72–4.

136. Streib EW, Sun SF. Distal ulnar neuropathy in meat packers. An occupational disease. J Occup Med 1984;26:842–3.

137. Swanson, AB, Biddulph SL, Baughman FA, et al. Ulnar nerve compression due to an anomalous muscle in the canal of Guyon. Clin Orthop 1972;83:64.

138. Tashima Y, Kimata Y. A case of ganglion causing paralysis of intrinsic muscles innervated by the ulnar nerve. J Bone Joint Surg Br 1961;43:153.

139. Taylor AR. Ulnar nerve compression at the wrist in rheumatoid arthritis. J Bone Joint Surg Br 1974;56:142.

140. Treece LG. Thrombosis of the ulnar artery. Aust N Z J Surg 1949;19:156.

141. Thomas CG. Clinical manifestations of an accessory palmaris muscle. J Bone Joint Surg Am 1958;40:929.

142. Thurman RT, Jindal P, Wolff TW. Ulnar nerve compression in Guyon's canal caused by calcinosis in scleroderma. J Hand Surg Am 1991;16:739–41.

143. Torok G, Giora A. Ulnar nerve lesion in the palm: entrapment neuropathy of the deep branch of the ulnar nerve. Isr Med J 1964;23:121–8.

144. Towfigh H, Schmidt G. Aneurysms. A rare cause of ulnar nerve compression in the palm. Handchir Mikrochir Plast Chir 1988;20:51–3.

145. Turner MS, Caird DM. Anomalous muscles and ulnar nerve compression at the wrist. Hand 1977;9:140.

146. Uriburu IJF, Morchio FJ, Marin JC. Compression syndrome of the deep branch of the ulnar nerve (piso-hamate hiatus syndrome). J Bone Joint Surg Am 1976;58:145–7.

147. Vance RM, Gelberman RH. Acute ulnar neuropathy with fractures at the wrist. J Bone Joint Surg Am 1978;60:692.

148. Vanderpool DW, Chalmers J, Whiston TB. Peripheral compression lesions of the ulnar nerve. J Bone Joint Surg Am 1968;50:792.

149. Watson-Jones R. Carpal semilunar dislocations and other wrist dislocations with associated nerve lesions. Proc R Soc Med 1929;22:1071.

150. Weeks PM, Young VL. Ulnar artery thrombosis and ulnar nerve compression associated with anomalous hypothenar muscle. Plast Reconstr Surg 1982;69:130–1.

151. White NB. Neurilemomas of the extremities. J Bone Joint Surg Am 1967;49:1605.

152. White WL, Hauna DC. Troublesome lipomata of the upper extremity. J Bone Joint Surg Am 1962;44:1353.

153. Woischnek D, Hussein S, Hollerhage HG. Bicycle rider's ulnar nerve paralysis. Neurochirurgia (Stuttg) 1993;36:11–13.

154. Wood VE. Nerve compression following opponensplasty as a result of wrist anomalies: report of a case. J Hand Surg Am 1980;5:279.

155. Worster-Drought C. Pressure neuritis of the deep palmar branch of the ulnar nerve. BMJ 1929;1:247.

156. Yoshii S, Ideda K, Murakamji H. Ulnar Nesci 1999;43:295–7.

157. Zahrawi F. Acute compression ulnar neuropathy at Guyon's canal resulting from lipoma. J Hand Surg Am 1984;9:238–9.

158. Zielinski CJ. Intraneural ganglion of the ulnar nerve at the wrist. Orthopedics 2003;26:429–30.

159. Zoega H. Fracture of the lower end of the radius with ulnar nerve palsy. J Bone Joint Surg Br 1966;48:514.

160. Gelberman RH, Eaton RG, Urbaniak JR. Peripheral nerve compression. Instr Course Lect 1994;43:31–53.

161. Grundberg AB. Ulnar tunnel syndrome. J Hand Surg Br 1984;9:72–4.

162. Packer NP, Fisk GR. Compression of the distal ulnar nerve with clawing of the index finger. Hand 1982;14:38.

163. Russell WR, Whitty CWM. Traumatic neuritis of the deep palmar branch of the ulnar nerve. Lancet 1947;1:828.

164. Subin GD, Mallon WJ, Urbaniak JR. Diagnosis of ganglion in Guyon's canal by magnetic resonance imaging. J Hand Surg Am 1898;14:640–3.

165. Binkjovitz LA, Berquiat TH, McLoed RA. Masses of the hand and wrist: detection and characterization with MR imaging. AJR Am J Roentgenol 1990;155:323–6.

166. Zeiss J, Jakab E. MR demonstration of an anomalous muscle in a patient with coexistent carpal and ulnar tunnel syndrome. Case report and literature summary. Clin Imaging 1995; 19:102–5.

167. Bordalo-Rodrigues M, Amin P, et al. MR imaging of common entrapment neuropathies at the wrist. Magn Reson Imaging Clin North Am 2004;12:265–79.

168. Ruocco MJ, Walsh JJ, Jackson JP. MR imagining of ulnar nerve entrapment secondary to an anomalous wrist muscle. Skeletal Radiol 1998;27:218–21.

169. Ziess J, Jakab E, Khimji T, et al. The ulnar tunnel at the wrist (Guyon's canal): normal MR anatomy and variants. AJR Am J Roentgenol 1992;158:1081–5.

170. DiBenedetto MR, Nappi JR, Ruff ME, et al. Doppler mapping in hypothenar syndrome: an alternative to angiography. J Hand Surg Am 1989;14:244–6.

171. Nakamichi KJ, Tachibana S, Kitajima I. Ultrasonography in the diagnosis of ulnar tunnel syndrome caused by an occult ganglion. J Hand Surg Br 2000;25:503–4.

172. Nakamichi K, Tachibana S. Ganglion-associated ulnar tunnel syndrome treated by ultrasonographically assisted aspiration and splinting. J Hand Surg Br 2003;28:177–8.

173. Ebeling P, Gilliat RW, Thomas DK. A clinical and electrical study of ulnar nerve lesions in the hand. J Neurol Neurosurg Psychiatry 1960;23:1.

174. Hacke W. Sensory conduction in the syndrome of Guyon's tunnel. J Neurol 1981;226:195–8.

175. Silver MA, Gelberman RH, Gellman H, et al. Carpal tunnel syndrome: associated abnormalities in ulnar nerve function and the effect of carpal tunnel release on these abnormalities. J Hand Surg Am 1985;10:710.

176. Ablove RH, Moy OJ, Peimer CA, et al. Pressure changes in Guyon's canal after carpal tunnel release. J Hand Surg Br 1996;21:664–5.

177. Zoch G, Meissl G, Millesi H. Results of decompression of the ulnar nerve in Guyon's canal. Handchir Mikrochir Plast Chir 1990;22:125–9.

178. Aguiar PH, Bor-Seng-Shu E, Gomes-Pinto F, et al. Surgical management of Guyon's canal syndrome, an ulnar nerve entrap-

ment at the wrist: report of two cases. Arq Neuropsiquiatr 2001;59:106–11.

179. Mondelli M, Mandarini A, Stumpo M. Good recovery after surgery in an extreme case of Guyon's canal syndrome. Surg Neurol 2000;53:190–2.

180. Brand RW. Tendon transfers for median and ulnar nerve paralysis. Orthop Clin North Am 1973;2:447.

181. Brown PW. Reconstruction for pinch in ulnar intrinsic palsy. Orthop Clin North Am 1974;2:323.

182. Bunnell S. Tendon transfers in the hand and forearm. Instru Course Lect 1949;6.

183. Omer GE Jr. Tendon transfers in combined nerve lesions. Orthop Clin North Am 1974;2:377.

184. Posner MA. Compressive neuropathies of the ulnar nerve at the elbow and wrist. Instru Course Lect 2000;49:305–17.

185. Riordan DC. Tendon transplantations in median nerve and ulnar nerve paralysis. J Bone Joint Surg Am 1953;35:312.

186. White WL. Restoration of function and balance of the wrist and hand by tendon transfer. Surg Clin North Am 1960;40:427.

187. Zancolli EA. Claw hand caused by paralysis of the intrinsic muscles: a simple surgical procedure for its correction. J Bone Joint Surg Am 1957;39:1076.

188. Szabo RM, Steinberg DR. Nerve entrapment syndromes in the wrist. J Am Acad Orthop Surg 1994;2:115–23.

B COMPRESSIVE NEUROPATHY OF THE ULNAR NERVE AT THE ELBOW

Martin A. Posner

INTRODUCTION

Ulnar nerve compression at the elbow is second only to median nerve compression in the carpal tunnel as the most common neuropathy in the upper limb. However, symptoms of ulnar nerve compression are more likely to be experienced than those of carpal tunnel syndrome. At one time or another most people have experienced numbness and paresthesias in their ring and little fingers after leaning on their elbows or keeping them flexed as when talking on the telephone or reading in bed. Certainly, almost everyone has had these symptoms after inadvertently striking their "funny bone." Fortunately, the numbness and paresthesias in these situations are transient and rarely progress to a neuropathy.

ANATOMY AND ETIOLOGIES

The boundaries for ulnar nerve compression in the elbow extend from approximately 10 cm proximal to approximately 5 cm distal to the medial epicondyle. Five potential sites for compression have been identified in this area.[1]

Sites for Potential Ulnar Nerve Compression at the Elbow

1. Arcade of Struthers to medial epicondyle
2. Medial epicondyle
3. Epicondylar groove
4. Entrance at flexor carpi ulnaris (FCU) (the cubital tunnel)
5. Flexor pronator aponeurosis

The most proximal site is the widest, begins at arcade of Struthers, and ends just proximal to the epicondyle (Fig. 16B–1). The arcade of Struthers is a 1.5- to 2.0-cm musculofascial band that, when present, courses obliquely and superficial to the ulnar nerve. It is primarily composed of superficial muscle fibers from the medial head of the triceps. Although the arcade has been identified in 70% of cadaver specimens, it is more of an anatomical curiosity than a cause of nerve compression.[2] The intermuscular septum and the medial head of the triceps are much more likely to cause compression at this site. The septum can cause compression if the nerve passes over its edge, particularly at its distal portion where it is thicker. This can occur following anterior dislocation of the nerve over the medial epicondyle, an unusual occurrence, or as a postoperative complication following ulnar nerve transposition if the septum had not been excised, also an unusual occurrence. The medial head of the triceps can cause compression when it is hypertrophied, a problem seen in some bodybuilders, or when it snaps over the epicondyle with elbow flexion, a problem that can mimic a dislocating ulnar nerve. Although the nerve in the latter condition does not dislocate, persistent snapping of the muscle often irritates the nerve.

The second site for potential ulnar nerve compression is at or just proximal to the medial epicondyle. Compression at this site develops as a consequence of a valgus deformity secondary to an old epiphyseal injury to the

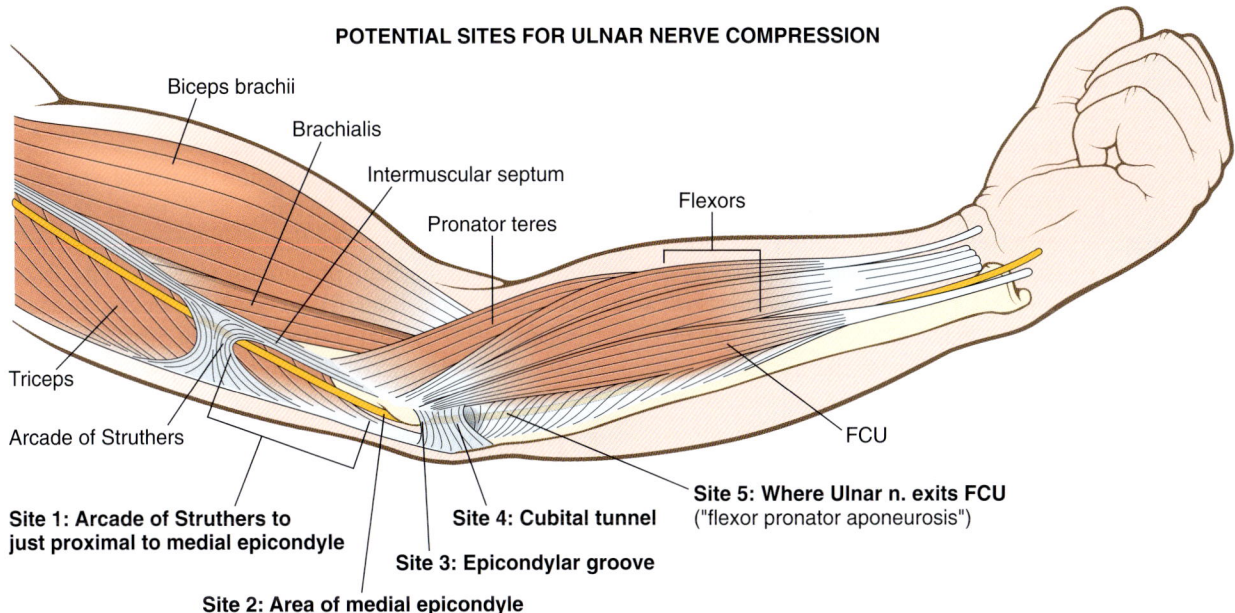

POTENTIAL SITES FOR ULNAR NERVE COMPRESSION

Biceps brachii

Brachialis

Intermuscular septum

Pronator teres

Flexors

Triceps

Arcade of Struthers

FCU

Site 1: Arcade of Struthers to just proximal to medial epicondyle

Site 4: Cubital tunnel

Site 5: Where Ulnar n. exits FCU ("flexor pronator aponeurosis")

Site 3: Epicondylar groove

Site 2: Area of medial epicondyle

Figure 16B–1 Sites for potential ulnar nerve compression at the elbow. (From Amadio PC. Anatomical basis for a technique of ulnar nerve transposition. Surg Radiol Anat 1986;8:158, with permission.)

lateral condyle or secondary to a malunited supracondylar fracture. Ulnar neuropathy following a humeral fracture was first described by Mouchet in 1914, and soon thereafter was known on the European continent as the "maladie de Mouchet." Two years later, Hunt introduced the term "tardy ulnar palsy" in the United States.

The third site for potential compression is the epicondylar or olecranon groove, a fibro-osseous tunnel bounded anteriorly by the medial epicondyle, laterally by the olecranon and ulnohumeral ligament, and covered by a fibroaponeurotic band. Compression at this site can be caused by a wide variety of lesions and conditions that can be grouped into three categories: lesions within the groove, conditions outside the groove, and conditions that predispose the nerve to displace from the groove.

Causes of Ulnar Nerve Compression in the Epicondylar Groove

Lesions within the Groove

1. Fracture fragments
2. Arthritic spurs arising from the epicondyle or olecranon
3. Soft tissue tumors
4. Bone tumors
5. Synovitis (e.g., rheumatoid arthritis)
6. Infections (e.g., tuberculosis)
7. Hemorrhage following trauma
8. Hemorrhage due to a bleeding disorder (e.g., hemophilia)

Conditions Outside the Groove (Most Common of the Three Categories)

1. Individuals who lean on their elbows for prolonged periods of time (e.g., patients confined to bed or in the left elbows of truck drivers who rest them on the window frame of their vehicles).
2. Improper positioning of the arm during surgery for unrelated problems. (Most of these patients already have subclinical nerve compressions that are aggravated rather than caused by the position of their arms during surgery.)
3. Anomalous anconeus epitrochlearis muscle that arises from the medial border of the olecranon and inserts into the medial epicondyle. (The muscle is probably atavistic in humans, and is replaced by a band, the epitrochleoanconeus ligament.)[3]

Conditions that Predispose the Nerve to Displace from the Groove

1. Congenital laxity of the fibroaponeurotic covering of the epicondylar groove
2. Traumatic tear in the covering
3. Congenital hypoplasia of the trochlea
4. Post-traumatic deformity of the medial epicondyle

An ulnar nerve subluxation or dislocation should not be confused with a hypermobile nerve, a condition that is usually bilateral, and is seen in approximately 20% of individuals.[4] While a hypermobile ulnar nerve is not a pathologic condition, the nerve frequently becomes irritated due to constant rubbing over the epicondyle. Since the ulnar nerve slips over the medial epicondyle with elbow flexion, it is at risk to become compressed when the elbow is immobilized in that position by a tight cast or splint for an unrelated problem. It is also at risk to be inadvertently injured by a steroid injection administered to treat medial epicondylitis.

The fourth site for potential compression is where the nerve passes between the two heads of the FCU muscle. This site and the third site, the epicondylar groove, are the most common sites for ulnar nerve compression at the elbow. The floor of the passageway through FCU is the medial collateral ligament of the elbow, and the roof is a fibrous band that is a continuation of the fibroaponeurotic covering of the epicondylar groove. The fibrous band has been referred to as Osborne's ligament, the triangular ligament, the arcuate ligament, or the humeroulnar arch. In 1958, Feindel and Stratford named this site the "cubital tunnel."[5] Although "cubital tunnel syndrome" is often used to describe any compressive ulnar neuropathy at the elbow, it more accurately refers to nerve compression at this specific site. The ulnar nerve is especially vulnerable for compression in the cubital tunnel because the contours of the tunnel change with elbow flexion. Osborne's ligament stretches (5 mm for every 45 degrees of flexion) and becomes taut, and the medial collateral ligament relaxes and bulges medially. The cross-sectional contour of the tunnel changes from an oval with the elbow in full extension to a flattened ellipse with the elbow in full flexion (Fig. 16B–2). As a consequence of these changes, pressure within the tunnel increases 7-fold with elbow flexion, and when contraction of the FCU muscle is added, the increase in pressure is 20-fold.[6] The result is mechanical deformation of the nerve that compromises its intraneural circulation.

The vascular effects of pressure on peripheral nerves have shown that at 20 to 30 mm Hg, circulation in the epineurial venules is impaired and intracellular axonal support is slowed. Capillary flow in the epineurium and perineurium remain unchanged until 60 to 80 mm Hg when it ceases and the nerve becomes ischemic. If that pressure is relieved within 2 hours, intraneurial circulation is rapidly restored although the nerve remains edematous for several hours due to increased permeability of the epineurial vessels. Prolonged compression results in permanent nerve damage.

The fifth site for compression is where the ulnar nerve penetrates a fascial layer as it leaves the FCU muscle to lie between the flexor digitorum superficialis and flexor digitiorum profundus muscles. The fascial layer has been referred to as the "flexor pronator aponeurosis."[7] Similar to the arcade of Struthers, it is a very rare site for nerve compression.

CLINICAL PRESENTATION AND EXAMINATION

Symptoms can range from mild numbness in the ring and little fingers to severe pain on the medial aspect of the elbow, with dysesthesias radiating distally into the hand and sometimes proximally into the shoulder and neck. In chronic cases, patients are usually aware of some muscle weakness that may manifest itself as loss of dexterity with fine motor activities or a sense of "clumsiness" when handling objects. A careful physical examination is critically important at arriving at a correct diagnosis and that examination should begin in the neck. Limited cervical spine motions may indicate disc pathology and/or arthritis. Axial compression on the cervical spine may reproduce radicular pain. With compression in the brachial plexus, the site(s) of tenderness should be localized by palpation and also by percussion over the supraclavicular and infraclavicular areas. Tenderness in these areas is often accompanied by a Tinel sign. Nerve compression can also be due to a thoracic outlet syndrome that is evaluated using a variety of provocative diagnostic tests that include the following:

1. Adson's maneuver (arm at side with head extended and rotated away from the affected side and then toward the affected side)
2. Wright's maneuver (arm abducted and externally rotated with the shoulders braced)
3. Costoclavicular maneuver (scapular retraction into a military brace position)
4. Roo's test or the overhead exercise test (arms above the head followed by rapid finger flexion and extension for 3 minutes)

All these tests are considered positive when they obliterate the radial pulse. However, this frequently occurs in normal individuals and a more significant finding is when the test reproduces the patient's symptoms.

The elbow is then inspected for any deformity and the ulnar nerve palpated, starting proximally in the upper arm and ending distally in the forearm, for any

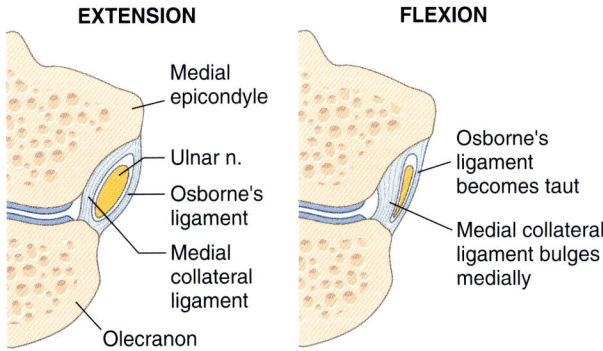

Figure 16B–2 Contours of the cubital tunnel in elbow extension and flexion. (From Adelaar RS, Foster WC, McDowell C. The treatment of cubital tunnel syndrome. J Hand Surg Am 1984;9:91, with permission.)

tenderness, enlargement (usually due to swelling), or a mass. The absence of tenderness or the absence of a Tinel sign is a significant finding, and may indicate that the problem is not due to a compressive neuropathy but rather to a demyelinating neuropathy for which surgery is contraindicated.[8] When the ulnar nerve is palpated in the epicondylar groove, the elbow is brought into flexion in order to determine if the nerve subluxates or dislocates. When the nerve does shift it is more likely to slip onto the tip of the epicondyle rather than dislocate anterior to it. A provocative test analogous to Phalen's test for median nerve compression in the carpal tunnel is the elbow flexion test. The elbow is positioned in full flexion and the wrist in full extension for 1 minute (up to 3 minutes is recommended by some clinicians). The test is considered positive when paresthesias and/or numbness develop in the ulnar nerve distribution of the hand. As with Phalen's test, the elbow flexion test is more sensitive than specific, and false positive results occur in approximately 10% of individuals.[9]

Numbness in the ulnar nerve distribution of the hand is a common finding that can vary in severity depending on the degree and duration of nerve compression. The sensory deficit often involves the entire anatomical distribution of the ulnar nerve (ulnar half of ring finger and entire little finger), or it may be confined to the little finger or even to just one side of that finger. The sensory deficit typically also involves the dorsoulnar side of the hand and dorsum of the little finger that are innervated by the dorsal sensory branch of the ulna nerve, which usually leaves the main body of the nerve 3 to 4 cm proximal to the ulnar styloid. When dorsal sensibility remains intact, nerve compression is more likely to be at the wrist in the canal of Guyon (ulnar tunnel syndrome) than at the elbow. In such cases, there will usually be some tenderness or a Tinel over the nerve in the canal of Guyon. Simultaneous ulnar nerve compression at both the elbow and wrist is common.

Regarding sensibility, the initial changes in nerve compression affect nerve threshold rather than innervation density. Therefore, vibratory perception and light touch (using Semmes-Weinstein monofilaments) are more likely to be affected than static or moving two-point discrimination. Innervation density is compromised when there is axonal degeneration, a condition that is usually seen with chronic neuropathies of year's duration. Muscle weakness generally appears later than sensory complaints, although occasionally a patient's inability to adduct the little finger (positive Wartenberg sign) is the presenting complaint. Muscle weakness affects the intrinsic muscles of the hand more commonly than the extrinsic muscles of the forearm due to the intraneural topography of the ulnar nerve in the epicondylar groove (Fig. 16B–3). The motor fascicles to the intrinsic muscles (as well as the sensory fascicles) are

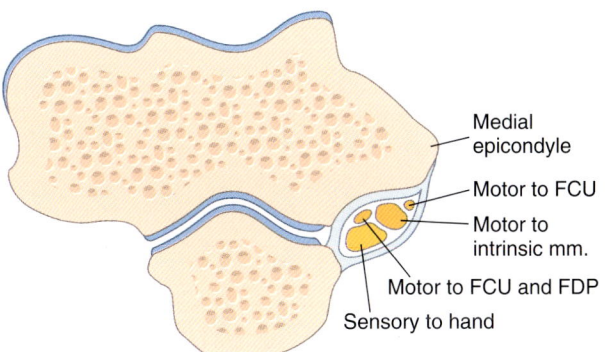

Figure 16B–3 Intraneural topography of the ulnar nerve in the epicondylar groove. (From Sunderland S. The intraneural topography of the radial, median and ulnar nerves. Brain 1945;68:243–99, with permission.)

situated in the medial or superficial portion of the nerve, and are therefore more vulnerable to compression than the fascicles to the extrinsic muscles. When intrinsic muscle weakness is severe and particularly when associated with atrophy, there is often clawing of the ring and little fingers, and weak pinch characterized by a positive Froment's sign (flexion of the interphalangeal joint of the thumb) and a positive Jeanne's sign (hyperextension of the metacarpophalangeal joint of the thumb). When there is extrinsic weakness, it always involves the flexor digitorum profundus (FDP) to the little finger and to a lesser degree the ring finger. The ring finger may not be affected due to the fact that its muscle is dually innervated by both median and ulnar nerves. Weakness of the FCU is rarely encountered.

IMAGING STUDIES

Radiographic examination of the elbow is always carried out. In addition to routine anterior–posterior and lateral views, a view profiling the epicondylar groove should be obtained in patients with traumatic and/or arthritic conditions whose nerve compression may be due to bone fragments or osteophytes in the groove. Magnetic resonance imaging is indicated when there is unusual swelling in the nerve or a palpable mass. However, it should not be used as the sole means to either diagnose the problem or to determine the appropriate treatment.

DIFFERENTIAL DIAGNOSIS

The differential diagnosis includes any lesion that affects the origins of the ulnar nerve in the cervical spine (C8–T1 nerve roots) and/or the medial cord of the brachial plexus. The medial cord can by compressed due to thoracic outlet syndrome or by a Pancoast tumor. Not infrequently, the ulnar nerve is compressed at more than one site, a condition commonly referred to as "double crush."[10] Occasionally, the nerve can be compressed in the cervical spine, elbow and wrist, resulting in a "triple crush." The differential diagnosis also includes systemic and metabolic disorders such as diabetes mellitus, hypothyroidism, alcoholism, malignant neoplasms, and vitamin deficiencies. The presence of any of these problems does not preclude the possibility of a concomitant compressive neuropathy.

ELECTRODIAGNOSTIC STUDIES

Electrodiagnostic studies are never a substitute for obtaining a complete history and conducting a thorough and careful examination. Although electrodiagnostic studies are commonly ordered when nerve compressions are suspected, they are not essential for primary cases, particularly when the clinical presentation is clear-cut. They can sometimes be misleading, and false negative and false positive results occur. Electrodiagnostic studies are most useful when the site of nerve compression is uncertain and may be located farther proximally in the brachial plexus or cervical spine, when a polyneuropathy is suspected, or when the neuropathy is due to a demyelinating disease that can mimic a compressive neuropathy. They are also useful when prior surgery was unsuccessful, particularly when they can be compared to the original studies.

Electrodiagnostic studies comprise motor and sensory conduction velocities, and electromyography. Motor conduction of the ulnar nerve at the elbow is measured over a 10- to 12-cm segment of the nerve with the elbow flexed. Conduction times measured with the elbow extended will yield false positive results; they can be almost 10 m/s slower than when they are correctly measured with the elbow flexed.[11] The reason for this is that it is difficult to measure the length of the nerve with the elbow extended because it is lax in that position and its length is frequently underestimated.

Motor conduction is generally considered to be absolutely slowed when it is less than 50 m/s and relatively slowed when it is more than 10 m/s slower across the elbow than it is farther distally in the forearm or farther proximally in the upper arm. The age of the patient must always be considered when evaluating results because motor conduction times can be as much as 10 m/s slower in the elderly. Sensory conduction studies are performed in a similar fashion as motor conduction studies by stimulating the nerve proximally and recording the action potential distally through an electrode placed on the little finger. Since this is opposite to the physiologic direction of sensory conduction, it is referred to as antidromic. Sensory conduction can also be performed in an orthodromic fashion; the sensory nerve fibers are stimulated from distal to proximal in the physiologic direction of their conduction. For the ulnar

nerve at the elbow, antidromic responses are easier to elicit than orthodromic responses.

Electromyography demonstrates axonal degeneration in muscles. Since these changes are seen in chronic neuropathies, electromyography is not as useful as conduction times for the diagnosis of early nerve compression. When muscle abnormalities are noted, they are usually initially seen in the intrinsic muscles, generally the first dorsal interosseous, followed in frequency by the muscles in the hypothenar eminence.

NONOPERATIVE TREATMENT

Ulnar neuropathies can be classified as acute, subacute, and chronic. Acute compressions result from a single traumatic episode such as blunt trauma to the medial aspect of the elbow or following a fracture. They also occur in substance abusers (drugs and/or alcohol) who may lie for prolonged periods of time in positions that put pressure on the nerves. Subacute compressions are typically seen in individuals who persistently rest on their elbows at work or at home, or in patients confined to bed because of a debilitating illness or following surgery. Acute and subacute compressions have been referred to as "external compression syndrome of the ulnar nerve."[12] Most cases resolve if the nerve irritation is reversed. This can frequently be achieved by simply instructing patients to avoid leaning on their elbows or keeping them flexed for prolonged periods of time. Alterations can sometimes be made in the workplace such as positioning a computer keyboard so that the operator's elbows are not acutely flexed. Elbow flexion is sometimes unavoidable for activities that involve precise manipulative skills that require individuals to work with their hands close to their bodies such as doing watch repair. However, some relief can usually be achieved if they avoid resting on the medial aspects of their elbows.

When symptoms are severe and have persisted for weeks, temporarily immobilizing the elbow in a moderated extended position will usually permit the local nerve irritation to subside. Although a short elbow splint may provide some improvement, a long-arm splint immobilizing the elbow in approximately 35 degrees of flexion and the wrist in neutral position is generally more effective. The wrist is immobilized in order to reduce the effects of contraction of the FCU that, as previously noted, results in a 20-fold increase in pressure on the ulnar nerve in its passage through the cubital tunnel. Patients are instructed to wear the splint day and night for 3 to 4 weeks. The splint is removed only to wash and bathe and during those few times each day, active range of motion exercises of the elbow and wrist are carried out to avoid joint stiffness. Nonsteroidal anti-inflammatory can also be prescribed, although splint immobilization is usually more effective. Corticosteroid injections around the nerve are almost never indicated. In most cases, splint immobilization will relieve pain and dysesthesias, although the improvement may not be permanent.

In patients with recurring symptoms, surgery is often necessary. There is never any urgency for such treatment unless there is muscle weakness. In the absence of muscle weakness, the timing for surgery is totally dependent on the severity of symptoms and the resultant disability, a situation that is best determined by the patient. Only when work and/or leisure time activities are significantly compromised is surgery recommended. Patients with no muscle weakness and whose disability does not warrant surgery are periodically re-examined to re-assess muscle strength. Weakness that develops is an indication for surgery even if there is no change in symptoms. Although repeat electrodiagnostic studies are usually obtained, the indication for surgery is determined more on the deterioration in muscle strength than the results of the studies that may or may not have changed. Mild weakness that persists for 3 to 4 months is also an indication for surgery.

OPERATIVE TREATMENT

Operative results depend on several factors that include the age of the patient, the duration of nerve compression, and the severity of numbness and muscle weakness. Young patients usually do better than elderly patients, and nerve compressions of several months' duration generally have a better prognosis than those that have been present for years. Surgery can be divided into two groups of procedures—decompression without transposition of the ulnar nerve and decompression with transposition of the nerve.

Decompressions without Ulnar Nerve Transposition

Decompression In Situ

Decompression without transposition of the ulnar nerve is often referred to as decompression in situ or "simple decompression." The procedure is usually reserved for localized problems either distal or proximal to the epicondylar groove. The nerve at either site is decompressed without releasing the fibroaponeurotic covering of the groove that will often result in subluxation of the nerve with elbow flexion. For decompression distal to the epicondylar groove where the nerve passes thru the two heads of the FCU (cubital tunnel), Osborne's ligament is simply sectioned. The procedure is ideally suited for patients who experience recurrent symptoms of nerve compression secondary to swelling of the FCU muscle with repetitive activities. This is sometimes

encountered in the left upper extremities of professional violinists who repetitively contract their wrist and digital flexors while maintaining their elbows in flexion. Decompression proximal to the epicondylar groove is performed for ulnar nerve compression due to marked hypertrophy of the medial head of the triceps, a situation encountered in some bodybuilders, or when there is snapping of the medial head of the triceps. Decompression for the latter problem is performed in conjunction with transferring the medial head of the triceps to the central tendon of the muscle.

Decompression in situ is the least complicated of all operations performed for ulnar compressive neuropathies. Since dissection of the nerve is very limited, there is no need for post-operative immobilization. The indications for the operation are few and it is contraindicated for cases when the effects of traction on the nerve must be reduced or when transposition of the nerve to a healthy tissue bed is necessary because of perineural scarring.

Medial Epicondylectomy

King and Morgan modified decompression in situ by excising the medial epicondyle.[13] Their rationale for the procedure was based on potential problems that they perceived with transpositions. They were concerned about scarring after a submuscular transposition and of persistent nerve irritation following a subcutaneous transposition if the nerve displaced posteriorly with elbow extension. They believed that the nerve did not necessarily have to shift back into the epicondylar groove for this to occur. Rather, it could be irritated by repeatedly slipping onto the apex of the medial epicondyle. By removing the epicondyle, proponents of the procedure believe that the prominence against which the nerve is compressed is eliminated and the nerve will then "seek it own course of least resistance."[14] Excision of a proper amount of bone is critically important; excising too much can damage the medial collateral ligament and result in valgus instability of the elbow and excising too little can compromise the outcome. The procedure has never become popular; it fails to relieve traction forces on the nerve, which limits its effectiveness.

Decompressions with Ulnar Nerve Transposition

Ulnar nerve decompressions with transposition of the nerve are far more frequently performed than decompressions without transposition, for two main reasons. The first is that the nerve is repositioned from a bed that is often scarred to a more favorable bed that is scar free, and the second reason is that by transposing the nerve, tension that normally occurs with elbow flexion is relieved since its new pathway is volar to the axis of elbow motion. The second reason is obviously important for the neuropathy that develops as a consequence of traction forces such as a valgus deformity of the elbow. Ulnar nerve transpositions are categorized into three groups: subcutaneous, intramuscular, and submuscular. Each surgical technique has its advocates, but only two are commonly accepted as effective procedures: subcutaneous and submuscular transpositions.

Subcutaneous Transposition

Subcutaneous transpositions are the most commonly performed of the three types of ulnar nerve transpositions. They are the procedures of choice for repositioning the nerve during operative reduction of acute elbow fractures and dislocations, during arthroplasties of the joint for arthritis, and for secondary ulnar neurorrhaphies when length is needed to overcome large gaps after the neuromas are excised. They are also the procedure of choice for many surgeons for the treatment of compressive neuropathies of the ulnar nerve, especially in obese patients whose arms have a thick layer of adipose tissue. The main disadvantage of the procedure is that the nerve remains vulnerable to repeated trauma, particularly in active individuals.

Intramuscular Transposition

While subcutaneous transpositions are the most commonly performed transposition operation, intramuscular transpositions are the most controversial. They were popularized by Platt in 1928 who recommended burying the ulnar nerve in a groove fashioned in the pronator teres muscle, a groove that he referred to as an "intramuscular gutter."[15] It is that technical part of the procedure that makes it so controversial. The groove is approximately at right angles to the transposed nerve. Consequently, repeated contraction of the muscle results in traction forces on the nerve that is likely to exacerbate the original problem. Although proponents of the operation report good results, complications are commonplace and are among the worst seen following ulnar nerve transpositions. It is a procedure that should be avoided.

Submuscular Transposition

Submuscular transposition, first described by Learmonth in 1942, has several advantages over the other two types of transpositions.[16] It ensures that all the potential sites for compression have been decompressed and, more importantly, it repositions the nerve to an unscarred anatomical plane that is not subject to any traction forces. Since the nerve is deep to the entire flexor–pronator muscle mass, it is well protected from external compressive forces, an important consideration in active individuals, particularly in serious amateur and

professional athletes. It is also the procedure that is recommended when other operations for ulnar nerve compression have failed. Since submuscular transposition is considered the most predictable of all operations for ulnar nerve compression at the elbow, it is the procedure that I favor for most cases. The procedure is generally contraindicated for arthritic elbows with limited mobility, in elderly patients with serious medical problems, and in very obese patients.

Surgical Techniques for Subcutaneous and Submuscular Transpositions

Regardless of the method used for transposition of the ulnar nerve, surgery is carried out using regional or general anesthesia and tourniquet control. The anesthetic preference is an infraclavicular block because it blocks the entire portion of the brachial plexus that innervates the upper extremity, including the intercostobrachial nerve that is often a cause of tourniquet pain. The pneumatic tourniquet is placed as far proximally as possible and the axilla is padded to prevent any irritation from the proximal edge of the tourniquet. It is not necessary to use a sterile tourniquet.

The surgical incision should be of sufficient length to ensure that the course of the transposed nerve will be relatively straight and does not abruptly loop volar to the medial epicondyle. The incision begins on the medial aspect of the upper arm, approximately 8 to 10 cm proximal to the epicondyle and directly over the medial intermuscular septum that can almost always be palpated except in obese patients. The incision is carried distally along the epicondylar groove, midway between the medial epicondle and the tip of the olecranon, and ends approximately 6 cm distal to the epicondyle over the ulnar nerve that can usually be palpated. The incision is carried down through the subcutaneous tissues, and care must be taken to identify and protect the posterior branch or branches of the medial antebrachial cutaneous nerve that innervate the skin over medial aspect of the elbow (Fig. 16B–4). The anatomic course of these sensory branches is variable; they cross the elbow anywhere from 6 cm proximal to the epicondyle to 6 cm distal to the epicondyle. Injury to these branches can result in annoying scar tenderness and dysesthesias.[17] Skin flaps are mobilized sufficiently to expose the intermuscular septum in the proximal portion of the operative field and the fascia over the flexor–pronator muscle farther distally. The fascia immediately posterior to the medial intermuscular septum is incised directly over the ulnar nerve at the proximal end of the operative field. Retracting the proximal end of the skin incision facilitates releasing the fascia even farther proximally. The neurolysis proceeds in a proximal to distal direction. The fascia over the nerve is released sequentially; first in the upper arm, followed by the

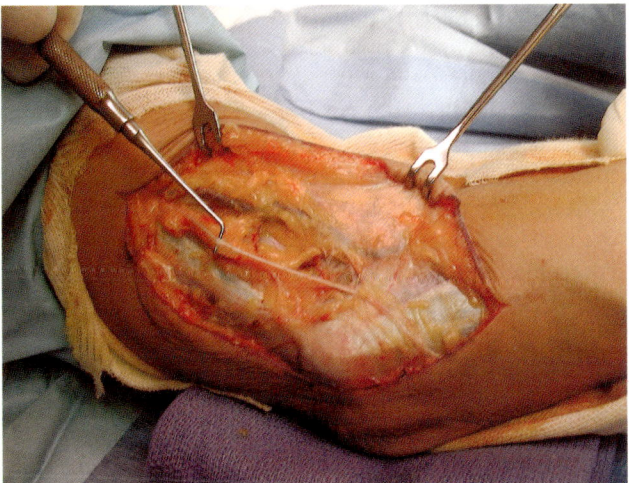

Figure 16B–4 Posterior (olecranon) branch of the medial antebrachial cutaneous nerve (under probe).

fibroaponeurotic covering over the epicondylar groove, then Osborne's ligament at the cubital tunnel, and finally, the fascia where the nerve passes between the two heads of the FCU (Fig. 16B–5 A to D). The medial intermuscular septum which is thicker and wider distally than it is proximally is then excised except for a 1- to 2-cm distal segment that is preserved to facilitate later reattachment of the pronator teres muscle following a submuscular transposition (Fig. 16B–6). The septum can be excised prior to the neurolysis rather than after; it makes no difference and is simply the surgeon's preference. Prominent vessels adjacent to the epicondyle that are part of the extensive collateral circulation of the elbow should be protected. Excising the medial intermuscular septum eliminates the possibility of nerve compression at that site following transposition. During mobilization of the nerve, manipulation and traction should be kept to a minimum to avoid any additional

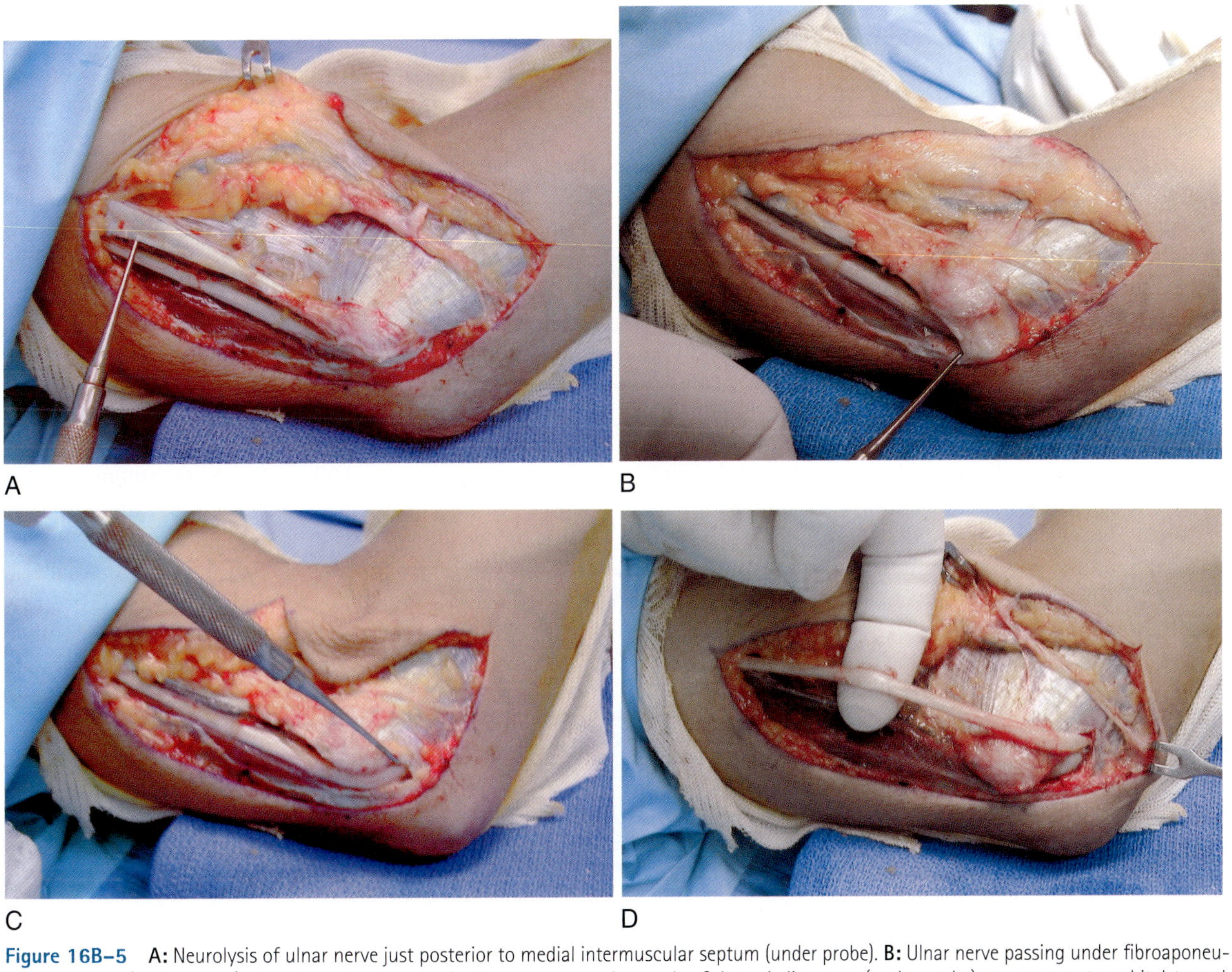

A

B

C

D

Figure 16B–5 **A:** Neurolysis of ulnar nerve just posterior to medial intermuscular septum (under probe). **B:** Ulnar nerve passing under fibroaponeurotic covering (under probe) of epicondylar groove. **C:** Ulnar nerve passing under Osborne's ligament (under probe) at entrance to cubital tunnel. **D:** Following release of the cubital tunnel and fascia between two heads of FCU, the nerve can easily be transposed.

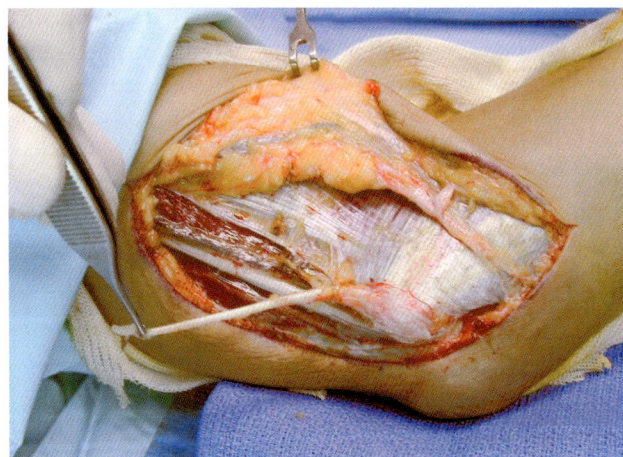

Figure 16B–6 Excision of medial intermuscular septum except for distal 1 to 2 cm.

damage. This can best be achieved by retracting the nerve with one's finger rather than using a metal retractor, Penrose drain, or vessel loop. The surgeon's finger is much more sensitive to the amount of traction being applied to the nerve than is any material or instrument. It may be necessary to cauterize a few small vessels in the mesoneurium when mobilizing the nerve, and this can be done safely without compromising its extrinsic blood supply. Generally, there is one or more small nerve branches that tether the nerve in or just proximal to the epicondylar groove. These branches are often thought to be articular branches that can readily be sacrificed. However, they are more likely to be motor branches to the FCU that should be preserved.[18] Regardless of function, nerve branches can be safely mobilized by interfasicular dissection. The ulnar nerve at the site of compression is often enlarged, its epineurium thickened, and its normal glistening white appearance altered. The faint transverse striations and longitudinal fascicles characteristic of a normal nerve are often absent. An epineurolysis at this site should be performed using loupe magnification.

When the nerve is transposed subcutaneously, it is stabilized at its new position by constructing a fasciodermal sling that will prevent it from slipping back into the epicondylar groove.[19] The flap, approximately 1.5 cm in width and length and based laterally, is elevated from the fascia over the flexor–pronator muscle and sutured to the subcutaneous tissues. The fascial flap is based laterally on the epicondyle rather than medially as described in the original description of the technique in order to position the smooth outer surface of the fascia against the nerve rather than the rougher inner surface (Fig. 16B–7 A to D). When suturing the flap to the subcutaneous tissues, care must be taken to ensure that the nerve is not kinked by the flap.

For a submuscular transposition, the entire origin of the flexor–pronator muscle is detached. Various techniques have been recommended, including leaving a small cuff of tissue on the epicondyle to permit reattachment after the nerve is transposed, dividing the muscle origin in a step-cut fashion in order to lengthen it, detaching the muscle via an osteotomy through the medial epicondyle, and then reattaching the epicondyle with a screw, and elevating the entire muscle origin from the bone and reattaching it directly to the bone.[20–24] The latter method is preferred because fixation is secure and dependable. The proximal margin of the pronator muscle is identified and the fascia is incised along that margin. The muscle is first elevated at that site in order to visualize the brachialis muscle, an important landmark in submuscular transpositions Fig. 16B–8 A and B). Identifying the brachialis prior to detaching the flexor–pronator muscle eliminates the possibility of inadvertently dissecting in an incorrect plane deep to the brachialis. The flexor–pronator muscle is then detached sharply from the bone using a scalpel. Attempting to remove the muscle with a periosteal elevator is likely to shred its fibrous origin and will compromise achieving a secure reattachment. Damage to the medial collateral ligament must be avoided and distinguishing the ligament from the muscle is determined by color rather than attempting to distinguish a difference by the direction of their fibers. The red flexor–pronator muscle is sharply elevated from the white medial collateral ligament that extends from the anterior aspect of the medial epicondyle to the ulna (Fig. 16B–9). The proximal 1- to 2-cm attachment of the FCU to the ulna distal to the insertion of the ligament is also released to ensure that the nerve is not kinked at that site. The median nerve is almost always visualized after the flexor–pronator muscle has been detached from its origin and retracted distally. The ulnar nerve is now positioned onto the bed of the brachialis muscle and it is important to ensure that its path from the proximal end of the operative field to the distal end is relatively straight (Fig. 16B–10). Reattachment of the flexor–pronator muscle is achieved by drilling four holes in the epicondyle in a sequential fashion beginning just proximal to the origin of the medial collateral ligament and going farther proximally (Fig. 16B–11). Occasionally, six holes are drilled when the epicondyle is unusually wide. The four drill holes accommodate two mattress sutures of a 0-grade braided synthetic suture material (or three sutures when six holes are drilled). It is important to place the sutures in the fibrous origin of the flexor–pronator muscle rather than in the thinner fibroaponeurotic covering of the epicondylar groove. Keith needles facilitate passage of the sutures through the bone. The fascia over the two heads of the FCU and the fascial covering of the epicondylar groove are then closed with 3-0 nylon horizontal mattress sutures (Fig. 16B–12). Reattaching the muscle origin in this fashion provides a secure fixation that

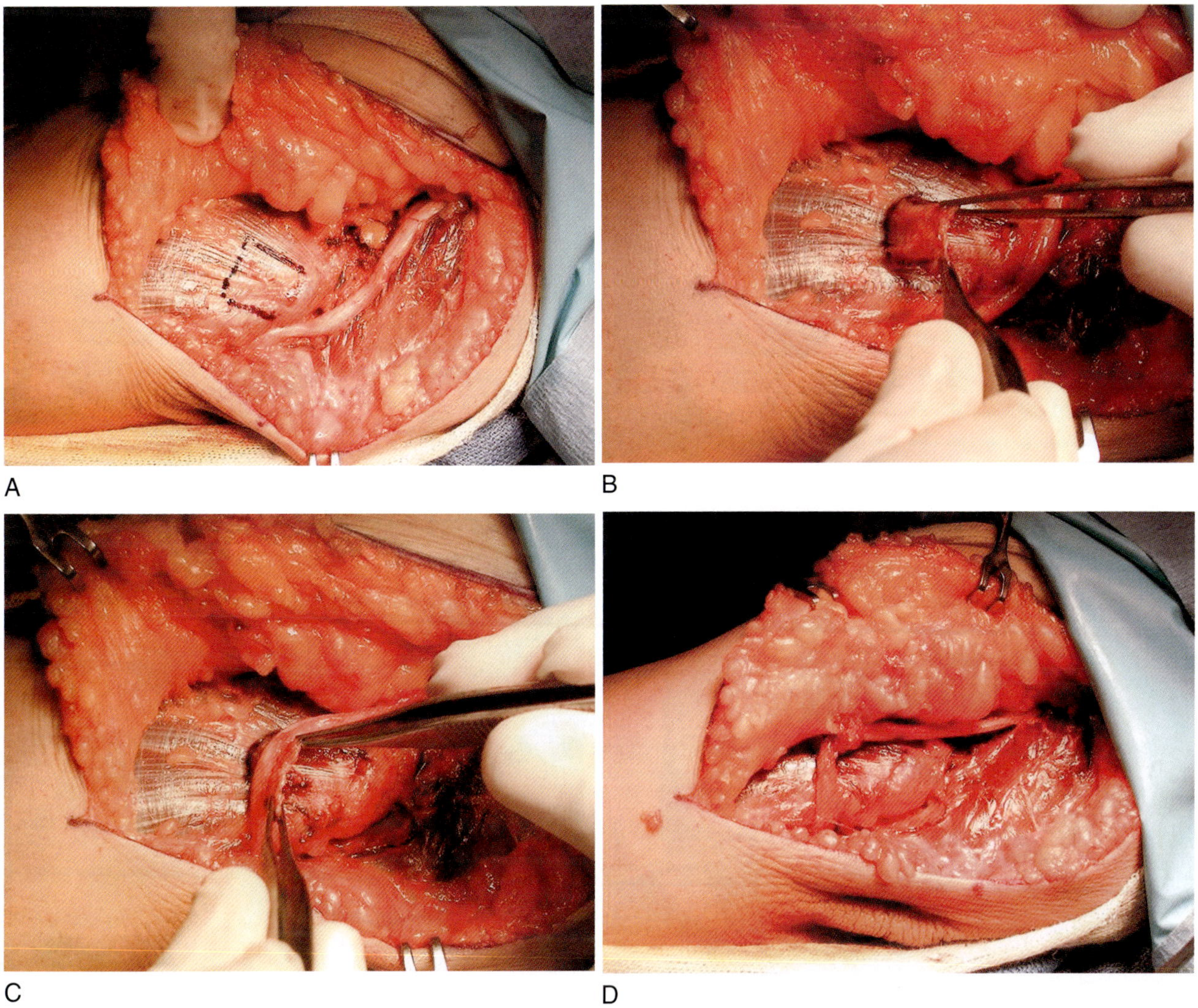

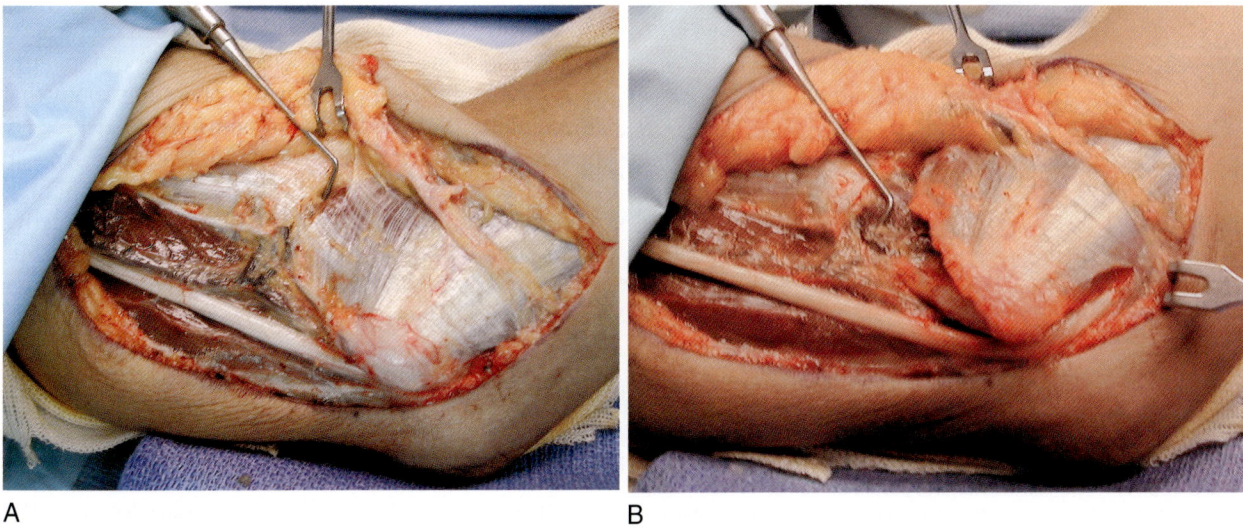

Figure 16B–7   **A:** Outline of laterally based flap (*ink line* between the parallel lines shows the length of the flap from the medial epicondyle). **B:** The flap elevated with forceps holding the medial edge. **C** and **D:** The flap is passed under ulnar nerve, and is sutured to the subcutaneous tissues.

Figure 16B–8   **A:** Identifying proximal margin of pronator teres muscle (probe). **B:** The muscle is first detached at this site in order to visualize the brachialis muscle.

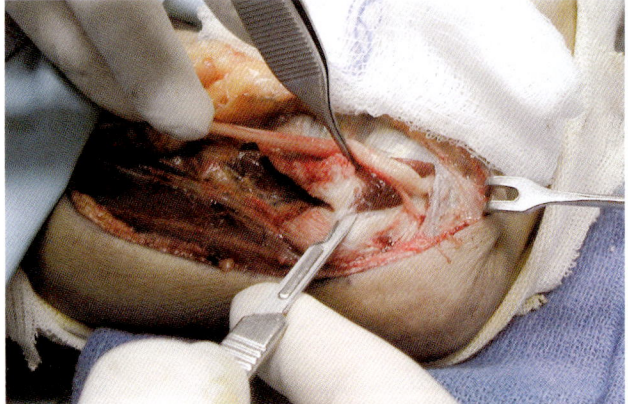

Figure 16B–9   Identifying and protecting medial collateral ligament.

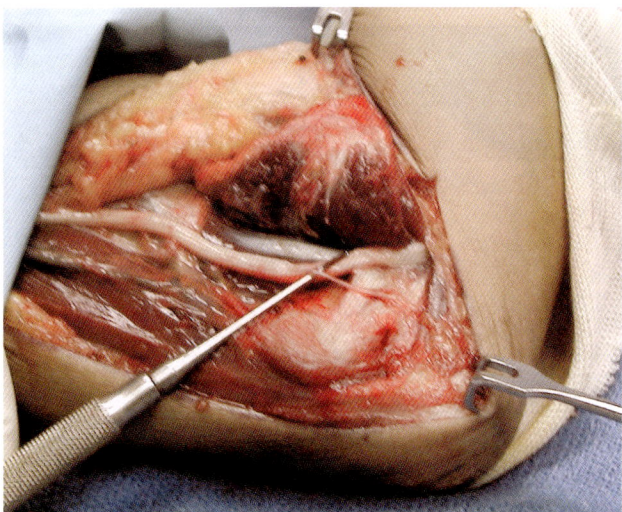

Figure 16B–10   The ulnar nerve is positioned on the brachialis muscle. A motor branch to the flexor carpi ulnaris (under probe) was mobilized by interfascicular dissection.

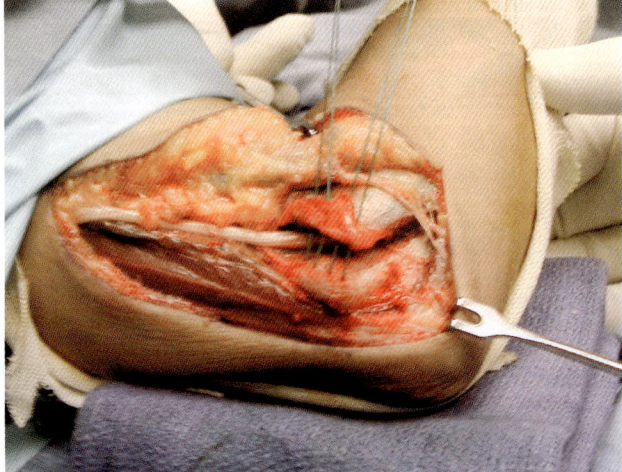

Figure 16B–11   Two mattress sutures passed though drill holes in the epicondyle. When the pronator teres has a proximal origin on the medial intermuscular septum, it is reattached to the septum.

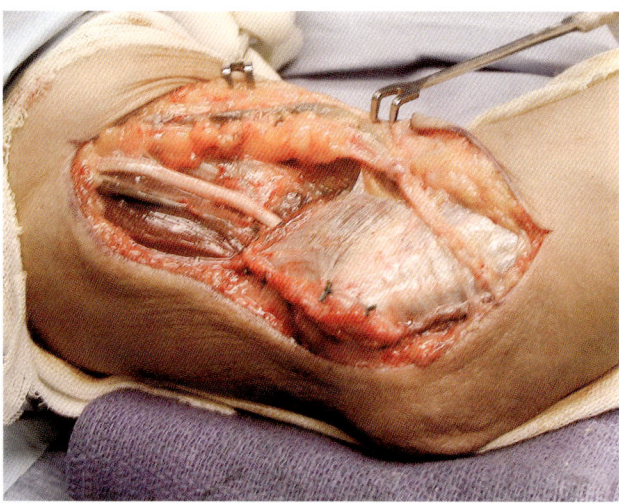

Figure 16B–12   3-0 Nylon sutures close the fibrous covering of the epicondylar groove and the fascia between the two heads of the flexor carpi ulnaris.

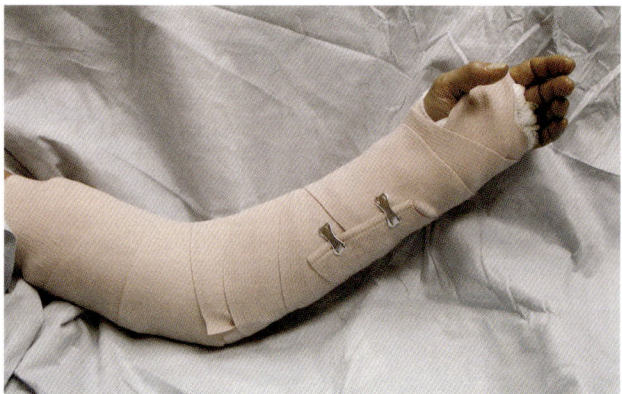

Figure 16B–13   Postoperative immobilization.

permits complete extension of the elbow without risk that the muscle will disrupt. The tourniquet is released to ensure that there are no small vessels that require cauterization or ligation. The subcutaneous tissues are closed with 4-0 absorbable sutures and the skin incision with a cutaneous 4-0 nylon suture. A posterior long-arm fiberglass splint is applied in the operating room that immobilizes the elbow in approximately 35 degrees of flexion, the forearm in neutral rotation and the wrist in neutral flexion-extension (Fig. 16B–13). The splint is maintained for 3 to 4 weeks, and during that time active range of motion exercises are encouraged for the digits and shoulder. Following removal of the splint active exercises are begun for the elbow, forearm, and wrist. Resistive exercises are instituted as soon as the patient regains complete mobility, and this usually occurs within a few weeks. In most cases, patients can resume full activities within several months, although for some strenuous activities such as professional baseball pitchers, approximately 9 months are necessary for complete recovery.

Operative Technique Sequence for Both Subcutaneous and Submuscular Transpositions

1. Skin incision: along medial intermuscular septum in upper arm and then distally along epicondylar groove to end approximately 5 cm distal to medial epicondyle over the ulnar nerve.
2. Identify and protect the posterior branches of the medial antebrachial cutaneous nerve.
3. Identify ulnar nerve just posterior to the medial intermuscular septum.
4. Neurolysis of ulnar nerve in a proximal to distal direction. Incise the following in sequence:
   a. Fascia posterior to intermuscular septum
   b. Fibroaponeurotic covering of the epicondylar groove
   c. Osborne's ligament at FCU (cubital tunnel)
   d. Fascia over nerve between two heads of FCU
5. Excise intermuscular septum (this can be performed prior to the neurolysis in Step 4).
6. Mobilize fascicles to FCU by interfascicular dissection and epineurolysis of nerve at area of compression (loupe magnification).

Subcutaneous Transposition

Construct fasciodermal sling based laterally on fascia over flexor–pronator muscle at epicondyle.

Submuscular Transposition

1. Identify proximal margin of pronator teres and incise fascia along that margin.
2. Identify brachialis muscle.
3. Sharply detach the entire flexor–pronator muscle from the medial epicondyle.
4. Identify and protect medial collateral ligament.
5. Release origin of FCU from ulna 1 to 2 cm distal to distal end of ligament.
6. Drill four (or six) holes in medial epicondyle.
7. Reattach flexor pronator muscle with 0-grade braided synthetic mattress sutures.
8. When the pronator teres has a proximal origin on the medial intermuscular septum, reattach the muscle to the septum.
9. Close fascia over FCU and fibroaponeurotic covering over epicondylar groove with 3-0 nylon horizontal mattress sutures.
10. Close subcutaneous tissues with 4-0 absorbable sutures.
11. Skin closure with a continuous 4-0 nylon.
12. Posterior fiberglass splint immobilizing the elbow in approximately 35 degrees of flexion, forearm in neutral rotation, and wrist in neutral position for 3 to 4 weeks.

RESULTS

Currently, there is no generally accepted grading system that evaluates the results of surgery for ulnar nerve compression. McGowan in 1950 proposed a system that is often cited in the literature but it focuses only on pre-operative ulnar nerve function.[25] Grade I (minimal) lesions are characterized as having paresthesias and numbness but no weakness; Grade II (intermediate) lesions as having numbness and intrinsic muscle weakness; and Grade III (severe) lesions, numbness and complete intrinsic paralysis. The system essentially grades preoperative intrinsic muscle function and does not compare that function with postoperative results.

A system that compares postoperative results with preoperative findings would obviously be more useful. While muscle strength can be objectively graded, it is difficult to grade subjective symptoms. What one patient may characterize as "mild" may be considered "severe" by another patient. In order to minimize that problem, a system was formulated that simply acknowledges the presence of a subjective complaint, but makes no effort to grade the severity of that complaint. The three most common symptoms of ulnar nerve compression at the elbow are evaluated: local pain including tenderness over the nerve, numbness anywhere in the ulnar distribution, and paresthesias in that same distribution. If only one of the three symptoms is present, regardless of severity, it is given a grade of S-1; two symptoms are graded S-2; and all three symptoms, S-3. For muscle strength, there are also three grades: M-1 represents mild weakness, M-2 moderate weakness, and M-3 severe weakness with intrinsic atrophy that may include clawing of the ring and/or little fingers. Postoperatively, the same two grading systems are used. For symptoms, the grade is reduced to zero if the patient notes an improvement in that symptom. For example, a patient with a preoperative grade of S-3 who reports that postoperative tenderness at the site of compression and paresthesias in the hand have improved, but numbness persists, is graded S-1. Reduction in grade(s) indicates a significant improvement in the symptom; it does not necessarily indicate complete elimination of the symptom.

In a series of more than 200 submuscular transpositions, approximately 75% of patients had all three symptoms preoperatively, and the two most common were tenderness over the nerve and numbness in the ulnar nerve distribution of the hand. Paresthesias were the least frequent reported symptom. Muscle weakness was present in more than 90% of cases, and usually affected the intrinsic muscles. Extrinsic muscle weakness was always associated with intrinsic weakness. Approximately 25% of patients had severe weakness and were graded M-3. Postoperatively, symptoms improved in all but five patients. In patients who had all three symptoms (S-3), each noted an improvement in at least one symptom, and more than 50% reported that all three symptoms had improved resulting in reduction of their preoperative S-3 grade to a postoperative S-0 grade. Regarding muscle strength, 25% of patients whose muscle weakness was graded M-3 preoperatively, regained complete strength postoperatively and were graded M-0. Approximately 5% of patients had no improvement in postoperative muscle strength; these were patients who has severe weakness preoperatively and whose nerve compression was of a year's duration. Although they did not improve, they were not made worse by the operation. Ulnar nerve transpositions are the most effective operation for the treatment of the majority of chronic ulnar nerve compressions at the elbow. For most patients, submuscular transposition is the preferred operative technique.

REFERENCES

1. Posner MA. Compressive ulnar neuropathies at the elbow. Part I. Etiology and diagnosis. J Am Acad Orthop Surg 1998;6:282–8.
2. Spinner M, Kaplan EB. The relationship of the ulnar nerve to the intermuscular septum in the arm and its clinical significance. Hand 1976;8:239–42.
3. Masear VR, Hill JJ, Cohen SM. Ulnar compression neuropathy secondary to anconeus epitrochlearis muscle. J Hand Surg Am 1988;13:720–4.
4. Childress HM. Recurrent ulnar-nerve dislocation at the elbow. Clin Orthop 1975;108:168–73.
5. Feindel W, Stratford J. The role of the cubital tunnel in tardy ulnar palsy. Can J Surg 1958;1:287–300.
6. Werne CO, Ohlin P, Elmqvist D. Pressures recorded in ulnar neuropathy. Acta Orthop Scand 1985;56:404–6.
7. Amadio PC, Beckenbaugh R. Entrapment of the ulnar nerve by the deep flexor pronator aponeurosis. J Hand Surg Am 1986;11:83–7.
8. Dhillon MS, Chu ML, Posner MA. Demyelinating focal motor neuropathy of the ulnar nerve masquerading as compression in Guyon's canal: a case report. J Hand Surg Am 2003;28:48–51.
9. Rayan GM, Jensen C, Duke J. Elbow flexion test in the normal population. J Hand Surg Am 1992;17:86–9.
10. Upton AR, McComas AJ. The double crush in nerve entrapment syndromes. Lancet 1973;2:359–62.
11. Kincaid J. The electrodiagnosis of ulnar neuropathy at the elbow. Muscle Nerve 1988;11:1005.
12. Wadsworth TG. The external compression syndrome of the ulnar nerve at the cubital tunnel. Clin Orthop 1977;124:189–204.
13. King T, Morgan F. The treatment of traumatic ulnar neuritis. Aust N Z J Surg 1950;20:33–42.
14. Froimson AI, Anouchi YS, Seitz WH, et al. Ulnar nerve decompression with medial epicondylectomy for neuropathy at the elbow. Clin Orthop 1991;265:200–6.
15. Platt H. The operative treatment of traumatic ulnar neuritis at the elbow. Surg Gyn Obstet 1928;47:822–5.
16. Learmonth JR. A technique for transplanting ulnar nerve. Surg Gyn Obstet 1942;75:792–3.
17. Dellon AE, Mackinnon SE. Injury to the medial antebrachial cutaneous nerve during cubital tunnel surgery. J Hand Surg Br 1985;10:33–6.
18. Watchmaker GP, Lee G, Mackinnon SE. Intraneural topography of the ulnar nerve in the cubital tunnel facilitates anterior transposition. J Hand Surg Am 1994;19:915–22.
19. Eaton RG, Crowe JF, Parkes JC III. Anterior transposition of the ulnar nerve with a non-compressing fasciodermal sling. J Bone Joint Surg Am 1980;62:820–5.
20. Leffert RD. Anterior submuscular transposition of ulnar nerves by the Learmonth technique. J Hand Surg Am 1982;7:147–55.
21. Dellon AL. Operative technique for submuscular transposition of the ulnar nerve. Contemp Orthop 1988;16:17–24.
22. Pasque CB, Rayan GM. Anterior submuscular transposition of the ulnar nerve for cubital tunnel syndrome. J Hand Surg Br 1995;20:447–53.
23. Mass DP, Silverberg B. Cubital tunnel syndrome: anterior transposition with epicondylar osteotomy. Orthopaedics 1986;9:711–15.
24. Posner MA. Compressive ulnar neuropathies at the elbow. Part II. Treatment. J Am Acad Orthop Surg 1998;6:289–97.
25. McGowan AJ. Results of transposition of the ulnar nerve for traumatic nerve neuritis. J Bone Joint Surg Br 1953;32:293–301.

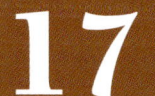

17

Compression Neuropathies of Radial Nerves

Robert W. Beasley

INTRODUCTION

This chapter is based on personal experience of treating 109 proved radial compression neuropathies with a minimal follow-up of 1 year. The reporting of upper limb compression neuropathies has increased dramatically in recent years. Is this an absolute increase in frequency of occurrence, or does it reflect greater awareness of the pathology to increase frequency of the diagnosis? No one knows; in fact, it is purely academic conjecture, for if the problem is discovered, it needs treatment.

Radial compression neuropathies have both common and different symptoms from those of the median and ulnar nerves. One commonality is that compression neuropathies do not occur at random locations but at specific sites where the anatomy is predisposed to it. Second, certain individuals have a constitutional predilection for such connective tissue disorders, which includes compression neuropathies. Clearly, there is an "itis" type, as was brought into focus by Nirschl in 1969.[1] He pointed out that a patient who has more than one connective tissue inflammatory disorder, such as carpal tunnel syndrome or lateral epicondylitis, has a very high probability of having other inflammatory disorders eventually. This is certainly confirmed, and in fact, I have observed that patients often may have more than one disorder simultaneously.

In considering upper limb inflammatory disorders, one needs to be aware that like direct compression, adhesions of nerves can disturb their conduction capacities by stretch rather than normal free gliding when joints are crossed. The most susceptible to this is the ulnar nerve passing through the cubital tunnel where in the adult nerve excursion is typically 5 to 6 cm.

LOCATIONS OF RADIAL NERVE COMPRESSION NEUROPATHIES

At no location does the radial nerve pass through a spherical conduit like the carpal or cubital tunnels. Therefore the term "radial tunnel syndrome" is a misnomer. In the middle of the arm above the elbow the radial nerve emerges through the intermuscular septum to pass distally along the lateral margin of the brachialis muscle but in soft subcutaneous tissues. About 3 cm proximal to the skin crease of the elbow, the radial nerve gives off branches that innervate the extensor carpi radialis longus (ECRL) and brevis (ECRB) muscles. Opposite the head of the radius there are some fibrous bands from the joint's capsule and immediately distal to this, the nerve is regularly crossed by several prominent veins, the "leash of Henry." Theoretically, the nerve could have minor compression

269

from either of these, but it just does not happen. I cut and ligate the veins, not for the fear of pressure, but for secure hemostasis even from the risk of their being torn by the subsequent essential use of retractors. Immediate distal to the leash of Henry, the radial nerve divides into two major divisions. Superficial is the superficial sensory branch (SBRN) of the radial nerve, while the deeper portion is designated as the posterior interosseous (PI) nerve (Fig. 17–1 and Fig. 17–4), which is said to be a motor nerve, but it also contains the sensory nerve branches from which by far the greater portion of pain from proximal radial nerve compressions is derived.

The SBRN, without giving off branches, passes distally on the undersurface of the brachioradialis muscle to the mid-forearm where it pierces the muscle's attachment to the radius to lie in the soft and mobile subcutaneous tissue, through which it crosses the styloid process of the radius where it is not infrequently damaged in operations for de Quervain's tenosynovitis. It begins divisions in that area, giving progressively smaller branches to innervate the hand's dorsal-lateral skin (Fig. 17–2).

The deep division of the radial nerve, the posterior interosseous (PI) nerve, passes distally and laterally under the proximal fibrous margin of the supinator

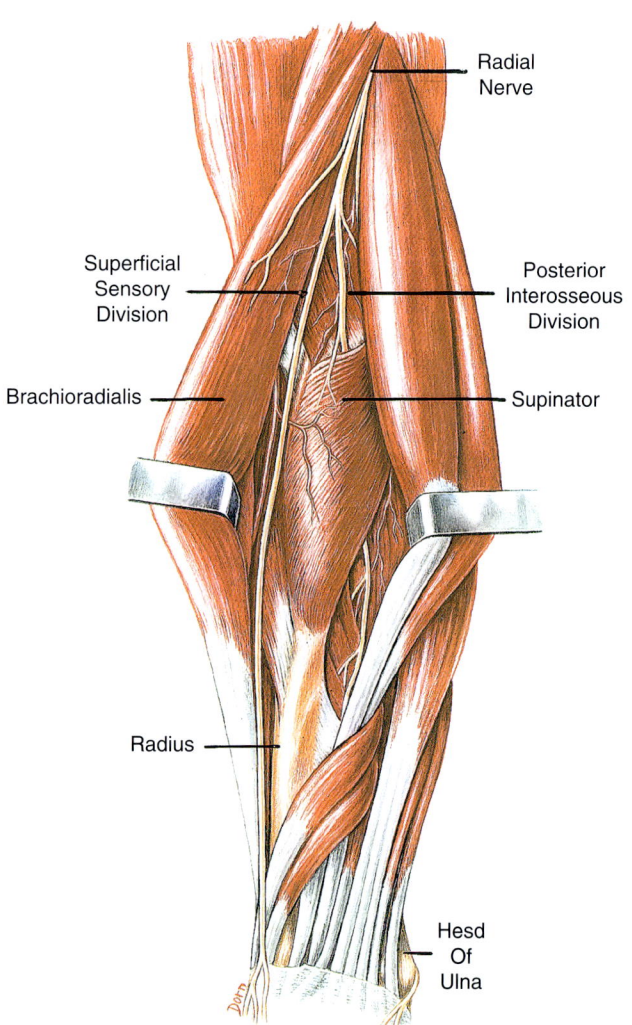

Figure 17–1 Basic anatomic pattern of the radial nerve with superficial sensory and posterior interosseous divisions at elbow. One must be alert for small individual variation from the illustrated basic pattern. The deeper posterior interosseous division passes medially and beneath the supinator muscle whose fibrous proximal margin is the sight of most radial nerve painful neuropathies in the absence of direct trauma damage to it. Branches of the radial nerve innervating the radial wrist extensor and the brachioradialis separate from the nerve well proximal to the elbow. (Courtesy of the Foundation for Hand Research, Inc.)

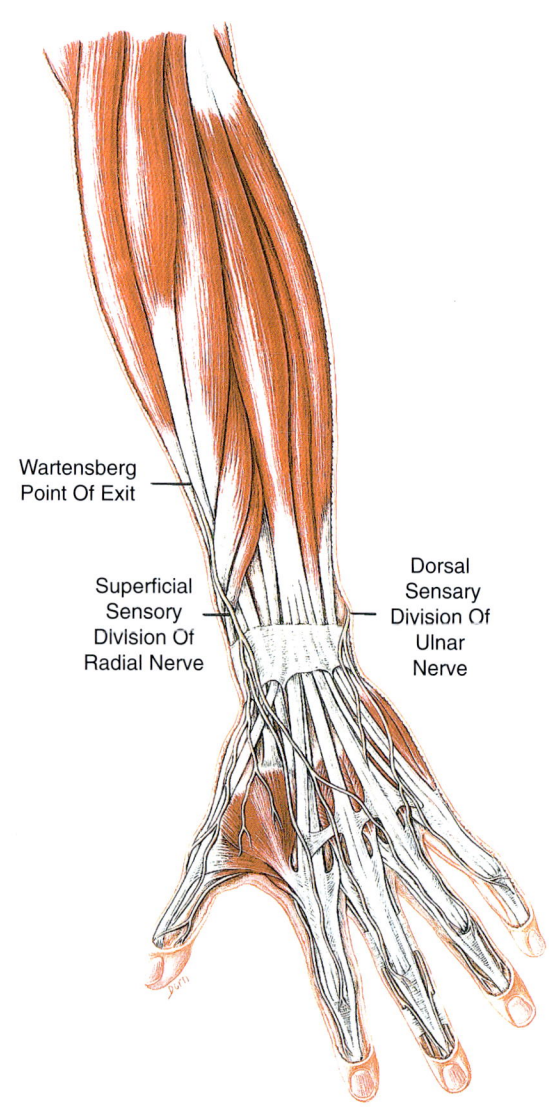

Figure 17–2 The superficial sensory division of the radial nerve passes distally of the undersurface of the brachioradialis muscle to the mid-forearm where it penetrates the muscle's attachment to the radius (site of Warternberg's compression syndrome). It continues distally in the soft subcutaneous tissues along the radius, and begins over the styloid process of the radius its highly variable pattern of progressive divisions to innervate the skin on the dorsal-lateral aspects of the hand proper. (Courtesy of the Foundation for Hand Research, Inc.)

muscle. It has multiple divisions, including branches to the digital extensor muscles, but in contrast to traditional teaching it incorporates sensory nerves. It should be examined carefully just proximal to the supinator muscle's margin, as it often divides there and one needs to be certain that all of it is decompressed (Figs. 17–1 and 17–5).

PATHOGENESIS

Today excessive and forceful use of the upper limbs is frequently credited with their developing various connective tissue inflammatory disorders, including compression neuropathies; the hand is analogous to a machine, which wears out with use. This is in contradiction to both long-standing and current observations, which indicate that it is disuse rather than overuse, that causes fibrosis and contraction of connective tissues. Such observations were most striking in the days when wrist fractures were treated primarily by plaster immobilization with weeks of poor muscular activity. As the return of venous blood to the heart depends on effect muscular "pumping" action, loss of that for any reason results in stagnation of venous blood in the tissues and edema (Fig. 17–3). The resulting gross thickening and contraction of connective tissues, most easily observed around small joints, made capsulectomies and collateral ligament excisions very frequently performed operations. Less dramatic but similar tissue changes are seen today along nerve sheaths, and most probably should be attributed to light and repetitive actions rather than excessively robust ones. This explains how any injury, perhaps to the hand or wrist, causing a long period of ineffective muscular function can cause connective tissue thickening and contraction at a distant location such as in the proximal forearm. With the pressure of oxygen- and nutrient-laden arterial blood being near zero at the terminal capillaries, it cannot displace the stagnant and nutritionally depleted venous blood from the tissues to deliver the needed arterial blood's contents to them.

Constant isometric contraction of prime movers against antagonist for the stabilization necessary for fine, precision movements impairs the venous portion of the circulatory cycle. These connective tissue problems were not seen until light-touch computer consoles replaced mechanical and even electric typewriters. I have yet to encounter a single person who types by the "hunt-and-peck" technique with these tissue changes. It

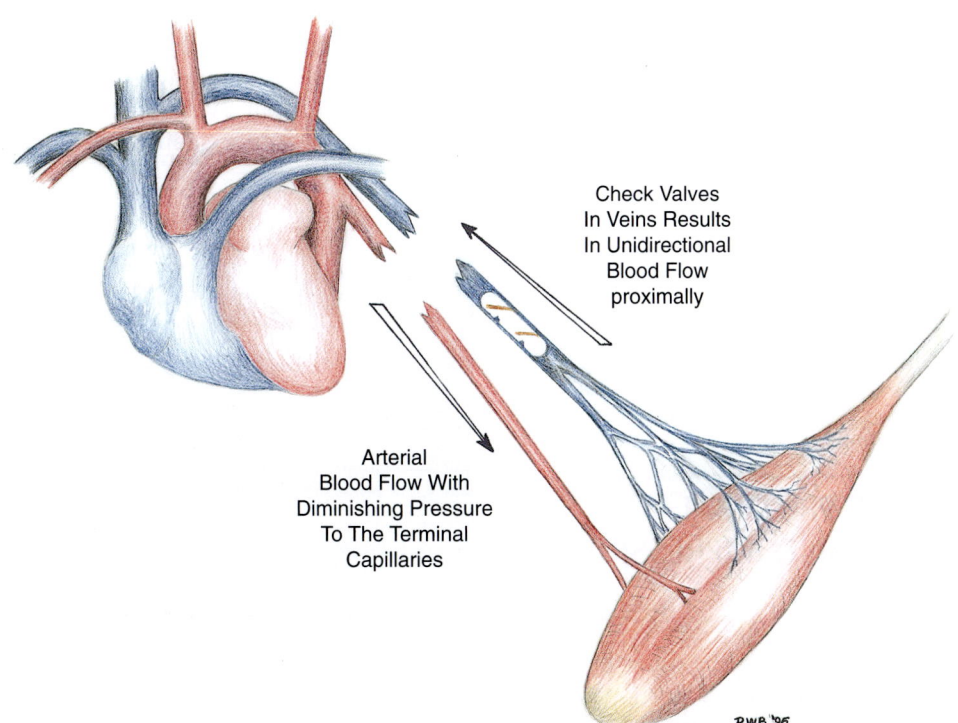

Check Valves In Veins Results In Unidirectional Blood Flow proximally

Arterial Blood Flow With Diminishing Pressure To The Terminal Capillaries

RWB '95

Figure 17–3 The old high school picture of the heart pumping blood in a complete circuit is incorrect. It pumps oxygenated and nutrient-filled blood to the tissues with pressure approaching zero at the terminal capillaries. The return of nutrient-depleted and carbon dioxide–laden blood to the heart's right atrium occurs via firm muscular activities pressing blood from the tissues into veins whose check valves permit the blood's movement only in proximal direction back to the heart. Thus, any condition causing a substantial period of poor muscle action is a setup for venous stagnation, local tissue nutritional deficiency, hypoxia, and chronic diffuse edema in the limb. (From Beasley RW. Beasley's Surgery of the Hand. New York: Thieme Medical Publishers, 2004,[2] with permission.)

appears that any prolonged activity causing poor venous return and chronic edema (even at low levels) is a setup in a susceptible individual to develop these connective tissue changes.[2]

DIAGNOSIS OF RADIAL COMPRESSION NEUROPATHIES

As with most of medicine, taking a detailed history followed by careful examination is fundamental to developing a working diagnosis. With the sole exception of Wartenberg's syndrome (compression of the SBRN where it emerges from beneath the BR muscle in the mid-forearm), a convincing history of single-incident proximal forearm trauma is almost never obtained. Basically, all patients relate two greatest complaints: (1) ill-defined pain and soreness in the radial innervated proximal forearm muscles with radiation of pain to the shoulder and/or neck, and (2) a sense of profound heaviness and fatiguing of the involved limb.

Physical examination for most reveals prominent soreness of the radial innervated proximal forearm muscles with digital pressure applied to the posterior interosseous nerve where it passes under the proximal margin of the supinator muscle causing a dramatic sudden accentuation of the chief complaints. Generally, a strong Tinel sign is present there, although radial innervated skin on the dorsum of the hand is disturbed in less than 20% of cases. Attempted supination of the forearm against resistance greatly accentuates the chief symptoms consistently. Testing of finger–thumb extension and the "third finger extension test" were consistently normal.

Electrophysiologic measurements or other tests available have proved to be of little benefit in establishing a diagnosis. Occasionally, EMG may demonstrate some increase in polyphasic patterns from a finger extensor muscle, but in general electrodiagnostic studies are of so little help as not to be obtained, unless the objective is to evaluate some other suspected problem.

TREATMENT OF PROXIMAL FOREARM RADIAL COMPRESSION NEUROPATHIES

For the great majority of patients, the onset of symptoms is heralded in by an insidious development of idiopathic soreness of the radial innervated proximal forearm muscle which with progression radiates pain into the shoulder and often the neck. This appears to be an inflammatory reaction, but rarely does it respond favorably to anti-inflammatory medications. However, with very mild symptoms spontaneous remissions may

occur, but usually only over a period of many months. Therefore, most patients are candidates for surgical decompressions, especially as the risk and morbidity is so low and the probabilities for a prompt resolution of symptoms so high.

TECHNIQUE OF SURGICAL DECOMPRESSION OF PROXIMAL RADIAL NERVES

I prefer a general anesthetic, as I do not like to inject around nerves already in trouble, but the operation can be done with local infiltration anesthesia. Tourniquet time is not a problem as most patients tolerate it well for 40 minutes or so, provided the arm has been completely exsanguinated prior to tourniquet inflation. A longitudinal incision is planned beginning about 2 cm distal to the transverse skin crease of the elbow and directly over the course of the SBRN for a distance of about 12 cm (Fig. 17–4). Dissection through the subcutaneous tissues is with as little damage to cutaneous nerve branches as possible. After opening the muscle fascia, the plane between the brachioradialis and the radial wrist extensors is readily identified with passive flexion and extension of the wrist. Blunt dissection down this plane to separate the muscles is essentially bloodless and atraumatic. The smooth white SBRN will be encountered, and with appropriate magnification a meticulous external neurolysis (never internal) is done proximally to about 2 cm proximal to the elbow's skin crease. This is easily accomplished with tissue retraction

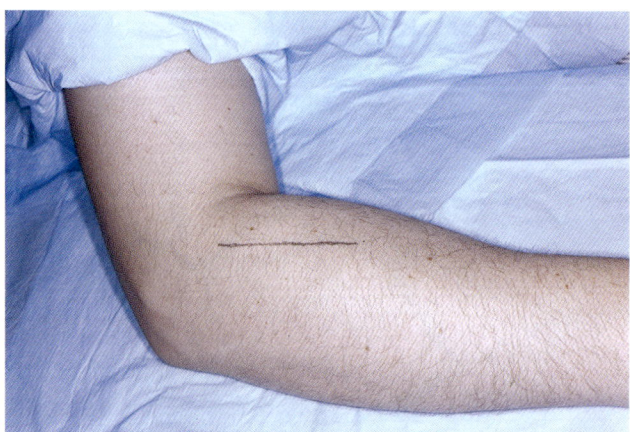

Figure 17–4 The incision for proximal forearm radial nerve decompressions should begin just distal to the skin creases of the elbow, and extend distally over the course of the superficial division of the nerve for a distance of only 10 to 12 cm. After fascia connecting the radial wrist extensors and the brachioradialis are incised, passive wrist flexion and extension illustrate the physiologic plane about these muscles. Their separation by essentially blunt dissection down to the superficial division of the radial nerve is very atraumatic.

without more proximal cutting of the skin. The same is done distally to well under the brachioradialis muscle. Even if the patient has some paresthesias in the radial nerve's distribution (less than 20%), even subtle gross constriction is rarely observed. The sensory nerve's disturbance is probably part of the "double crush" phenomena first described in England by Upton.[3] Briefly stated, this was the observation that a nerve with prominent inflammation in it at one area would often show evidence of inflammation along its whole course. Such mild secondary symptoms clear up spontaneously once the primary pathology is resolved.

Next, attention is directed to identification of the posterior interosseous (PI) division of the nerve, which separates off its deeps surface. With retraction of the SBRN, the PI is identified proximal to the fibrous proximal margin of the supinator muscle that the nerve passes under in a deep and lateral direction (Fig. 17–5). Often it will have divided into two or more branches before passing under the supinator muscle, so very careful and thorough exploration is indicated to be certain that all parts will be decompressed. Occasionally, the swelling of a neuroma-in-continuity will be encountered immediately proximal to the PI nerve's passing under the supinator (Fig. 17–6), but in the majority of cases no gross pathology is identified until the muscle has been split (the pathology is under it). The fibrous margin of the supinator crossing the PI nerve is severed, after which the muscle proper is split longitudinally along the radius (Fig. 17–7) until closed Littler scissors can be passed freely without resistance along the branches of the nerve. As stated, up to this stage nerve pathology is rarely apparent, as the pathology is primarily under the muscle and exposed only after the supinator muscle has been split. Then subtle but definite indentation of the nerve usually can be

observed at the area where the nerve was under the supinator muscle by comparing it to the normal nerve proximal to the muscle (Fig. 17–8).

Meticulous hemostasis is observed through the operation. Rarely is an artery encountered, but if so, it is cut and its ends ligated. About 1 cm proximal to the supinator muscles, the whole radial nerve will consistently be crossed by several 2- to 3-mm veins, known as the "leash of Henry." As previously noted, these do not contribute to nerve compression, but severing and ligating them prevents them from being torn by essential tissue retractions. I do not use an electric cautery, which needlessly damages tissues with no possibility of every small venule being coagulated. These small veins will all coagulate after the tourniquet is deflated to activate the

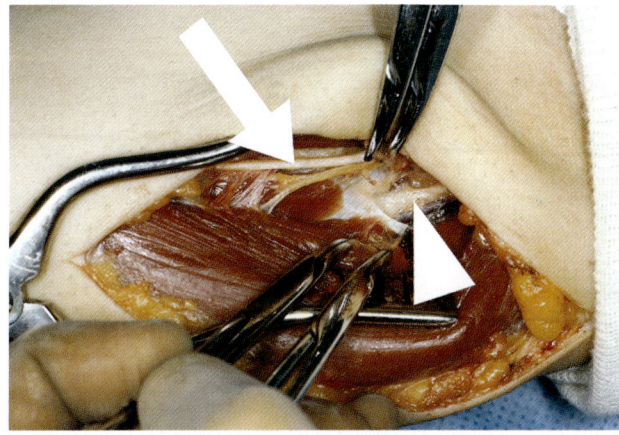

Figure 17–6 The pathology of even very symptomatic proximal forearm radial nerve compressions is usually subtle, and often no gross pathology can be seen until after the supinator muscle has been split longitudinally. The basic pathology lies beneath the muscle, especially at its proximal fibrous margin. Occasionally, a neuroma-in-continuity will be encountered *(pointer)* immediately proximal to the nerve's passing under the supinator. The normal superficial sensory division *(arrow)* is seen passing over the supinator muscle.

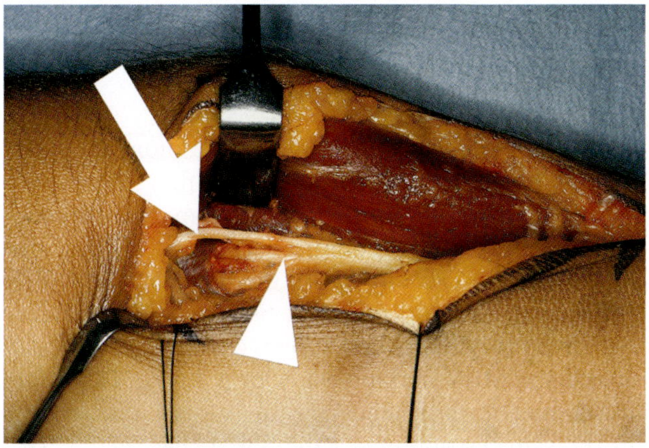

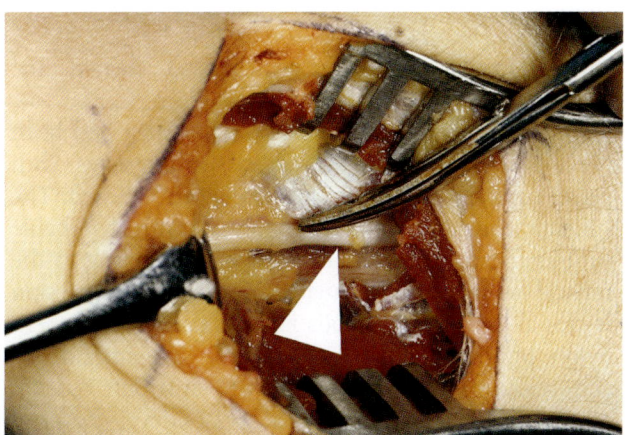

Figure 17–5 Immediately distal to the elbow, the radial nerve divides into the superficial sensory division *(arrow)* and the posterior interosseous *(pointer)* division. The pattern of the PI nerve's subsequent bifurcations is highly variable, but usually some division of it begins before it passes under the supinator muscle.

Figure 17–7 As the supinator muscle is split longitudinally along the radius, a subtle indentation of the PI nerve can be appreciated by comparing the segment under the muscle with the normal nerve to the left.

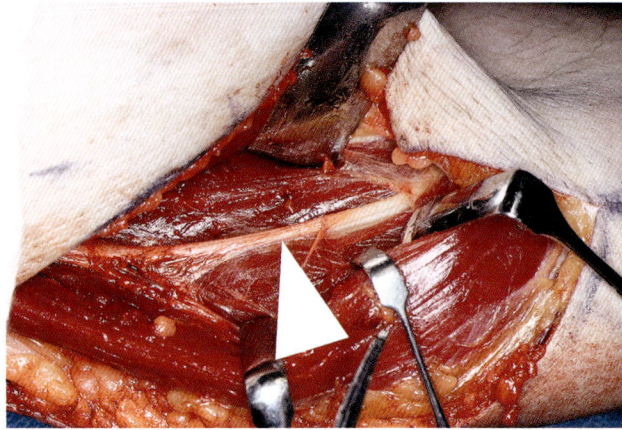

Figure 17–8 With wide exposure of the PI nerve under the supinator muscle, the long segment of nerve with reduced diameter *(pointer)* demonstrates that compressions are not limited to the segment of the nerve under the thick fibrous proximal margin of the muscle.

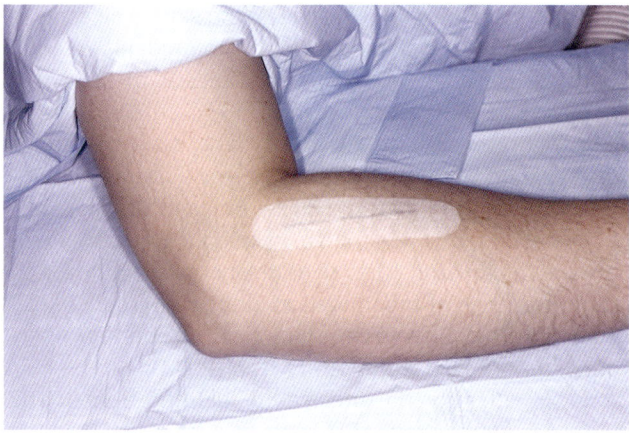

Figure 17–10 After removal of the pull-out suture, the wound should be protected continuously from longitudinal (not transverse) tension for at least 2 months, simply using a strip of 3M paper tape and appropriate skin adhesive. This is remarkably effective, and the only thing that minimizes skin scar hypertrophy.

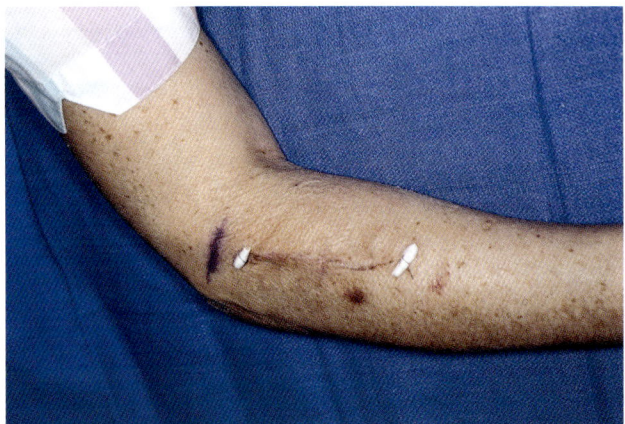

Figure 17–9 With wound closure, the fascia that had united the BR and wrist extensor muscles are not repaired, but the subcutaneous tissues are coated with interrupted sutures to prevent postoperative scar "puckering" from skin scars having healed to the muscle fascia. Skin margins are approximated with a continuous monofilament nylon suture, with each end being tied around the tip of an applicator stick to distribute pressure evenly, and obviate stitch abscesses even if in place for more than 2 weeks.

clotting factors. After the acidosis has cleared, the tourniquet is reinflated for wound closure.

Drains are used only if tissue in the area had been previously damaged, and scar tissue interferes with vessel contraction. The muscle fascia is not closed. The subcutaneous tissues are approximated with absorbable sutures to prevent the scar of the skin adhering to the muscle fascia to pucker unattractively. Usually the skin is closed with a continuous intradermal monofilament nylon pull-out suture with its end tied around the cotton end of an applicator stick to distribute tension on the skin broadly. No stitch abscesses develop even if the suture is in place for 3 weeks or more (Fig. 17–9). Carefully fitted sterile dressings are placed and supported with strong cloth adhesive tape, but no attempt

at immobilization is made. Postoperative elevation of the arm above heart level is required for 2 days, and longer if there is throbbing pain. Elevation should be continued at night for at least 2 weeks, while free use of the hand is encouraged.

Scar hypertrophy is effectively minimized or obviated by longitudinal (not transverse) taping of the wound continuously for a minimum of 2 months.[4] A skin adhesive is painted on the skin and allowed to dry. A single strip of paper tape is then cut to proper length and simply pressed onto wound (Fig. 17–10). Usually it requires replacement only every 3 to 4 days even when the patient takes normal showers. If the tape is applied with tension, skin irritation or even blistering could develop. In fact, most of what is called "tape allergy" is the result of application of tape to the skin under traction. Longitudinal taping of wounds has dramatically reduced scar hypertrophy (Fig. 17–11).

WARTENBERG'S SYNDROME

This is a special situation that—unlike proximal radial nerve compressions—involves only the SBRN, and invariably is preceded by direct trauma to the mid-forearm area. It is a compression neuropathy of the SBRN as it exits from beneath the brachioradialis (BR) muscle into the subcutaneous tissues along the distal half of the radius. The condition is characterized by pain at the site of its entrapment with a strong Tinel sign there, and a variable degree of sensory disturbance in the skin distribution of the SBRN (Fig. 17–2). The diagnosis is clinical and the treatment is surgical decompression.

A short longitudinal incision is made directly over the area of the strong Tinel sign. Initial exploration is

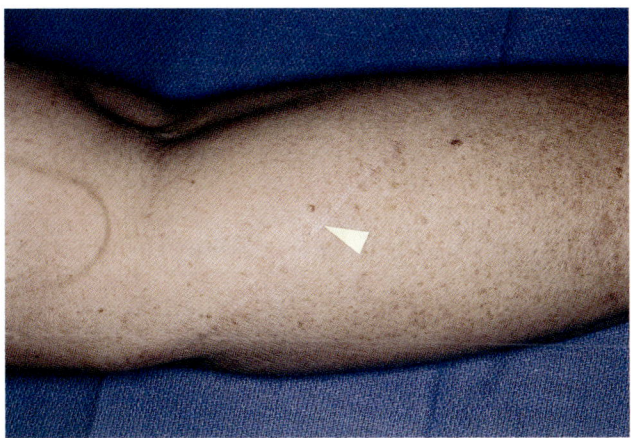

Figure 17–11   Scar of proximal forearm radial nerve decompression *(pointer)*, treated post-suture removal from 2 months of constant longitudinal taping, seen 1 year later. This is the only thing known to predictably minimize scar hypertrophy, and the results for most cases are astonishing.

distal to this to identify the SBRN in the normal subcutaneous tissues there. Dissection is then from distal to proximal until the nerve is seen to penetrate from beneath the brachioradialis muscle (BR) at its thick fibrous attachment to the radius. This margin of the BR muscle should be severed in a vertical fashion at intervals of about 5 to 6 mm. The fibrous muscle margin directly over the nerve exit is excised.

As with treatment of proximal lesions, the tourniquet should be deflated briefly to activate the clotting factors, after which it is reinflated and the wound closed as one prefers. Again, immobilization is not required, but elevation of the hand for 48 hours after the operation is important.

RESULTS

Evaluation of treatment is difficult for two reasons. First, it has to be based essentially on subjective information from the patient, and second, about half of the patients will concurrently have other connective tissue or inflammatory disorders, with many being unable to accurately assign the source of symptoms. Rinker et al.[5] in 2000 undertook a critical evaluation of the results of 79 prox-

imal radial nerve decompressions that I had performed. This chapter is essentially a condensation and extension of that study, with the number of patients evaluated 1 year or more after treatment increased to 109.

We judged results to be excellent if all of the preoperative major symptoms attributable to proximal radial nerve compression were resolved. These symptoms were forearm soreness, chronic pain radiating from the forearm to the shoulder and/or neck, and a sense of profound heaviness of the arm. This expanded series followed almost exactly the pattern of evaluation by Rinker et al.[5] with 80% of patient judged to have excellent results. The four cases of Warternberg's syndrome in the series all had immediate and lasting excellent results. Interestingly, in almost every instance, the relief followed the operation promptly with many stating "it's gone" as they awoke from anesthesia. A consistent finding was that if there were visual evidence of pathology, it often involved the posterior interosseous nerve. Clearly, pain and the other basic symptoms were predominantly derived from the posterior interosseous nerve, although classically it has been designated as a "motor nerve."

Our rating of good results required that the patient be relieved of forearm soreness most of the time, consistently relieved of heaviness and pain radiating to the shoulder and/or neck, and that they returned to their original job or other gainful employment. Seventeen percent of the patients were assigned to this category.

Three percent were assigned a rating of poor results, meaning that while all were improved from symptoms that were reasonably attributable to radial nerve compression, they continued to have multiple and changing complaints as well as inability to resume their job and regular activities.

REFERENCES

1. Nirschl RP. Mesenchymal syndrome. Va Med J 1969;:96–659.
2. Beasley RW. Beasley's Surgery of the Hand. New York: Thieme Medical Publishers, 2004.
3. Upton ARN, et al. The double crush in nerve compression syndromes. Lancet 1973:359–62.
4. Reiffel RS. Prevention of hypertrophic scars by long-term paper tape application. Plast Reconstr Surg 1995;1715–18.
5. Rinker B, Effron CR, Beasley RW. Proximal radial compression neuropathy. Ann Plast Surg 2004;52:174–80.

Double Crush Syndrome

Jeffrey Yao and A. Lee Osterman

INTRODUCTION

Originally described by Upton and McComas in 1973,[1] the double crush syndrome is the coexistence of compressive lesions along the course of a single peripheral nerve.[1–12] Nemoto et al.[5] labeled the phenomenon "double lesion neuropathy" to describe the situation when individually, two or more lesions are insufficient to disrupt nerve function, but together have a synergistic effect resulting in nerve conduction failure. Likewise, it has become widely accepted that a partial lesion of a nerve at one site makes the nerve more susceptible to compression at another site. Finally, a corollary of the double lesion neuropathy occurs when an intrinsically impaired nerve (i.e., as a result of peripheral neuropathy) becomes more susceptible to extrinsic compression.[13–23]

Clinical examples of the double crush syndrome include carpal tunnel syndrome (CTS) in the face of a cervical radiculopathy, ulnar nerve compression at both the elbow and the wrist, and thoracic outlet syndrome (TOS) with concomitant compression of a peripheral nerve. The purpose of this chapter is to address the historical perspectives, pathophysiology, experimental basis, common clinical examples, and treatment of the double crush syndrome.

PATHOPHYSIOLOGY

The pathophysiology of peripheral nerve dysfunction has been studied extensively.[10,24–30] Acute and transient neuropraxia is most commonly attributable to metabolic, ischemic, or transient traumatic causes. More chronic neuropathy is attributable to metabolic, immune, or structural causes, such as sites of compression. Structural changes of nerves at sites of compression include segmental demyelination, nodal intussusception, and bulbous myelin lesions with internodal narrowing. The extent of mechanical changes depends directly on the degree and duration of compression.[9,31,32]

In the double crush syndrome, one lesion along the course of a peripheral nerve affects nerve function elsewhere along its course. Explanations for this interaction have included:

1. Impairment of axonal flow from a lesion with subsequent structural changes both distally *and* proximally along the axon
2. Endoneural edema from a site of compression affecting distal intraneural circulation and axonal flow

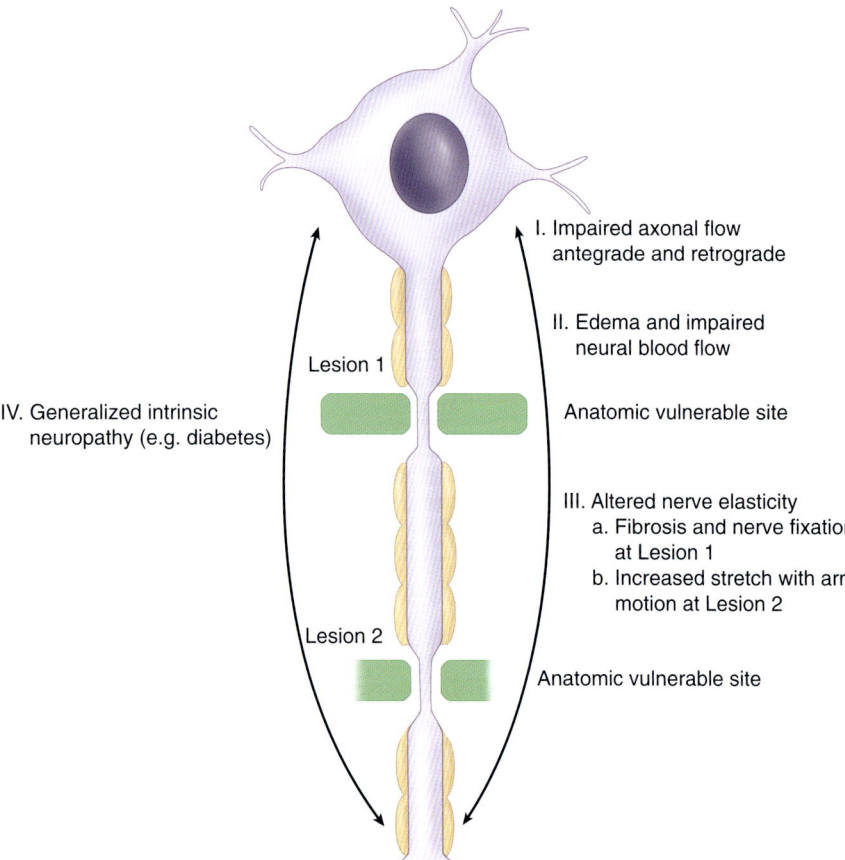

I. Impaired axonal flow
antegrade and retrograde

II. Edema and impaired
neural blood flow

Lesion 1

IV. Generalized intrinsic
neuropathy (e.g. diabetes)

Anatomic vulnerable site

III. Altered nerve elasticity
  a. Fibrosis and nerve fixation
    at Lesion 1
  b. Increased stretch with arm
    motion at Lesion 2

Lesion 2

Anatomic vulnerable site

Figure 18–1 Pathophysiology of the double crush syndrome. The mechanisms are multifactorial and interrelated. **I:** Impaired antegrade and retrograde axonal flow. **II:** Edema, impaired vascular flow, and subsequent ischemia. **III:** Altered biomechanical properties with fibrosis and fixation at one site leading to decreased excursion and stretch at the second site. **IV:** Intrinsic nerve susceptibility as seen in diabetic neuropathy.

3. Intrinsic susceptibility of a nerve to compression secondary to an underlying neuropathy (i.e., diabetic, autoimmune, genetic) or connective tissue disorder (systemic lupus erythematosus, scleroderma)
4. Altered nerve elasticity[7] (Fig. 18–1)

IMPAIRMENT OF AXONAL FLOW

Antegrade axonal flow from the cell body to the synapse provides neurotransmitter and structural proteins essential for the function of the axon. This transport involves two systems: fast transport for transmitter components and slow transport for cytoskeletal elements.[7] It has been found that compressive pressures as low as 15 to 20 mm Hg can impair the flow of these essential axonal components along the nerve.[26] Therefore, it is intuitive that an area of compression at one site along a nerve can lead to an increased susceptibility to compression at another site. This phenomenon was studied experimentally by Dellon, MacKinnon, and Seiler.[24,33–37] Using a rat model, bilateral sciatic nerves were banded with a silicone band for 4 months. No physiologic changes were identified. A second band was placed more distally on one sciatic nerve only. Four months later, the

double-banded side revealed a significantly prolonged conduction latency and decrease in impulse amplitude. Similarly, this experiment was repeated to show that both antegrade and retrograde flow was disrupted by these sites of compression. This confirmed that two sites of compression, each insufficient to produce a conduction disturbance alone, could impair function when present simultaneously.

Nemoto et al.[5] quantified these findings in their study using dog sciatic nerves. They found that complete conduction block did not occur in any nerves with a single site of compression, but conduction velocity was reduced to 39% of the preoperative values. When two compression clamps were used, complete conduction block was observed in 50% of nerves by 6 weeks, and conduction velocity was reduced to 34%. Lastly, they found that if the second site of compression was added 3 weeks after the first, complete conduction block also occurred in 50%, but velocity was reduced to 14%. Histologically, they found increased axonal degeneration distal to the second sites of compression.

Lundborg et al.[34] proposed a theory of a "retrograde double crush," postulating that retrograde flow of axonal elements was also important to axonal function, and that the disturbance of this retrograde flow made the proximal nerve more susceptible to compression. This was supported by the findings of Cragg and Thomas, who found that conduction velocity of the median nerve was slowed up to 40 to 50 cm proximal to the carpal tunnel in patients with carpal tunnel compression.[38] Similarly, Anderson et al. found chronic retrograde histologic changes following more distal compression of the median nerve in guinea pigs,[39] and Anastasopoulos and Chroni found F-wave data on EMG to suggest proximal conduction slowing secondary to a distal compression of the median nerve at the wrist.[40]

ENDONEURAL EDEMA AND IMPAIRMENT OF INTRANEURAL BLOOD FLOW

Functional impairment of a nerve has also been linked to ischemia. Sites of compression lead to a blockage of venous flow, at pressures as low as 20 to 30 mm Hg as shown by Rydevik et al.[36] This occlusion can lead to an impairment of the delivery of nutritional and neural elements along the axon both primarily and secondarily due to the increase in endoneural fluid pressure and development of endoneural edema. Lundborg et al. found a threefold increase in the endoneural pressure following compression of 30 mg after 8 hours.[34] Pressures of 15 to 30 mm Hg is comparable to that found in human compression neuropathy.[35,36] Spencer et al. showed that blockage of energy dependent axonal transport, leading to localized defects in energy metabolism can lead to pathologic changes that culminated in distal axonal degeneration.[41] Therefore, it is subsequently intuitive that the nerve distal to a site of compression would be less resilient to further injury.

INTRINSIC SUSCEPTIBILITY SECONDARY TO UNDERLYING NEUROPATHY/CONNECTIVE TISSUE DISORDER

Intrinsic abnormalities of a peripheral nerve make it more susceptible to developing a compressive neuropathy. Etiologic examples include diabetic neuropathy, uremic neuropathy, hypothyroidism, genetic abnormalities such as hereditary neuropathy, Dejerine-Sottas and Charcot-Marie-Tooth diseases, Friedreich's ataxia, myxedema, pyridoxine deficiency, chronic alcoholism and connective tissue disorders (vasculitis, scleroderma). Likewise, these disorders are similarly implicated in compressive neuropathies.[13,14,16,18,20,21,23,42–45] It is clear that nerves affected by an intrinsic neuropathy are predisposed to developing subsequent compressive lesions, as seen in the double crush syndrome.

Diabetes mellitus represents the most commonly encountered cause of intrinsic neuropathy. Therefore, diabetic nerves have been shown to be highly susceptible to compressive neuropathy.[13,14,16,20,21,42,43,45] Causes of this susceptibility are linked to the diabetic-related changes in the vaso nervorum, leading to decreased perfusion and subsequently increased intraneural pressure.[17] Also implicated is the altered glucose metabolism, which increases the water content in the endoneurial space. This increases the endoneurial pressure, thus reducing axoplasmic flow.[31] As discussed previously, these changes lead to impaired axonal function, again leading to susceptibility to multiple sites of compression. The level of neuropathy is directly related to the age of the patient and duration of the diabetes. Brown and Asbury found entrapment neuropathies in 15 of 38 diabetic patients.[14] The incidence of diabetes in patients who require surgical release for CTS ranges from 4% to 20%.[14,16,20,21,43]

Similarly, patients with chronic renal failure on hemodialysis are susceptible to developing uremic neuropathy, likely due to the presence of uremic neurotoxins and β-2-microglobulin amyloid deposition. Patients with chronic renal failure have been found to have a high incidence of compression neuropathy, ranging from 3% to 32%.[19,44]

Hereditary neuropathy, an autosomal dominant disorder with variable penetrance, is characterized by focal myelin thickening, with recurrent and multiple compression neuropathy at anatomically vulnerable sites.[23,42] Most commonly affected nerves are the ulnar, radial, median, and peroneal. Once diagnosed, the best treatment is activity modification and avoidance of positions that produce symptoms. Operative management should only be considered in those with unrelenting symptoms.

With intrinsic neuropathy, the incidence of compressive neuropathies of multiple peripheral nerves increases. Baba et al.[13] reported a 16% incidence of simultaneous CTS and cubital tunnel in diabetics. This is compared to the 6% incidence of ulnar neuropathy at the elbow in patients with isolated CTS as reported by Kuntzer.[46] Kenzora found that 20% of patients with uremic neuropathy had compressed median and ulnar nerves at the wrist.[19]

Treatment for these patients should be directed at medical management of the cause for the underlying neuropathy, and simple release of the site of compression when symptoms are unrelenting.

ALTERED NERVE ELASTICITY

Nerves are elastic and glide throughout a full range of motion of the extremity. Nerve elasticity and resistance to stretch are functions of the perineurium. The epineurium similarly provides resistance to externally applied forces such as compression. Injury to a nerve may lead to extraneural and intraneural fibrosis, and ultimately to stiffer nerves by reducing elasticity. Entrapment neuropathy restricts excursion by tethering a nerve extrinsically as well as thickening the nerve connective sheaths intrinsically. This restricted excursion predisposes a nerve to both proximal and distal stretch, even with through a normal range of motion. This abnormal stretch makes the nerve susceptible to further compression injury, both distally and proximally. As shown by Lundborg and Rydevik, intraneural circulation is directly affected by the amount of stretch on a nerve.[47] They showed that blood flow was impaired by an elongation of a nerve by a mere 8%, and that it was completely occluded with elongation of as low as 11%. This decreased blood flow has been previously discussed as impairing neural function. This combined with the abnormal epineurium, increases susceptibility of a nerve to compression at multiple sites.

COMMON CLINICAL EXAMPLES

The double crush syndrome can affect any peripheral nerve, but the most common clinical examples in the upper extremity are discussed below (Fig. 18–2).

Median Nerve Double Crush

Clearly, double crush of the median nerve is the most commonly encountered. The median nerve originates from the C6–T1 nerve roots, with C6 and C7 being the major contributors. At the brachial plexus level, all trunks and the lateral and medial cords form the median nerve. Prior to entering the carpal canal, the median nerve gives off its anterior interosseous and palmar cutaneous branches. It then terminates in the recurrent motor branch and the digital sensory branches.

CTS is the most common compressive neuropathy. Cervical radiculopathy is also a common entity, with classical symptoms of neck pain, stiffness, and radiating arm pain and parasthesias. It is common to see some symptom overlap in patients with CTS and cervical radiculopathy, leading to potential improper diagnoses or incomplete diagnoses. Upton and McComas initially believed that 75% of patients with CTS had a coexistent radiculopathy.[1] Hurst et al.[3] retrospectively reviewed 1000 cases of CTS and found a significant correlation between clinically and radiographically diagnosed cervical arthritis and CTS. Yu et al.[48] found an 11% incidence of electrodiagnostically-proven cervical radiculopathy in patients with electrodiagnostically-proven CTS. Osterman found prospectively that 18% of patients with CTS had concomitant cervical radicu-

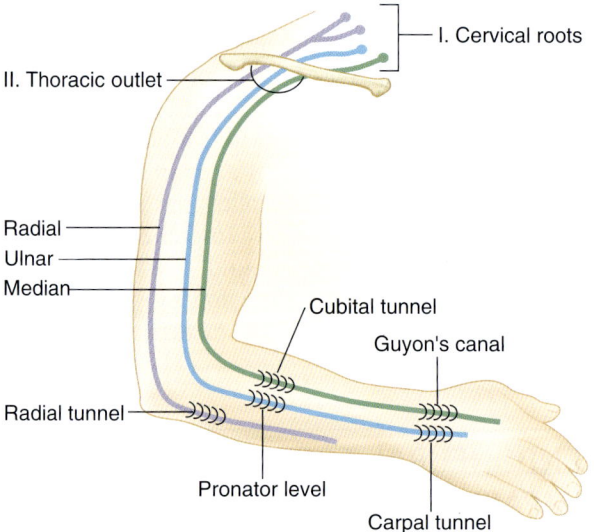

Common Double Crush Syndromes

Median

Cervical radiculopathy and carpal tunnel syndrome
Thoracic outlet and carpal tunnel syndrome
Pronator syndrome and carpal tunnel syndrome

Ulnar

Cervical radiculopathy and carpal tunnel syndrome
Thoracic outlet and carpal tunnel syndrome
Cubital tunnel and Guyon's canal syndrome

Radial

Cervical radiculopathy and radial tunnel syndrome

Figure 18–2 Common sites of double crush and multiple crush entrapment.

lopathy, and the mean age for these double crush patients was over a decade older than those with CTS or cervical radiculopathy alone.[6] It was also found that parasthesias were more common in the double crush group than the CTS group, but numbness and night symptoms were less common. On physical examination, the only significant finding was weaker grip strength in the double crush group. Radiographs of the cervical spine revealed increased disc space deterioration at the C5–C6, C6–C7, and C7–T1 levels in the double crush group. However, the correlation between electrodiagnostic studies and the radiographic findings were not found to be statistically significant. This confirms another study that found no correlation between radiographic findings in symptomatic and asymptomatic patients.[49] Interestingly, Osterman found that while motor latency and EMG findings were similar for the CTS and double crush groups, sensory latency was more significantly increased in the CTS over the double crush group.[6] This supports the theory that less compression of the median nerve at the carpal tunnel is required to produce symptoms in patients who have a concomitant lesion more proximally (i.e., double crush). Surgical release of the carpal tunnel was found to be less successful in the patients with double crush than those with isolated CTS. Thirty-three percent of those patients viewed surgery as a failure, compared to 7% in the isolated CTS group, and postoperative grip and pinch strength values remained lower. While 84% of the CTS patients returned to their original jobs, only 58% of the double crush group did.[6]

Therefore, in patients with median nerve compressive symptoms who present with any cervical complaints, with more parasthesias than numbness, less severe night symptoms, and only mildly increased sensory latency, a diagnosis of double crush should be suspected. Electrodiagnostic studies of these patients should include the cervical roots. Cervical radiographs are not usually helpful and not routinely obtained. Treatment should also be directed at both lesions. Although some relief should be expected, poorer surgical prognosis should be anticipated by the patient and physician following carpal tunnel release alone. A trial carpal tunnel injection may be helpful in these patients. Often a successful response to an injection will predict a similar surgical improvement. In a double crush patient with a poor response to a carpal tunnel injection, the primary pathology may be originating more proximally, and hence the surgical release may be deferred.

Treatment for cervical radiculopathy is generally nonoperative, although the advent of less invasive cervical decompression and fusion has made surgical intervention more common in recent years.

Double crush of the median nerve may also occur at the pronator level and at the carpal tunnel. Breidenbach and Tsai[50] reported on 21 of these patients, and concluded that these patients benefited from surgical decompression at both levels.

Radial Nerve Double Crush

Radial tunnel syndrome is a subtle entity, diagnosed both clinically and electrodiagnostically. This syndrome is classically a pain-only syndrome, where the radial nerve is compressed as it enters the forearm. Common sites of compression include the arcade of Frohse, radial recurrent vessels, medial border of the extensor carpi radialis brevis (ECRB) and the supinator. As with the median nerve, compression of the radial nerve may be potentiated by another more proximal lesion (cervical radiculopathy).[50] In our series of 78 patients with "refractory lateral epicondylitis," 27% had proven cervical radiculopathy, 23% had radial tunnel syndrome (72% diagnosed clinically alone, 28% confirmed electrodiagnostically), and 8% had evidence of both. Seventeen patients underwent radial tunnel release and 84% of the radial tunnel patients noted improvement, whereas only 50% of the double crush patients noted improvement. This failure of distal treatment alone is

indicative that a more proximal lesion will contribute to the residual symptoms.[65]

Ulnar Nerve Double Crush

As is true with the other peripheral nerves of the upper extremity, the ulnar nerve is similarly affected by the double crush syndrome. Proximal sites of compression may be at the low cervical/thoracic root level, or the inferior brachial plexus levels. Distal sites include the intermuscular septum, arcade of Struthers, cubital tunnel, Osborne's ligament, the heads of the FCU and Guyon's canal. Leffert found that 10% of patients with cubital tunnel syndrome had simultaneous findings of TOS.[51] To date, there are no studies that evaluate the prevalence of ulnar nerve double crush at the cubital tunnel and Guyon's canal levels. However, the entity exists and should be kept in mind when the ulnar nerve is decompressed at the elbow. Transposition may put additional stretch on the nerve, potentiating a site of compression elsewhere along the nerve (i.e., Guyon's canal).

Role of Thoracic Outlet Syndrome in Double Crush

A mention of TOS is appropriate in any discussion of the double crush syndrome. TOS is the most common cause of brachial plexopathy, when the plexus is compressed as it exits the neck on its way to the axilla. Sites of compression include the scalene musculature, and/or the first or anomalous cervical ribs. This presence of this entity would predispose a patient to a distal site of entrapment or compression. Multiple studies have shown a relationship between TOS and distal neuropathies, most commonly CTS, cubital tunnel, median nerve entrapment at the pronator, and radial tunnel.[50,52-55] Narakas et al. reported a 30% incidence of CTS and a 10% incidence of cubital tunnel syndrome in patients with TOS.[53] Similarly, Wood and Biondi[56] and Wood et al.[55] reported that 44% of their patients with TOS had double crush. However, Carroll and Hurst found that the incidence of combined occurrences of TOS and CTS was extremely low. They believed that CTS in the face of TOS is rare, not related and certainly not a case of double crush.[57] The controversy continues, as it is difficult to elucidate symptomatology surrounding TOS with concomitant CTS versus CTS with proximally referred symptoms. TOS is often a difficult clinical diagnosis. Subjective symptoms often exceed physical findings. Physical examination is often nonspecific, with the Roos, Adson, and Wright tests being nonspecific and difficult to interpret. Objective electrical criteria are often lacking. Indeed, current neurologic literature (Raps and Rubin[8] and Anastasopoulos and Chroni[40]) confirms the entity of double crush seen with cervical radiculopathy and simultaneous median nerve compression at the carpal tunnel, but cannot confirm the role of TOS in the double crush syndrome. It is our opinion that in patients who suffer from double crush with components of TOS with a distal site of compression, conservative measures should be exhausted first. Should nonoperative measures fail, and surgery is contemplated, the distal site of compression should be addressed first. Distal decompression is more predictable and less risky. Proximal decompression for TOS (scalenectomy, rib resection, or both), has a high risk for complications, and is often unnecessary as patients frequently improve with the distal release alone. Proximal decompression should be reserved for a last resort situation.

CONCLUSION

Double crush syndrome is a proven entity, occurring when a lesion anywhere along the course of a nerve, whether mechanical or intrinsic (metabolic, etc.) makes that nerve susceptible to another lesion somewhere else along that nerve, either distally or proximally. The pathophysiology of double crush is multifactorial, and to this day is still not fully elucidated. The common theme persists that axoplasmic flow up and down an axon is essential to the normal function of a nerve, and any impairment of that flow may lead to a nerve susceptible to compression. Any peripheral nerve may be affected by double crush, and the nerves most commonly encountered are the median, ulnar and radial. Patients with double crush must be identified initially, as treatment of one lesion alone is typically unsatisfactory and the patient's ultimate prognosis is dependent on the diagnosis and treatment of *both* lesions.

REFERENCES

1. Upton ARM, McComas AJ. The double crush in nerve entrapment syndromes. Lancet 1973;2:359–62.
2. Benarik J, Kadanka Z, Vohanka S. Median nerve mononeuropathy in spondylotic cervical myelopathy: double crush syndrome? J Neurol 1999;246:544–51.
3. Hurst LC, Weissberg D, Carroll RE. The relationship of the double crush syndrome to carpal tunnel syndrome, an analysis of 1000 cases of carpal tunnel syndrome. J Hand Surg Br 1985;10:202–4.
4. Massey W, Riley T, Pleet B. Coexistent carpal tunnel syndrome and cervical radiculopathy (double crush syndrome). South Med J 1981;74:957–9.
5. Nemoto K, Matsumato N, Tazakik, et al. The double lesion neuropathy: an experimental study and clinical cases. J Hand Surg Am 1987;12:552–9.
6. Osterman AL. The double crush syndrome: cervical radiculopathy and carpal tunnel syndrome. Orthop Clin North Am 1988;19:147–55.
7. Osterman AL. Double crush and multiple compression neuropathy. In: Gelberman RH, ed., Operative Nerve Repair and Reconstruction. Philadelphia: J.B. Lippincott, 1991:1211–29.
8. Raps SP, Rubin M. Proximal median neuropathy and cervical radiculopathy: double crush revisited. Electromyogr Clin Neurophysiol 1994;34:195–6.
9. Seiler WA, Schleged R, Mackinnon SE, et al. The double crush syndrome: development of a model. Surg Forum 1983;34:596–8.
10. Shuman J, Osterman AL, Bora FW. Compression neuropathies. Semin Neurol 1987;7:76–87.
11. Simpson RL, Fern SA. Multiple compression neuropathies and the double-crush syndrome. Orthop Clin North Am 1996;27:381–8.
12. Wilbourn AJ, Gilliatt RW. Double crush syndrome: a critical analysis. Neurology 1997;49:21–9.
13. Baba M, Ozaki I, Watahiki Y, et al. Focal conduction delay at the carpal tunnel level and the cubital fossa in diabetic polyneuropathy. Electromyogr Clin Neurophysiol 1987;27:119–23.
14. Brown MJ, Asbury AK. Diabetic neuropathy. Ann Neurol 1984;15:2–12.
15. Clayburgh RH, Beckenbaugh RD, Dobyns JH. Carpal tunnel release with diffuse peripheral neuropathy. J Hand Surg Am 1987;12:380–3.
16. Comi G, Lozza L, Galardi G, et al. Presence of carpal tunnel syndrome in diabetes: effect of age, sex, diabetes duration and polyneuropathy. Acta Diabetol Lat 1985;22:259–62.
17. Dahlin LB, Meiri KF, McLean WG, et al. Effects of nerve compression on fast axonal transport in streptozotocin-induced diabetes mellitus in the rat sciatic nerve. Diabetologia 1986;29:181.
18. Gilliatt RW, Willison RG. Periphereal nerve conduction in diabetic neuropathy. J Neurol Neurosurg Psychiatry 1962;25:11–8.
19. Kenzora J. Dialysis carpal tunnel syndrome. Orthopaedics 1978;1:195–203.
20. Leffert RD. Diabetes mellitus presenting as peripheral neuropathy in the upper limb. J Bone Joint Surg Am 1969;51:1005–10.
21. Mulder DW, Lambert EH, Bastron JA, et al. The neuropathies associated with diabetes: a clinical and electromyographic study of 103 unselected diabetic patients. Neurology 1961;11:275–84.
22. Roos D, Thygesen P. Familial recurrent neuropathy. Brain 1972;95:235–48.
23. Rosen SA, Wang H, Cornblath DR, et al. Compression syndromes due to hypertrophic nerve roots in hereditary sensory neuropathy type I. Neurology 1989;39:1173–7.
24. Dahlin LB, Rydevik B, Lundborg G. Pathophysiology of nerve entrapment and nerve compression injuries. In: Hargens AR, ed., Tissue Nutrition and Viability. New York: Springer, 1986:135–60.
25. Gelberman RH, Rydevik BL, Pess GM, et alG. Carpal tunnel syndrome: a scientific basis for clinical care. Orthop Clin North Am 1988;19:115–24.
26. Gelberman RH, Szabo RM, Hargens AR. Pressure effects on human peripheral nerve function. In: Hargens AR, ed., Tissue Nutrition and Viability. New York: Springer, 1986:161–83.
27. Neary O, Ochoa J, Gilliatt RW. Subclinical entrapment neuropathy in man. J Neurol Sci 1976;24:283–9.
28. Ochoa J, Fowler JJ, Gilliatt RW. Anatomical changes in peripheral nerves compressed by pneumatic tourniquet. J Anat 1972;113:433–55.
29. Stewart JD, Aquayo AJ. Compression and entrapment neuropathies. In: Dyck PJ, Thomas PK, Lambert EH, eds., Peripheral Neuropathy, 2nd ed. Philadelphia: W.B. Saunders, 1984:1435–57.
30. Szabo RM, Gelberman RH. The pathophysiology of nerve entrapment syndromes. J Hand Surg Am 1987;12:880–4.
31. Dellon AL, MacKinnon SE. Basic scientific and clinical applications of peripheral nerve regeneration. Surg Annu 1988;20:59–100.

32. MacKinnon SE, Dellon AL. Multiple crush syndrome. In: MacKinnon SE, Dellon AL, eds., Surgery of the Peripheral Nerve. New York: Thieme Medical Publishers, 1988:347–92.

33. Dahlin LB, McLean WG. Effects of graded experimental compression on slow and fast axonal transport in rabbit vagus nerve. J Neurol Sci 1986;72:19.

34. Lundborg G, Myers R, Powell H. Nerve compression injury and increased endoneurial fluid pressure, a "miniature compartment syndrome." J Neurol Neurosurg Psychiatry 1983;46:1119–24.

35. Rydevik B, Brown MD, Lundborg G. Pathoanatomy and pathophysiology of nerve root compression. Spine 1984;9:2–15.

36. Rydevik B, Lundborg G. Effects of graded compression on intraneural blood flow. J Hand Surg Am 1981;6:3–12.

37. Rydevik B, Lundborg G, McClean WG, et al. Blockage of axonal transport induced by acute graded compression of the rabbit vagus nerve. J Neurol Neurosurg Psychiatry 1980;43:690–8.

38. Cragg BG, Thomas PK. Changes in conduction velocity and finger size proximal to peripheral nerve lesions. J Physiol [Lond] 1961;157:315–22.

39. Anderson M, Fullerton P, Gilliatt R, et al. Changes in the forearm associated with median nerve compression at the wrist in the guinea pig. J Neuro Neurosurg Psychiatry 1970;33:70–9.

40. Anastasopoulos D, Chroni E. Effect of carpal tunnel syndrome on median nerve proximal conduction estimated by F-waves. J Clin Neurophysiol 1997;14:63–7.

41. Spencer PS, Sabri MI, Schaumburg HH. Does a defect of energy metabolism in the nerve fiber underlie axonal degeneration in polyneuropathies? Ann Neurol 1979;5:501–7.

42. Behse F, Buchtahal F, Carlsen F, et al. Hereditary neuropathy with liability to pressure palsies: electrophysiologic and histopathological aspects. Brain 1972;95:777–94.

43. Chaudhuri K, Davidson AR, Morris IM. Limited joint mobility and carpal tunnel syndrome in insulin-dependent diabetes. Br J Rheumatol 1989;28:191–4.

44. Gilbert MS, Robinson A, Baez A, et al. Carpal tunnel syndrome in patients who are receiving long-term renal dialysis. J Bone Joint Surg Am 1988;70:1145–53.

45. Thomas JE, Lambert EH, Czeuz KA. Electrodiagnostic aspects of the carpal tunnel syndrome. Arch Neurol 1967;16:635–41.

46. Kuntzer T. Carpal tunnel syndrome in 100 patients: sensitivity, specificity of multi-neurophysiological procedures and estimation of axonal loss of motor, sensory and sympathetic median nerve fibers. J Neurol Sci 1994;127:221–9.

47. Lundborg G, Rydevik B. Effects of stretching the tibial nerve of the rabbit, a preliminary study of the intraneural circulation and the barrier function of the perineurium. J Bone Joint Surg Br 1973;55:390–401.

48. Yu J, Bendler EM, Mentari A. Neurological disorders associated with carpal tunnel syndrome. Electromyogr Clin Neurophysiol 1979;19:27–32.

49. Friedenberg ZB, Miller WT. Degenerative disc disease of the cervical spine. J Bone Joint Surg Am 1963;45:1171–8.

50. Breidenbach W, Tsai TM. Ipsilateral Pronator Teres and Carpal Tunnel Compression of the Median Nerve. Paper presented at annual meeting of the American Society for Surgery of the Hand, Las Vegas, 1985.

51. Leffert RD. Thoracic outlet syndromes. Hand Clin 1992;8:285–97.

52. Dale WA, Lewis MR. Management of thoracic outlet syndrome. Ann Surg 1975;181:575–85.

53. Narakas A, Bonnard C, Egloff DV. The cervicothoracic outlet compression outlet syndrome: analysis of surgical treatment. Ann Chir 1986;5:195–207.

54. Williams HT, Carpenter NH. Surgical treatment of the thoracic outlet syndrome. Arch Surg 1978;113:850–2.

55. Wood VE, Twito R, Vereska JM. Thoracic outlet syndrome: the results of first rib resections in 100 patients. Orthop Clin North Am 1988;19:131–46.

56. Wood VE, Biondi J. Double crush nerve compression in thoracic outlet syndrome. J Bone Joint Surg Am 1990;72:85–7.

57. Carroll RE, Hurst LC. The relationship of thoracic outlet syndrome and carpal tunnel syndrome. Clin Orthop 1982;164:149–53.

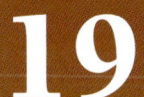

19 Thoracic Outlet Syndrome

Rashid M. Janjua, Gabriel C. Tender, Robert L. Tiel, and David G. Kline

INTRODUCTION

Achy burning pain of an arm that is usually but not always confined to the medial border of the arm and hand, sometimes but not always associated with elevation of the arm or activity of the extremity, and sometimes associated with vasomotor changes of the extremity usually evokes the specter of thoracic outlet syndrome (TOS). Few syndromes generate as much controversy and emotion, both pro and con as the TOS. To understand the passions that this syndrome evokes, a knowledge of the history and evolution of the entity must be appreciated.

What can be appreciated is that various groups and disciplines have discovered different etiologies for similar symptoms. As a result most authors have divided TOS into different categories:

1. Neurogenic or true neurogenic TOS
2. Disputed neurogenic TOS
3. Arterial TOS
4. Venous TOS

HISTORY

TOS has been and continues to be a controversial topic in thoracic and vascular surgery and in neurosurgery. The existence of cervical ribs was known at the time of Galen, but Hunald[1] did not describe the cervical rib and its symptomatology until 1742. This was followed by Sir Astley Cooper in 1818, who reported a woman with an ischemic limb attributed to "a projection of the lower cervical vertebrae towards the clavicle and consequent pressure on the subclavian artery."[2] The first surgical intervention was reported by Coote[3] in 1861, who removed an exostosis of the transverse process of the seventh cervical vertebra to treat a weak, ischemic hand followed by Paget's description in 1875 of an axillary vein thrombosis.[4] The initial emphasis focused on cervical ribs being the culprit for symptoms presumably produced by vascular compromise of the upper limb. In 1907, Keen[5] reviewed 42 cases of cervical rib resection from the literature, and by 1910, Murphy[6] reported a follow-up of 3 months after a surgical procedure for first rib resection in patients without cervical ribs but TOS-like symptoms. Halsted postulated that vascular turbulence was the etiology for poststenotic aneurysms and then described his series of 716 cases of cervical ribs.[7] The first rib was felt to be the responsible structure for the TOS.

Adson and Coffey[8] promulgated the phrase "cervical rib syndrome" in their series of 31 patients who underwent rib resection, and had what was then a novel operation, scalenotomy. These authors also acknowledged the "frequent complications of rib resection." This was followed by Telford and Mottershead,[9] who re-emphasized the important role that both the first and cervical rib play in neurovascular compression.

Ochsner et al.[10] in 1935 were the first to coin the phrase "scalenus anticus syndrome," as they reviewed reports of the anterior scalene abnormalities. A similar term "cervicobrachial syndrome" was used by Aynesworth[11] in 1940 to encompass all causes of TOS. Peet et al.[12] are to be credited for using the current term of TOS in 1956, when they used this to express pain, numbness, and other symptoms in the upper extremity. In their series of 55 patients, 71% improved with conservative management alone.

The pendulum swung back towards first rib resection when Clagett advocated removal of that rib as the optimal treatment as opposed to the scalenotomy.[13] His description of a posterior approach for rib resection was an adaptation from the old tuberculosis surgical literature. His impetus arose from a dissatisfaction with the high recurrence rate after procedures involving scalenotomy alone. Following this description, Roos[14] described the transaxillary route for the first rib resection.

Ever since, selection of either a supraclavicular or transaxillary approach has been dictated by the personal preference of the surgeons.

DEFINITION OF THE THORACIC OUTLET

Generally, the area called the "thoracic outlet" is anatomically defined as the area that is bounded inferiorly by the lung apex, posteriorly by the spine, and laterally by the first rib. The mediastinum forms the medial border. Superiorly, the outlet continues to the level of the fifth cervical spinal nerve where it becomes more cone shaped (Fig. 19–1) (Table 19–1).

For many anatomists, the thoracic "outlet" is felt to be the site of communication between the thorax and abdomen (inferior thoracic aperture).[15] The area between the scalene muscles and the first rib-clavicle area is as a result called the "thoracic inlet." Be that as it may, the definition of inlet and outlet is, at least for vessels with blood flow, determined by the direction of their flow. Therefore, from the perspective of a subclavian vein, this region of interest is an inlet whereas for the artery it is an outlet. Interestingly enough, for the nerves that suffer from compression, it is neither an inlet nor an outlet when viewed from the perspective of the

TABLE 19–1
Contents of the Thoracic Outlet
The anterior and middle scalene
Five cervical spinal nerves and their trunks
Nerves: Phrenic, long thoracic, dorsal scapular, suprascapular
Stellate ganglion and sympathetic fibers
The subclavian artery and vein
The thoracic duct
Lymph nodes
Apex of the lung

thorax, as the afferent and efferent nerve fibers pass through this region towards the upper extremity. Since the term TOS is so prevalent, it still seems best to use it. One can then further refine the diagnosis by adding the neurogenic or vascular as adjectives.

ANATOMIC ASPECTS

All facets of the anatomy of the thoracic outlet in the setting of TOS need to be well understood. The outer margin of this region can be subdivided into three regions with respect to the sites of compression: the scalene triangle, the costoclavicular space and the pectoralis minor space. The most common site of compression is the scalene triangle (Fig. 19–2), followed in frequency by the costoclavicular space.

Many anatomic variations can be the source of compression at these sites. Roos[16] described nine different compressive bands at various locations which may cause neurovascular compression. In our series, the Roos Type 7 involving the middle scalene was the most commonly found variation but sometimes, no specific structure was found. In TOS patients undergoing reoperation, scar tissue was sometimes implicated as a compressive element of the plexus. After Roos's description, Poitevin[17] described three separate restrictive bands that crossed over the region of Sibson's fascia where plexus compression may be present.

Although plexus compression in the costoclavicular space is infrequent, the neurovascular bundle may be compromised by bony pathology involving the clavicle and/or first rib. The costoclavicular region is a triangular space bordered anteriorly by the medial portion of the clavicle, the underlying subclavius muscle with its tendon and the costocoracoid ligament. This space is bordered posteromedially by the first rib and the insertion of the anterior and middle scalene muscles. Posterolaterally it is bordered by the upper scapula. Congenital abnormalities such as a straight first rib and/or a straight clavicle can compromise this space. A tight subclavius muscle with a prominent ligament can restrict the available space and directly impinge upon the trunks and

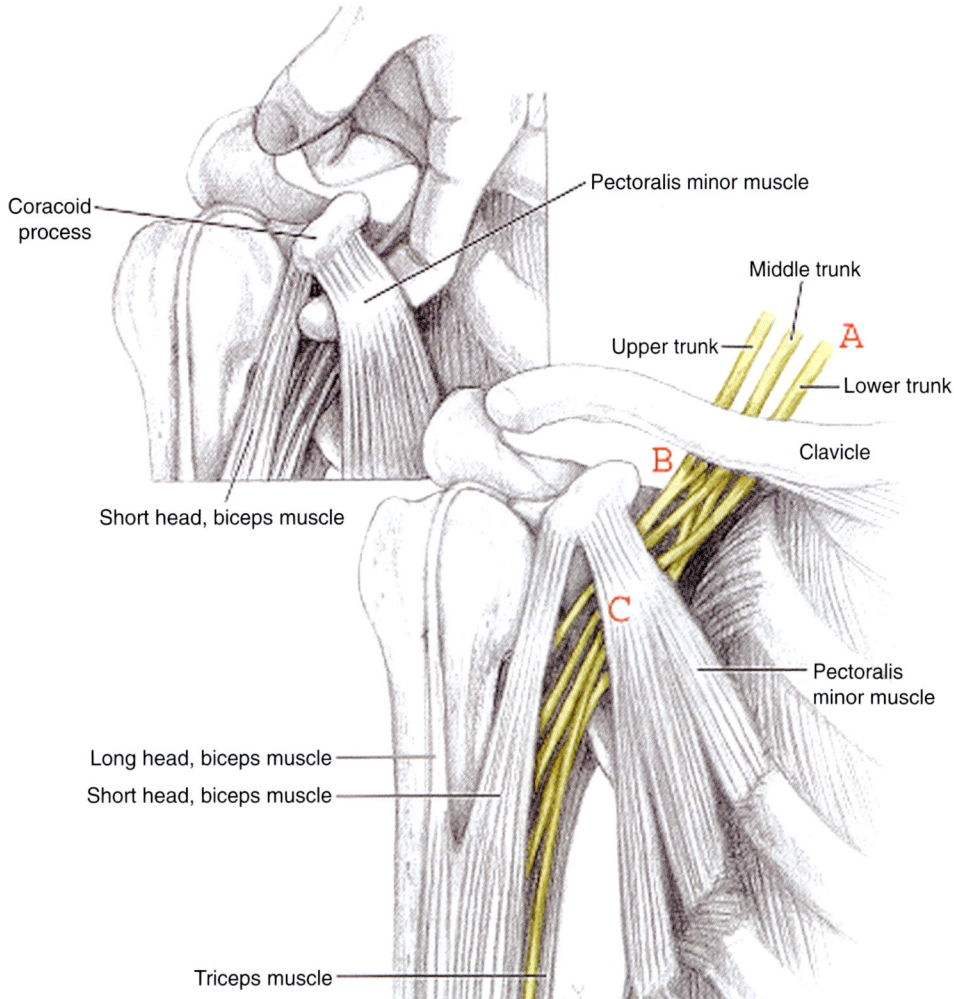

Figure 19–1   Three regions of possible compression. **A:** Scalene triangle. **B:** Costoclavicular space. **C:** Pectoralis minor space. (From Kline DG, Hudson AR, Kim DH. Atlas of Peripheral Nerve Surgery. Philadelphia: W.B. Saunders, 2001,[34] with permission.)

their divisions. Similarly, a fractured clavicle with excessive callus formation can lead to TOS at this level.

Patients who have droopy shoulders, whether habitual or secondary to an external cause, may also experience some compromise of the available space in this region.

During abduction of the shoulder, depression of the coracoid process and scapula can lead to impingement of the neurovascular bundle against the subclavius muscle and/or ligament. This maneuver, albeit rarely, may also be a causative factor in the irritation of the nerve bundle against the lower edge of the pectoralis minor in the subpectoral minor space.

PATHOPHYSIOLOGIC CONSIDERATIONS

Nerve compression can distort the blood—nerve barrier and cause demyelination or even axonal loss, depend-

ing on the severity and duration of compression and susceptibility of the patient.[18] Excellent reviews of the successive histologic changes are provided elsewhere.[18–21]

In patients with TOS, compression at the "outlet" can be an isolated phenomenon or it can occur in combination with other more peripheral entrapment syndromes.[21,22] This is an extremely important factor in those patients as a "double crush,"[23] "reverse double crush,"[24] or "multiple crush"[21] phenomenon can require additional investigation and treatment. Upton and McComas[23] introduced the "double crush theory," which suggested nerve compression proximally could lead to increased susceptibility distally due to interruption or dampening of the axoplasmatic flow. The initial compression site may be asymptomatic, but when combined with distal pathology, both sites may cause symptoms. Lundborg[24] subsequently argued that a similar phenomenon could occur proximally if distal compression was present (reverse double crush). The incidence

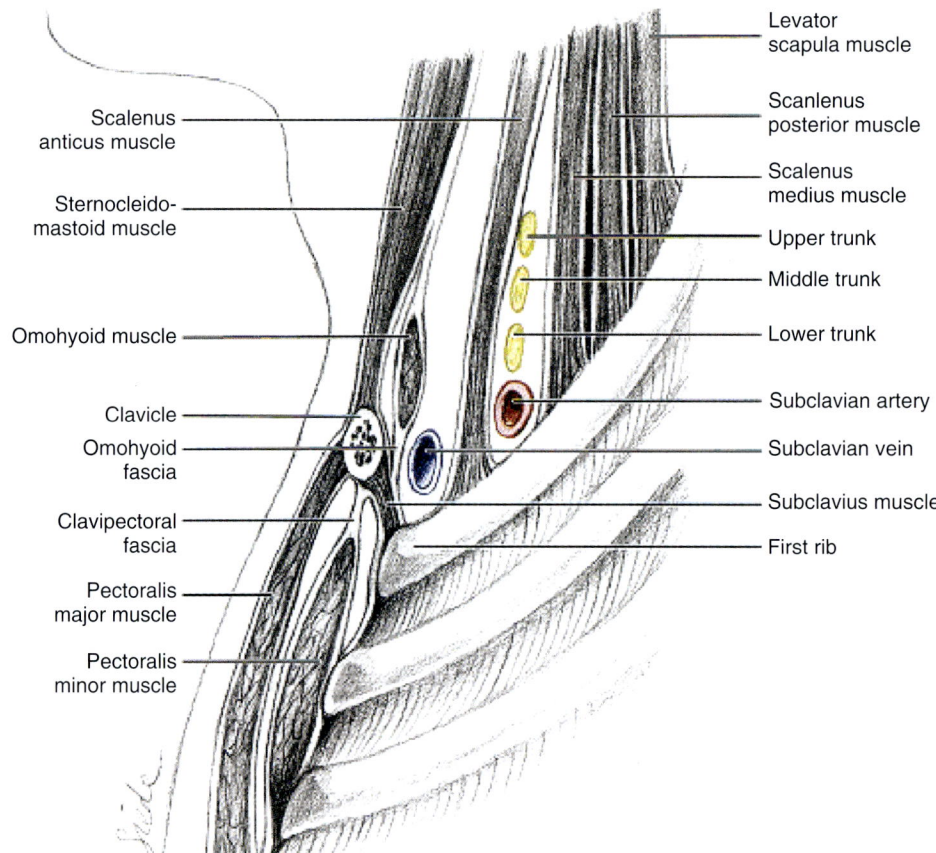

Figure 19–2   Scalene triangle. The brachial plexus elements are bound medially and anteriorly by the anterior scalene muscle, and laterally and posteriorly by the middle scalene muscle. (From Kline DG, Hudson AR, Kim DH. Atlas of Peripheral Nerve Surgery. Philadelphia: W.B. Saunders, 2001,[34] with permission.)

of double crush has been reported to be as high as 44% in TOS cases.[25] The precise pathogenesis is as yet unclear. The factors leading to compromise can be biologic (diabetes, metabolic diseases of the peripheral nervous system, etc.),[26] structural (i.e., compression),[27–30] or vascular.[26] On a cellular level, this compression may result in proximal endoneurial edema. This edema may lead to an impairment of the distal neural microcirculation,[31] disruption of the lymphatic and/or venous outflow in the region of nerve compression,[32] and a decreased number of neurofilaments.[28]

In patients with TOS, release of a concomitant distal cubital or carpal tunnel entrapment may improve axonal flow, and subsequently obviate the need to decompress the plexus at the outlet. As a result, there may be significant improvement in symptoms and the potential morbidity associated with a first rib resection can be avoided.

The scalene muscles can exhibit fibrosis, which is sometimes related to cervical injury. Spasm and resultant shortening of these muscles places them at an ergonomical disadvantage which in turn can lead to dysfunctional and painful neck muscles. This excessive stress leads to an imbalance in other muscle groups such as the trapezius.[33]

We reviewed a 30-year experience with neurogenic TOS at the Louisiana State University.

PATIENTS AND METHODS

Patient data were gathered on 135 patients operated on over the previous 30 years. Patients were placed into three categories: spontaneous TOS, postinjury TOS, and recurrent TOS. The patient's age, mechanism of injury, symptoms, physical examination, and operative findings and outcomes were recorded. Preoperatively, radiographs were reviewed and electrophysiologic studies performed. During surgery, observations regarding potential areas of compression were noted, and nerve action potentials were elicited by stimulating spinal nerves and recording from more distal trunks and their divisions. All patients had at least 1 year of postoperative follow-up.

RESULTS

A total of 125 patients underwent 133 operations: 66 were approached via an anterior (50%) and 67 via a

TABLE 19–2	
Patient Demographics	
Unilateral TOS patients	117
Bilateral TOS patients	8
Total patients operated	125
Total Operations	133
Anterior Approach	66
Posterior Approach	67
Gender	
Males	48
Females	77
Age range	
10–20	13
20–30	25
30–40	55
40–50	22
50–60	14
60–70	3
Pain and Paresthesias	111
Prior cervical operation	56
History of trauma	36
Gilliat-Sumner Hand	33

TABLE 19–3		
Prior Operations		
Operation	**Subsequent Anterior Approach**	**Subsequent Posterior Approach**
Transaxillary first rib operation ×1	18	23
Transaxillary first rib operation ×2	2	2
Cervical rib removal	2	6
Scalenectomy	6	5
Anterior neurolysis	5	3
Thrombectomy	1	1
Sympathectomy	2	2
Cervical laminectomy	0	2
Anterior cervical fusion	3	2
Pulmonary lobectomy	0	2
Clavicle plating	1	2
Ulnar transposition	7	3
Carpal tunnel release	6	3
Needle biopsy of plexus	6	3
Clavicle resection	1	0

TABLE 19–4	
Intraoperative NAP Recordings	
Patients with abnormalities	91
Decreased amplitude T1 to LT	39
Decreased CV T1 to LT	45
Flat T1 NAP trace	10
Decreased amplitude C8 to LT	31
Decreased CV C8 to LT	30
C7 to MT abnormality	9
NAP abnormal on all elements	1
NAP on patients with prior serious plexus injury	7
(–) NAP's → Grafts	4
(+) NAP's → Neurolysis	1
(+) and (–) NAP's → Split or partial graft repairs	2

CV, conduction velocity; LT, lower trunk; MT, middle trunk; (+), positive; (–), negative.

posterior approach. The male to female ratio was 1 : 1.6, with the most common complaint consisting of pain and paresthesias (83%). Only 36 patients (28%) had a history of trauma to the shoulder or neck. Patient demographics are listed in Table 19–2. Fifty-six patients (45%) had either a previous exploration of their brachial plexus or a prior first rib resection for suspected TOS before undergoing surgery at our institution (Table 19–3).

The anterior approach (Fig. 19–3 A to F) consisted of a supraclavicular exposure of the brachial plexus elements through a horizontal incision. A careful dissection of the nerves and especially the vessels, which may be displaced considerably, can identify the offending structure. In our practice, this approach is not used for first rib removal. The posterior approach (Fig. 19–4 A to E) uses a posterior corridor to gain access to the proximal plexus elements after division of the rhomboids, inferior trapezius and posterior scalene muscles. This is a safe route in experienced hands, particularly for exposure of the inferior part of the plexus. An extensive step by step description of these procedures is provided in the *Atlas of Peripheral Nerve Surgery*.[34]

All patients underwent intraoperative nerve action potential (NAP) recordings (Table 19–4). The most commonly encountered findings were decreased NAP amplitude and velocity when stimulating from the T1 and C8 spinal nerves and recording from the lower trunk. In ten patients no NAP could be elicited from the T1 root. Typically, the upper plexus elements, such as the C5 and C6 to upper trunk and its divisions, were unaffected. In nine patients, the C7 spinal nerve to the

middle trunk showed slowing of the conduction velocity. Upper element recordings served as a control to those performed on the lower elements. Most of the patients were found to have slowing of the nerve conduction near the spine at a spinal nerve level as opposed to more distally. Forty-two plexuses (32%) had normal NAP recordings.

The most common finding in patients operated on through an anterior approach was an elongated transverse process of C7 with or without a displaced and somewhat fibrous middle scalene (n = 23). The next most common finding was that of a thickened middle

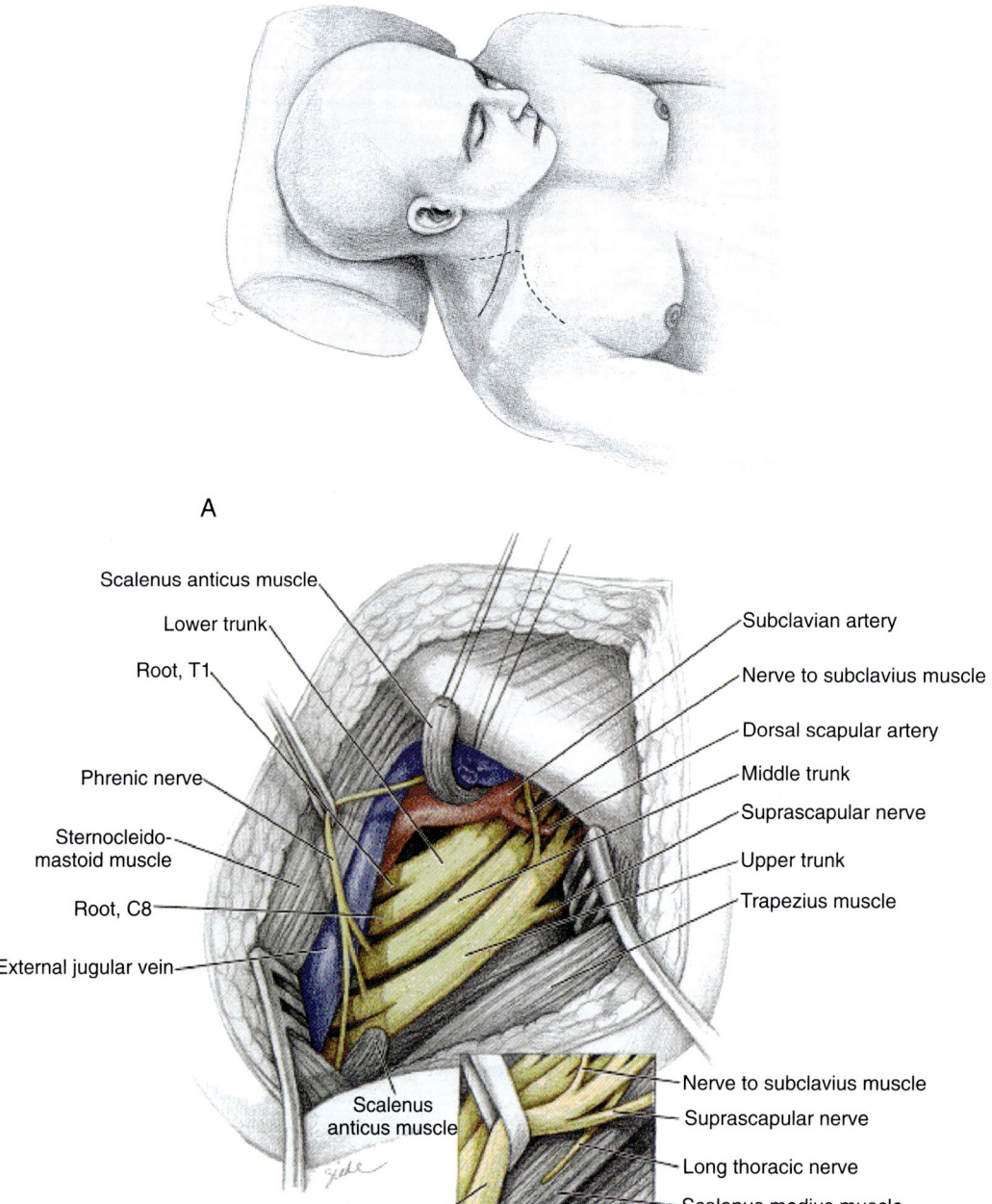

A

Scalenus anticus muscle

Lower trunk

Root, T1

Phrenic nerve

Sternocleido-mastoid muscle

Root, C8

External jugular vein

Subclavian artery

Nerve to subclavius muscle

Dorsal scapular artery

Middle trunk

Suprascapular nerve

Upper trunk

Trapezius muscle

Scalenus anticus muscle

Upper trunk

Nerve to subclavius muscle

Suprascapular nerve

Long thoracic nerve

Scalenus medius muscle

B

Figure 19–3 Anterior approach. **A:** Positioning for the supraclavicular approach. A transverse incision is made 1 in superior to the clavicle. Occasionally, a classic brachial plexus incision is necessary *(dotted line)* to obtain infraclavicular exposure. This may be necessary due to patient habits or for decompression of infraclavicular plexus elements. **B:** It is usually not necessary to dissect much of the C5 or C6 spinal nerves. However, the more distal upper trunk and its divisions should be dissected and gently retracted laterally by Penrose drains. This permits a good view of C7 and its extension into the middle trunk, and from there, one can advance the dissection medially to the lower trunk and eventually to the C8 and T1 spinal nerves.

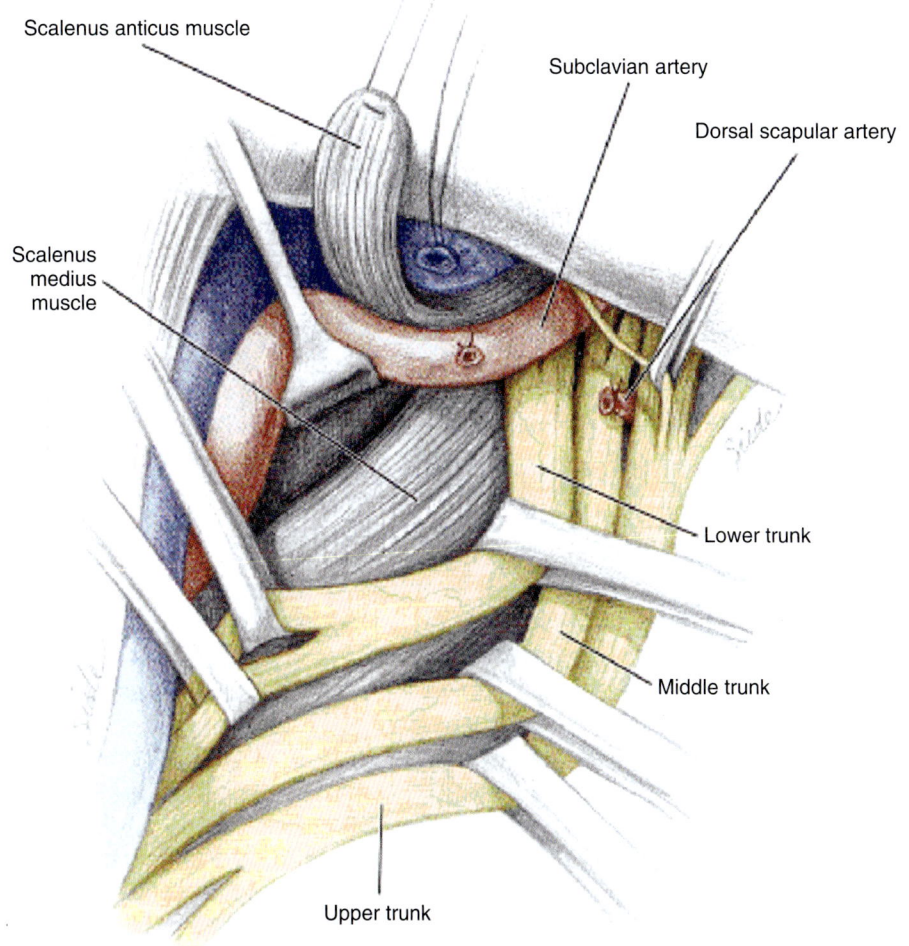

Scalenus anticus muscle

Subclavian artery

Dorsal scapular artery

Scalenus medius muscle

Lower trunk

Middle trunk

Upper trunk

C

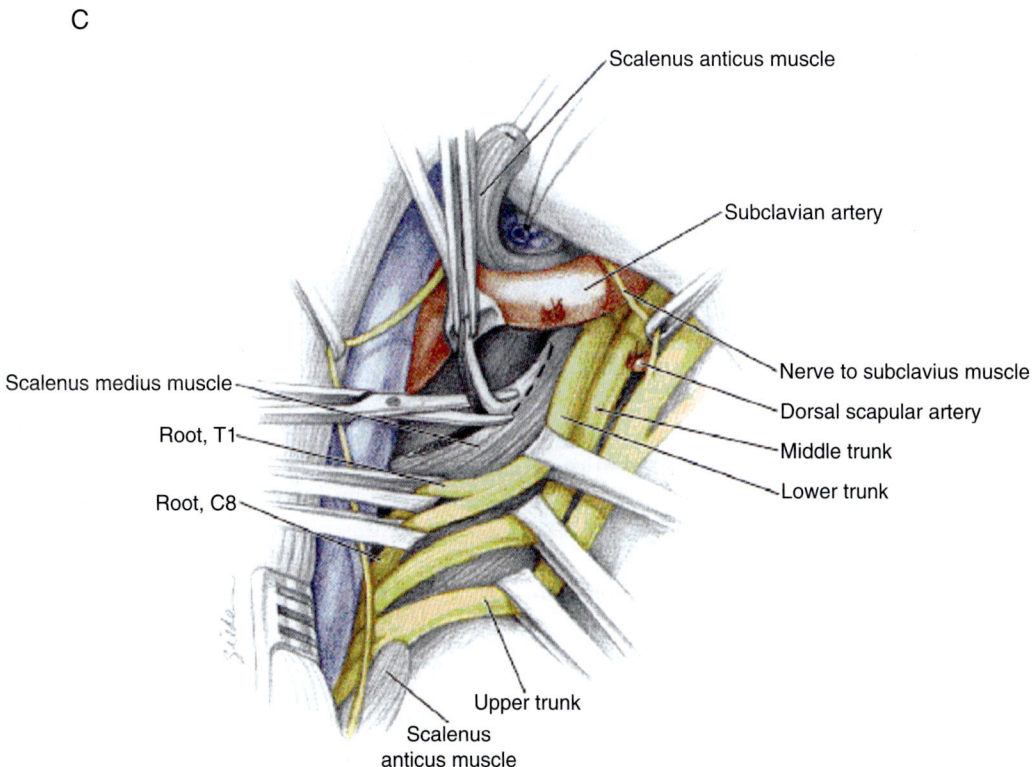

Scalenus anticus muscle

Subclavian artery

Scalenus medius muscle

Nerve to subclavius muscle

Root, T1

Dorsal scapular artery

Middle trunk

Root, C8

Lower trunk

Upper trunk

Scalenus anticus muscle

D

Figure 19–3—Cont'd   Anterior approach. **C:** After identification of the individual elements, Penrose drains are used for retraction. A segment of the anterior scalene is usually resected. The subclavian artery is mobilized and retracted anteriorly to expose the inferior elements better. This allows exposure of the medial edge of the middle scalene muscle. **D:** The dissection is carried out to the foramina of C7, C8, and T1. The elements are followed distally and all fibrotendinous bands are divided. In this instance a fibrous medial edge of the middle scalene is resected.

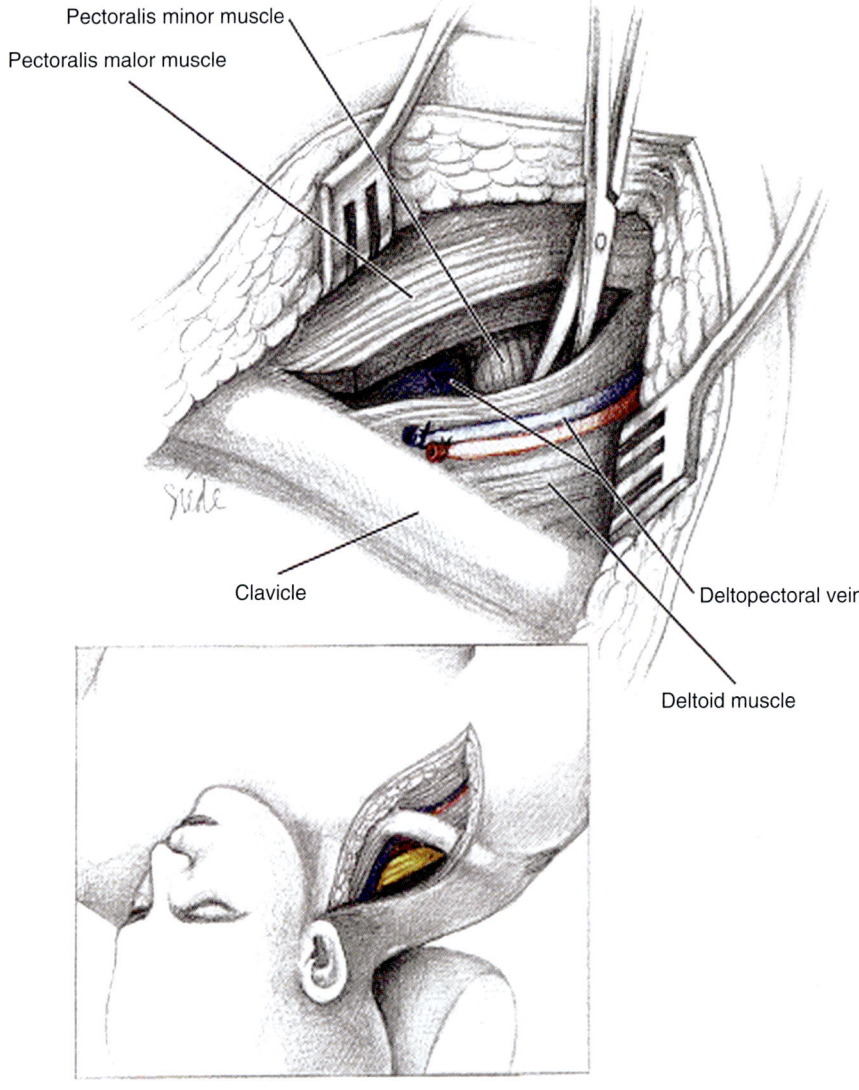

Pectoralis minor muscle

Pectoralis malor muscle

Clavicle

Deltopectoral vein

Deltoid muscle

E

Figure 19–3–Cont'd   Anterior approach. **E:** Occasionally, an infraclavicular exposure is necessary. The supraclavicular vessels are divided and the pectoralis major muscle is split along the delto-pectoral groove. Additional exposure can be gained by passing moist sponges under the clavicle thus encircling and elevating it. This allows for better exposure of the medial cord.

scalene muscle, usually with a fibrous edge (n = 19), in addition to scar tissue related to a prior operation (n = 16). The latter was found most commonly in patients operated on through the posterior approach (n = 29) (Table 19–5).

Postoperatively, following an anterior approach (Table 19–5), 37 patients had complete resolution of their pain or paresthesias. Another 21 patients had a decrease in their symptoms. Nine patients had serious residual pain. One had a new deficit. Table 19–6 lists the complications, which include pleural opening in 3, phrenic paralysis in 4, and chylothorax in 1 patient. Of the 67 patients operated on from a posterior approach, 34 experienced resolution of their pain with an additional 27 experiencing some relief. There was a new

deficit in 1 patient, a pleural opening in 4, phrenic paralysis in 3, and 1 case of a wound infection. It should be kept in mind that most of these patients had undergone previous surgery.

CLINICAL ASPECTS

Patients who are felt to be suffering from entrapment or compression at the thoracic outlet can present with various symptomatology. This can range from headaches and facial pain to the more common symptoms of pain and tingling along the medial side of the arm and even frank atrophy in the hand musculature.[35] Of our patients, 89% (111/125) presented with pain or paresthesias. We

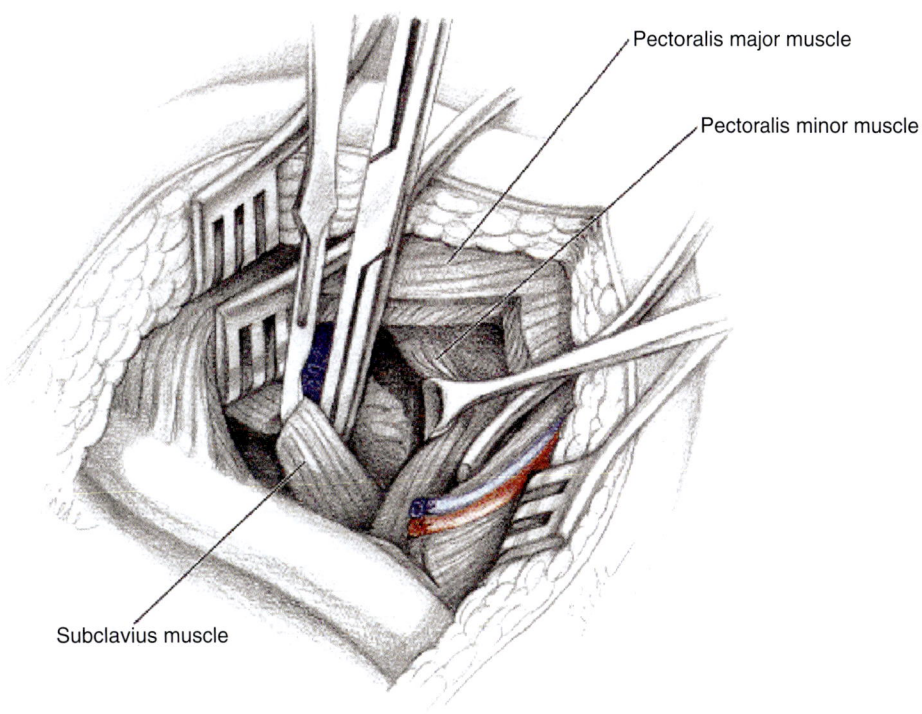

Pectoralis major muscle

Pectoralis minor muscle

Subclavius muscle

F

Figure 19–3—Cont'd   Anterior approach. **F:** By division of the subclavius muscle, better subclavicular visualization is obtained. (From Kline DG, Hudson AR, Kim DH. Atlas of Peripheral Nerve Surgery. Philadelphia: W.B. Saunders, 2001,[34] with permission.)

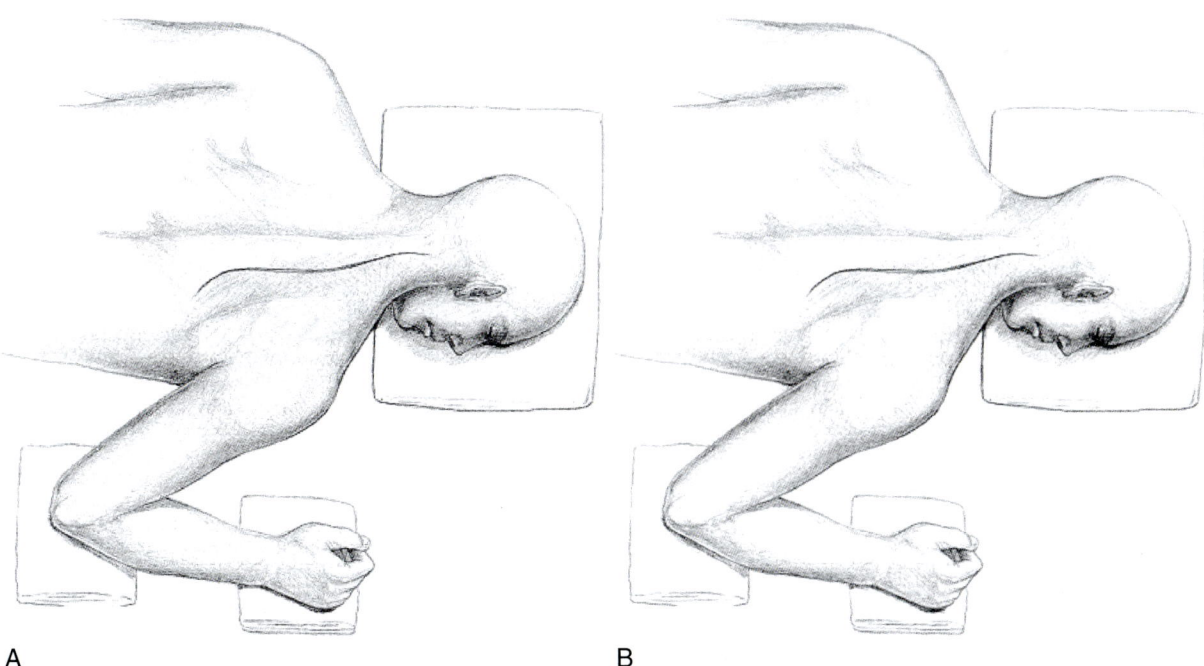

A   B

Figure 19–4   Posterior approach. **A, B:** Positioning for the posterior subscapular approach. The patient is placed in the prone position with the ipsilateral shoulder abducted and the flexed elbow and forearm placed on an adjacent Mayo stand. The position of the operating table is raised or lowered to move the scapula more or less out of the surgical corridor. The incision is curved along the medial edge of the scapula, lateral to the spinous processes of the thoracic spine. It extends superiorly to the posterolateral aspect of the lower neck. Care is taken to pad the elbow and hand to protect against pressure neuropathy. **C:** The trapezius is divided halfway between the medial edge of the scapula and the spine.

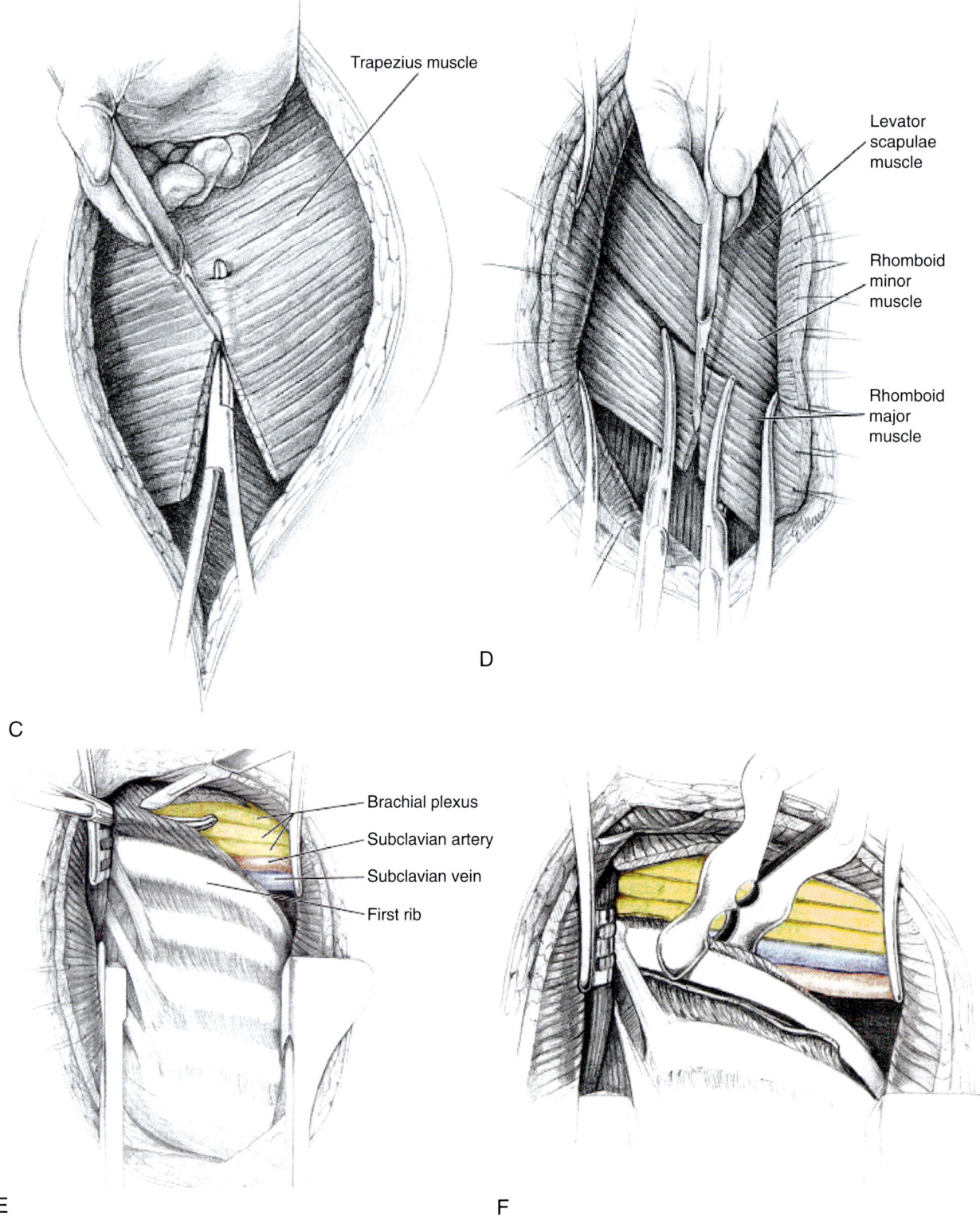

Trapezius muscle

C

Levator scapulae muscle

Rhomboid minor muscle

Rhomboid major muscle

D

Brachial plexus

Subclavian artery

Subclavian vein

First rib

E

F

Figure 19–4–Cont'd   **D:** After division of the trapezius muscle, the rhomboids are clamped by Serat's and divided. The muscle edges on both sides are marked with sutures so that at the end of the procedure opposing sides can be better approximated. **E:** With a chest retractor, the posterior surface of the ribs is exposed and the posterior scalene divided and retracted to expose the spinal nerves. **F:** Using Leksell rongeurs, the first rib and its transverse process are resected. (From Kline DG, Hudson AR, Kim DH. Atlas of Peripheral Nerve Surgery. Philadelphia: W.B. Saunders, 2001,[34] with permission.)

have previously published the findings in one subset of these patients who had a Gilliat-Sumner hand or true neurogenic TOS (Table 19–7).[36]

In our approach to patient selection, we reserve operative treatment for those patients who have symptomatology that is associated with either abnormal radiographic findings and/or electromyographic studies or those who have failed conservative management. In patients who present with progressive neurological loss, operative management should be the first line of treatment. The operative approach, whether anterior or posterior is individualized for each patient. The posterior approach was usually selected for patients in whom there were large cervical ribs or other sizable bony abnormalities or for patients who had a failure following a prior anterior or transaxillary operation.

Full resolution of the sensory symptoms was obtained in 53% (71/133) of our patients, with partial improvement seen in an additional 36% (48/133). These results closely match those published by Sanders and Hammond[37] and Nannapaneni and Marks.[38]

In 1989, Sanders and Pearce[30] published a comparison of transaxillary first rib resections (111 cases), anterior and middle scalenectomy (279 cases), and combined supraclavicular first rib resection with scalenectomy (278 cases). At a mean follow-up of 15 years, the results obtained were almost identical with each of these surgical approaches.

Disputed TOS

Patients with complaints of vague medial arm pain and a plethora of other complaints are often diagnosed as having TOS. Further investigation through physical examination and ancillary testing typically yield no hard findings that are indicative of neural compromise at the brachial plexus level. The proper diagnosis in those of patients having a "disputed TOS" has been a source of debate among many treating physicians. These considerations make TOS a diagnosis of exclusion that is entertained only after entities such as a cervical spondylosis and disc disease, nerve entrapments and diabetic neuropathies are excluded.

TABLE 19–5

Gross Operative Findings

Finding	Anterior Approach	Posterior Approach
Cervical rib	4	5
Residual cervical rib	3	6
Residual first rib	2	8
C7 elongated with or without band	23	6
Medial scalene bands	19	7
Other bands	8	8
Sibson's fascial band	3	3
Tight or taut plexus element(s)	5	23
Scar involving plexus element(s)	16	29
Prior serious operative plexus injury	4	5

TABLE 19–6

Results and Complications

Result	Anterior Approach	Posterior Approach
No pain/paresthesias	37	34
Partial improvement pain	21	27
Serious residual pain	8	6
Re-operation for pain	1	2
Mild motor deficit improved	9	10
Mild motor deficit unchanged	7	2
Severe motor deficit improved	7	7
Severe motor partially improved	7	10
Severe motor deficit unchanged	3	7
New deficit produced	1	1
Pleural opening	3	4
Phrenic paresis	4	3
Wound infection	0	1
Scapular winging	0	4
Chylothorax	1	0
Subsequent diagnosis of syrinx	0	1
Chest tube	0	2
Postop thoracentesis	2	3

TABLE 19–7

Recent Studies with Results from True Neurogenic Thoracic Outlet Syndrome

Study	# operations	Method of diagnosis	% Patients with resolved pain Sx	% Patients with decreased pain Sx	Complication rate %	Approach
Nannapaneni 2003	59	Radiographic	60	20	0	Scl
Sanders 2002	65	Radiographic	59	13	N/A	Scl, TA
Current group	133	Radiogr. and EMG	53	36	24	Scl, Psc

The majority of the patients who are operated on for TOS fall into the category of disputed TOS. Surgeons who believe in this clinical entity believe that it can be caused by either compression or stretch of the brachial plexus, which leads to chronic irritation of the plexus and subsequent complaints. Thoracic outlet decompression therefore, is felt to be the solution. Despite the fact that many clinical tests such as the Adson and Roos tests and electrodiagnostic testing such as somatosensory studies are felt by some to have predictive value, they have failed to demonstrate merit upon scientific scrutiny.

Clinical symptoms complicating disputed TOS can be subdivided into four groups:

1. Concomitant cervical plexopathy: posterior, lateral, and anterior neck pain; trapezial ridge pain; ear pain; temporomandibular pain; occipital pain ("migraine headache"); trapezius muscle spasm
2. Sympathetic or central nervous system dysfunction: facial and neck swelling; eye pain; blurred vision; eyelid droop; nonfocal syncope; hyperactive reflexes; reflex sympathetic dystrophy with livido reticularis; limb swelling; joint contractures; movement disorders (inability to initiate movement, tremor, spasms, dystonic posture); pain spread to ipsilateral lower and contralateral upper extremities
3. Inability of plexus elements to move or glide smoothly, secondary to anomalous structures or plexus/periplexus scarring: cervical radiculopathies; ulnar neuropathies at the elbow and hand; posterior interosseous nerve compression at the forearm; median neuropathies at the elbow and wrist (carpal tunnel syndrome)
4. Abnormal posture (excessive descent of the scapula; forward displacement of the shoulder): impingement syndrome (rotator cuff tear); trapezius spasm; biceps tendinitis; trigger points; lateral epicondylitis

Some or all of these symptoms are all felt to originate from TOS, but no solid evidence has been provided for such. A study performed in Washington State among worker's compensation patients demonstrated higher medical costs and a three to four times greater likelihood of disability in 50% of the patients who underwent surgery for TOS. Consequently, the diagnosis of TOS has not been recognized in many areas of that state.

It is our belief that in consideration of the lack of evidence for this entity, surgical treatment should be reserved for some but not all patients. Those patients in whom the differential diagnoses has been excluded yet have persistent symptoms despite a lengthy trial of physical and occupational therapy may be candidates for an operation, provided there are clear cut clinical, radiographic, or electrodiagnostic findings. Other patients may achieve good results following physical therapy.[39]

Arterial TOS

Arterial complications in the thoracic outlet occur from long-standing and intermittent vascular compression. In the vast majority of cases, cervical ribs are present. Fusion of the cervical rib to the first rib or the presence of a fibrous band arising from a hypertrophic scalene muscle causes displacement of the supraclavicular course of the artery. Initially, this vascular compression is asymptomatic but it is followed by minor thromboembolic symptoms (small punctuate lesions in the fingers and thumb). In more advanced cases or in cases of delayed diagnosis, major arterial occlusion and potentially limb-threatening ischemia can occur. The more proximal the arterial insult, the better it is tolerated due to collateral blood supply downstream. Other reported symptoms include Raynaud's phenomenon, with episodic pallor, cyanosis, chronic pain, coldness, and paresthesias.

The initial diagnosis is made by physical examination through the presence of a pulsatile mass in the supraclavicular area as a result of displacement and/or prestenotic dilatation of the artery. Auscultation can be useful as a bruit can often be heard. A thrill may be felt with careful palpitation. Hyperabduction tests such as the Adson test can reveal a decrease in arterial pressure. The Roos test, which was originally developed to diagnose vascular compression,[16] can be used to detect exercise-induced ischemia. In the occasional patient, skin pallor, coldness of the hand or finger(s), atrophy, hair loss, and, in later stages, atrophy of the intrinsic hand muscles, may be seen.

In the workup, a chest and cervical spine x-ray are important in the diagnosis of cervical ribs, an elongated transverse process of C7 and other abnormalities such as callus formation following an old clavicular fracture. Once the an arteriogram performed with the arm initially at the side and then abducted, produces the most reliable information with regards to compromise of the subclavian artery.

Treatment relies on the obliteration of the offending structure, that is, bands, cervical ribs, fracture callus, and so on. Occasionally, the vessel may be damaged to such an extent that primary arterial grafting may be necessary in order to preserve vascular flow. This can usually be performed through a supraclavicular approach.

Venous TOS

Also known as Paget-Schroetter syndrome, the subclavian vein can be compromised upon its entry into the supraclavicular space where it empties into the innominate vein. It is located medial to the anterior scalene muscle. It may be thrombosed spontaneously (primary) or secondary to an anatomic constraint or following multiple iatrogenic manipulations during the insertion of a subclavian catheter. Contrary to arterial TOS, venous TOS manifests as swelling and cyanosis of the extremity.

The diagnosis of venous TOS can be confirmed with duplex/Doppler, but dynamic venography that is performed with the arm in first a neutral then abducted position, is the gold standard. Treatment options are variable and dependent on the age of the thrombosis and the structural abnormality of the vessel, as well as the need for the removal of any potentially constrictive structures.

REFERENCES

1. Tyson RR, Kaplan GF. Modern concepts of diagnosis and treatment of the thoracic outlet syndrome. Orthop Clin North Am 1975;6:507–19.
2. Cooper A. On exostosis. In: Cooper A, Travers B, eds., Surgical Essays, Part 1. London: Cox and Son, 1818:159–61.
3. Coote H. Exostosis of the left transverse process of the seventh cervical vertebra, surrounded by blood vessels and nerves: successful removal. Lancet 1861;1:360–1.
4. Paget J. Clinical Lectures and Essays. London: Longman, Greens, and Co., 1875.
5. Keen WW. The symptomatology, diagnosis and surgical treatment of cervical ribs. Am J Med Sci 1907;133:173–218.
6. Murphy T. Brachial neuritis caused by pressure of first rib. Aust Med J 1910;15:582–5.
7. Halsted WS. An experimental study of circumscribed dilation of an artery immediately distal to a partially occluding band and its bearing on the dilation of the subclavian artery observed in certain cases of cervical rib. J Exp Med 1916;24:271–86.
8. Adson AW, Coffey JR. Cervical rib: a method of anterior approach for the relief of symptoms by division of the scalenus anticus. Ann Surg 1927;85:839–57.
9. Telford ED, Mottershead S. The costoclavicular syndrome. BMJ 1947;1:325–8.
10. Ochsner A, Gage M, DeBakey M. Scalenus anticus (Naffziger) syndrome. Am J Surg 1935;28:669–95.
11. Aynesworth KH. The cervicobrachial syndrome: a discussion of the etiology with report of twenty cases. Ann Surg 1940;111:724–42.
12. Peet RM, Hendrickson JD, Anderson TP, et al. Thoracic outlet syndrome: evaluation of a therapeutic exercise program. Mayo Clin Proc 1956;31:281–7.
13. Clagett OT. Presidential address: research and prosearch. J Thorac Cardiovasc Surg 1962;44:153–66.
14. Roos DB. Transaxillary approach for first rib resection to relieve thoracic outlet syndrome. Ann Surg 1966;163:354–8.
15. Ranney D. Thoracic outlet: an anatomical redefinition that makes clinical sense. Clin Anat 1996;9:50–2.
16. Roos DB. Congenital anomalies associated with thoracic outlet syndrome. Am J Surg 1976;132:771–8.
17. Poitevin L. Proximal compression of the upper limb neurovascular bundle: an anatomic research study. Hand Clin 1988;4:575–81.
18. Mackinnon SE, Dellon AL, Hudson AR, et al. Chronic nerve compression: an experimental model in the rat. Ann Plast Surg 1984;13:112–20.
19. Dellon AL, Mackinnon SE. Human ulnar neuropathy at the elbow: clinical, electrical and morphometric correlations. J Reconstr Microsurg 1988;4:179–84.
20. Mackinnon SE, Dellon AL. Experintental study of chronic nerve compression: clinical implications. Hand Clin 1986;2:639–50.
21. Mackinnon SE. Double and multiple crush syndromes. Hand Clin 1992;8:369–80.
22. Novak CB, Mackinnon SE, Patterson GA. Evaluation of patients with thoracic outlet syndrome. J Hand Surg Am 1993;18:292–9.
23. Upton ARM, McComas AJ. The double crush in nerve-entrapment syndromes. Lancet 1973;2:359–62.
24. Lundborg G. Nerve injury and repair. New York: Churchill-Livingstone, 1988.
25. Wood V, Biondi J. Double crush nerve compression in thoracic outlet syndrome. J Bone Joint Surg Am 1990;72:85–7.27.
26. Hebl JR, Horlocker T, Pritchard DJ. Diffuse brachial plexopathy after interscalene blockade in a patient receiving Cisplatin chemotherapy: the pharmacologic double crush syndrome. Anesth Analg 2001;92:249–51.
27. Chaudhary V, Clawson L. Entrapment of motor nerves in motor neuro disease. Does double crush occur? J Neurol Neurosurg Psychiatry 1997;62:71–6.
28. Horluchi Y. Experimental study of a peripheral nerve lesion: compression neuropathy. J Jpn Orthop Soc 1983;75:789.
29. Katz JN, Simmons BP. Carpal tunnel syndrome. N Engl J Med 2002;346:1807–12.
30. Sanders RJ, Pearce WH. The treatment of thoracic outlet syndrome: a comparison of different operations. J Vasc Surg 1989;10:626–34.
31. Golovchinsky V. Double crush syndrome in the lower extremities. Electromyogr Clin Neurophys 1998;38:115–20.
32. Sunderland S. Nerves and Nerve Injuries, 2nd ed. Edinburgh: Churchill-Livingstone, 1978.
33. Mackinnon S. Thoracic outlet syndrome. Curr Probl Surg 2002;39:1070–145.
34. Kline DG, Hudson AR, Kim DH. Atlas of Peripheral Nerve Surgery. Philadelphia: W.B. Saunders, 2001.
35. Gilliatt RW, LeQuesne PM, Logue V, et al. Wasting of the hand associated with a cervical rib or band. J Neurol Neurosurg Psychiatry 1970;33:615–24.
36. Tender GC, Thomas AJ, Thomas N, et al. Gilliat-Sumner hand revisited: a 25-year experience. Neurosurgery 2004;55:883–90.
37. Sanders RJ, Hammond SL. Management of cervical ribs and anomalous first ribs in the management of neurogenic thoracic outlet syndrome. J Vasc Surg 2002;36:51–6.
38. Nannapaneni R, Marks SM. Neurogenic thoracic outlet syndrome. Br J Neurosurg 2003;17:144–8.
39. Lindgren KA. Conservative treatment of thoracic outlet syndrome: a 2 year follow-up. Arch Phys Med Rehabil 1997;78:373–8.

20 Adult and Obstetrical Brachial Plexus Injuries

Vincent R. Hentz

INTRODUCTION

In the early 20th century, surgeons published encouraging results of brachial plexus reconstruction.[1] However, little else was published regarding reconstruction of the brachial plexus until the late 1970s when surgeons began to apply the methods described by Millesi[2] to brachial plexus birth and traumatic brachial plexus injuries.

In the late 1980s and early 1990s, advances occurred in diagnostic techniques, refinement of surgical techniques and procedures, new surgical procedures, and experimental nonoperative treatments. In the late 1990s, very aggressive reconstruction, using extraplexal sources for reinnervation of vascularized muscle transfers, was reported for complete brachial plexus palsies in adults.

Since the first reported attempts at repair by Kennedy[1] in 1903, the role of surgical reconstruction in infants has been more controversial than for adults. The principal reasons behind the controversy are the lack of a uniform system of evaluation, and lack of agreement about what level of function is necessary to qualify as a good result. Children are difficult to examine thoroughly before the age of 3.5 to 4 years, when they can cooperate with muscle strength testing. Many studies lack reliable data on the initial clinical picture and report 80% to 95% "good" results, but there is no consensus on what constitutes a good result.

Full recovery of function after brachial plexus reconstruction in adults and infants still remains unachievable, but probably not permanently so. The exciting developments of the past several years have considerably improved surgical outcomes, and future directions for research are promising.

DESCRIPTIVE ANATOMY

We define five segments of the brachial plexus: roots, trunks, divisions, cords, and branches.[3] Note that numerous variations of the brachial plexus are possible, perhaps the most common of which are pre- and post-fixed plexuses. The most common anatomy will be described (Figs. 20–1 to 20–3).

Roots

Brachial plexus nerves are cervical nerves consisting of dorsal and ventral spinal nerves emerging from the subarachnoid space. The root actually consists only of the anterior primary ramus of the spinal nerve. The posterior primary ramus branches dorsally after

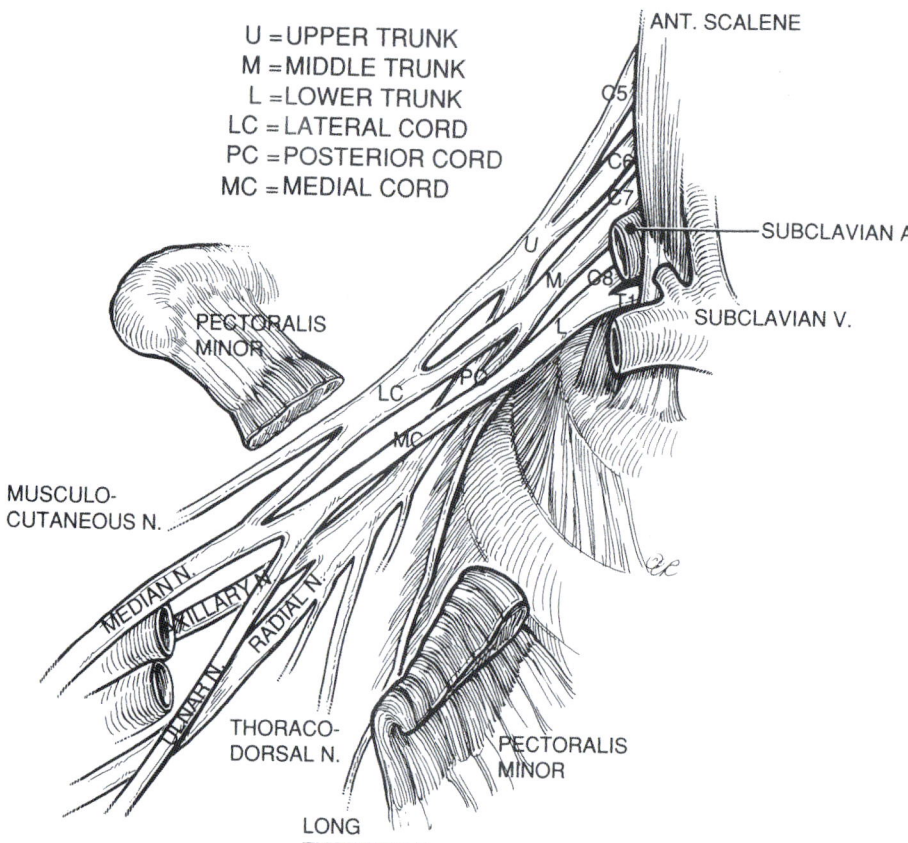

U = UPPER TRUNK
M = MIDDLE TRUNK
L = LOWER TRUNK
LC = LATERAL CORD
PC = POSTERIOR CORD
MC = MEDIAL CORD

ANT. SCALENE

SUBCLAVIAN A.

SUBCLAVIAN V.

PECTORALIS MINOR

MUSCULO-CUTANEOUS N.

MEDIAN N.

AXILLARY A.

RADIAL N.

ULNAR N.

THORACO-DORSAL N.

PECTORALIS MINOR

LONG THORACIC N.

Figure 20–1 The standard anatomy of the supraclavicular and infraclavicular brachial plexus is illustrated. The clavicle is removed and the pectoralis minor is depicted as divided to expose all elements of the plexus, including the five roots (C5–T1), three trunks (U, upper; M, middle; L, lower), the anterior and posterior divisions (not labeled), the three cords (LC, lateral cord; PC, posterior cord; MC, medial cord), and the principal branches as shown.

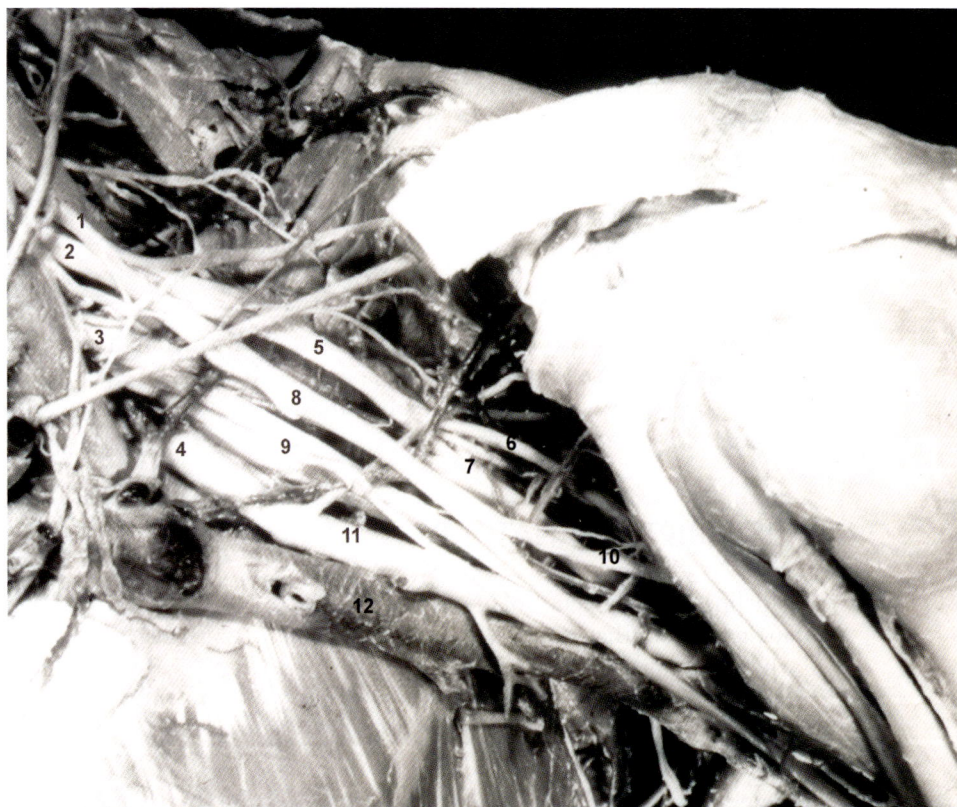

Figure 20–2 An anatomic dissection of a left brachial plexus illustrates the structures depicted in fig. 20–1 The clavicle has been removed along with the pectoralis major, pectoralis minor, and deltoid muscles. (1) C5 root. (2) C6 root. (3) C7 root and middle trunk. (4) Inferior trunk (just visible beneath middle trunk). (5) Posterior cord. (6) Axillary nerve. (7) Continuation of posterior cord (radial nerve). (8) Lateral cord. (9) Medial cord. (10) Musculocutaneous nerve. (11) Subclavian to axillary artery. (12) Subclavian to axillary vein.

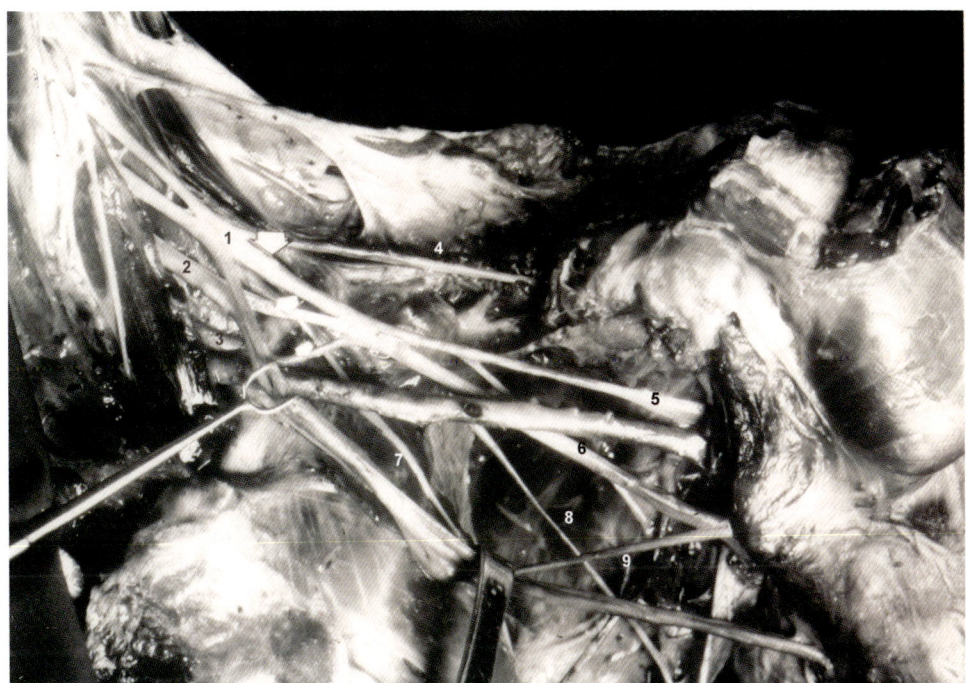

Figure 20–3   The posterior divisions from the upper, middle, and lower trunks as they form the posterior cord and its multiple branches. The anterior division structures are reflected inferiorly by the retractor. *(1)* Superior (upper) trunk. *(2)* Middle trunk. *(3)* Inferior (lower) trunk. *(4)* Suprascapular nerve. *(5)* Axillary nerve. *(6)* Continuation of the posterior cord (radial nerve). *(7)* Long thoracic nerve. *(8)* Thoracodorsal nerve to subscapularis muscle.

emerging from the dura at the transverse process to innervate skin and muscles of the dorsal neck.

The upper roots, consisting of C5, C6, C7, and occasionally C4 in the prefixed plexus, run a similar course in the proximal plexus. Emerging from intervertebral foramina behind the vertebral artery, the roots pass between the anterior and posterior tubercles of the C5–C7 cervical transverse processes. Traveling forward and downward from their respective troughs, the upper roots emerge between the anterior and middle scalene muscles. Note that C5 and C6 may also be found piercing through the anterior scalene muscle (Figs. 20–1 and 20–2).

There are a few key nerve branches coming off the upper roots. The long thoracic nerve arises from roots C5–C7, with C6 generally contributing the most. The long thoracic crosses the first rib and descends behind the brachial plexus to innervate the serratus anterior muscle. The phrenic nerve, which supplies the diaphragm, pericardium, and mediastinal pleura, comes mostly off root C4, but also receives contributions from C3 and C5. Finally, the dorsal scapular nerve arises from C5 to innervate the major and minor rhomboids.

The lower brachial plexus roots, consisting of C8, T1, and occasionally T2 in the postfixed plexus, are situated much deeper than the upper roots and pose greater difficulty in the surgical approach. Both C8 and T1 are situated behind the cervical pleura and subclavian vessels and wrap around the neck of the first rib. The C8 root

is located above the first rib, while T1 is located below the first rib. Therefore, T1 must travel upwards to join C8 and form the lower trunk. C8 travels obliquely and over the first rib, passing behind the inferior cervical or stellate sympathetic ganglion. The complex and deep arrangements of nerve roots and vessels make lower root surgical access more difficult than upper root access.

Trunks

Further distally, the five brachial plexus roots become three trunks. C5 and C6 join at "Erb's point," located on the surface of the scalenus medius approximately 2 to 3 cm above the clavicle, to become the superior or upper trunk. In a prefixed plexus, C4 would join C5 proximal to Erb's point. C7 does not join with any other root and continues on as the middle trunk. C8 and T1 join on the inner border of the first rib and become the inferior or lower trunk. Spatially, the trunks can be found just deep to the omohyoid inferior belly and the suprascapular artery, with the upper trunk more superficial to the middle and lower trunks. The three trunks extend outwardly below the clavicle to enter the axilla. As they pass the clavicle, the trunks split into anterior and posterior divisions to eventually form the terminal cords of the brachial plexus.

Two nerves can be seen branching from the upper trunk. The suprascapular nerve arises from the superolateral border of the upper trunk and travels posterior to the inferior omohyoid and anterior to trapezius. The suprascapular nerve passes underneath the superior transverse scapular ligament through the suprascapular notch. The nerve continues deep to supraspinatus and rounds the notch of the scapular neck into the infraspinous fossa, innervating both supraspinatus and infraspinatus. The other upper trunk nerve branch, nerve to subclavius, is not clinically important. Middle and lower trunks do not give rise to any nerve branches.

Divisions

Each trunk splits into anterior and posterior divisions while passing under the clavicle. The anterior divisions of upper and middle trunks form the lateral cord, while the posterior divisions of upper and middle trunks form the major portion of the posterior cord. The anterior division of lower trunk continues on as the medial cord, while the thinner posterior division of lower trunk contributes weakly to the posterior cord. As the divisions give way to cords, the plexus has entered the axilla. The divisions do not give rise to any nerve branches (Figs. 20–2 and 20–3.)

Cords

The posterior, lateral, and medial cords receive their respective names from their spatial orientation to the second part of the axillary artery. A few specific nerves emerge from the lateral and medial cords. The lateral pectoral nerve branches from the lateral cord superficial to the first part of the axillary artery and vein, sends a branch to the medial pectoral nerve, and continues on to innervate pectoralis major. The medial pectoral nerve arises from the medial cord, passes forward between the axillary artery and vein, and branches to complete a nerve loop with the lateral pectoral nerve in front of the axillary artery. The medial pectoral nerve continues on to innervate pectoralis minor, actually piercing pectoralis minor to also supply the overlying pectoralis major.

Also stemming from the medial cord are the medial cutaneous nerves of the arm and forearm. The medial brachial cutaneous nerve runs medially along the axillary vein and innervates the skin of the medial arm. The medial antebrachial cutaneous nerve arises between the axillary artery and vein and courses medial to the brachial artery. Piercing the deep fascia along with the basilic vein, it innervates the skin of the medial forearm as far as the wrist.

In contrast, several nerves classically emerge from the posterior cord. The upper subscapular nerve arises from the posterior cord to innervate the upper portion of subscapularis. The lower subscapular nerve supplies the lower subscapularis and teres major by traveling down-

ward behind the subscapular vessels. The thoracodorsal nerve arises between the two subscapular nerves, runs behind the axillary artery, and travels along with the thoracodorsal artery to innervate the latissimus dorsi.

Branches

Generally, the posterior cord innervates the posterior structures in the arm and forearm (Fig. 20–3). After giving off subscapular and thoracodorsal branches, the posterior cord terminates relatively rapidly into two branches: the axillary and radial nerves. The lateral and medial cords mostly innervate structures in the anterior arm and forearm. The lateral cord gives off the terminal musculocutaneous nerve, which pierces the coracobrachialis muscle and innervates coracobrachialis, biceps brachii, and brachialis. The musculocutaneous nerve continues on as the lateral antebrachial cutaneous nerve. The medial cord terminates principally as the ulnar nerve, which does not branch in the arm and continues to innervate most of the hand muscles. Finally, the lateral and medial cords combine to terminate as the median nerve. The median nerve also does not branch in the arm and innervates almost all wrist flexor muscles and some hand muscles.

ETIOLOGY

Essentially, all brachial plexus birth and most traumatic injuries of the brachial plexus are due to traction.[4] Low-energy stretching injuries, not severe enough to cause rupture or avulsion, typically cause more or less reversible injuries such as neuropraxia (Sunderland I)[5] or various degrees of axonotmesis (Sunderland II to IV). High-energy injuries are associated with more significant damage to the plexus, including rupture of peripheral nerve at any plexus level (neurotmesis/Sunderland V) or avulsion of nerve roots from the spinal cord (Fig. 20–4).

Brachial Plexus Injuries in the Adult

The typical candidate for microneural reconstruction is the young man who is thrown from his motorcycle. Although his helmet saves his life, it cannot prevent his shoulder from being driven downward and posteriorly and his neck driven in the opposite direction as he lands. If his shoulder–neck angle is forcibly widened by downward traction of his arm, damage is imparted first to the upper roots and trunk; if the scapulohumeral angle is forcibly widened, damage is imparted first to C8 and T1 roots and the inferior trunk. If the impact is extreme, all levels will sustain damage. The T1 and C8 roots are more likely to be avulsed from the spinal cord,

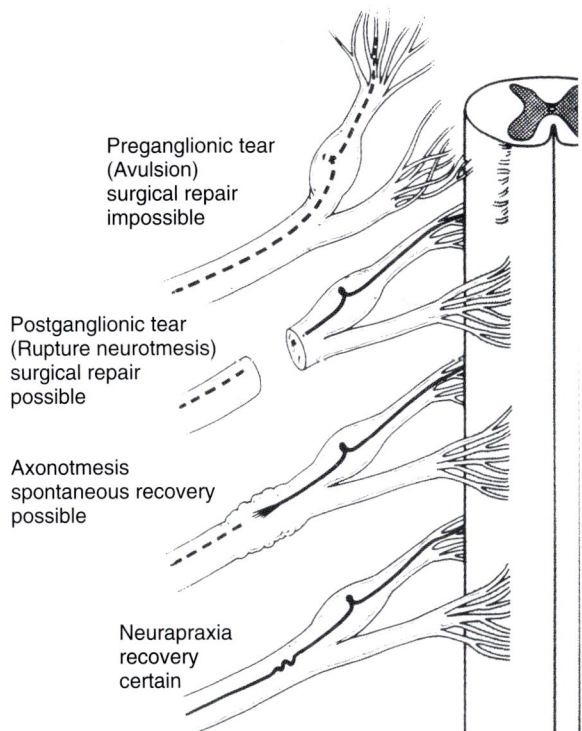

Figure 20–4 Types of pathology affecting the roots and trunks of the brachial plexus during traction injuries. Preganglionic injuries are avulsions of the rootlets from the spinal cord. Postganglionic ruptures are classical neurometic (Seddon) or Sunderland Type V injuries. Traction without complete rupture is classified as axonotmesis (Seddon) or Sunderland Type II, III, or IV injury. Traction that causes no tissue breakage but edema of the nerve sufficient to block conduction is termed neuropraxia (Seddon) or Sunderland Type I injury.

while the C6 and C5 roots are more likely to stretch or rupture in continuity after exiting the neural foramina. The principal factors determining the extent of injury are the energy of the blow and, to a lesser degree, the direction and the relationship of arm to body.

Obstetrical Injuries

Historic obstetric teachings regarding brachial plexus birth palsy (BPBP) have stated that essentially all brachial plexus injuries result from excessive traction and flexion exerted on the infant's neck during delivery, thereby tearing or avulsing the cervical nerve roots from the spinal cord. From the earliest operative experience of Sever[6] and Kennedy[1] until today, surgeons have essentially universally accepted that birth trauma was responsible for essentially all babies with brachial plexus injuries, and that the trauma was associated with the maneuvers of the birth attendant, maneuvers made necessary because of the presence of one or several predisposing circumstances.

Most published studies of BPBP are consistent in their identification of such predisposing factors as macrosomia, defined as birth weight greater than 4,000 grams. A related association is maternal diabetes. Other associated assumed predisposing factors include infant–maternal cephalo-pelvic disproportion, maternal obesity, and increased maternal age. The most important assumed factor is a delivery complicated by shoulder dystocia and other signs of birth trauma, such as fracture of the clavicle during delivery.[7]

While there are similarities between adult and infant plexus injuries as regards mechanisms of injury and the pathologic consequences, there are significant differences in terms of indications, evaluation, and management between these two injuries. Therefore, they will be discussed separately.

Adult Injuries: Indications and Timing

Most of the modern series describing the experience in brachial plexus reconstruction attest to the inverse relationship between time from injury to operation to outcome. In cautious and skilled hands, exploration seldom results in extension of the injury. Even when total palsy exists, less than 20% of patients demonstrate avulsions of all five roots of the plexus, which means that for the great majority, the surgeon will find something to repair or graft and, if this is not possible, to reinnervate by nerve transfer from an extraplexal source of motor and sensory nerves. If nerve transfer is included, then virtually 100% of patients might theoretically benefit from microneural reconstruction. These factors imply that when there is a strong suspicion of significant damage to the plexus, in the form of root avulsions and nerve ruptures, surgical exploration is warranted.

Immediate Surgery

Immediate surgery is indicated for essentially any patient with a plexus injury of almost any degree of severity secondary to a penetrating injury such as a stab wound, or following an iatrogenic injury such as known or suspected injury to the plexus at the time of first rib resection for the treatment of thoracic outlet syndrome. There are many good arguments against immediate reconstruction of the plexus in traction injuries. Most surgeons feel that some period of time must pass to permit delineation of injured from noninjured nerve.

Early Surgery (3 Weeks to 3 Months)

Early surgery is indicated for patients who present with total or near total palsy, or an injury associated with high energy levels. It is also indicated for gunshot wounds to the plexus. The presence or absence of an advancing Tinel's sign can be a useful guide. The absence of a Tinel's sign in the supraclavicular fossa in the face of a nearly complete C5–C6 level palsy is a poor prognostic sign for spontaneous recovery and warrants an early exploration with the likelihood that C5 and C6 nerve roots may be avulsed. In this case, nerve transfer will be necessary.

Delayed Surgery

For those injuries associated with lower levels of energy and those associated with partial upper level palsy, it is preferable to follow the course of recovery for 3 to 6 months, leaning toward operation if recovery seems to plateau as determined by several successive evaluations carried out at monthly intervals.

Controversial Indications

An occasional patient presents with a partial C8 and complete T1 lesion, with some finger flexors working, but with essentially an intrinsic palsy and anesthesia in the C8 and/or T1 distribution. This represents somewhat of a dilemma in decision making, because it seems almost impossible to recover intrinsic muscle function in the adult and, when injured, the C8 and T1 nerve roots are so often avulsed from the spinal cord that it is unlikely that anything repairable or even worth repairing will be found.

Surgical Technique

Patient Preparation and Informed Consent

The surgeon must discuss the expected outcome of surgery in detail, and compare it with the expected outcome if surgery is not performed. The patient and family must be made aware of the long period of time necessary for reinnervation of muscles, when essentially nothing happens that the patient can appreciate.

Prior to surgery, the patient should be taught the exercises necessary to maintain normal passive range of motion, rather than depending on the therapist to perform these exercises for him. The therapist can record progress, teach, and advise, but the patient must accept responsibility for performing the exercises. If the patient has had a previous subclavian artery reconstruction, a unit of autologous blood should be donated prior to surgery. The need for intraoperative or postoperative transfusion is rare. Otherwise, no special preoperative preparations are necessary.

Positioning of Patient and Microscope

If possible, the electrodes for intraoperative corticosensory or spinal evoked potentials are placed prior to the patient's arrival in the operating room. This permits the neurologist or technician to test the equipment, electrodes, and electrode placement.

The nature of the case, especially the indeterminate length of the procedure and the need to perform intra-

operative stimulation and recordings, are discussed with the anesthesiologist prior to induction of anesthesia. This allows the anesthesiologist to alter techniques and agents in order to avoid giving a long-acting paralytic agent and those agents that depress cortical response sufficient to compromise corticosensory recordings. The anesthesiologist is also reminded of the need to reposition the patient's head periodically to avoid causing scalp ischemia and hair loss.

The patient is positioned in the supine position and a small pillow, placed beneath the ipsilateral scapula brings the shoulder forward. The head is turned to the opposite side and the arm is abducted on an arm board. The ipsilateral or bilateral (if the contralateral C7 nerve root may be transferred), neck, mandible and hemithorax, and ipsilateral axilla, entire upper extremity, and both lower extremities (for possible nerve grafts) are prepared and draped. The arm is prepared and draped freely so that the response to nerve stimulation can be observed and so that traction can be applied during the procedure. The surgeon should be prepared to expose both supraclavicular and infraclavicular portions of the brachial plexus. If nerve grafts are required, sural nerve, radial nerve, or vascularized ulnar nerve is harvested depending on the length and diameter of the nerve graft. All donor nerve can be harvested in the supine position, avoiding the need for positional change during operation. A bipolar microcoagulator, nerve stimulator, magnifying loupes, and operative microscope should be available. Well-padded tourniquets are placed on both thighs, and both legs are draped free to the tourniquet, in preparation for harvesting sural nerve grafts.

SURGICAL APPROACHES TO BRACHIAL PLEXUS

There are two main surgical approaches to the brachial plexus, suprasclavicular and infraclavicular exposures, using a zig-zag skin incision (Fig. 20–5 A and B). The classical supraclavicular approach begins at the angle of the jaw and drops vertically to the midclavicle along the posterior border of the sternocleidomastoid, and the infraclavicular approach begins at the insertion of the sternocleidmastoid medially and extends to the deltopectoral groove laterally. These incisions may be connected if the widest exposure is preferable. However, the connecting incisions have a risk of scar hypertrophy, and recently most surgeons prefer to use the separate the transverse skin incisions as described below.

Preferred Approaches

We use two basic approaches. The upper roots are exposed through a transverse cervical skin incision, and

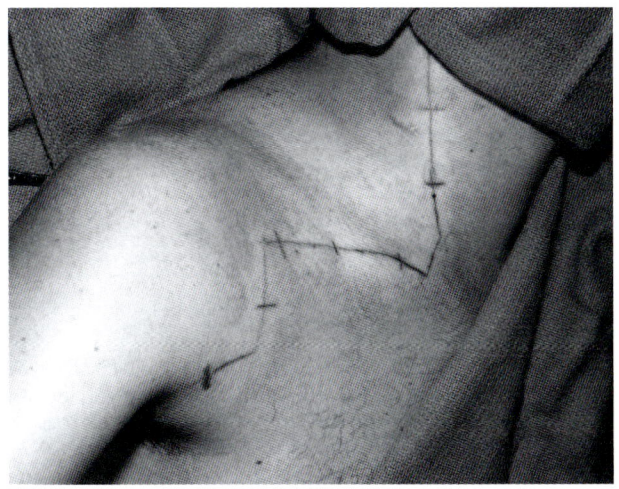

A

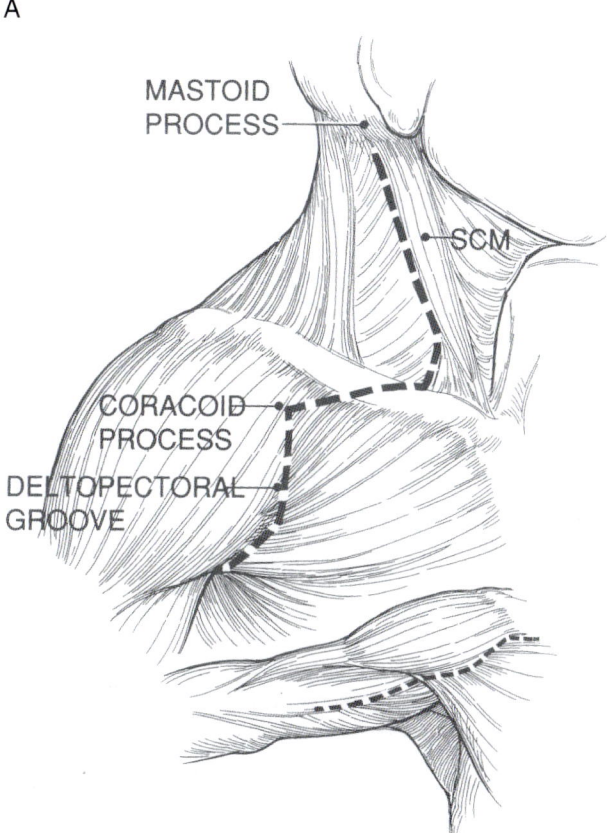

MASTOID PROCESS

SCM

CORACOID PROCESS

DELTOPECTORAL GROOVE

B

Figure 20–5 **A** and **B:** An incision designed to expose the entire brachial plexus is depicted. The superior vertical limb parallels the posterior margin of the sternocleidomastoid. The horizontal limb first parallels and then crosses the clavicle. The lower vertical limb follows the deltopectoral groove and then turns into the axilla by paralleling the anterior axillary crease. The key muscle and bony landmarks are illustrated in **B.**

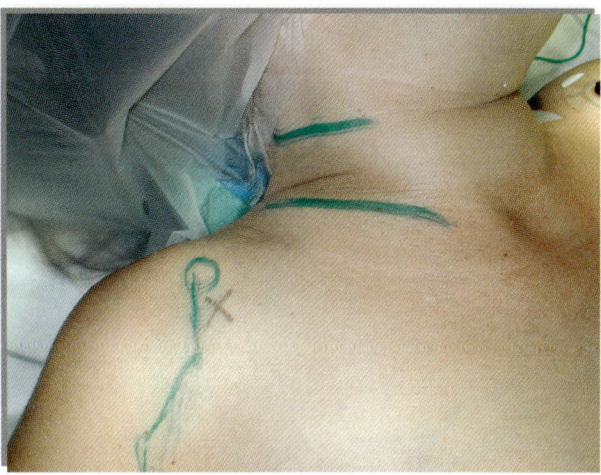

Figure 20–6 A more cosmetically appropriate series of incisions is depicted. In adult injuries, it may be necessary only to make the two inferior incisions to provide adequate exposure. The higher incision may be indicated when the C5 root is difficult to identify or if there is a prefixed plexus.

lower roots and brachial plexus exposure through transverse clavicular skin incision for supraclavicular lesion of the brachial plexus to minimize the operative scar. For infraclavicular lesion, the traditional exposure through the transverse clavicular and deltopectoral approaches are utilized (Fig. 20–6).

Supraclavicular Lesions

The upper cervical roots C5 and C6 are explored through the transverse cervical skin incision, between the posterior tubercle of C5 transverse process and anterior tubercle of C6 transverse process, which can be palpated easily, running along the transverse cervical skin folds (Fig. 20–7). The skin incision is infiltrated with a vasopressor agent to decrease bleeding. Following skin incision, the platysma muscle is incised in the same line, and the cutaneous branches of the cervical plexus are identified and protected, as is the spinal accessory nerve, which lies beneath the sternocleidomastoid muscle at the apex of the wound. The external jugular vein, on the surface of the sternocleidomastoid muscle, is dissected and retracted with a tape. Dissection proceeds along the lateral margin of the sternocleidomastoid muscle, which is retracted medially. Underneath the sternocleidmastoid muscle, the cutaneous branches of the cervical nerves, the supraclavicular nerve, which arises from the C4 cervical root, is traced proximally, and the phrenic nerve, which is easily distinguished by contraction of diaphragm following electric nerve stimulation, is found as it branches from the C4 nerve root and runs distally on the anterior scalenus muscle. The internal jugular vein is protected. Dissection is carried under the anterior scalenus muscle, identifying the palpable posterior tubercle of the C5 transverse process

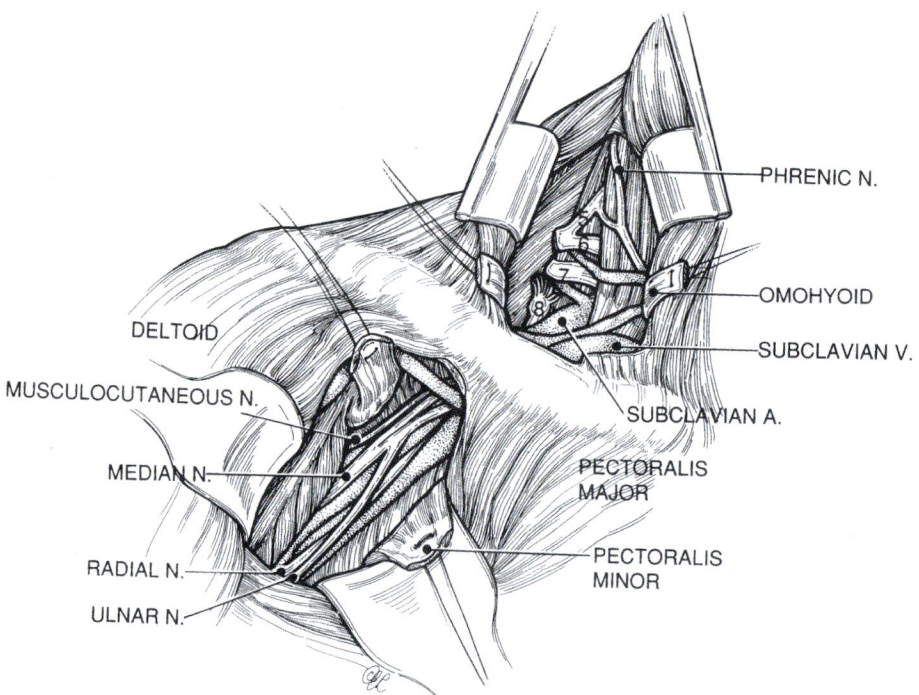

PHRENIC N.

OMOHYOID

SUBCLAVIAN V.

DELTOID

MUSCULOCUTANEOUS N.

SUBCLAVIAN A.

MEDIAN N.

PECTORALIS
MAJOR

RADIAL N.

PECTORALIS
MINOR

ULNAR N.

Figure 20–7 The completely exposed plexus is illustrated. The omohyoid and superficial crossing vessels are divided. The phrenic nerve is a key guide to the C5 root. The transverse scapular artery crosses just under the origin of the C7 root. The subclavian artery is the guide to the C8 and T1 roots. Through an extended dectopectoral incision, the pectoralis minor muscle is divided between suture markers to provide complete visualization of the infraclavicular plexus.

and anterior tubercle of the C6 transverse process, and the proximal stump of each root can be identified if it exists. There are many variable conditions of these nerve roots, from only scarred tissue to normal appearance of nerve root depending on the level of injury. If the nerve root exists in situ, the nerve root is traced distally to find the lesion, and electric stimulation is applied to the proximal side of the lesion. If contraction of the proximal muscles such as rhomboid or serratus anterior muscle occurs, the lesion should be at the postganglionic level and the nerve root is repairable. If more distal muscles such as the supraspinatus or deltoid are contracted by electric stimulation, the lesion is more distal, and is an infraclavicular lesion. If no muscular contraction occurs, the lesion may be preganglionic, or intraforamainal, which is unrepairable.

The lower three cervical roots, C7, C8, and T1, and upper trunk of the brachial plexus, are explored through the transverse supraclavicular skin incision, beginning at the infraclavicular fossa proximally, and running transversely on the clavicle to the supraclavicular distally along with the skin fold, which is usually connected to the deltopectoral incision for exposure of the infraclavicular lesion. The platysma muscle is cut in the same line of skin incision.

For exploration of C7, C8, and T1, and upper trunk, dissection proceeds into the supraclavicular fossa, identifying and retracting the external jugular vein and supraclavicular nerve. The clavicular head of the sternocleidmastoideus muscle is detached from the clavicle. The omohyoid muscle is usually divided and beneath the omohyoid muscle the superficial cervical

(transverse cervical) and suprascapular vessels traverse the brachial plexus perpendicularly. They may be preserved if possible; however, they are usually ligated and cut for better exposure of the brachial plexus. Underneath these vessels, the upper trunk of the brachial plexus (if present) is visualized. The suprascapular nerve, arching posteriorly away from the upper trunk, is preserved. C7 and the middle trunk are found dorsal and caudal to the C5 and C6 roots between the anterior and middle scalene muscles. The caudal roots course in a more horizontal, less oblique direction than the cranial roots. C8 and T1 roots are hidden partially behind the arching third part of the subclavian artery. The exposure of the inferior trunk is facilitated by identifying the medial cord through the infraclavicular approach and following it in a central direction. Without cutting the clavicle, maximal lifting of the clavicle increases the space for access. If further exploration of T1 root is necessary, the clavicle should be predrilled for ultimate plating and then osteotomized and retracted and this will require the additional infraclavicular approach described below. In total paralysis with postganglionic injury of C5 root and preganglionic injuries of other lower roots, or upper type paralysis, supraclavicular exposure without osteotomy of clavicle is enough to examine the lower roots by division of the scalenus anterior muscle (protecting the phrenic nerve), and mobilization and gentle retraction of the subclavian artery inferiorly.

If the upper roots are avulsed, the rootlets and swollen dorsal root ganglion may be found twisted, and lying either behind the clavicle or slightly above it in the region of the C8 root. If the upper roots or superior trunk and/or the middle trunk are ruptured, the distal ends typically lie behind the clavicle. The avulsed (often) or ruptured (infrequently) TI structures are usually found much closer to their respective foramina than is the case with C5 or C6.

Any combination of injuries may occur, including avulsion, rupture, and neuroma-in-continuity. The supraclavicular dissection usually allows the surgeon to determine the type(s) of injuries. However, if the supraclavicular findings favor some type of reconstruction by nerve grafting, the surgeon must complete the infraclavicular exploration, because two-level injuries are common, and an untreated distal injury can diminish the results of the surgical treatment of a proximal injury. For example, rupture of the superior trunk is often seen in combination with avulsion of the axillary nerve from the deltoid, or rupture of the musculocutaneous nerve at the level of the shoulder.

Infraclavicular Lesions

The infraclavicular approach to the brachial plexus is designed to expose the cords and branches. The skin incision is transverse parallel to the clavicle described above, and follows the deltopectoral groove, beginning proximally at the clavicle extending over the coracoid, to the axillary crease distally. The deltopectoral interval is developed, exposing the cephalic vein and thoroacoacromial artery and its concomitant veins, which are isolated and reflected with a vascular tape if free muscle transfer or vascularized nerve graft is planned. The clavicular origin of the pectoralis major muscle is detached and the subclavius is isolated. By lifting the clavicle with a retractor, the infraclavicular brachial plexus is exposed. The lower plexus is explored by detaching the tendinous origin of the pectoralis minor from the coracoid process. The clavipectoral fascia is incised, exposing the lateral cord superficial and lateral to the axillary artery. The posterior cord is slightly lateral and deep to the artery and the medial cord medial and deep to the axillary artery. Care should be taken to preserve the medial and lateral pectoral nerves that arise at this level. If there is extensive scarring, exploration should begin as far distally as necessary to locate normal tissue before proceeding proximally. Distally, the lateral cord can be identified by following the median nerve proximally. At this point, the musculocutaneous nerve can be seen branching laterally and piercing the coracobrachialis muscle. The medial root of the median nerve is followed to the medial cord, which is then followed distally to the ulnar, medial brachial cutaneous, and medial antebrachial cutaneous nerves. Medial and deep to the axillary artery and vein, coursing laterally, is the radial nerve. It is followed proximally to the posterior cord and axillary nerve, which is seen branching from the posterior cord.

Different anatomic structures can be marked using different colors of vessel loops. We have found it useful to bring a sterilized drawing of the normal plexus, and to make a sketch of the operative findings on this. We use this map to plan priorities in reconstruction, and to describe what reconstruction was performed. It is a mistake to depend on memory to dictate the operative notes.

Intraoperative Evoked Potentials

After we have visualized the plexus, we perform intraoperative corticosensory or spinal evoked potentials on the nerve roots to determine if they are in-continuity with the spinal cord. The root is placed on electrodes and 64, 128, or 256 stimulations are performed and averaged (Fig. 20–8). We rely on this examination to differentiate between an avulsion from the spinal cord and a rupture. Following an intraforaminal avulsion, the root may still be present in its sleeve, or, more commonly, the root sleeve is empty. Intraoperative somatosensory evoked potential recording (SSEP) enables the integrity of the intraforaminal part of the sensory tract to be evaluated. However, not even indirect information can be obtained as to the condition of the anterior motor root. This limitation is important, considering that there are dissociated intraforaminal lesions of both the motor and the sensory roots. Somatosensory evoked potential is easily affected by depth of anesthesia, and technical failures cannot be neglected.

Practical Tips: Intraoperative Decisions and Priorities of Repair

We have followed the recommendations of Narakas[8] and others in developing a sequence of reconstruction based on functional priorities and the ability to achieve the function by neural repair/reconstruction. The microneural reconstruction performed depends on the intraoperative assessment of the damage and the following list of priorities. These priorities have been chosen for three reasons: first is functional significance; second is the likelihood of regaining the function by nerve reconstruction (proximal muscles are reinnervated more successfully than distal muscles); and third is the degree of difficulty in achieving the function by secondary surgery. For example, in the adult there are few reliable muscle tendon transfers to restore horizontal abduction of the shoulder.

For the patient with a total brachial plexus palsy, the priorities of repair include:

1. Elbow flexion by biceps/brachialis muscle reinnervation
2. Shoulder stabilization, abduction, and external rotation by suprascapular nerve reinnervation

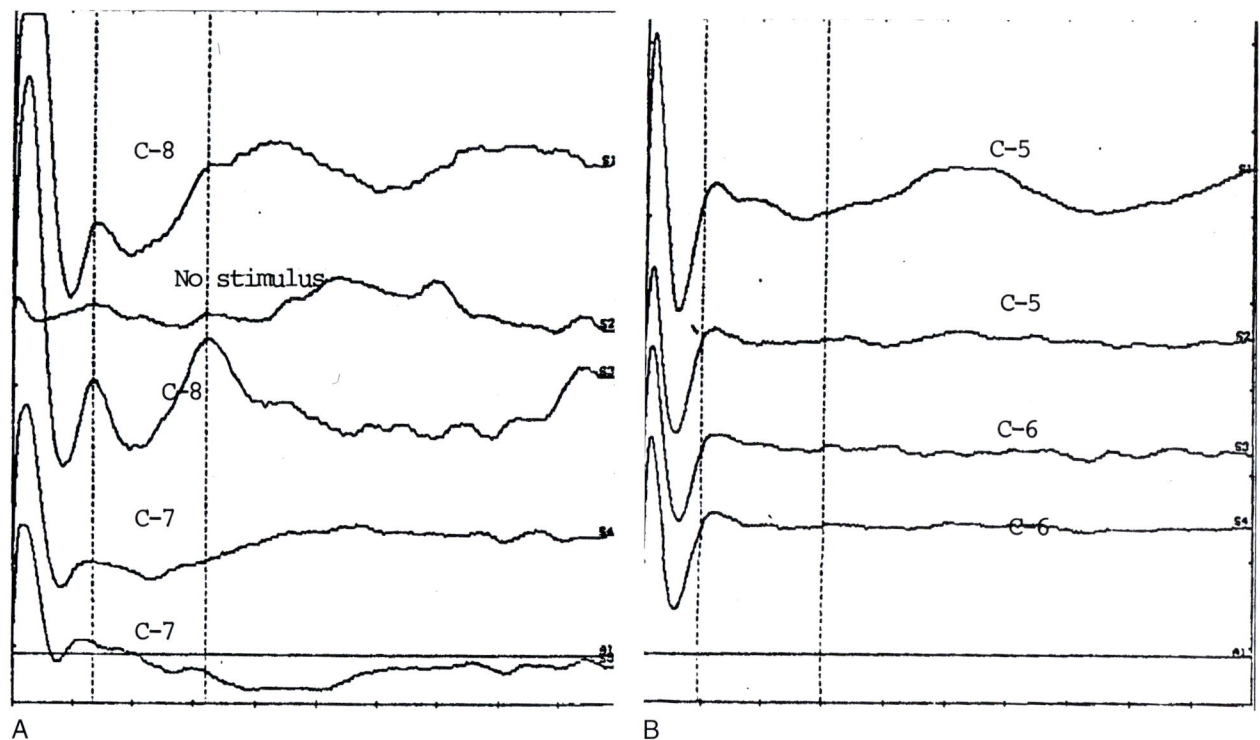

Figure 20–8   A, B: Intraoperative evoked potentials help identify roots still in continuity with the spinal cord (sensory elements). In **A,** stimulation of the C8 root elicits a sizable cortical response, indicating continuity of the root with the spinal cord. Two series of stimulations of the C7 root yielded no cortical response, indicating that the root was avulsed.

3. Brachiothoracic pinch (adduction of the arm against the chest) by reinnervation of the pectoralis major muscle
4. Sensation below the elbow in the C6–C7 area by reinnervation of the lateral cord
5. Wrist extension and finger flexion by reinnervation of the lateral and posterior cord

For the patient with an injury limited to the upper roots (C5, C6), regaining elbow flexion and shoulder stability (numbers 1 and 2 above) are priorities. In addition, we will attempt to help the patient recover wrist extension (number 5). The decisions regarding the rare patient with an injury limited to the lower elements of the plexus have already been discussed.

NEUROLYSIS, REPAIR, AND RECONSTRUCTION

Indications

Exploration of the brachial plexus and supplemental examination such as imaging, electrodiagnosis, and biochemical assay provide the exact level of injury. In a postganglionic injury involving a lesion of the lower cervical roots one should consider whether to primarily repair with nerve grafting or proceed to immediate reconstruction such as a Steindler procedure,[9] shoulder

arthrodesis, or muscle transfer. This decision is influenced by the age of the patients and time interval between injury and operation. In young patients, less than 3 or 4 months after injury, operative exploration of the brachial plexus and nerve grafting is indicated. In patients older than 40 years, and in whom the chance of nerve regeneration are poor, or longer than 6 months after injury even if young, an immediate reconstruction procedure is the better choice.

Operative Procedure

Exploration of the brachial plexus is as described above and each lesion should be meticulously examined concerning the level of lesion (preganglionic or postganglionic), degree of the lesion (Sunderland's classification; degree 1~5 and mixed lesion[5]), and continuity of lesion by macroscopic findings and supplemental electrophysiology with nerve action potentials and compound motor action potentials.

When discontinuity of the nerve is found, the decision is to proceed with nerve repair, although the proximal stump should be examined by the electrophysiological testing, biochemical assay, and imaging described above in order to rule out a more proximal or intraforaminal lesion. Lesions in continuity are treated by initial microsurgical neurolysis. First, the nerve is liberated from adhesions to neighboring tissue at the level of the epineurium (external neurolysis). Next, electrical stimulation is applied to the proximal side of the lesion, and when no contraction from muscle distal to the lesion occurs or no compound motor action potential can be measured, the lesion is one of discontinuity of the nerve fibers and excision of the neuroma is indicated. When contraction or compound motor action potentials are found from the muscles distal to the lesion, internal neurolysis is indicated under the microscope. Longitudinal incisions are made in the fibrotic layers of the epineurium and epifascicular epineurium and all fascicles are completely separated, removing the surrounding scar tissue. If any fascicles are found to be divided or scarred, they are cut and repaired with interfascicular nerve grafting. There are many occasions when it is difficult to decide whether neurolysis alone or further neurotomy and nerve repair should be selected, especially in the presence of positive contraction of the distal muscles by electric nerve stimulation, because continuity of a few fascicles is not enough to achieve useful function, yet will provide muscle contraction. In such situations, the preoperative clinical condition should be considered and when electromyographic recovery was poor longer than 3 or 4 months after injury, neurotomy and nerve repair are recommended depending on the condition of scar tissue.

Priority of Nerve Repair

In the presence of a partial nerve injury in the distal brachial plexus, division, cord, and branches, and when it is a short defect, we prefer to reestablish continuity to all injured parts, using every available donor nerve. For longer defects in the distal plexus and proximal nerve injury at the level of the root and trunk, this approach becomes impossible because there is not enough autologous donor nerve tissue available to restore continuity to all parts of the brachial plexus and the priorities of repair nerve should be considered.

The shorter the length between the site of nerve suture and the neuromotor unit of the target muscle, the better the final outcome. Therefore, the more proximal muscles should be selected as the target muscle for nerve repair. Traditionally, most previous surgeons selected the musculocutaneous nerve as the first priority, and then suprascapular nerve and axillary nerve for shoulder reconstruction. The musculocutaneous nerve can be successfully reconstructed by intercostal nerve transfer or by partial ulnar nerve transfer; however, the suprascapular nerve can be repaired only by spinal accessory nerve transfer, which is also an important innervator of the trapezius muscle and a donor nerve for musculocutaneous neurotization or free muscle transfer. We prefer to select the suprascapular nerve as the first choice of repair, and the second is the musculocutaneous.

The axillary nerve can be ignored in most severe plexus injuries, since simple axillary nerve palsy does not result in serious paralysis of shoulder function.

The serratus anterior muscle also has a very important function and, if possible, the long thoracic nerve is neurotized. The triceps brachii muscle is also a unique and useful muscle for antagonist of elbow flexion in reconstruction of distal function and is a potential donor muscle for secondary transfer to the biceps. The radial nerve, especially the branches to the triceps brachii muscle, is the next priority. Attempt to recover the forearm musculature is of lower priority because the chance of their recovery is minimal and useless for voluntary finger function and provides at best only academic satisfaction, except the median nerve for digital sensibility.

Donor Nerves

Conventional fascicular nerve graft (nonvascularized) is commonly used to repair the nerve defect of the brachial plexus; however, a vascularized nerve graft is indicated when the segment to be grafted is excessively long (15 to 20 cm; excessive length encourages fibroplasia to exceed and overcome the rate of axonal regeneration), and when the diameter of the graft is large.

When coapting both nerve stumps with sural nerve grafting, different fascicular patterns are matched individually to lead the generating axons to the proper motor fascicles of the distal nerve. Epiperineurial suture between the proximal nerve and each nerve graft and epineurial suture between the distal nerve and each nerve graft are commonly used under microscope magnification of using with 8-0 to 10-0 nylon sutures. Tissue adhesive can simplify the approximation of multiple strands of nerve graft proximally to a single large root stump or distally to a trunk or cord (Fig. 20–9).

CONTROVERSIES

The functional results of brachial plexus repair in adults continue to be somewhat disappointing. This has been attributed to two potential causes. First is the diffusion of motor and sensory axons when nerve grafts are used to connect mixed (sensory and motor) proximal to mixed distal targets. Insufficient numbers of appropriate axons reach key muscles, or axons innervate incorrect muscles. The second potential cause is that the time required for regeneration of axons over long distances exceeds the time consistent with successful functional muscle recovery.

This has led to an evolution of the concept of nerve transfer from one that is an adjunct to conventional nerve repair, toward one that substitutes for repair. Those who advocate this shift in emphasis argue that, in selected patients, nerve transfers should be used preferentially because the technique allows better targeting of motor to motor axons, thus reducing the diffusion of

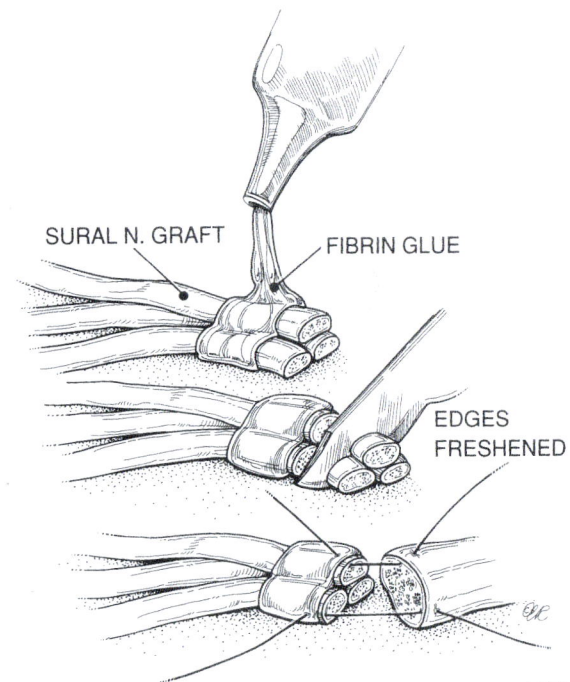

SURAL N. GRAFT   **FIBRIN GLUE**

EDGES FRESHENED

Figure 20–9 Nerve grafts may be sutures into place or fixed into position with tissue adhesives such as fibrin glue, or a combination of techniques used.

axons toward inappropriate targets, and the nerve junctures can be frequently performed much closer to the muscle to be reinnervated, thus reducing the time the muscle remains paralyzed. Operative times are significantly reduced. For example, in circumstances where there exists good evidence of C5–C6 avulsion, those advocating nerve transfer would recommend the following:

- Transfer of the SAN (spinal accessory nerve) to the suprascapular nerve via a limited supraclavicular approach
- Transfer of the radial nerve innervation to the long head of the triceps to the axillary nerve
- Transfer of a motor fascicle of the ulnar nerve to the musculocutaneous nerve (MCN) branch to biceps, referred to as the Oberlin procedure[10]

Additional transfers reported include:

- Either the C5 or the C6 contribution to the long thoracic nerve to suprascapular nerve
- Transfer of the thoracodorsal nerve to an appropriate target
- Transfer of a motor element of the median nerve in the upper arm to MCN branches
- Thorascopic harvest of the phrenic nerve to innervate motor elements of the median nerve in the distal part of the upper arm

Some would argue that these procedures, where technically feasible, should supplant the conventional direct

repair approach that has guided treatment for the past 40 years. While there are significant numbers of cases of the Oberlin[10] procedure now studied, this is not yet the case for most of the other nerve transfer procedures more recently introduced.

SALVAGE PROCEDURES

Free Muscle Transfer

Free muscle transfer is a feasible procedure in reconstruction of brachial plexus injury, not only for secondary salvage in delayed or failed cases, but prehensile reconstruction in recent cases.[11,12] Many have been described but the most commonly performed include:

- Free muscle transfer for elbow flexion in delayed cases
- Double free muscle transfer for prehensile function in cases with complete avulsions
- Multiple muscle transfer for reconstruction of glenohumeral function

Shoulder Arthrodesis

Shoulder arthrodesis is a well-established operative procedure that involves fusion of the humeral head to the glenoid.[13] The indications include total brachial plexus paralysis and upper type paralysis.

Obstetrical Palsy

Indications and Timing

The approach to the infant who has suffered a traction injury of the brachial plexus differs somewhat from the adult though the mechanism of injury is very similar, i.e., excessive direct traction on the brachial plexus associated typically with a difficult delivery or perhaps by compression of the plexus by the first rib (Fig. 20–10). Since the first reported attempts at repair in 1903,[1] the role of surgical reconstruction has been far more controversial than for the adult cases and remains so to this day. Renewed interest in operating on infants has been stimulated primarily by a better appreciation of the natural history of spontaneous evolution following injury provided by longitudinal studies[14] which determined that:

Complete recovery seems possible only if the biceps and deltoid demonstrate some level of function by the 2nd month.

The results, although still good, are nevertheless incomplete, if initial contracting of these two muscles requires 3 to 3.5 months.

If the biceps is not contracting strongly by 5 months, the results will be highly unsatisfactory.

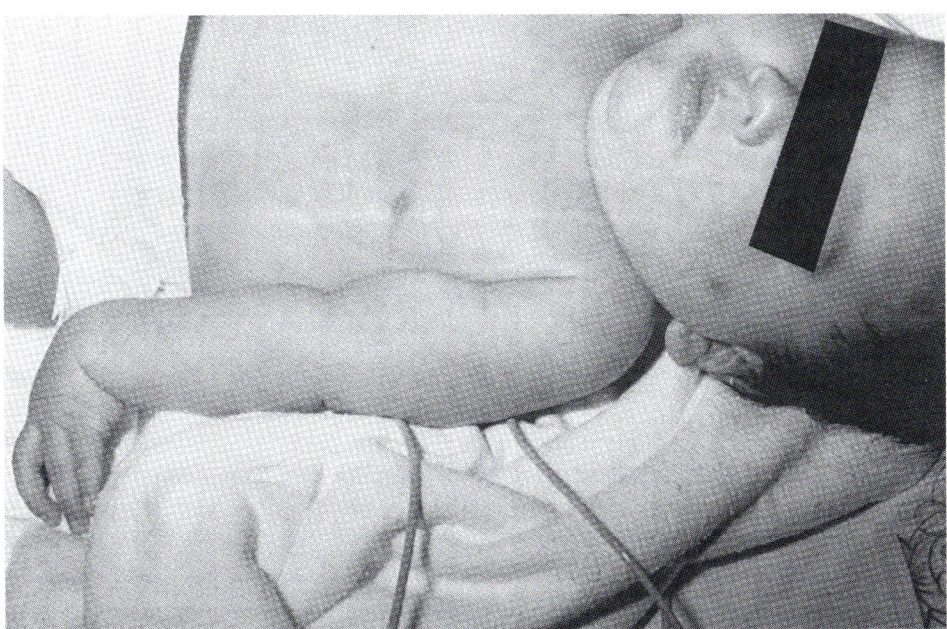

Figure 20–10 The typical appearance of a baby with an upper plexus (Erb's) palsy. The arm is adducted by the side and the elbow is held extended, the forearm is pronated and the wrist is held in flexion (waiter's tip position).

Gilbert[15] recommended using the rate of biceps recovery as a means of determining which baby should have early plexus exploration (3 to 4 months of age). More recently published and presented longitudinal studies have questioned whether the rate of recovery of the biceps is sufficiently predictive. Michelow et al.[16] found that biceps recovery incorrectly predicted recovery in 13% of patients. Clark and Curtis[17] recommend combining scores for elbow flexion with scores for wrist, finger, and thumb extension. These were predictive in almost 95% of 61 patients allowed to evolve without nerve surgery.

Preoperative Evaluation

The posture of the newborn is frequently diagnostic with either a flail limb indicating complete palsy or an internally rotated, adducted limb with the forearm pronated and the wrist flexed indicating an upper root problem (Fig. 20–10). Gilbert et al.[18] use a simple muscle testing scheme for these infants, where M0 is no contraction, M1 represents contraction without movement, M2 slight movement, and M3 complete movement. Clark and Curtis[17] recommend a somewhat more complicated analysis using seven grades for each movement. With gravity eliminated, the grades are 0=no contraction, 1=contraction, no motion; 2, motion range, 3=motion > range, and 4=full motion. Against gravity, the grades are 5=motion range, 6=motion range, and 7=full motion.

The sensory exam is even less precise; the examiner tests the reaction to pinching the skin only. Other signs to be observed include evidence of trophic changes such as differences in hair growth or color, and the presence of a Horner's sign. Electromyographies (EMGs) are not obtained until later.

The infant is reexamined at 1 month of age. Recovery may already be evident, and if present will probably ultimately be complete. For the remaining babies, several presentations are evident:

If the palsy is still total and is associated with a Horner's sign, the outlook for spontaneous recovery is poor and early surgery is indicated.

If the hand is recovering but no biceps or shoulder recovery is evident, there is still a chance for spontaneous recovery. A third evaluation prior to 3 months of age will be necessary to determine indications for surgery.

At 3 months of age, the child is retested. If any biceps function is evident, surgery is not recommended. For those without biceps function, an EMG is scheduled, although the results of EMG have been difficult to correlate with final outcome. However, total absence of electrical evidence of reinnervation at this time indicates avulsion of the corresponding roots. Cervical myelography was previously recommended. Today less invasive magnetic resonance imaging, when skillfully performed can give almost equivalent sensitivity and reliability.

Gilbert[19] today firmly adheres to his previously published guidelines regarding early surgery depending on biceps recovery. Others wait until 6 months or later to make a decision. No firm consensus exists at present.

Operative Technique

Once neural surgical exploration and reconstruction have been recommended and accepted (about 10% of parents decline surgery even when strongly recommended), the baby is evaluated by the pediatric anesthesiology staff, primarily to alert them that we will be performing intraoperative evoked potentials and to allow them to plan their anesthetic regimen accordingly. Until recently, a themoplastic head–chest splint was constructed in advance of surgery. We have abandoned its use in the last 2 years and have seen no difference in early outcome.

If the infant is cooperative, scalp electrodes for somatosensory evoked potentials (SSEP) studies are attached in the preoperative preparation area; otherwise, they are attached once anesthesia is induced. A stimulating electrode is placed on the volar wrist of both the affected and unaffected side, and a recording electrode is placed at Erb's point in the supraclavicular fossa. A spinal electrode is placed just below the occiput. After anesthetic induction, the initial electrophysiologic studies are performed, with stimulation of both the involved and uninvolved sides. Stimulating the normal side allows us to determine whether the equipment is functioning properly, and gives some idea regarding the effects of the anesthetic agents on signal properties. Even the normal nerves of the infant are incompletely myelinated, and therefore conduction velocities and signal amplitudes are reduced. Once these initial electrophysiologic studies are performed, the wrist and Erb's point electrodes are removed. Occasionally, stimulating at the wrist on the affected side will result in some intrinsic muscle contractions that were not noted on the preoperative physical exam.

The baby's head is placed in a gel-head rest, making certain that the occiput does not "bottom out." We have had two incidences of significant alopecia when we failed to follow this regimen conscientiously. Anesthetic levels can be adjusted so that there is sufficient depth of anesthesia to perform the initial exploration and then adjusted to as light a plane as possible for the second set of SSEP studies. The head is turned away from the operative side. Most of these infants, especially the chubby ones, have little or no neck to speak of and it is difficult to discern what are true skin creases versus folds of fatty skin. The proposed transverse supraclavicular incision is marked, and then injected with 0.5% bupivicaine with epinephrine 1:200,000 units per mL. The neck, shoulder, and entire arm and both legs are prepped. For infants, we no longer use thigh tourniquets to harvest sural nerve grafts. With the infant supine and the leg fully elevated, as is necessary to harvest grafts, bleeding is minimal. Skin staples assist in maintaining drapes in place.

The supraclavicular fossa is explored through a transverse incision made just above the clavicle (Fig. 20–6). We switched from the more deforming longitudinal incision recommended in earlier communications (as have most others) without noticeable loss of visualization. If the epinephrine has had time to be effective, this incision is bloodless. The platysma is essentially nonexistent at this age. The external jugular vein, if encountered, can be mobilized laterally and never needs dividing. The supraclavicular sensory nerves are encountered lying on the superficial layer of the deep cervical fascia and, in general, can be stretched out of the way. The lateral border of the sternocleidomastoid (SCM) muscle is visualized and dissected. Scalpel dissection is preferred to this point. Spreading and cutting with scissors distorts the elegant virginal tissue planes. A small vein or two will be encountered as the dissection along the lateral border of the SCM proceeds proximally. These identify the origins of the supraclavicular sensory branches of the cervical sensory plexus, and serve to warn the surgeon to move more cautiously at this point.

The SCM is retracted slightly medially, and the submuscular layer of the superficial fascia is opened in a vertical direction (Fig. 20–7). This will expose the omohyoid muscle, crossing the surgical field transversely, the lymphatic-rich fatty layers that lie between the superficial and deep cervical fascia, and the transverse cervical artery and accompanying vein. These vessels are ligated using vascular clips. The omohyoid muscle is typically divided between two marking sutures placed into the muscle. The muscle and the fatty-lymphatic pad will be approximated at the time of closure. Clamps on either end of these two marking sutures help with retraction. An appropriately sized self-retaining retractor is placed transversely. A second retractor can then be placed at right angles to the first. The lymphatic tissues are grasped between a forceps and a bipolar stimulating forceps and, with cautery, this layer is pulled apart. The temptation to simply retract this layer from medial to lateral should be avoided, as one will pull a never-ending amount of fatty-lymphatic tissues out of the mediastinum. The underlying scalene muscle, the phrenic nerve and plexus, or neuroma-in-continuity remain protected by the injury thickened deep layer of the deep cervical fascia. At this point, a key landmark—the phrenic nerve—is identified. Close to the clavicle, this nerve is much farther medial than one expects. Therefore, it is important to begin this search higher in the neck. The phrenic nerve is the surgeon's guide to the C5 root. Once identified, it is stimulated with a portable nerve stimulator to confirm that it is functioning. If this nerve is nonfunctional at this early phase of exploration, or if stimulation results in minimal contraction of the diaphragm, the C5 root is almost surely avulsed, and quite likely the C4 root is also avulsed. We

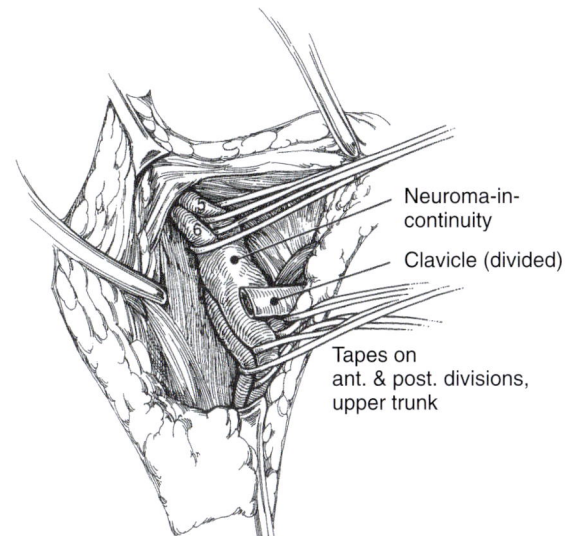

Neuroma-in-
continuity

Clavicle (divided)

Tapes on
ant. & post. divisions,
upper trunk

Figure 20–11 A typical intraoperative finding in an infant with a global palsy is illustrated. A large neuroma-in-continuity is located at the confluence of the C5 and C6 roots. The C7 root and its continuation as the middle trunk are fixed to this neuroma. The clavicle is pictured divided. It is unusual to need to divide the clavicle in obstetrical palsy operations.

have seen this only in babies with global palsies, and in babies who suffer upper root injuries associated with breech or cesarean deliveries.

The phrenic nerve is followed superiorly and carefully protected if functioning. Permanent surgical injury to the phrenic nerve has led, although thankfully rarely, to significant postoperative respiratory complications. If present, the C5 root will be encountered passing obliquely over the middle scalene muscle. More typically, just lateral to the phrenic nerve will lie a large neuroma-in-continuity at the confluence of the C5 and C6 roots and the superior trunk (Fig. 20–11). If one begins at the more normal superior part of the C5 root, the root can be more easily dissected into the neuroma-in-continuity.

The C6 root lies deeper in the neck in relation to the C5 root and its proximodistal course is less transverse than the C5 root (which has a more exaggerated sigmoid course than the C6 root). The C6 root, if present is invariably larger than the C5 root. At this point, we dissect carefully the phrenic nerve–C5 root relationship, searching for evidence of a large element coming from C4 (typically as part of the phrenic nerve), and then joining the C5 root. This is termed a pre-fixed plexus. The typical findings are a branch of some size exiting the phrenic nerve and joining the C5 root and then, almost immediately, a smaller branch exiting the C5 root to rejoin the continuing course of the phrenic nerve.

If a large neuroma-in-continuity is present, it can be rapidly dissected along its medial border in a proximal to distal direction. Dissection along its lateral margin should proceed with some care so that too deep a dis-

section does not risk injury to the C6 contribution, if existing, to the long thoracic nerve of Bell. As the clavicle is approached, the neuroma-in continuity will give off the suprascapular nerve, another key landmark. This is dissected distally and surrounded with a rubber vascular loop. The traction of the birth injury will have displaced this nerve more distally and laterally than normal. Finding this branch allows rapid dissection of the anterior and posterior divisions of the superior trunk. These are also surrounded with a vascular loop. If a neuroma-in-continuity is present, this part of the dissection can be performed rapidly and safely. If the C5 and or C6 roots are avulsed or completely ruptured and retracted proximally, dissection can be tedious, and missteps, such as confusing a band of scalene muscle for a nerve root, frequent.

The C7 root can be identified using several landmarks. It lies even deeper in the neck, and its course is even less transverse than the C6 root. If the transverse scapular artery, a branch of which accompanies the suprascapular nerve can be identified, it can be followed medially. It will cross immediately under or occasionally over the C7 root as it becomes the middle trunk. The neuroma-in-continuity, if present, can be elevated and retracted laterally to expose the interval between anterior and middle scalene muscles. The C7 root lies deep in this interval. The foramen of exit of the C7 root lies much more superiorly than anticipated. The C7 root, in my experience, is better hidden in these injuries than the C6 or C8 roots. If present, this root is circled with a rubber loop and dissected proximally and distally. The C7 root and middle trunk will often be confluent with the large neuroma-in-continuity, and separating middle from superior trunk will be difficult as there is no longer an anatomic plane. These two elements become one because axonal sprouting will have occurred from one into the other. For example, we have systematically noted that babies who, at the time of surgical intervention, have begun to show flickering of their biceps, will demonstrate this same flicker of activity after surgery, even when the C5 and C6 root neuroma, or superior trunk neuroma, are resected, and C5 and C6 reconnected to distal targets via nerve grafts. In these infants, pre-neuroma resection, stimulation of the C7 root, when present, or even the C8 root, will result in a contraction of the biceps that is much more forceful than can be appreciated on the preoperative clinical exam. These findings convince us that the reason why the majority of babies, even unoperated babies with severe upper trunk injuries, achieve biceps reinnervation is because of collateral (side-to-end) sprouting from adjacent healthier roots.

The subclavian artery is a useful guide to the C8 root and the inferior trunk. The C8 root lies posterior to the curve of the subclavian artery. Even if injured, the C8 root is rarely bound to the artery by scar and if present, is typically more easily identified than the C7 root and middle trunk. The T1 root is not always easily dissected. Frequently, it emerges from so deep within the interval between anterior and middle scalene muscles that what appears to be the C8 root is actually the inferior trunk. If the baby has a global palsy, and particularly if there is a Horner's sign present, it is senseless, in our opinion, to dig deep into this interval because the T1 root, in these cases, is typically avulsed. We have never grafted onto a ruptured T1 root stump, having no faith that any motor regeneration will result. We have seen babies in whom a Horner's sign is present, and who, at exploration have a perfectly normal appearing C8 and T1 root. However, stimulation of the inferior trunk results neither in motor movement nor SSEPs. We have judged these roots to be avulsed at the intraforaminal level. All of this dissection can take place through the supraclavicular incision.

SURGICAL DECISION MAKING

Once the pathoanatomy has been identified, systematic electrical stimulation of each root, or trunk is performed (Fig. 20–4). We try to alert the anesthesiologist as this time is approaching so that anesthetic agents or levels can be adjusted. The contralateral side is again stimulated to determine that spinal and cortical signals are obtainable. We compare these with those signals obtained prior to any deeper planes of anesthesia that might have been necessary to allow dissection of the plexus. If there is a large difference, the anesthesiologist is asked to reduce the level of anesthesia to the minimum necessary to avoid extraneous muscle-generated noise. As a practical matter, electrically noisy operating room equipment unnecessary for the moment is unplugged. In our experience, the most significant source of electrical "noise" is the warm-air "Baer-hugger" warmer.

Depending on findings, both nerve-to-nerve and nerve-to-brain (or spinal cord) studies are performed. We begin by stimulating the most superior root identifiable, almost always the C5 root. If we see a large motor response in appropriate muscles, and a good cortical signal, we will then stimulate the C5 root and record in turn from the suprascapular nerve (SSN), the anterior division of the superior trunk (ADST), and the posterior division of the superior trunk (PDST). Each root is stimulated using signal averaging techniques, and this is repeated to confirm that the response is reproducible and real (not artifact). We judge the response on a 0 to 3 scale, with 0 being no discernible (above noise level) response, 1 being an easily seen and reproducible response, 2 being a response equal to at least 50% of the contralateral side, and 3, a response equal or nearly equal to the opposite side.

If we see motor movement, and a clear signal that does not require any signal averaging, we will strongly consider simple neurolysis of the involved area of root, trunk, division, or cord. This is a more common circumstance in older babies, and rarely occurs in babies who have global palsies and who meet our operative indications. Once all recordings are accomplished, decisions regarding how to manage each level of injury can be made and reconstruction can proceed.

RECONSTRUCTIVE GOALS

For babies with lesions restricted to the upper roots, reconstructive goals are similar to adults with traumatic brachial plexus injuries. We focus on restoring function to shoulder movers, particularly abduction and external rotation, elbow flexion, and wrist extension. These babies have several typical pathoanatomic patterns. The most common, as mentioned above, is a large neuroma at the confluence of the C5 and C6 roots as they form the superior trunk. Exiting the neuroma will be the suprascapular nerve (SSN) and the anterior and posterior divisions of the superior trunk (ADST, PDST). Usually, the C7 root or the middle trunk will be adherent to this neuroma. If both the C5 and C6 roots are identifiable, we use the SSEP studies as a guide to determining which is likely to be the healthier root. If the studies indicate poor regeneration across the neuroma-in-continuity, the neuroma is excised proximally in a stepwise fashion using the operating microscope to study the cut face of the root for characteristics of a healthy root. If both roots have a favorable appearance and good response on SSEP studies, both will be used to reinnervate the distal elements. The suprascapular nerve and anterior and posterior divisions are dissected superiorly into the neuroma as far as they remain recognizable. These elements are sectioned at this level and their cut facies are examined under the operating microscope. Additional distal sectioning is performed as necessary.

In babies with global palsies, the goals of neural reconstruction differ from those recommended for adults with traumatic brachial plexus injuries. For these babies, restoring hand function is of paramount importance. The next priority is restoring elbow flexion, followed by shoulder stabilization and shoulder adduction. Some ingenuity is required to address the variety of injury presentations.

It is rarely possible to perform direct nerve coaptation, and, as in the adult, nerve grafts are almost universally necessary and nerve transfers frequently necessary. We preferentially harvest one or both sural nerves, and no longer use thigh tourniquets in our babies. The assistant fully flexes the leg at the hip, and so elevated, there is very little bleeding. A stocking-seam

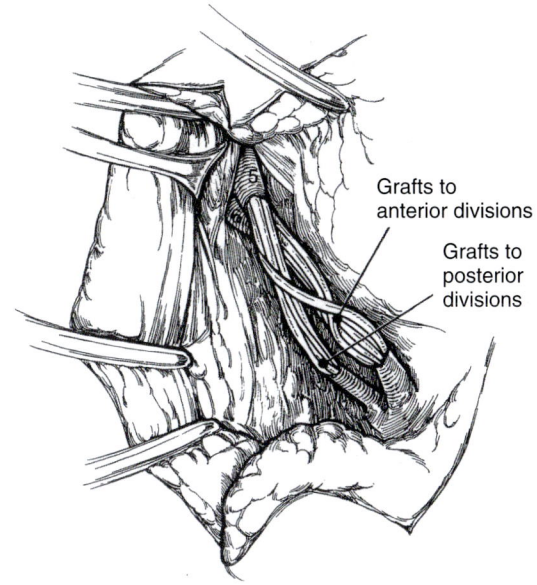

Figure 20–12 A typical reconstruction by multiple nerve grafts to the anterior and posterior divisions of the superior trunk, and the suprascapular nerve.

Grafts to anterior divisions

Grafts to posterior divisions

incision is used, extending from lateral malleolus to the flexion crease at the popliteal fossa. A careful dissection is needed in order to identify the anatomy of the sural nerve and its contributions from the popliteal (or sciatic) nerve and a frequently large contribution from the peroneal nerve. If additional graft is needed, we harvest the medial brachial and antebrachial cutaneous nerves through an incision extending from axilla to mid-humeral level. Leg incisions are closed in layers with absorbable sutures and dressings supported by elastic wraps.

The placement of nerve grafts is determined by the anatomic findings (Fig. 20–12). For reinnervation of the elements of the superior trunk (suprascapular, anterior and posterior divisions) we respect the anterior–posterior aspects of the C5 and C6 root (if both are available), placing grafts bound for the SSN and PDST on the posterior aspect of the root and grafts destined for the ADST on the anterior aspects. The typical sequence is first to determine how many grafts can be placed on each available root, and how many grafts can be accepted on each target. A map is sketched, to assist with operative dictation, and distances from root to target measured. Nerve grafts are cleared of unnecessary connective tissue and are sectioned into appropriate lengths. The posterior grafts are set into place on the appropriate root and their distal ends segregated in an accessible site for later distal placement. The anteriorly designated grafts are layered on top of the previously placed grafts and their distal ends segregated from the posteriorly directed grafts. Fibrin glue is used to fix the grafts to the proximal root stumps (Fig. 20–9). Occasionally, the graft is constructed on the back table and a few sutures are used

to approximate the construct to the proper target. We now rarely suture grafts in place unless exposure of the target root is so poor that gluing is not feasible. Once the fibrin glue has solidified, any excess is sharply trimmed and the root–graft junctures inspected. The distal ends of the grafts are then distributed according to the plan of reconstruction. Typically, the posterior division is reconstructed first, then the anterior division, and finally the SSN.

For babies with global palsies, nerve grafts are placed according to findings and reconstructive goals. Several common scenarios have been encountered, including avulsions of C8 and presumably T1, based on clinical presentation and intraoperative SSEP determinations and ruptures of C5, C6, and C7. In such a case, if the C7 root has a healthy appearance and reasonable SSEP signals, and stimulation of the C8 root results in no SSEPs, we will divide the C8 root as high as possible into its foramen, and then can suture this directly onto the C7 root stump. If the C7 root is also avulsed, we try to connect the anterior aspect of the healthiest root to reinnervate the C8 root or lower trunk. The more severe the injury, the more likely we are to use nerve transfers, particularly the distal branches of the spinal accessory nerve leading to the SSN and, rarely, the phrenic nerve to the anterior division of the superior trunk. We have not used the contralateral C7 root as a source of axons in our babies. On only three occasions have we transferred motor fascicles of the ulnar nerve to directly innervate nerve branches to the biceps to reinnervate the biceps. All were breech-born babies and, at exploration, were found to have relatively uninjured appearing C5 and C6 roots, but totally unstimulatable and lacking any SSEP signals. We judged these root to have suffered intraforaminal avulsions.

Special Circumstances

We have rarely had to divide the clavicle in babies. We have never had to divide the clavicle in babies with isolated upper root injuries, and have had to do so in less than 20% of babies with global palsies. If necessary, an additional infraclavicular incision is made, beginning just below the outer third of the clavicle and curving into the deltopectoral groove. The lateral origin of the pectoralis major muscle is elevated off the clavicle, and a small area of clavicle is cleared and two reciprocal periosteal flaps elevated. A bone cutter will usually suffice to section the clavicle. The sharp point of a self-retaining (Gelpi-type) retractor can be placed into the end of each side of the divided clavicle and opened progressively. The subclavius muscle can be divided to expose the sub- and infra-clavicular portions of the plexus. Once reconstruction is completed, a heavy absorbable suture is used to approximate the clavicular elements.

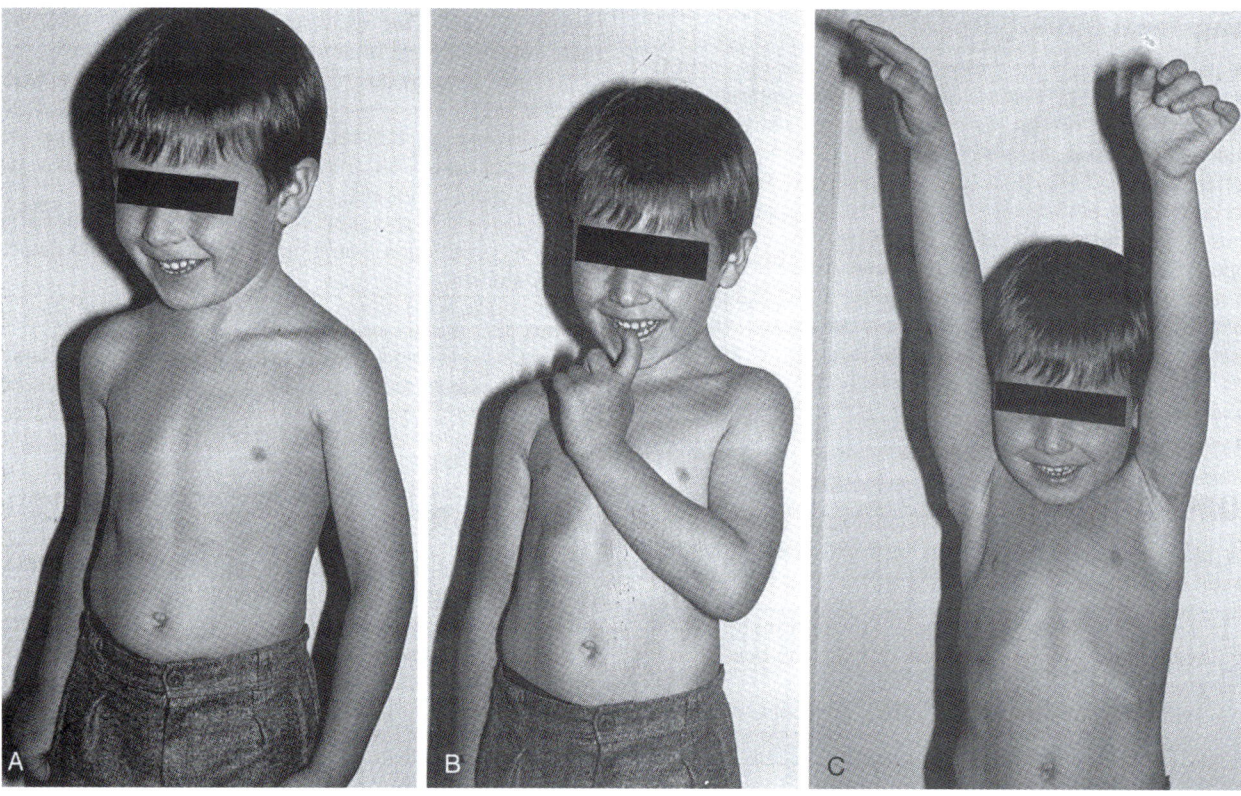

Figure 20–13   An excellent recovery of function in a child with ruptures of C5 and C6, and elongation of C7 treated with multiple nerve grafts as depicted in Fig. 20–12.

Following wound closure with absorbable sutures and skin tape, a soft cotton "T-shirt" is applied and the affected arm is adducted and wrapped against the chest with an elastic bandage. We no longer use a prefabricated head immobilizer. We have learned the value of modifying the infant's car seat from our colleague, Dr. Jose Borrero. Babies usually stay overnight and are discharged the next day. No babies have required transfusion. The average operative time, including SSEP studies is about 4 hours (Fig. 20–13).

COMPLICATIONS

This intervention has been associated with few complications. We have never had to transfuse a baby undergoing this procedure. We have experienced no postoperative infections. We have not lost pre-existing function except, for several months, the small amount of shoulder and elbow movement present in some older babies. These minimal pre-existing movements, the consequence of neural regeneration deemed inadequate according to time since birth, will be lost in babies with global palsies since all available nerve roots are used to reinnervate the plexus.

The phrenic nerve must be carefully protected if functioning. Permanent surgical injury to the phrenic

nerve has led, although thankfully rarely, to significant postoperative respiratory complications. Two babies suffered an inadvertent injury to a preoperatively functioning phrenic nerve, as manifest by decreased O_2 saturation in the recovery room and by a complicated recovery following later-derived respiratory infections. Both recovered within several months.

The incision sites for sural nerve harvest frequently demonstrate scar hypertrophy, especially for the first 2 years following surgery.

Salvage Procedures

Many babies who suffer BPBP will benefit from secondary (non-neural) surgery, which may include:

1. Release of an internal rotation contracture of the shoulder combined with transfer of one or two internal rotators to a position of external rotation
2. Muscle tendon transfers (typically trapezius and levator scapula) to improve horizontal shoulder abduction
3. Neural transfers (Oberlin procedure[10]) to restore elbow flexion
4. Release of elbow flexion contracture
5. Relocation of dislocated radial head
6. Rerouting of biceps to restore forearm pronation
7. Transfers to restore wrist/finger extension

WHAT WE NOW BELIEVE

1. There are nonobstetrical etiologies for this condition.
2. It is becoming less clear that neural surgery for babies with isolated C5–C6 palsies (babies who have absolutely normal functioning wrists and hands) leads to a better functional outcome than allowing spontaneous recovery with plans for early secondary shoulder surgery and, for the rare baby with poorly recovering biceps, an Oberlin[10] type biceps (boost) procedure.
3. All babies with global palsies should have neural surgery.
4. Surgery can be well performed without complications, and without loss of pre-existing function by most competent plastic and orthopaedic surgeons, and good outcomes can be obtained in circumstances other than a high-volume specialized "centers."
5. A good functional result at 4 years of age may become less so as the child ages. This argues for more longer-term studies of operated and nonoperated children with obstetrical brachial plexus injuries.
6. The loss of passive external shoulder rotation should be operated as early as possible.
7. Follow-up and dedicated therapy are needed throughout the child's growing years and probably beyond.
8. Contrary to the claims of litigators and their well-paid physician and nonphysician "experts," these children are not, as a rule, made susceptible as adults, to a lifetime of secondary problems, such as nerve entrapments or shoulder arthropathies.

REFERENCES

1. Kennedy R. Suture of the brachial plexus in birth paralysis of the upper extremity. Br Med 1903;1:298.
2. Millesi H. Surgical management of brachial plexus injuries. Hand Surg 1977;2:367–79.
3. Hentz V, Hong M. The surgical anatomy of the brachial plexus. In: Doyle J, Botte M, eds., Surgical Anatomy of the Hand and Upper Extremity. Philadelphia: Lippincott, 2002:297–315.
4. Hentz VR, Meyer RD. Brachial plexus microsurgery in children. Microsurgery 1991;12:175–85.
5. Sunderland S, ed. Nerves and Nerve Injuries, 2nd ed. Edinburgh: Churchill-Livingstone, 1978.
6. Sever JW. Obstetric paralysis: report of eleven hundred cases. JAMA 1925;85:1862–5.
7. Gilbert A, Hentz VR, Tassin JL. Brachial plexus reconstruction in obstetric palsy: operative indications and postoperative results. In: Urbaniak JR, ed., Microsurgery for Major Limb Reconstruction. St. Louis: C.V. Mosby, 1987:348–64.
8. Narakas AO. Brachial plexus surgery. Orthop Clin North Am 1981;12:303–23.
9. Steindler A. Tendon transplantation in the upper extremity. Am J Surg 1939;44:534–44.
10. Oberlin C, Beal D, Leechavengvongs S, et al. Nerve transfer to biceps muscle usin a part of ulnar nerve for C5-C6 avulsion of the brachial plexus: anatomical study and report of four cases. J Hand Surg Am 1994;19:232–7.
11. Doi K, Kuwata N, Sakai K, et al. A reliable technique of free vascularized surga nerve grafting and preliminary results of clinical applications. J Hand Surg Am 1987;12:677–84.
12. Doi K, Muramatsu K, Hattori Y, et al. Restoration of prehension with the double free muscle technique following complete avulsion of the brachial plexus. Indications and long-term results. J Bone Joint Surg Am 2000;82:652–66.
13. Barr JS, Freiberg JA, Colonna PC, et al. A survey of end results on stabilisation of the paralytic shoulder. J Bone Joint Surg Am 1942;24:699–707.
14. Tassin J. Paralysies obstetricales du plexus brachial: Evolution spontanee, resultats des interventions reparatrices process. Paris: Universite Paris VII, 1983.
15. Gilbert A. Etiology and Pathology of Obstetrical Brachial Plexus Palsy—A Review of 100 Operated Cases. Paper presented at 39th annual meeting of American Society for Surgery of the Hand, San Antonio TX, American Society for Surgery of the Hand, 1984.
16. Michelow BJ, Clarke HM, Curtis C, et al. The natural history of obstetrical brachial plexus palsy. Plast Reconstr Surg 1994;93:675–80, discussion 681.
17. Clarke HM, Curtis CG. An approach to obstetrical brachial plexus injuries." Hand Clin 1995;11:563–80, discussion 580–1.
18. Gilbert A, Hentz V, Tassin J, et al. Brachial plexus reconstruction in obstetric palsy: operative indications and postoperative results. In: Urbaniak J, ed., Microsurgery for Major Limb Reconstruction. St. Louis: C.V. Mosby, 1987:384–64.
19. Gilbert A. Long-term evaluation of brachial plexus surgery in obstetrical palsy. Hand Clin 1995;11:583–94, discussion 594–5.

21

Electrodiagnostic Testing of the Upper Extremity

David J. Slutsky

INTRODUCTION

The treatment of nerve disorders of the upper extremity has become a highly specialized area. There has been an evolution in the electrodiagnostic (EDX) approach for evaluating patients with these disorders. Differential latency testing can aid in the diagnosis of dynamic nerve entrapment disorders such as radial tunnel syndrome. Comparative latency testing increases the test sensitivity in the diagnosis of carpal tunnel syndrome, and cubital tunnel and ulnar tunnel syndrome. Digital nerve conduction testing can detect isolated digital nerve lesions and can be used to monitor the adequacy of reinnervation following a nerve repair.[1] Nerve conduction studies are not a panacea, however, especially in recurrent carpal tunnel syndrome.[2,3]

The electrodiagnostic evaluation consists of nerve conduction studies (NCS) and electromyography (EMG). Although these tests are invaluable extensions of the physical examination, many physicians are unable to interpret the test results, and so they base their operative decisions on electromyographers' impressions. Techniques for recording the electrophysiologic events in nerve and muscle carry with them a number of potential pitfalls. This may lead to false-positive or false-negative results, which in turn lead to erroneous conclusions.[4] A systematic approach to the interpretation of the NCS/EMG allows surgeons to determine the nature and location of lesions as well as the degree of involvement and the viability of the affected nerve and muscles.[5] The foundation for this approach can be gained through an understanding of the electrophysiology of nerve and muscle as well as the methodology underlying the electrodiagnostic test.[6]

NERVE ELECTROPHYSIOLOGY

The nerve cell membrane is composed of a lipid bilayer that has hydrophilic (water loving) and hydrophobic ends. When placed in an aqueous medium, the phospholipids arrange themselves so that the hydrophilic ends are facing outwards and the hydrophobic ends are inside. This leads to an ionic separation across the nerve axon that results in a charge separation. Although there are a number of charged proteins, the electrical gradients are mostly due to the difference in concentrations between sodium (Na^+) and potassium (K^+) ions. Minute changes in these concentrations lead to a change in the membrane potential, even though there is relatively little actual ion flow.

Various membrane channels consist of proteins embedded in the phospholipid bilayer that have a neutral charge and allow the passive flow of charged ions. There are separate channels for Na^+, K^+, and calcium (Ca^{+2}) ions. The interior of the axon has a charge of approximately −90 millivolts (mV), with a relatively greater concentration of K$^+$ ions with respect to the outside. There is a passive leak of K$^+$ ions out and Na$^+$ ions in, which causes the interior of the axon to become less negative with regard to the outside. There is an ATP dependent Na$^+$/K$^+$ pump which imports K$^+$ and exports Na$^+$ in a ratio of two K$^+$ for every three Na$^+$. This maintains the normal resting membrane potential, and prevents spontaneous depolarization. Since maintaining the ionic charge separation across the membrane requires energy, this mechanism stops when the energy supply is interrupted. In other words, local nerve ischemia will prevent depolarization. This is one of the mechanisms for the conduction block that occurs with nerve compression.

When the resting membrane potential reaches −50 mV, the membrane depolarizes. This generates an action potential, which is the electrical wave due to the flow of ions. The Na$^+$ channels open in response to depolarization allowing an influx of Na$^+$ ions down their concentration gradient. The Na$^+$ channels then close and become refractory to opening for a finite period of time. The Na$^+$/K$^+$ pump then pumps out the Na$^+$ in exchange for K$^+$ ions, restoring the membrane potential. The K$^+$ channels open after the Na$^+$ channels and remain open longer. This continued efflux of K$^+$ leads to transient hyperpolarization of the axon interior. An inward K$^+$ leak ultimately restores the baseline potential.

NERVE ANATOMY

Schwann cells are specialized satellite cells that separate the axon from the endoneurial fluid. They provide trophic support and aid in maintaining the periaxonal environment. In unmyelinated nerves, a single Schwann cell incorporates multiple axons into longitudinal invaginations of its cytoplasm. In myelinated nerves, a single Schwann cell surrounds one axon and lays down sphingomyelin. The myelin acts as a capacitor in that it is an insulator that has a high resistance to the flow of electrons. This allows a charge separation to develop on either side of the axonal membrane. The Schwann cells are arranged longitudinally along the axolemma. Each Schwann cell territory delineates an internode. At the junction between adjacent Schwann cells, the axon is exposed at a gap called the node of Ranvier. Local currents exit only at the nodes, where the myelin sheath thins down and disappears. A conductive material called "gap substance" coats the axon membrane and facilitates the flow of ions. There is also a higher concentration of Na$^+$ channels at the nodes, and a relative paucity in the membrane underneath the myelin. In this way, there is increased resistance to the flow of ions (current) except at the nodes.

Depolarization—Unmyelinated Nerves

Depolarization is an all or nothing phenomenon, and cannot be stopped once it starts. The membrane does not allow ion flow except in areas with Na$^+$ channels. In unmyelinated nerves, the Na$^+$ channels are spread out along the membrane, and signal conduction is uniform and successive. Once an action potential (AP) is generated, there is sequential depolarization along the membrane. As the AP propagates down the axon, each section of the membrane must be depolarized in turn. This not only takes time, but also diminishes the residual amount of current available to spread down the interior of the axon, which becomes attenuated faster. This leads to slow conduction velocities in the range of 10 to 15 m/s.

Depolarization—Myelinated Nerves

In myelinated nerves, the resistance of the axon interior to current flow is much less than the myelinated membrane, which results in preferential ionic flow down the axon. There is also a relative paucity of Na+ channels except at the internodes. The current flows down the axon, stopping only at the nodes of Ranvier. The Na$^+$ channels open, allowing the node to depolarize. The depolarizing current then flows down the axon interior to the next node. Depolarization thus jumps from node to node (saltatory conduction) rather than sequentially depolarizing each section of the membrane. This markedly speeds up the conduction velocities, which are in the range of 90 to 100 m/s.

Speed of Conduction

The electrical resistance to current flow varies inversely with diameter. Larger nerves conduct faster than smaller nerves. In order to survive, organisms must be able to react quickly to their environment; hence, nerve conduction must be fast. In complex organisms with billions of axons, increasing the nerve diameter is not a viable option. Myelination solves this problem by increasing impulse conduction without the need to increase the fiber diameter. The result of myelination is a 50 times decrease in nerve diameter with a 4 times increase in the conduction velocity.[7]

WAVEFORM GENERATION

Recording electrodes detect the small voltage changes associated with a nerve or muscle AP and convey them to an amplifier. Following amplification, the signal is filtered to remove extraneous electrical activity that can distort the waveform. Newer machines change the analogue signal into a binary signal (digital) through a to large, less dextrous muscles such as the gastrocnemius (1,934 fibers per motor unit).[38]

NORMAL ELECTRICAL POTENTIALS IN MUSCLE

Spontaneous Activity

In a normal muscle at rest, the isoelectric line should be silent except when the electrode is close to a neuromuscular junction. There are two types of spontaneous potentials that can be recorded from the end plate. When the tip of the needle rests near a muscle end plate, mechanical irritation of the nerve terminals provokes miniature end-plate potentials (MEPPs). These are non-propagating, irregular, mono- or bi-phasic negative waveforms of 10 to 50 μV that last 1 to 3 milliseconds. They sound like a dull roar ("distant ocean waves"). End-plate potentials (EPPs) are thought to be due to needle-tip impalement of the end plate. They also originate from the neuromuscular junction, but are larger than MEPPs (Fig. 21–5). They are initially negative, irregular/continuous, biphasic potentials of 100 to 300 μV, lasting 2 to 4 milliseconds. They have a high-pitched "rat-a-tat-tat" similar to a fibrillation.

End-plate spikes (EPS) are short (3 to 5 milliseconds), irregularly firing, biphasic initially negative waves of 100 to 200 μV, which are thought to be sub-threshold end-plate APs from a single muscle fiber. They may also be bi- or tri-phasic, initially positive waves, and mistaken for positive sharp waves or fibrillation potentials.[39] They most likely occur when the needle tip touches one of the small terminal branches of an intramuscular nerve near the neuromuscular junction, which then leads to the subsequent contraction of a muscle fiber. Since the needle is usually recording from the muscle fiber and not the neuromuscular junction, the waveform is initially negative.

MUAPs are distinguished from spontaneous potentials in that they are more regular and have slower rates. The MUAP disappears when the needle is moved slightly or the antagonist muscle is contracted. EPPs and EPS do not disappear, but their rate may slow if the needle is not moved. In a suspected denervated muscle when the electromyographer is unable to record muscle activity or a compound motor nerve action, spontaneous end plate activity would indicate that some axons are intact. In other words, MEPPs, EPPs, and EPSs will not be detected following denervation. If a patient presents paralysis, and MEPPs or EPPs are detected, the patient is malingering.

ABNORMAL SPONTANEOUS POTENTIALS IN MUSCLE

Fibrillation Potentials

Denervation results in muscle membrane instability, which may lead to spontaneous depolarization. The instability of the muscle fiber membrane is theorized to result from oscillations of the membrane potential, which becomes less negative until threshold is reached. Once threshold is reached, a propagating AP is induced, which is referred to as a fibrillation potential.[40] These are spontaneous depolarizations of a single muscle fiber. This process regularly repeats on a time interval that is dependent on the depolarization to threshold turn-around time.[41] They may also be precipitated by needle movement when introduced into denervated or myopathic muscle. The regularly occurring fibrillation potentials fire in a cyclical pattern, with periods of quiescence. Fibrillations may be seen after direct muscle injury. This can make it difficult to localize a coexisting nerve lesion, such as a radial nerve palsy after a humeral fracture.[42]

Fibrillation potentials are regular, biphasic (occasionally triphasic) waveforms with a positive wave and negative phase. They have a duration of 1 to 5 milliseconds, and an amplitude ranging from 20 to 1,000 μV.[43] Fibrillation potentials may also fire irregularly up to 50% of the time. They fire at rates of 1 to 50 times per second (cycles per second equal hertz) and have a high-pitched "manual typewriter" sound. They usually are associated with axonal denervation, but they may also occur in upper motor neuron lesions and myopathies. Fibrillations decrease as muscle tissue becomes fibrotic, whereby all electrical activity stops. Clinically, it is not possible to determine the extent of damage solely based on the number of fibrillations. Fibrillation potentials can be differentiated from end-plate potentials in that they are usually regular and the rate of firing (1 to 30 Hz) is usually slower than EPPs or EPSs (2 to 100 Hz).

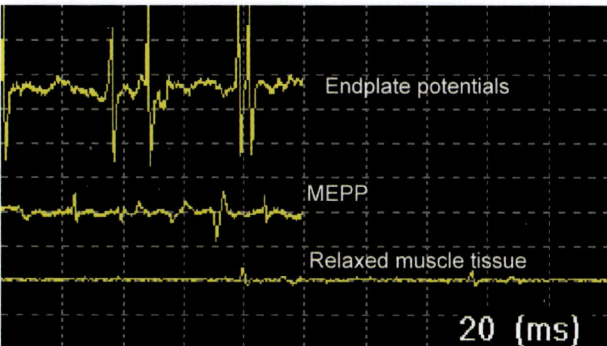

Figure 21–5 Spontaneous potentials. MEPP, mini end-plate potential. (From Slutsky D. Electromyography in hand surgery. J Am Soc Surg Hand 2004;4:176–86, with permission.)

Fibrillation potentials and positive sharp waves are graded on a 1 to 4 scale (Table 21–2).[44] This is an ordinal (density) scale rather than a ratio scale. In other words, 4+ fibrillations are not twice as bad as 2+.[45] The presence of 4+ fibrillation potentials does not by itself indicate that the entire muscle is denervated, but rather only a specific region of the muscle surrounding the needle electrode. One must look for MUAPs and examine multiple areas of the muscle before concluding that it is completely denervated. In addition, comparison of fibrillation numbers from one exam to another is not reliable.[46] Axon loss is better evaluated by a loss of recruitment and a drop in the distal CMAP.

Positive Sharp Waves

This potential consists of a primary initial positive monophasic wave, although there may be a small negative phase (biphasic). They have a duration of 2 to 100 milliseconds, with amplitudes of 100 to 1,000 μV, and a regular firing rate of 1 to 50 Hz.[47] The origin of positive sharp waves (PSWs) and their relationship to fibrillation potentials has not been clearly identified. PSWs are thought to have the same significance as fibrillation potentials, but often appear a few days earlier. They may be seen in distal muscles of normal subjects and have

no clinical significance. They may also occur after local muscle trauma.[43]

Muscle relaxation or contraction will abolish MUAPs, but will not have any effect on the spontaneous potentials. The time necessary for membrane instability is length dependent. The greater the distance between the lesion and the muscle, the longer it takes. Nerve lacerations close to the end-plate region may require only a few days for the onset of fibrillations/PSW, compared to cervical lesions, which may take weeks. This is the rationale behind waiting 10 days or more following injury to distinguish between neurapraxia versus axonotmesis/neurotmesis. Other abnormal spontaneous potentials that may be seen include complex repetitive discharges, myokemic potential, myotonic discharges, and fasciculation potentials (Table 21–3).

ELECTROMYOGRAPHIC EXAMINATION

The EMG examination has three parts: (1) observing the muscle at rest, (2) insertional activity, and (3) analyzing the morphology and recruitment of motor units at minimal to moderate voluntary muscle contraction.

Muscle at Rest

The examination starts with an observation of the muscle at rest, looking for any spontaneous electrical activity not under voluntary control. Healthy muscle is electrically silent.

Insertional Activity

A needle is sequentially advanced into the muscle to three successive depths. The needle is then withdrawn and redirected along a different line at four regions of the muscle, for a total of 12 sampling sites. Insertion of a needle electrode mechanically depolarizes muscle

---

TABLE 21–2

Fibrillation Grading Scale

Fibrillation Potentials	Grade
Absent	0
Persist over 1 second in 2 areas	1+
Persist over 1 second in 3 or more areas	2+
Intermittent in all areas	3+
Continuous in all areas	4+

Source: Daube JR. Needle examination in clinical electromyography. Muscle Nerve 1991;14:685–700,[44] with permission.

TABLE 21–3

Abnormal Spontaneous Potentials

Abnormal Potential	Description	Conditions
Complex repetitive discharge	Runs of regular spike patterns, abrupt onset and cessation	Myopathies, neuropathies, normal muscle
Myotonic discharge	Brief positive spikes that wax and wane	Myopathies, peripheral neuropathy
Fasciculations	Irregular normal or complex MUAP	Exercise-induced, lower motor neuron disorders, peripheral/metabolic neuropathy
Myokemic discharges	Regular persistent firing of normal MUAPs/occasional abrupt cessation	Chronic nerve compression, radiculopathy, multiple sclerosis

Source: Slutsky D. Electromyography in hand surgery. J Am Soc Surg Hand 2004;4:176–86,[5] with permission.
MUAP, motor unit action potential.

tissue. With normal insertional activity, the muscle produces brief bursts of high-frequency positive and negative spikes that sound somewhat like static.[48] The activity stops after cessation of needle movement. Increased insertional activity is present if the potentials persist for more than 300 milliseconds. The needle may also provoke transient or sustained fibrillation potentials or PSWs, before they are seen at rest. This is often but not invariably a sign of membrane instability. Decreased insertional activity occurs in myopathies, when muscle tissue is ischemic or has undergone fibrosis and is no longer capable of electrical activity.

Minimal to Moderate Voluntary Contraction

This is done to observe the MUAP morphology. Since MUAP amplitude varies with respect to the distance between the recording electrode and the muscle fiber, the MUAP should only be analyzed when the needle electrode is close to the muscle fiber under examination. A nearby MUAP sounds crisp and loud and has a short rise time, whereas a distant MUAP sounds like a muffled thud and has a long rise time. In general, 20 different MUAPs are analyzed for amplitude, duration, and phases.

Recruitment is the successive activation of motor units with increasing strength of muscle contraction. Minimal muscular effort results in the repetitive firing of 1-2 motor units, which are low amplitude, slow twitch (Type I) muscle fibers.[49] With stronger effort, the already activated motor units must fire more rapidly in order to maintain the strength of contraction. New high amplitude, fast twitch motor units (Type II) are then recruited (Fig. 21–6 A and B). With maximum contraction, many rapidly firing motor units ultimately run together, interfering with the recognition of individual MUAPs, that is, a full interference pattern (Fig. 21–7). Generally, after one MUAP fires at a rate of 10 times per second, a second MUAP is recruited. The recruitment ratio is the frequency of the fastest-firing MUAP divided by the number of different MUAPs seen. A normal recruitment ratio is close to five.[50] For example, if the fastest MUAP is firing 15 times per second, there should be three different MUAPs on the screen (Fig. 21–6 B).

In neurogenic disorders, there are fewer viable motor units, but there is no change in the number of muscle fibers. The remaining motor units must fire faster in an attempt to maintain the force of contraction. Too few MUAPs firing very rapidly leads to decreased recruitment (Fig. 21–8). In myopathies, the number of motor units is unchanged, but each motor unit contains fewer muscle fibers. Since the patient feels weaker, he or she tries to compensate by stimulating the remaining motor units to fire earlier and faster. When more MUAPs fire at a faster rate, increased recruitment results.

CLASSIFICATION OF NERVE INJURY

Physiologic Conduction Block

Lundborg and Dahlin described a physiologic conduction block that is due to either intraneural ischemia or a metabolic (ionic) conduction block, with little or no fiber pathology.[12] Intraneural ischemia would impair the ATP-dependent Na^+/K^+ pump, which would stop any nerve impulse transmission. An example of this would be the reversible compression of the sciatic nerve that one may experience with prolonged sitting at a movie theater. Sensory and motor conduction across the compressed segment is blocked by this loss of circulation, but immediately recovers once the compression is released. With more prolonged ischemia, intraneural edema develops; hence, recovery occurs over days or weeks. Axonal transport is also energy dependent; thus, extended ischemia may affect the nerve cell body function and viability.[51] Irreversible nerve fiber damage occurs if the ischemia lasts more than 6 to 8 hours.[52]

Neurapraxia

Initial Phase

The nerve connective tissue remains intact, but there is focal demyelination, which allows current leakage. The time for the AP to reach threshold at successive nodes is consequently prolonged. Partial lesions demonstrate slowing due to the loss of faster conducting fibers or demyelination of surviving fibers. The more protracted the compression, the slower the NCV due to repeated episodes of demyelination and subsequent remyelination. More extensive demyelination results in complete conduction block. The blocked nerve conduction prevents muscle fiber depolarization, which simulates axonal loss. Amplitude drops of more than 20% over a distance of 25 cm or less are abnormal. With stimulation proximal to the lesion, the potential is smaller or absent. Although there may be a sensory and motor loss, nerve conduction distal to the lesion is always normal. There is no axonal loss, and no Wallerian degeneration has occurred.

The most apparent finding on the EMG is reduced recruitment, due to a reduced number of motor unit potentials firing more rapidly than normal. The clinical correlate is that of muscle weakness without denervation, but fibrillation potentials may occasionally be seen (Fig. 21–9).[53]

Recovery Phase

Clinical recovery may occur in a patchy fashion, rather than proximal to distal. The nerve conduction should ultimately revert to normal if myelination is complete.

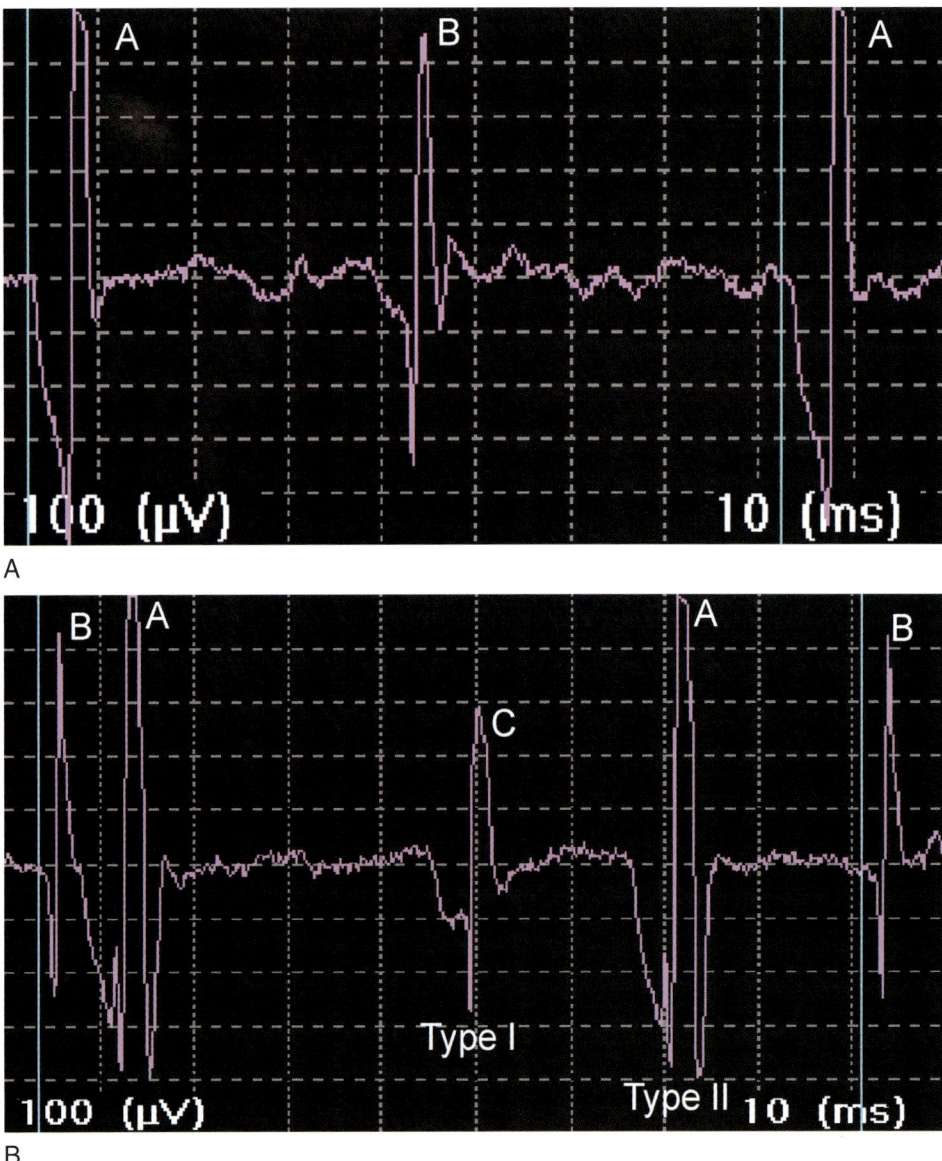

Figure 21–6   **A:** Normal recruitment. Motor unit action potential (MUAP) (A) fires every 80 milliseconds (eight grids at 10 ms/grid). The firing rate is thus 1,000/80 = 12.5 cycles/s (Hz). As MUAP (A) starts firing more than 10 Hz, a second MUAP (B) is recruited. The recruitment ratio (RR) is 12.5/2 = 6.25. **B:** Normal recruitment. The RR for fastest firing MUAP (A) is 1,000/60, 16.6 Hz. According to the rule of fives, there should be three different MUAPs on the screen. Both Type I and Type II MUAPs are firing. RR is 5.5. (From Slutsky D. Electromyography in hand surgery. J Am Soc Surg Hand 2004;4:176–86, with permission.)

Axonotmesis

Initial Phase

The axons are disrupted but the surrounding stroma is intact. Initially, the nerve segments distal to the lesion remain excitable and demonstrate normal conduction, but this ultimately wanes. Amplitude drops by more than 50% within the first few days are suggestive of an axonal injury.[30] Axonotmesis cannot be distinguished from complete severance of the nerve (neurotmesis) until sufficient time has passed for Wallerian degeneration to occur. Proximal stimulation results in an absent or small response from distal muscles.

Recovery Phase

The conduction velocity of the nerve proximal to the lesion returns to normal after 200 days if the target organ is reinnervated. The NCV distal to the nerve lesion only reaches 60% to 90% of its preinjury value (see Neurotmesis section).[54]

Partial lesions usually represent axonotmesis, where recovery depends on both axonal sprouting and nerve fiber regeneration. With an incomplete axonal injury, loss of motor units results in reduced recruitment. As axonal sprouting occurs, innervation of noncontiguous muscle fibers results in increased waveform duration,

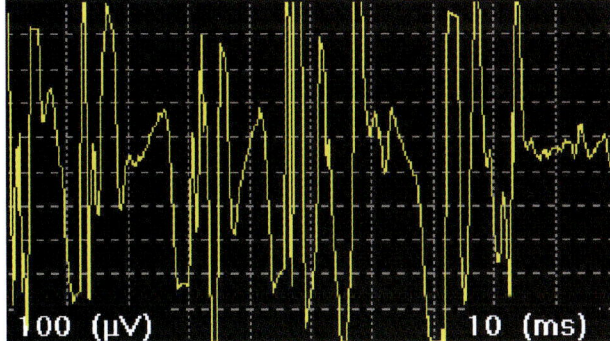

Figure 21–7 Full interference pattern. The baseline is completely obliterated by the motor unit action potentials. (From Slutsky D. Electromyography in hand surgery. J Am Soc Surg Hand 2004;4:176–86, with permission.)

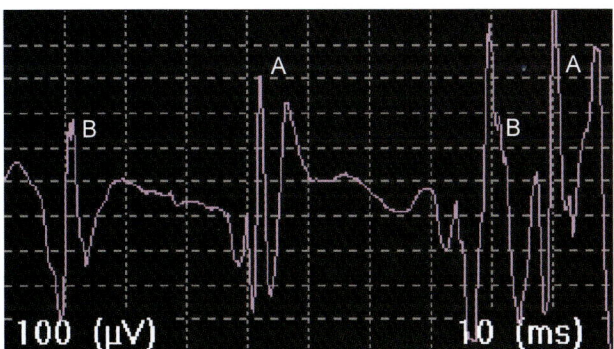

Figure 21–8 Decreased recruitment. Motor unit action potential (MUAP) (A) is firing at 16.6 Hz. There should be three different MUAPs on the screen, but there are only two. Recruitment ratio is 8.3. (From Slutsky D. Electromyography in hand surgery. J Am Soc Surg Hand 2004;4:176–86, with permission.)

polyphasia, and an increased MUAP amplitude. With time the polyphasia diminishes, but the increased amplitudes remain (see Motor Unit Action Potential Pathology section). There may be a biphasic pattern of recovery due to early axonal sprouting followed by late end organ reinnervation.

Neurotmesis

Initial Phase

The nerve is no longer in continuity, but the myelin remains intact until the axon degenerates. There is a preservation of the fastest conducting fibers until complete failure of the NAP. The latency and NCV remain unchanged until the end. Neuromuscular junction transmission fails before nerve excitability since the motor end plate degenerates before Wallerian degeneration is complete. As a consequence, one sees a disappearance of the CMAP by 3 to 5 days following nerve transection.[55] The SNAP amplitude is preserved until day 5 to 7, and sensory nerve conduction persists until day 11.[56]

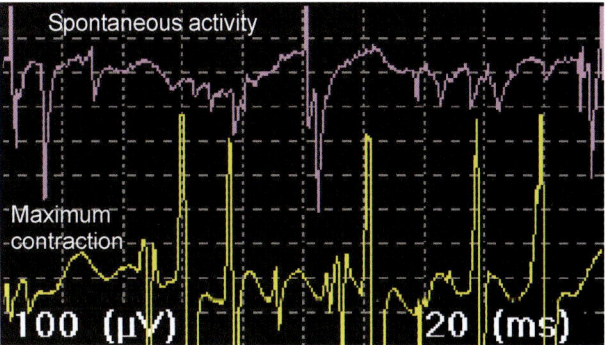

Figure 21–9 Partial ulnar nerve injury at 3 months. The **top** tracing shows trains of positive sharp waves obliterating the baseline. The **bottom** tracing shows only one rapidly firing motor unit action potential at maximum contraction, which reflects a loss of motor units. There is no polyphasia, indicating an absence of axonal sprouting (reinnervation). (From Slutsky D. Electromyography in hand surgery. J Am Soc Surg Hand 2004;4:176–86, with permission.)

Although it is dependent upon the length of the distal nerve stump, Wallerian degeneration typically occurs by 10 to 14 days.[56] Membrane instability is manifested by the appearance of fibrillation potentials and positive sharp waves. The appearance of the positive sharp waves may, however, predate fibrillation potentials by 2 to 3 days.[43] Fibrillations decrease in number as muscle reinnervation progresses. This also occurs in the absence of reinnervation due to a loss of viable muscle fibers secondary to fibrosis. The amplitude of the fibrillation potentials can be used to estimate the duration of the pathology, since it decreases with time. They may be 1,000 μV in acute conditions, but it is rare to find any larger than 100 μV after 12 months (Fig. 21–10 A and B).[57]

Recovery Phase

When the nerve is completely divided, recovery is dependent solely on axonal regeneration. The conduction velocity of the nerve proximal to the lesion remains at 60% to 70% if nerve continuity is not reestablished.[54] This occurs in part because the axon relies on retrograde transport of neurotrophic factors for maximal conductivity. Following nerve regeneration, remyelination is incomplete. The regenerating Schwann cells revert back to their shorter embryonic internodal length, which is a 2:1 to 3:1 ratio as compared to normal nerve. The regenerated nerve diameter slowly decreases distal to the lesion due to a failure to completely reexpand the endoneurial tube. These factors explain why the NCV distal to the nerve lesion only reaches 60% to 90% of preinjury value even though there may be full clinical recovery.

The EMG is initially silent, followed by the appearance of small, long duration, unstable, and polyphasic *nascent potentials* (Fig. 21–11). They usually precede the

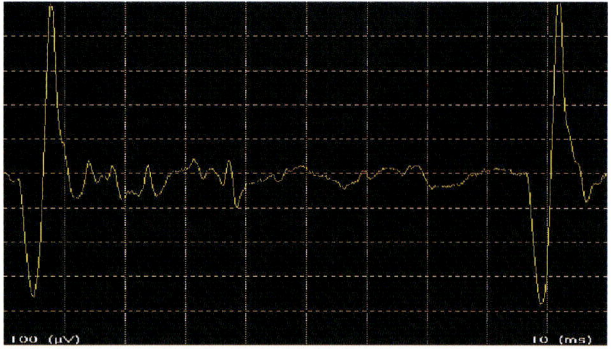

A

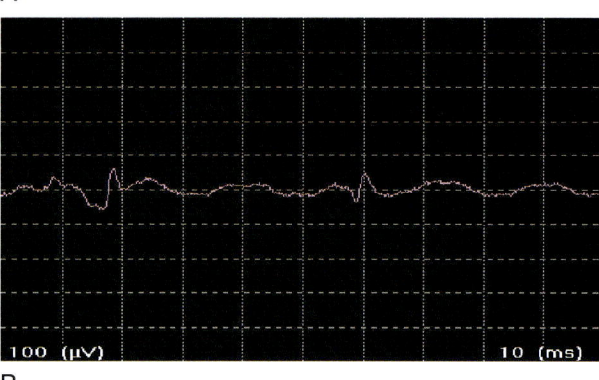

B

Figure 21–10 Fibrillation potentials. **A:** Recent denervation. The fibrillation potentials are of large amplitude. **B:** Chronic denervation. Note the small amplitude fibrillation potentials. (From Slutsky D. Electromyography in hand surgery. J Am Soc Surg Hand 2004;4:176–86, with permission.)

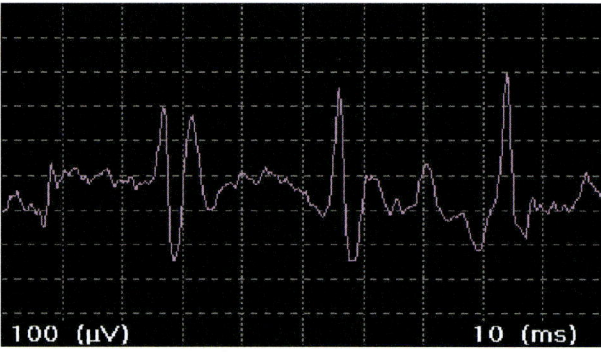

Figure 21–11 Early reinnervation of first dorsal interosseous following nerve repair. (From Slutsky D. Electromyography in hand surgery. J Am Soc Surg Hand 2004;4:176–86, with permission.)

onset of clinically evident voluntary movement.[46] It is prudent to wait 2 to 4 months and then look for evidence of reinnervation in previously completely denervated muscles.[58] As a general rule, nerve regrowth occurs at approximately 1 in per month.[59] Motor end plates degrade at about 1% per week; hence, the maximum length that a nerve can grow to restore motor function is approximately 13 to 18 in. Lesions that have spontaneous recovery are treated nonoperatively,

whereas those without recovery are explored. Repairs at the brachial plexus level rarely result in the recovery of any intrinsic muscle function. Sensory end organs, however, remain viable and can be reinnervated even after many years.[60]

COMPRESSIVE NEUROPATHIES

Standard electrodiagnostic studies often fall short in the assessment of many of the nerve disorders seen in a typical hand surgical practice.[4] There are, however, a number of specific techniques that have special application for hand surgeons.

MEDIAN NEUROPATHIES

Carpal Tunnel Syndrome

The standard nerve conduction studies should include sensory latencies to the thumb, index, and middle fingers, with comparative latencies to the radial sensory and ulnar sensory nerves.[17] The thumb is a more sensitive indicator for carpal tunnel compression, followed by the middle finger and then the index.[61] In mild carpal tunnel syndrome (CTS), the only test abnormality may include a prolongation of the transcarpal latency, or an abnormal comparative latency. The incidence of Type I errors (false positive) increases with multiple sensitive tests.[62] This had led some investigators to devise a comparative sensory index (CSI).[63] This consists of the sum of the thumb median–radial difference, the ring median–ulnar difference and the median–ulnar, mid-palmar orthodromic difference. A normal value is less than 1.0 milliseconds. The CSI is more sensitive and more specific, since it hinges on three parameters, which diminishes the technical error associated with making the diagnosis on one specific test.[64] The CSI is also temperature independent, since all of the nerves are examined under identical local conditions of conductivity, temperature, and digit circumference.

There are some caveats for nerve conduction studies in CTS. First, sensory abnormalities usually occur before motor abnormalities. In other words, the distal sensory latencies often slow before the distal motor latency. This is not surprising since 94% of the axons in the median nerve at the wrist level are sensory.[65] The sensory nerve axons are larger than the motor axons, and hence more susceptible to compression. If the DML is abnormal in the presence of normal SNAPs, extra care must be taken to rule out anterior horn cell disease or a C8 radiculopathy. Isolated recurrent motor branch compression, however, has been reported.[66] Second, the nerve conduction studies may not return to normal following decompression due to retrograde fiber degeneration or incomplete remyelination, even in the presence of a full clinical recovery.

Large myelinated and small unmyelinated fibers can be affected differently. Connective tissue changes follow with focal nerve fiber changes. The large myelinated nerves undergo segmental demyelination, while the small unmyelinated nerves undergo degeneration and regeneration. Normal fascicles are adjacent to abnormal fascicles. The nerve conduction study only tests the faster conducting fibers. This explains the seeming paradox of the patient who has established carpal tunnel syndrome but yet normal electrodiagnostic studies. It is the worst fascicles which produce symptoms, but it is the best fascicles which account for the normal nerve conduction studies.[67]

The nerve conduction study can yield useful information, but the severity of the pre-operative nerve conduction deficit does not provide significant data for prediction of the final outcome or return to work after carpal tunnel release.[68–70]

Recurrent Carpal Tunnel Syndrome

Electrodiagnostic studies are not a gold standard in recurrent CTS, which can be very difficult to evaluate. There is a difference between persistent CTS (persistent nerve entrapment) versus recurrent CTS (recurrent nerve entrapment). If there is a question of an incompletely released transverse carpal ligament (TCL), the NCS may be of use to determine if there has been significant change pre- and postoperatively and to rule out other sites of compression.[71] A traction neuropathy may be the cause of recurrent CTS symptoms rather than compression. Symptoms typically occur at 1 to 2 years following a carpal tunnel release (CTR).[72] In these cases, the NCS will be normal since conduction is unimpaired until an elongating force is applied to the tethered nerve. Provocative maneuvers to place traction on the nerve while measuring distal median motor latencies may increase the diagnostic yield.[73,74] Inching techniques across the carpal canal may also be useful in localizing an area of focal nerve compression.[18]

EXAMPLE

A 30-year-old administrative manager presented with a 2-year history of numbness and tingling of his right thumb, and index and middle fingers. Pre-operative nerve conduction studies were consistent with CTS. His symptoms did not improve following a CTR performed elsewhere. Upon reevaluation 1 year later, he was found to have a localized Tinel's sign, a negative Phalen's test, and normal two-point discrimination. Wrist x-rays and a metabolic screen were normal. Repeat electrodiagnostic studies demonstrated prolongation of the DML

with low amplitudes and prolonged SNAPs. At the time of a repeat right carpal tunnel release, an incompletely divided TCL, and a marked hourglass constriction of the median nerve were found. An epineurolysis and a hypothenar fat pad flap were performed.

Despite the complete TCL release, the patient's symptoms persisted. A repeat NCS at 1 year postop demonstrated improvement in the distal motor latency and amplitudes. An EMG of the APB demonstrated some polyphasia but no fibrillation potentials. Over the course of the following year, the patient developed a further loss of sensation with an increased frequency of symptoms. Two-point discrimination testing was now more than 25 mm in the median nerve distribution. A new NCS revealed absent sensory nerve potentials. The patient was taken back to the operating room where repeat exploration demonstrated generalized fibrosis with a focal region of compression of the sensory fascicles distal to the motor branch. After a neurolysis of this segment, the nerve was covered with a reverse pedicled radial fascial flap. At the time of examination 2 years later, the patient complained of continuous numbness and painful paresthesiae despite an improvement in the DML and SNAPs (Table 21–4).

Carpal Tunnel Syndrome and Pregnancy

CTS that occurs during pregnancy is most common in primiparas with generalized edema.[75] The electrophysiologic findings reveal that motor or sensory conduction blocks are more frequent than those observed in

TABLE 21–4

Recurrent Carpal Tunnel Syndrome

Date of Testing	Distal Motor Latency Onset/ Amplitude	Sensory Latency Peak/Amplitude
3/96 (preoperative)	5.0 ms/10 mV	4.7 ms/40 μV
5/97 (after incomplete release)	9.6 ms/3.0 mV[a]	5.9 ms/30 μV[a] (2 pd = 5 mm)
7/98 (after 2nd release)	5.0 ms/9.4 mV	5.1 ms/16 μV
5/99	5.1 ms/13.5 mV	No response[b] (2 pd >25 mm)
8/02 (after 3rd release)	4.8 ms/3.1 mV	3.9 ms/6.2 μV

[a] Note the increase in the distal motor latency and drop in amplitude.
[b] Absence of the distal sensory latency.
2 pd, two point discrimination.

TABLE 21–5

Carpal Tunnel Syndrome in Pregnancy

	Distal Motor Latency Onset/ Amplitude	Sensory Latency Peak/ Amplitude
During pregnancy	6.9 ms /3.8 mV[a]	5.5 ms/11 µV[a]
Postpartum (nonlactating)	4.1 ms/8.3 mV	5.2 ms/50 µV

[a] Note the prolonged latencies and low amplitudes, which improve in the postpartum period.

idiopathic CTS. They are thought to result from acute compression of the median nerve due to a hormone-dependent tenosynovitis.[76] CTS severe enough to warrant surgery occurs infrequently in pregnancy and generally resolves spontaneously postpartum.[77] This is reflected in pre- and post-partum nerve conduction studies (Table 21–5). The NCS, however, may not return to normal for 6 to 20 months.[78] Some patients may even develop recurrent symptoms and ultimately require a CTR.[79] Carpal tunnel syndrome that develops in association with breastfeeding appears to be a different condition.[80] These women do not typically have peripheral edema and their symptoms usually resolve after weaning.[81]

Pronator Syndrome

The more proximal of the median nerve compression neuropathies is the pronator syndrome. It is often associated with pain in the proximal volar forearm and paresthesiae in the median nerve distribution. Phalen's test is notably negative. The syndrome is classically associated with any of four potential areas of compression including the ligament of Struthers, the lacertus fibrosis, the aponeurotic fascia of the superficial or deep head of the pronator teres (PT) or the flexor digitiorum sublimus (FDS) arch.[82] It is imperative to exclude CTS and anterior interosseous nerve entrapment.[83]

Electrophysiologically, one might find a prolongation of the distal median sensory latencies and a reduced amplitude of the CMAP to the APB. The median NCV over the forearm segment may be abnormal, but this finding is not consistent.[84,85] Sequential needle stimulation of the median nerve in 1-cm increments while recording from the APB may identify an area of focal conduction block in or about the pronator teres muscle.[86] Nerve conduction studies during provocative maneuvers such as elbow flexion, forearm pronation and middle finger flexion against resistance do not increase the yield.[87] Patients with normal NCS seem to fare better following nerve decompression than patients with abnormal studies, which may be related to the severity of the compression.[88]

NCS are rarely diagnostic for pronator syndrome, but needle EMG is often of some value.[89] Membrane instability can be anticipated in all median-innervated muscles including the pronator teres, flexor carpi radialis, and flexor digitorum sublimus.

Anterior Interosseous Nerve Syndrome

The anterior interosseous nerve (AIN) is a purely motor branch that arises from the median nerve 5 to 8 cm distal to the medial epicondyle. It innervates the flexor pollicus longus (FPL), the flexor digitorum profundus (FDP) to the index and middle finger (which can be ulnar innervated), and the pronator quadratus (PQ). The AIN may be compressed by fibrous bands on the superficial or deep heads of the PT, the fibrous arch of the FDS, tumors, or enlarged bursae. It can also be compressed by aberrant muscles, especially Gantzer's muscle.[82] The patient typically presents with proximal forearm pain and an inability to flex the thumb interphalangeal joint or the distal phalanx of the index and/or the middle fingers. A positive tenodesis effect will rule out attritional tendon rupture. Of note is that finger sensation in the median nerve distribution is normal, and there is no weakness of the APB.

Electrophysiologically, all SNAPs in the affected upper extremity are normal. If an abnormal SNAP is found, it is due to some other lesion.[30] The most appropriate technique involves recording the CMAP from the pronator quadratus. The active surface electrode is placed in the midline dorsally, 3 cm proximal to the ulnar styloid. The median nerve is stimulated at the cubital fossa. The mean onset latency for the PQ is 3.6 ± 0.4 milliseconds, with a side-to-side difference of 0.4 milliseconds. Normal amplitudes range from 2.0 to 5.5 mV.[90] Side-to-side comparative latencies are helpful in establishing the diagnosis.[86] EMG testing of the PQ and FPL muscles should demonstrate signs of membrane instability.

If a Martin-Gruber anastomosis is present, the anatomic communication between the median and ulnar nerve is via a communicating branch from the AIN 91% of the time.[91] This may explain the presence of fibrillation potentials in the intrinsic muscles even though a coexisting ulnar nerve lesion has been ruled out. A brachial plexopathy may initially present with signs that are suggestive of AIN compression.[92] For this reason, EMG sampling of more proximal muscles should be performed in every case.

EXAMPLE

A 56-year-old male presented with a 6-month history of inability to flex his thumb and index fingers. This occurred after 3 days of repetitively lifting 25-lb boxes at work. He had no sensory complaints. Relevant physical findings included 0/5 power of the FPL and FDP$_{index}$ (Fig. 21–12 A), but 5/5 power of the APB, a negative Tinel's test, and a negative Phalen's test.

An NCS/EMG performed by the treating neurologist revealed normal median motor and sensory latencies and amplitudes, as well as normal forearm conduction velocities. An EMG of the APB was reported as showing large amplitude motor units with increased duration and decreased recruitment. There was no evidence of membrane instability in the intrinsics, flexor carpi radialis, flexor carpi ulnaris, brachioradialis (BR), biceps, triceps, deltoid and cervical paraspinal muscles. There was no electrodiagnostic testing of the PQ or FPL. The report conclusion was that of moderate right CTS.

This example emphasizes the importance of an adequate history and physical exam. The patient's presentation was classic for an AIN palsy. There was no clinical evidence of CTS. The normal median SNAPs ruled out more proximal median nerve compression. The lack of membrane instability of the upper limb muscles and cervical paraspinals ruled out a brachial plexopathy or anterior horn cell disease. On further electrodiagnostic testing, the latency to the PQ was prolonged with low

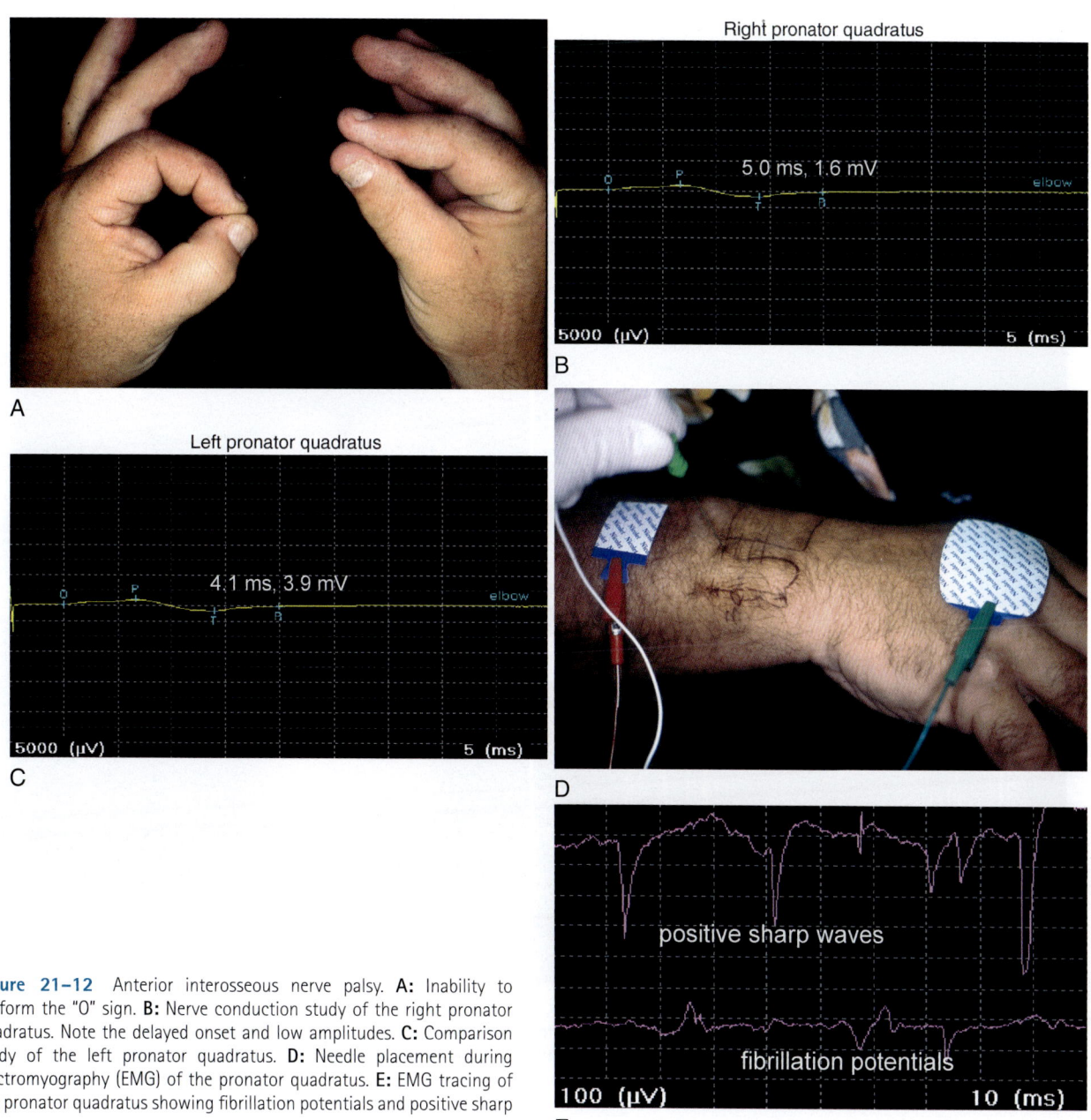

Figure 21–12 Anterior interosseous nerve palsy. **A:** Inability to perform the "0" sign. **B:** Nerve conduction study of the right pronator quadratus. Note the delayed onset and low amplitudes. **C:** Comparison study of the left pronator quadratus. **D:** Needle placement during electromyography (EMG) of the pronator quadratus. **E:** EMG tracing of the pronator quadratus showing fibrillation potentials and positive sharp waves.

amplitudes and marked slowing as compared to the opposite side (Table 21–6) (Fig. 21–12 B and C). EMG testing of the PQ and FPL showed signs of acute denervation manifested by increased insertional activity, with large amplitude fibrillation potentials (Fig. 21–12 D and E).

Preoperative elbow x-rays and MRI were normal. Intraoperatively, there was entrapment of the AIN branches by a fibrous proximal arch of the sublimus muscle (Fig. 21–13 A and B). Intraoperative stimulation of the AIN after decompression demonstrated a normal NAP as well as normal CMAPs of the PT and FPL (Fig. 21–13 C). At 8 months postoperatively, the patient had recovered active flexion of his index FDP_{index} (Figure 21–13 D), but still had no active contraction of his FPL. Repeat electrodiagnostic studies showed polyphasic MUAPs of the FDP_{index} that were consistent with reinnervation (Fig. 21–13 E). There was, however, still no improvement in the latencies of the PQ or FPL, and no EMG evidence of reinnervation.

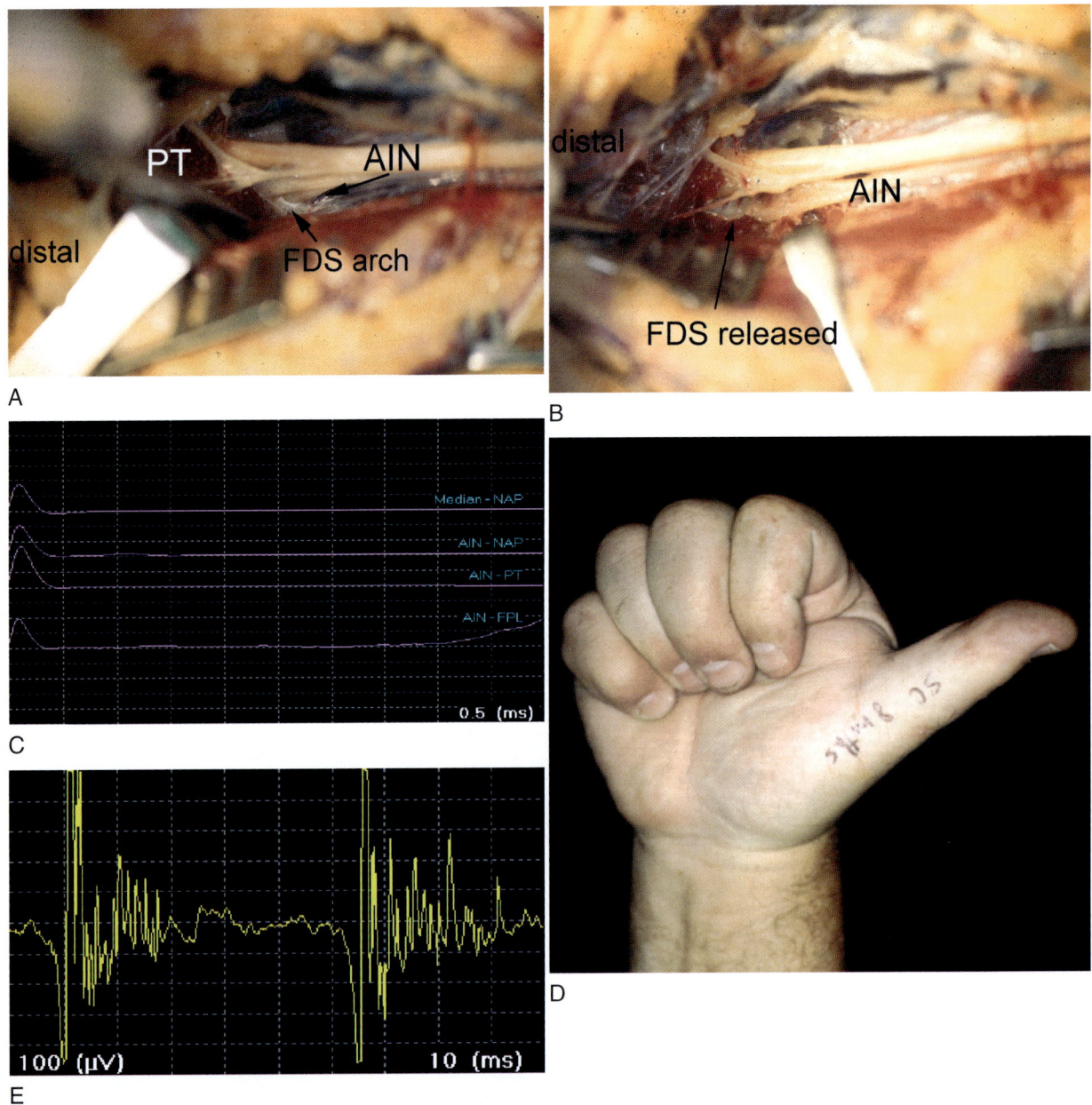

Figure 21–13 Anterior interosseous nerve (AIN) compression. **A:** Anterior approach to the AIN. Note the fibrous border of the sublimus muscle. **B:** Following release of the sublimus arch (flexor digitiorum sublimus). **C:** Tracing demonstrating a nerve action potential and compound motor action potentials to the flexor pollicus longus and pronator teres. **D:** Clinical photo at 8 months showing active flexion of the distal phalanx of the index but no active thumb interphalangeal joint flexion. **E:** Electromyography of the flexor digitorum profundus index demonstrating polyphasic motor unit action potentials, which are consistent with reinnervation.

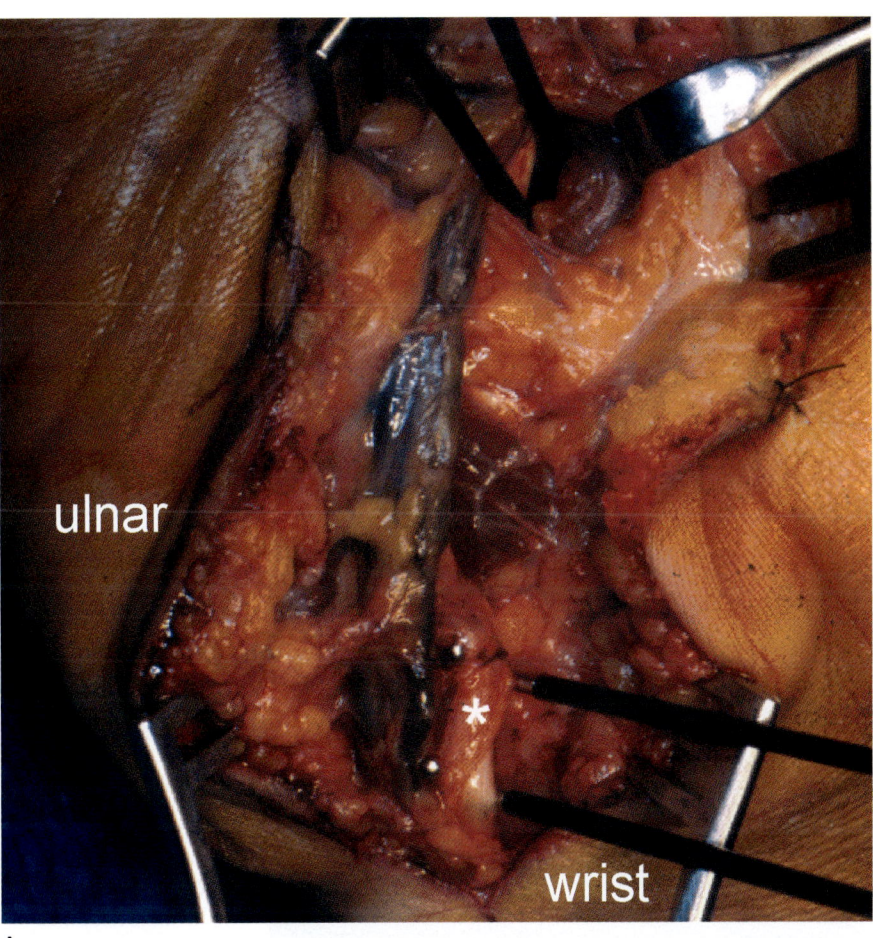

Figure 21–15 Distal ulnar nerve decompression. **A:** Intraoperative stimulation of the deep motor branch of the ulnar nerve (*).

A

TABLE 21-9		
Short Segment Incremental Studies		
Distance (cm)	**Latency (ms)**	**Amplitude (mV)**
−1	5.78	2.60
Wrist crease	7.89	1.80
1	5.31	2.21
2	5.31	2.03
3	3.05	1.51
4	NR	NR

Note: The right deep ulnar motor branch response is universally delayed in onset (left side >3.2 ms) and of low amplitude (left side >6.5 mV).
Source: Slutsky DJ. Nerve conduction studies in hand surgery. J Am Soc Surg Hand 2003;3:152–69, with permission.
NR, no response.

superficial to the nerve (Osborne's ligament, arcade of Struthers). The internal topography of the ulnar nerve at the elbow explains the relative sparing of the flexor carpi ulnaris and flexor digitorum profundus, since their motor fibers lay deep within the nerve.[97] The intrinsics are often uninvolved until the late stages of compression for similar reasons, whereas the superficially located sensory fibers are more susceptible to early compression.

Conduction velocities can be misleading if the surface measurement of the nerve is off, even by 1 cm. Testing inaccuracies also occur following ulnar nerve transposition, since the nerve no longer follows its anatomic course. Ulnar nerve conduction velocity is recorded as being faster with elbow flexion preoperatively, and with elbow extension postoperatively, when the skin measurement used for the distance is kept constant. Postoperatively the most valid measurement of ulnar nerve conduction is with a skin distance that is measured posterior to the medial epicondyle with the elbow extended.[98] With longer conduction distances, an area of focal block may be missed since it tends to be averaged out. Segmental stimulation of the ulnar nerve skirts these pitfalls, and is a sensitive method for determining focal conduction abnormalities. Measurement errors are minimized since the nerve is localized at each stimulation site. If the nerve is stimulated in 1-cm segments, a jump in NCV of more than 0.40 milliseconds is indicative of a focal abnormality. If the nerve is stimulated in 1-in increments, a jump of more than 0.75

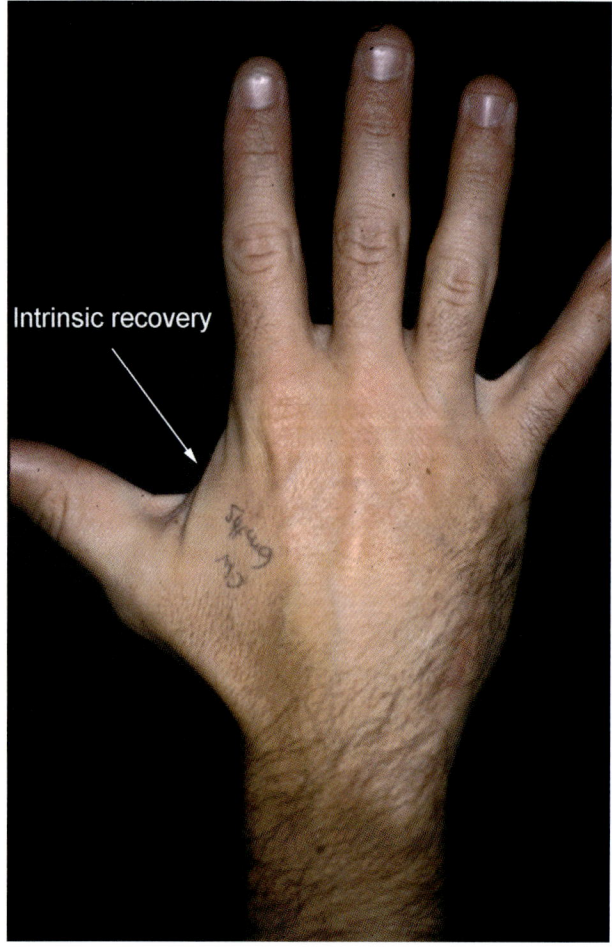

B

Figure 21–15—Cont'd Distal ulnar nerve decompression. **B:** Six months after operation. Note the normal bulk of the dorsal interossei and the active index finger abduction. (From Slutsky DJ. Nerve conduction studies in hand surgery. J Am Soc Surg Hand 2003;3:152–69, with permission.)

TABLE 21–10

Incremental Ulnar Nerve Stimulation at Elbow

Site (Right/Left)	Onset (ms)	Amplitude (mV)	Δ–O (ms)[a]
−2 cm	7.03/7.11	5.75/7.50	
−1 cm	7.19/7.27	5.79/7.39	0.16/0.16
Epicondyle	7.42/7.58	5.43/7.28	0.23/0.31
+1 cm	**7.81**/7.66	5.58/7.31	**0.39**/0.08
+2 cm	**7.81**/*7.81*	5.66/7.33	**0.00**/0.16
+3 cm	7.89/*7.81*	5.56/7.32	0.08/**0.00**
+4 cm	8.20/8.13	5.38/7.25	0.31/0.31

[a] Difference in onset.
Note: The identical latencies difference between 1–2 cm proximal to the epicondyle on the right (bold) and 2–3 cm on the left (in bold italic), most likely represent arcing of the current with depolarization proximal to the actual site of stimulation.
Source: Slutsky DJ. Nerve conduction studies in hand surgery. J Am Soc Surg Hand 2003;3:152–69, with permission.

are more than 50 m/s. Combining ulnar motor and sensory techniques adds useful information in complex cases, where clinical exam fails to localize the lesion. Conduction to the dorsal cutaneous branch of the ulnar nerve can be measured.[103] This test is relatively insensitive for detecting proximal ulnar nerve compression, since it is abnormal in only 55% of patients with cubital tunnel syndrome.[104] As in CTS, the patient's clinical findings and response to conservative measures should be a major determinant in the surgical decision making. Patients who have paresthesiae only, with no motor or sensory abnormalities (McGowan Stage I) can still benefit from an in situ release of the ulnar nerve, even if the NCS are normal.[105]

EXAMPLE

A 47-year-old male grocery clerk presented with a history of bilateral submuscular ulnar nerve transpositions 2 years previously. He complained of a 1-year history of recurrent tingling of the small and ring fingers bilaterally, exacerbated by use of a bottom scanner at work. He had a normal ulnar motor and sensory exam. He had a positive Tinel's sign over the ulnar nerves bilaterally. His elbow flexion test was equivocal. The referring neurologist's report indicated that the NCS were normal, yet there was a more than 40% drop in amplitude across the cubital tunnel bilaterally! Incremental stimulation of the ulnar nerves across the elbow localized the exact course of the nerve, reducing any measurement errors. There was no focal conduction slowing (i.e., <0.40 milliseconds), or any significant amplitude drops on either side (Table 21–10).

milliseconds is abnormal.[99] Segmental nerve conduction studies significantly improve the detection of an ulnar mononeuropathy at the elbow, and should be considered when routine studies are negative and clinical suspicion remains high.[100]

There is a poor correlation between the area of focal conduction block and the site of entrapment at time of surgery. This is likely due to the fact that if there is a partial conduction block, it is necessary to turn up the gain on the stimulation in order to obtain a response. With increasing current, the current flow tends to arc ahead of the stimulation, resulting in depolarization ahead of the applied stimulus site (Table 21–10).[101]

Across elbow sensory nerve studies have also been described.[102] The above and below elbow stimulation sites are the same as S2 and S3 for the motor studies, but in this case the SNAPs are recorded from ring electrodes placed on the small finger. Normal NCV values

TABLE 21–11

Differential Latency Testing of Radial Nerve

	Trial 1 (ms)	Trial 2 (ms)	Trial 3 (ms)
AE NCV in neutral[a]	5.16	4.77	4.53
AE NCV in pronation	4.92	4.61	4.61
AE NCV in supination	4.69	4.61	4.50
Δ (difference in latency)	0.55	0.16	0.08

[a] Note the abnormal latency difference between the AE NCV in neutral versus supination.
Source: Slutsky DJ. Nerve conduction studies in hand surgery. J Am Soc Surg Hand 2003;3:152–69, with permission.
AE, above elbow; NCV, nerve conduction velocity.

Across elbow sensory conduction velocities were normal bilaterally. Lumbrical interosseous latency testing and NCV differences from the ADM to the FDI were also normal. Based on this testing, continued conservative treatment with activity modification was recommended, rather than repeat surgery.

RADIAL NEUROPATHIES

Upper Arm

In the arm region, the radial nerve is often injured in association with some form of unconsciousness. In a Saturday night palsy, an obtunded patient sits with their arm over a chair back or rests his/her head on the lateral surface of their arm.[106] Alternatively, the radial nerve can be compressed in the groove between the brachialis and forearm muscles when one person rests their head on the middle third of the arm of another i.e., honeymooner's palsy.[30] The NCS typically demonstrates the absence of the superficial radial SNAP. Motor recordings are more difficult since no muscle is sufficiently isolated from other radially innervated muscles. A surface electrode over the EIP results in a volume conducted response from the adjacent radial innervated muscles, which makes side-to-side amplitude comparisons difficult. Radial nerve recordings using needle electrodes in the EIP are more common as a result, which makes it difficult to approximate the degree of axonal loss by assessing the amplitudes.[107] The EMG, however, is quite useful, and permits a relatively accurate localization of the lesion. In a spiral groove lesion, for example, all three heads of the triceps should be normal, with denervation of the brachioradialis and all muscles distal to it.

Forearm

Entrapment of the posterior interosseous nerve (PIN) at the elbow can result in two separate clinical syndromes.

Although the same nerve is compressed, the clinical presentation may be different and merely represents two ends of the spectrum of PIN compression. In the posterior interosseous nerve syndrome, the presenting symptoms are weakness and/or paralysis of the extensor muscles, which result in a wrist or finger drop. The presenting complaint for radial tunnel syndrome is proximal forearm pain often coexisting with lateral epicondylitis, without sensory nor motor loss.[108]

As it travels distally through the radial tunnel, the PIN may potentially be entrapped by fibrous bands anterior to the radiocapitellar joint, the radial recurrent leash of vessels, the fibrous edge of the extensor carpi radialis brevis (ECRB), and the proximal border of the supinator (i.e., the arcade of Frohse or the distal edge of the supinator muscle).

Radial Tunnel Syndrome

Classically, the NCS is normal in radial tunnel syndrome. Some authors have postulated that this syndrome reflects a dynamic entrapment of the posterior interosseous nerve. If the ECRB develops a fibrous edge, the PIN can be entrapped by a scissoring action between this edge and the arcade of Frohse during repetitive forearm supination and pronation. This can lead to intermittent PIN compression. Differential latency testing is based on this premise.[109] Across elbow radial motor nerve conduction is performed with the elbow extended, and the forearm positioned in neutral, pronation, and supination for 30 seconds. The testing is then repeated. An abnormal latency difference of more than 0.30 milliseconds is indicative of radial tunnel entrapment.

EXAMPLE

A 50-year-old female presented with a 3-year history of right proximal forearm pain. A lateral epicondylectomy 1 year previously failed to relieve her symptoms. She was tender over the distal border of the supinator and the lateral epicondyle. She had a positive middle finger extension test and pain with simultaneous wrist flexion, pronation, and ulnar deviation. A local anesthetic block of the posterior interosseous nerve on two separate occasions relieved her pain completely. Standard nerve conduction studies revealed normal radial motor conduction velocities. EMG testing of radial innervated muscles was normal. The results of differential latency testing revealed an abnormal latency difference in the first trial (Table 21–11). Based on the clinical exam and this testing, a radial tunnel decompression was performed. The PIN was normal in appearance at the time of surgery (Fig. 21–16 A and B).

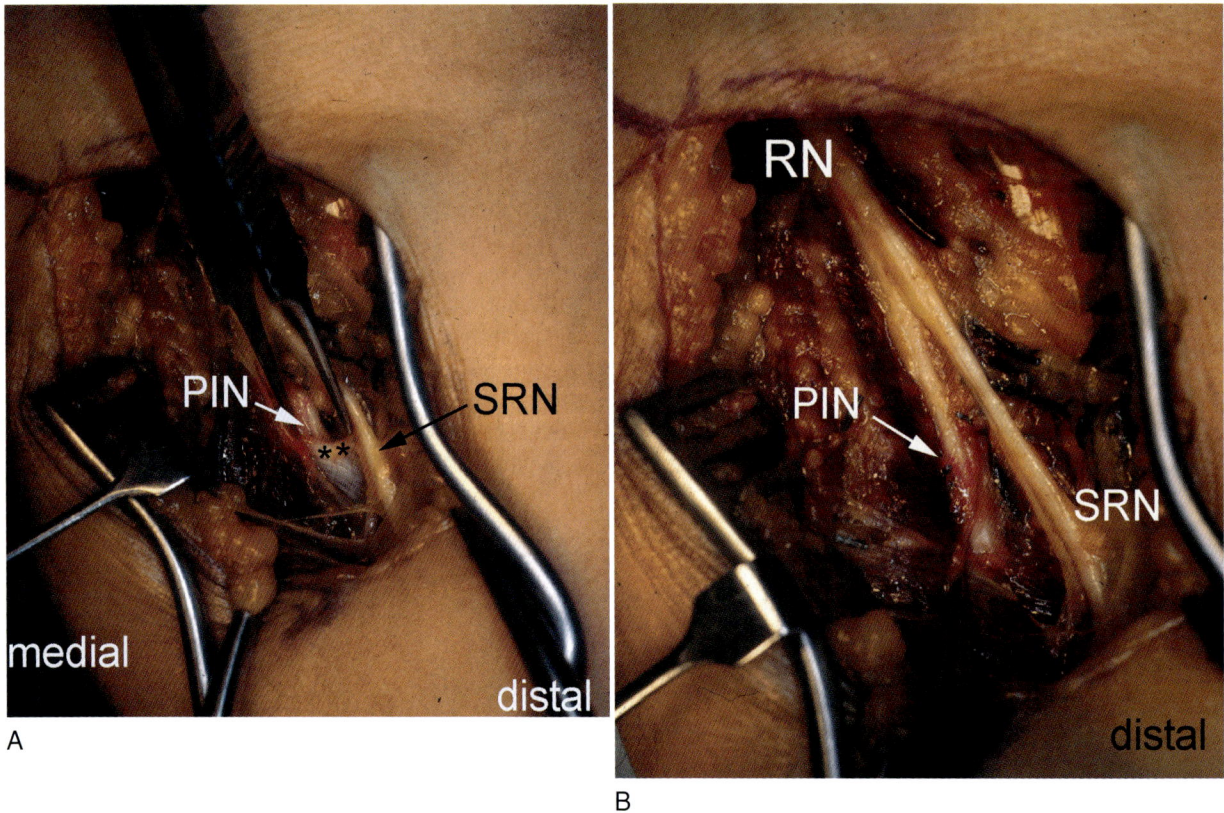

Figure 21–16 Radial tunnel syndrome. **A:** Anterior approach with a view of the proximal volar forearm demonstrating the arcade of Struthers (*). **B:** After release of the arcade. Note the normal appearance of the posterior interosseous nerve. PIN, posterior interosseous nerve; RN, radial nerve; SRN, superficial radial nerve.

Posterior Interosseous Nerve Entrapment

PIN lesions do not affect the superficial radial SNAP, which should be normal. The compound motor action potential of PIN innervated muscles may show a drop of conduction velocity or amplitude, but this is difficult to assess with surface electrodes. Needle EMG is the best technique for localization, especially with partial lesions.[30] In acute denervation, decreased recruitment, increased insertional activity, and fibrillation potentials and/or positive sharp waves are present. In chronic lesions seen after 3 to 6 months, decreased recruitment may still be seen along with giant motor unit potentials and polyphasia due to peripheral axonal ingrowth.

EXAMPLE

A 46-year-old laborer presented with an 8-month history of progressive weakness of wrist and finger extension after falling and striking the lateral aspect of his elbow. Electrodiagnostic studies demonstrated fibrillation potentials in muscles innervated by the PIN. During surgery, there was an hyperemic region of the PIN underneath the radial recurrent vessels (Fig. 21–17 A and B).

Superficial Radial Nerve Entrapment

The superficial radial nerve (SRN) can be injured in the distal forearm or at the wrist by tight bracelets or watch bands, handcuffs, radius fractures, lacerations, venous cutdown, and blunt trauma. The SRN may also be entrapped as it exits the fascia between the tendons of the BR and ECRB. Physical examination includes altered touch perception, moving two-point discrimination more than 15 mm, static two-point discrimination that is 5 mm greater than the contralateral first web space, a positive Tinel's sign over the SRN, and aggravation of the patient's symptoms with forced forearm pronation and wrist ulnar flexion.[110] Either partial or complete overlap of the lateral antebrachial cutaneous nerve (LABCN) with the SRN occurs up to 75% of the time. If a response is recordable from radial sensory recording electrodes while stimulating the musculocutaneous nerve, an intact LACBN may mask injury to the radial sensory nerve. Damage to the LABCN may be a concomitant finding in patients with an injury to the SRN.[111]

When there is extensive overlap in the nerve territories, special electrodiagnostic studies are required to establish the diagnosis of radial sensory nerve entrapment. The recording electrode (E1) is placed over a palpable branch of the SRN where it crosses the extensor

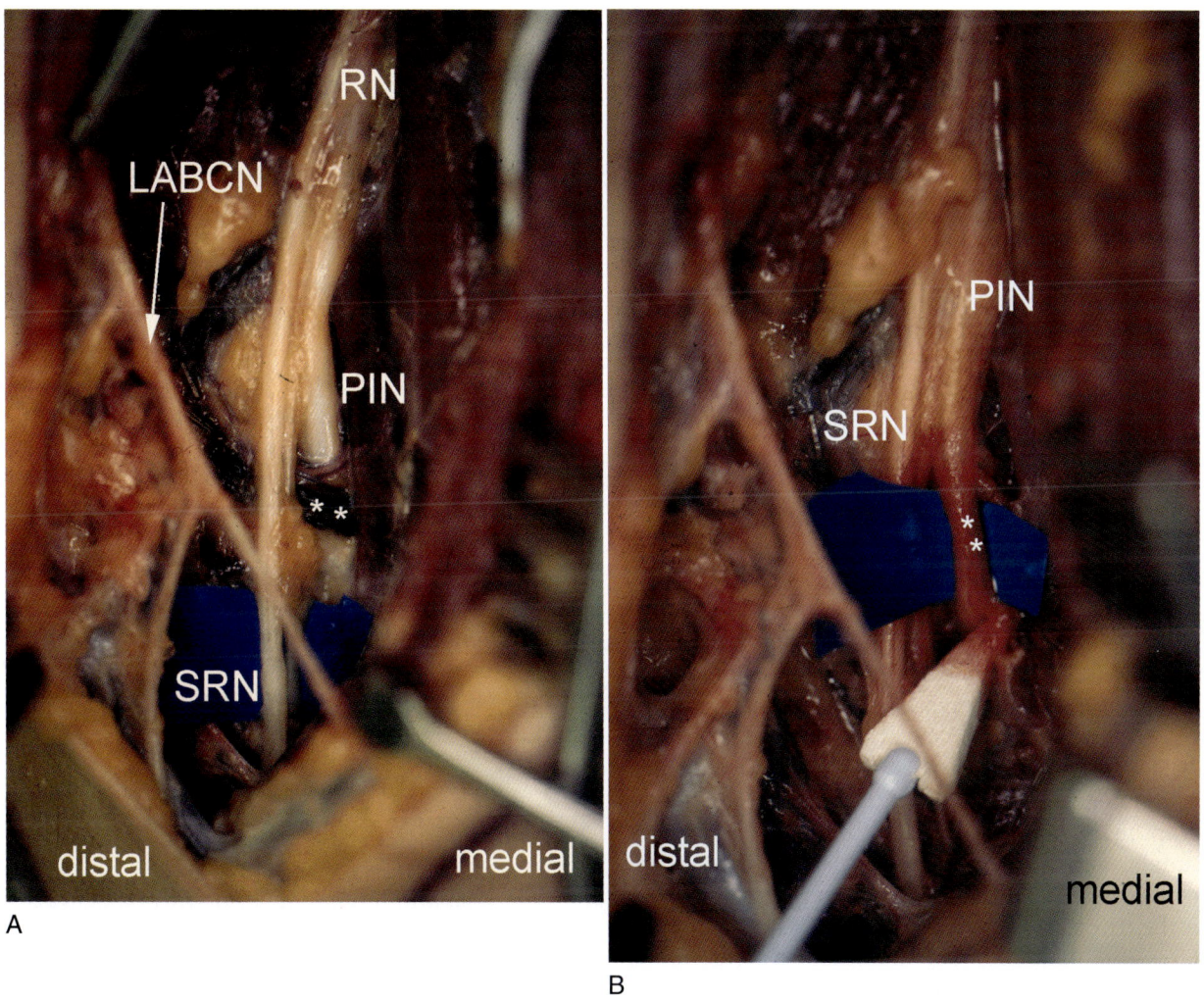

Figure 21–17   Posterior interosseous nerve (PIN) compression. **A:** Note the radial leash of vessels (*) crossing over the PIN. **B:** After ligation of the radial recurrent vessels. Note the hyperemia of the PIN (*). LACBN, lateral antebrachial cutaneous nerve. SRN, superficial radial nerve.

pollicus longus (EPL) tendon. The reference electrode is placed 4 cm distally, over the thumb. The SRN is first stimulated (S1) 10 cm proximal to E1 over the radius. The radial nerve is then stimulated in the antecubital fossa along the medial border of the brachioradialis (S2). In obese patients, needle stimulation at the elbow is required. Conduction velocities in the distal segment are determined by dividing the 10 cm distance by the distal latency. Forearm conduction is calculated by dividing the distance between S2 and S1 by the difference between the proximal and distal latencies. Normal values are 56.4 ± 4.0 m/s with amplitudes of 30.5 ± 5.0 µV for the wrist–first web space and 61.4 ± 3.1 m/s with amplitudes of 19.2 ± 6.4 µV for elbow–wrist, with a right–left difference of 1.8 ± 1.6 m/s.[112] The LACBN latencies are performed by stimulating the musculocutaneous nerve lateral to the biceps tendon, while record-

ing the SNAP 12 cm distally. Normal LACBN velocities from the elbow–wrist are 61.7 ± 2.9 m/s. A normal LACBN–SRN difference in the same arm is 1.9 ± 1.6 milliseconds.

The distal radial sensory latency may be normal even in the presence of abnormal forearm conduction. This commonly occurs with nerve entrapment due to segmental conduction velocity slowing. In mild cases, comparison studies with the ipsilateral LACBN and with contralateral SRN conduction can increase the diagnostic yield. The diagnosis of radial sensory nerve entrapment in the presence of an overlapping normal LABCN is made by comparing values obtained for each of these nerves with each other and with normative data.[113] In more advanced cases, slowing or a complete block of the distal SRN occurs. If the response is absent, it is difficult to localize the lesion.

RADICULOPATHY

A myotome consist of all of the muscles of a limb that are innervated by a specific nerve root level. Because of the multilevel innervation of limb muscles, each muscle belongs to more than one myotome. Anterior (efferent) and posterior (afferent) nerve roots arising from the spinal cord fuse to form the spinal nerve, which in turn divide into the anterior and posterior primary rami. Efferent motor fibers from the anterior cervical rami fuse to form the brachial plexus. Afferent sensory fibers from the posterior root fuse to form the dorsal root ganglion outside the neural foramen, where the sensory nerve cell bodies reside. Nerve root compression may result in subjective sensory abnormalities, although the SNAPs will remain normal. This is because the distal sensory nerve axons remain connected to healthy cell bodies in the dorsal root ganglion, which are distal to the lesion at the foraminal level. Cell bodies of the motor fibers are located in the ventral horn of the spinal cord. Radicular lesions thus lead to a loss of motor axons and Wallerian degeneration, with the subsequent appearance of fibrillation potentials and PSWs.

It is necessary to examine at least two or three muscles per myotome in both the anterior and posterior primary rami distribution. In a C6 lesion, for example, denervation potentials may be seen in the biceps, extensor carpi radialis, and pronator teres, but not the triceps, abductor pollicus brevis, or first dorsal interosseous muscles. For uncertain reasons, EMG abnormalities may occasionally be seen in only one or two limb muscles. It is not uncommon for patients to have both a C6–C7 cervical radiculopathy and carpal tunnel compression, or a C8–T1 radiculopathy and cubital tunnel syndrome. A nerve conduction study should therefore always be performed.

PARASPINAL EMG

If abnormalities are noted in the paraspinal muscles as well as the upper limb, the lesion must be as far proximal as the root level, since both the anterior and posterior first rami are affected. Approximately 25% to 40% of patients with a radiculopathy may demonstrate fibrillation potentials only in the paraspinal muscles.[114] Radiculopathies are one possible cause of paraspinal abnormalities, but any disorder of the anterior horn cell, posterior rami, or the muscle fibers themselves can produce membrane instability such as motor neuron disease, myopathies, diabetes, and so on.

BRACHIAL PLEXUS LESIONS

An axonal lesion distal to the origin of the posterior primary ramus, such as a brachial plexus lesion, should not affect the paraspinals. Since the plexus is distal to the dorsal root ganglion, the SNAP amplitudes should be decreased due to the loss of afferent sensory fibers. The EMG findings reflect the loss of motor axons as above. Lesions of the plexus may occur due to compression while lying on the side or with prolonged traction as a result of abnormal limb position while in an obtunded state secondary to drugs, alcohol, or general anesthesia.

EXAMPLE

A 48-year-old auto mechanic presented with a history of an alcohol-induced coma 3 months previously. After sleeping in a chair for 3 to 4 hours, he was moved to the floor where he lay recumbent for another 4 hours. He awoke with a flail upper extremity. It was noted that the patient also had a 10-year history of right-hand numbness that was precipitated by gripping. At the time of the initial consultation, the patient had regained some elbow flexion. The exam demonstrated 3/5 biceps and 3/5 brachioradialis power. He had 0/5 deltoid, 0/5 supraspinatus, 0/5 infraspinatus, 5/5 rhomboids, and 5/5 latissimus strength (Fig. 21–18 A). There was no scapular winging, and Horner's syndrome was absent. Sensory testing was normal.

A cervical MRI revealed no evidence of root avulsion, but there was significant hematoma in the anterior and posterior cervical triangles (Fig. 21–18 B). The NCS showed prolonged distal median motor latencies (due to superimposed CTS) with normal radial and ulnar motor conduction. There were generalized abnormalities of the SNAPs of the median, ulnar, and radial nerves. EMG testing demonstrated widespread denervation in the muscles innervated by the upper trunk with partial middle trunk involvement (Fig. 21–18 C). There was sparing of the lower trunk muscles (Table 21–12). There were some voluntary polyphasic CMAPs in the deltoid despite the absence of a palpable muscle contraction (Fig. 21–18 D). The cervical paraspinal EMG was normal, indicating that the lesion was distal to the posterior primary rami. Based on these findings, it was recommended that the patient undergo nerve transfers to restore shoulder abduction in addition to a carpal tunnel release.

Brachial Plexopathy

Brachial plexopathy (Parsonage-Turner syndrome, neuralgic amyotrophy) typically occurs after a viral illness. The most common pattern appears to be either a single mononeuropathy or multiple mononeuropathies affecting primarily the suprascapular, long thoracic, or axillary nerves.[115] Additionally the phrenic and anterior interosseous nerves may involved. The differentiating

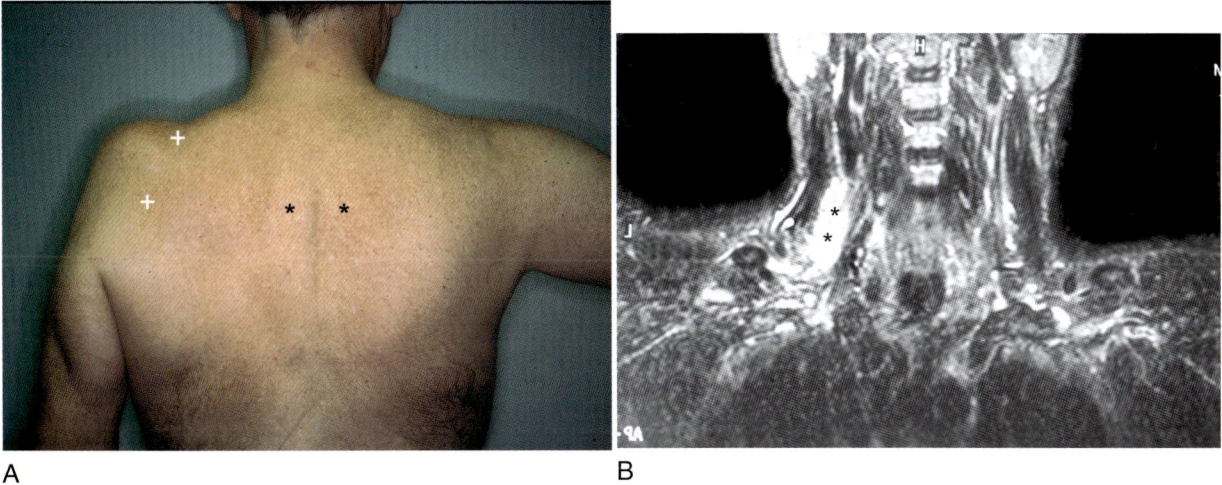

Figure 21–18 Upper/middle trunk palsy. **A:** Attempted left shoulder abduction. Note the wasting of the shoulder girdle muscles (+) but the normal rhomboids (*). **B:** Cervical magnetic resonance image demonstrating hematoma in the cervical triangle (*).

TABLE 21–12				
Upper/Middle Trunk Palsy				
Muscle	**Nerve**	**Root**	**Rest Activity**	**Recruitment**
Abductor pollicus brevis	Median	C8-T1	Silent	Normal
Flexor pollicus longus	Median	(C7),C8,T1	Silent	Normal
Flexor carpi radialis	Median	C6,C7,(C8)	4+ Fibs/PSW	Reduced
1st Dorsal interosseous	Ulnar	C8,T1	Silent	Normal
Pronator teres	Median	C6,C7	4 Fibs/PSW	Reduced
Extensor carpi radialis	Radial	C6,C7,(C8)	Silent	Normal
Brachioradialis	Radial	C5,C6	4+ Fibs/PSW	Absent
Biceps	MCN	C5,C6	4 Fibs/PSW	Reduced
Triceps	Radial	(C6),C7,C8	Silent	Normal
Deltoid	Axillary	C5,C6	4 Fibs/PSW	Reduced
Suprapinatus	Suprascapular	C5,C6	4+ Fibs/PSW	Absent
Infraspinatus	Suprascapular	C5,C6	4+ Fibs/PSW	Absent
Rhomboids	Dorsal scapular	C(4),C5	Silent	Normal
Trapezius	Spinal accessory	C3,C4	2+ Fibs/PSW	Reduced
Cervical paraspinals	Rami	C4–C7	Silent	Normal

Fibs, fibrillations; MCN, musculocutaneous nerve; PSW, positive sharp wave.

feature hinges on the demonstration of widespread EMG abnormalities outside of the AIN innervation. If the cervical paraspinals are affected, one must rule out a radicular lesion.

COMBINED NERVE INJURY

Combined nerve palsies can be a challenge to sort out. It can be quite difficult to differentiate this from a brachial plexus lesion or a brachial neuritis purely by clinical means. Electrodiagnostic studies are often necessary to establish the diagnosis.

EXAMPLE

A 50-year-old male presented with an 8-week history of left hand numbness and weakness after an intravenous heroin overdose. The patient was unsure as to whether he released the arm strap that he was using as a tourniquet before passing out. The NCS/EMG diagnosis by the treating neurologist was that of severe CTS and ulnar nerve compression at the wrist. On the presenting physical exam, it was noted that the patient held his wrist in an extended and supinated position. The wrist and finger joints were supple. The forearm

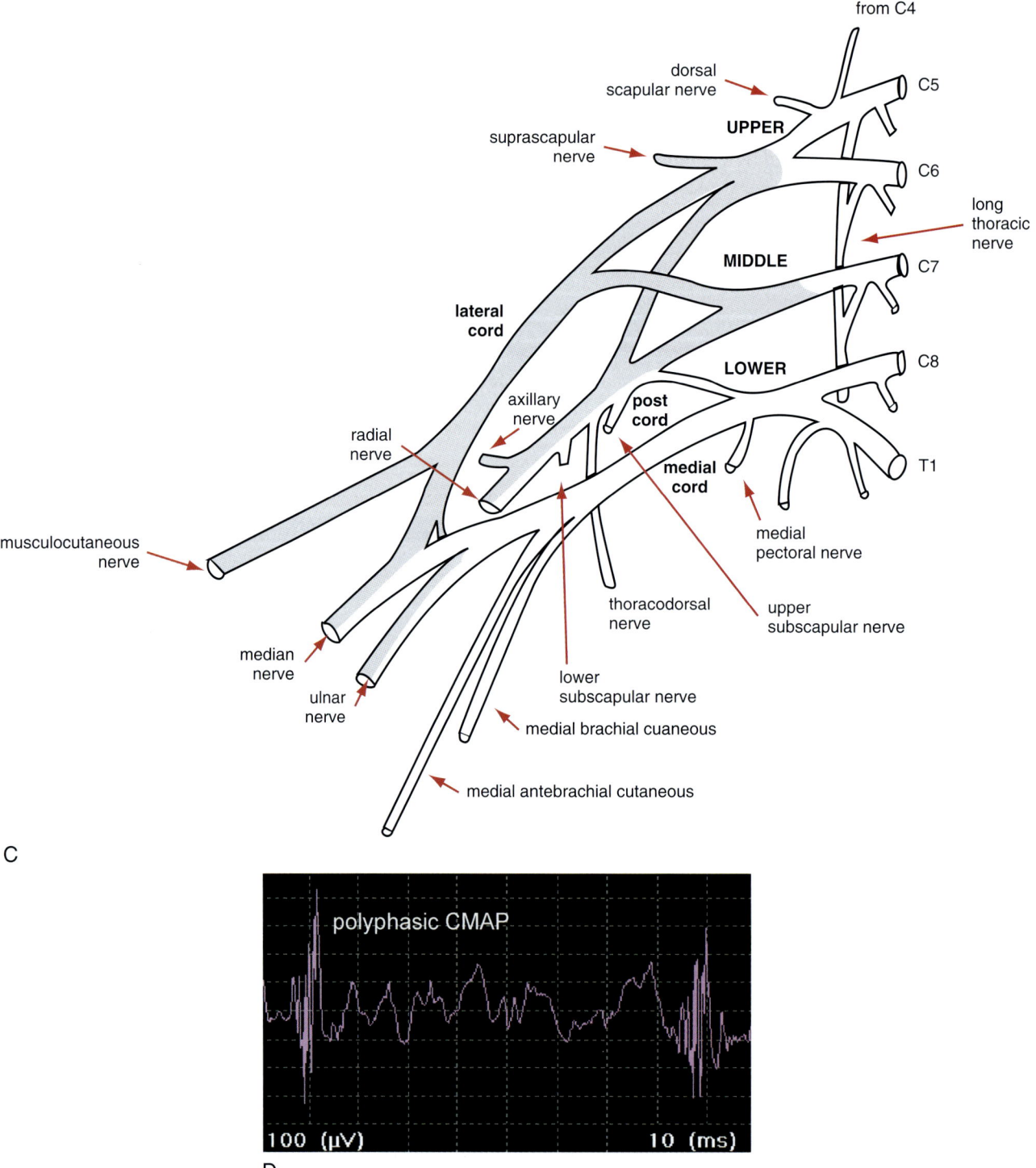

C

D

Figure 21–18–Cont'd   Upper/middle trunk palsy. **C:** Brachial plexus drawing illustrating the pattern of denervation found in a lesion affecting the upper and middle trunks. **D:** Electromyography of the deltoid demonstrating sparse, low-amplitude (600 μV), polyphasic compound motor action potentials with maximum voluntary contraction.

TABLE 21–13

Combined Nerve Palsy

Muscle	Nerve	Root	Rest Activity	Recruitment
Abductor pollicus brevis	Median	C8-T1	4+ Fibs/PSW	Absent
Flexor pollicus longus	AIN	(C7),C8,T1	4+ Fibs/PSW	Absent
Pronator quadratus	AIN	C7-T1	4+ Fibs/PSW	Absent
Flexor digitorum sublimus	Median	C7-T1	2+ Fibs/PSW	Reduced
1st Dorsal interosseous	Ulnar	C8,T1	4+ Fibs/PSW	Absent
Flexor digitorum profundus (III and IV)	Ulnar	C7-T1	4+ Fibs/PSW	Absent
Extensor indicis proprius	PIN	C7,C8	2+ Fibs/PSW	Reduced
Extensor digitorum communis	PIN	C7,C8	2+ Fibs/PSW	Reduced
Brachioradialis	Radial	C5,C6	2+ Fibs/PSW	Reduced
Biceps	MCN	C5,C6	Silent	Normal
Triceps	Radial	(C6),C7,C8	Silent	Normal
Deltoid	Axillary	C5,C6	Silent	Normal
Cervical paraspinals	Rami	C6-T1	Silent	Normal

Fibs, fibrillations; MCN, musculocutaneous nerve; PSW, positive sharp wave.

compartments were soft without evidence of Volkman's ischemia. There was a 1-cm eschar and indentation of the posteromedial arm (Fig. 21–19 A). There was a positive Tinel sign over the ulnar and median nerves, but a negative Tinel's over the radial nerve and the supraclavicular fossa. There was atrophy and paralysis of the APB, the intrinsics, FPL, PQ, PT, FCR, and FCU (Fig. 21–19 B). He had 3/5 sublimus power, 4/5 ECRB/L, 4/5 EDC, and 4/5 BR power. There was 5/5 strength of the biceps, triceps, deltoids, pectorals, latissimus suprapinatus, infraspinatus, rhomboids, and trapezius. The patient had no scapular winging and an absent Horner's sign. Two-point discrimination was more than 25 mm for the thumb and all of the fingers. The patient was numb along the course of the medial antebrachial cutaneous nerve (MABCN), but he had normal sensation in the distributions of the medial brachial cutaneous nerve, SRN, and LABCN.

The NCS showed a complete motor and sensory conduction block of the median and ulnar nerves, which made localization of the lesion difficult. There were normal radial distal motor latencies and normal radial motor CV across the elbow with no significant loss of amplitude. The distal radial sensory latency was only marginally prolonged. EMG testing revealed extensive denervation in the median and ulnar nerve distribution with some membrane instability of the radial innervated muscles distal to the spiral groove despite the normal radial motor nerve conduction (Table 21–13). There were no fibrillation potentials in the sternocostal head of the pectoralis or the latissimus. The diagnosis was that of a combined high median and ulnar nerve palsy

with a MABCN neuropraxia and partial involvement of the radial nerve distal to the spiral groove.

With a history of prolonged unconsciousness, one must be suspicious of a plexus injury. In fact, there are many features of this case that mimic a lower trunk lesion with involvement of the medial and posterior cords. The EDX findings ruled against this, however. The absence of membrane instability of the sternocostal head of the pectoralis muscle and the latissimus established that the lesion was distal to the takeoff of the medial pectoral and thoracodorsal nerves. The sensory innervation to the thumb, and index and middle fingers is through the median nerve by way of the upper and middle trunks (C5, C6, C7). Motor innervation to the thenar muscles, however, was through the lower trunk. As a result, axonal injury to the lower trunk results in denervation of the thenar and hypothenar muscles, but spares sensation to the thumb, and index and middle fingers. In order to account for the patient's sensory loss of the thumb, and index and middle fingers, there would have to be either upper trunk or lateral cord involvement, but there was no electrodiagnostic evidence to support this.

At the time of surgery, there was a region of swollen, grayish brachialis muscle with secondary ulnar nerve constriction by the tense overlying fascia (Fig. 21–19 C and D). The median nerve appeared normal. At the 10-month follow-up, the patient had a positive Tinel's sign along the course of the median and ulnar nerves into the fingertips. He had regained 5+ power of the PT, FCR, FCU, and FPL as well as 5+ power of the FDS and FDP to all of the fingers. He had normal 2 point discrimination of 5 mm for the thumb and fingers and normal sensation of the MABCN. However, he still had no return of intrinsic muscle function with 0/5 power of the APB, ADM and FDI.

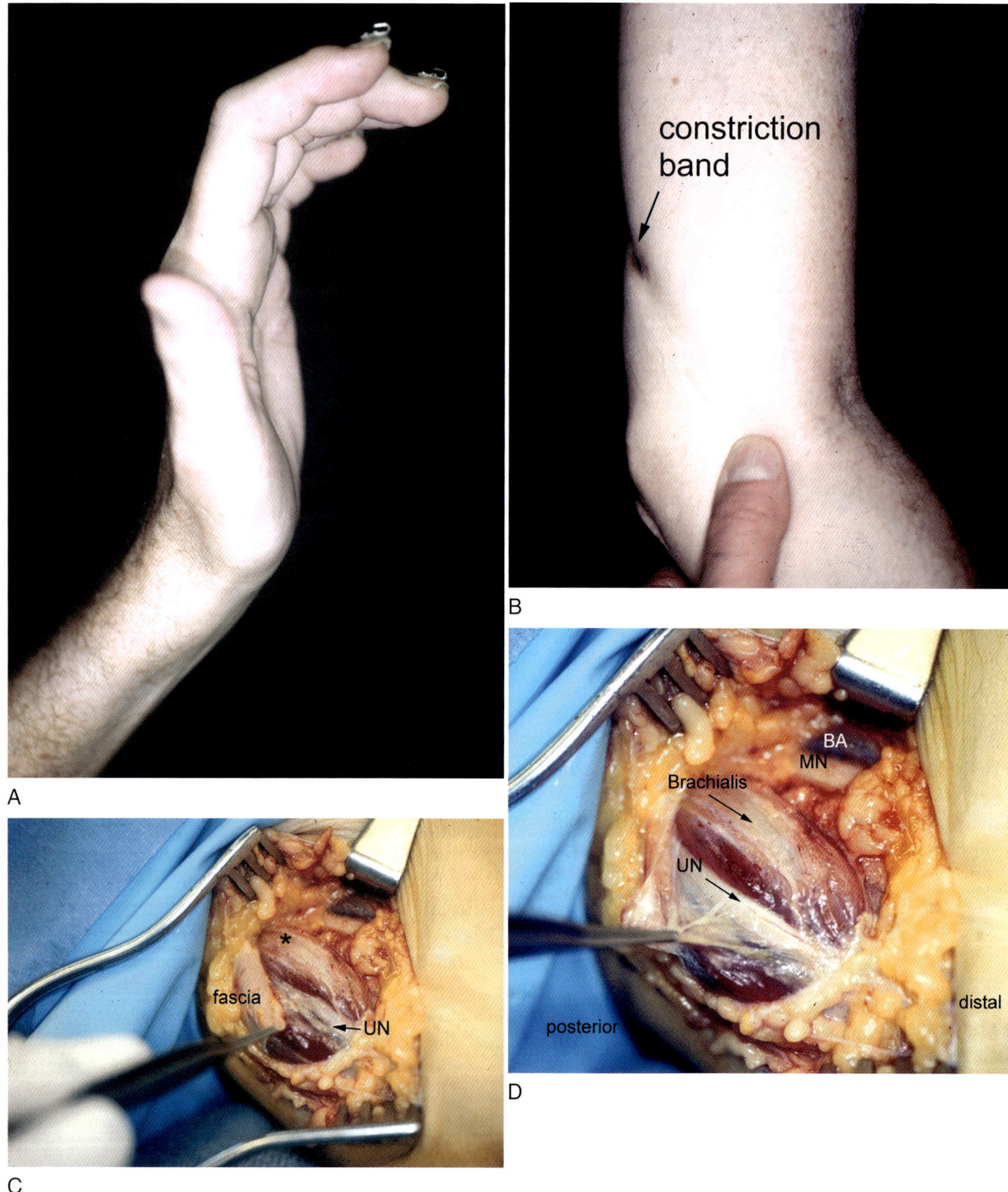

Figure 21–19 Combined nerve palsy. **A:** There is an eschar along with indentation of the posteromedial border of the arm. **B:** Observe the marked thenar and intrinsic muscle atrophy. **C:** Swollen and nonviable medial brachialis muscle (*) with tense overlying fascia. **D:** Note the interruption of the longitudinal epineurial vessels of the ulnar nerve. BA, brachial artery; MN, median nerve; UN, ulnar nerve.

Essential Components of the Electrodiagnostic Report

One study of a 100 reports revealed widespread inadequacies.[116] In order to be able to adequately interpret test results, a number of parameters must be included in the nerve conduction report. These include the distances between the recording electrodes and the stimulation sites (since reference values are based on standardized distances), the amplitude of the waveform, conduction velocities, limb temperature, and normal reference values. The EMG report should list the type of needle used, the insertional activity with the muscle at rest, and the presence of spontaneous potentials. An analysis of the MUAP configuration, amplitude, and duration with minimal and maximal contraction, as well as the recruitment pattern, should be included. A list of the muscles along with their segmental innervation facilitates a localization of the lesion.

NERVE CONDUCTION STUDY PITFALLS

There are a number of factors that affect the nerve conduction study. Certain potential pitfalls must be looked for such as volume conduction. Placing an electrode on the skin over a specific muscle does not ensure that the only response detected will arise from the desired tissue.[30] If the nerve in question has a partial or complete block, it is usual to turn up the gain (current). At some point, an adjacent nerve will be stimulated which can lead to a false waveform (Fig. 21–20 A and B). Often, the only clue is the morphology of the waveform plus a high index of suspicion. Error may also arise when the onset marker is erroneously positioned, which commonly occurs with the double-peaked ulnar CMAP. This leads to falsely prolonged distal motor latencies and lower amplitudes. The newer digital machines set the markers automatically, so it is good practice to quickly review the waveforms before looking at the data.

Falsely low amplitudes can be secondary to temporal dispersion.[117] Any given nerve is composed of faster and slower conducting axons. The NAP is the summation of thousands of individual fibers. When there is a longer distance between the site of nerve stimulation and the recording electrodes, such as with above elbow stimulation, there is less synchronous arrival of action potentials due to a marked variation in conduction velocities between the individual nerve fibers. Less "in-phase" summation of similar waveform aspects leads to phase cancellation and amplitude reduction. This leads to a wave with a longer duration. Temporal dispersion occurs more with sensory than motor nerves due to their faster conduction velocity. It can lead to falsely low amplitudes that may be interpreted as axonal loss. This

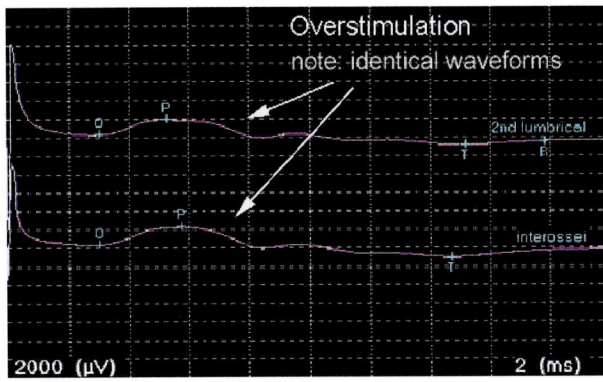

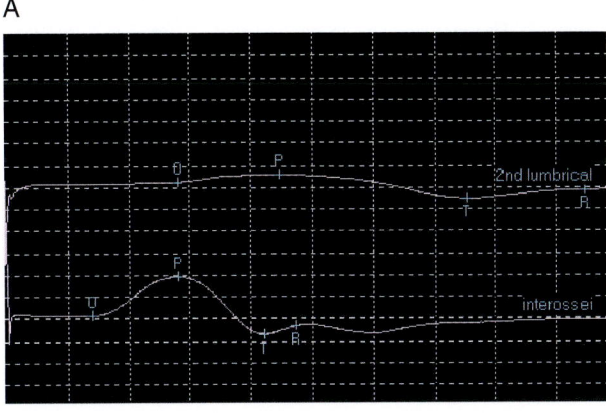

Figure 21–20 Lumbrical–interosseous recording in severe carpal tunnel syndrome. **A:** Median nerve overstimulation also depolarizes the ulnar nerve. The second palmar interosseous compound motor action potential replaces the second lumbrical response. The result is identical waveforms. **B:** As the median nerve stimulus is decreased, a delayed and low amplitude second lumbrical response is unmasked. Note the difference in the waveform morphology. (From Slutsky DJ. Nerve conduction studies in hand surgery. J Am Soc Surg Hand 2003;3:152–69, with permission.)

can be suspected by calculating the area under the waveform, which will be normal in temporal dispersion, and reduced with axonal loss.

Temperature effects can affect the values considerably; hence, it is important to measure the hand temperature during testing. The conduction velocity changes 5% for each 1°C change in temperature.[118] The distal latencies may increase and conduction velocities may decrease when the hand is cool.[119] In general, the hand should be at least 30°C. The need for rewarming should be indicated on the report.

ELECTROMYOGRAPHY PITFALLS

False Positive

Insufficient Muscles Examined

Radicular injuries are diagnosed not only by documenting abnormalities in a particular myotome, but

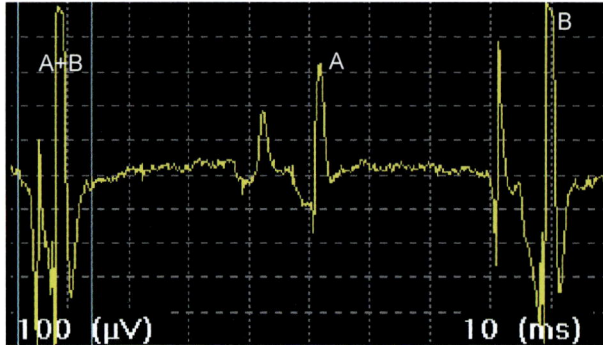

Figure 21–21 Pseudopolyphasia. Motor unit action potential (MUAP) (A) and (B) run together, producing an artificially polyphasic MUAP. (From Slutsky D. Electromyography in hand surgery. J Am Soc Surg Hand 2004;4:176–86, with permission.)

demonstrating a distinct lack of abnormalities in other myotomes, especially of the opposite limb.

Misidentification of Normal Potentials

End-plate spikes that fire irregularly at high rates may be mistaken for fibrillation potentials, which fire regularly at slower rates.

Overinterpretation of Normal Variants

Trains of PSWs may last longer than anticipated after needle insertion or movement, which is a normal variant, and is not diagnostic of any nerve or muscle disorder.[120]

Motor Unit Action Potential Overlap

MUAPs that run together may appear polyphasic and of increased duration (Fig. 21–21). This can be minimized by using a trigger and delay line on the EMG trace to ensure that the same MUAP is being examined.

False Negative
Time of Study

Generally, the peak of fibrillations and PSWs is 2 to 4 weeks. An exam performed within the first 7 to 10 days may be falsely negative.

Temperature

Decreased temperature suppresses the firing rates and the number of fibrillation potentials and PSWs.

Instrumentation Defects

Defective EMG needles may lead to faulty recordings.

Motor Unit Action Potential Parameters

MUAP amplitude varies with respect to the distance between the recording electrode and the muscle fiber. An MUAP should only be analyzed when the distance between the needle electrode an the muscle tissue is optimal so that the needle is close to the fiber that its recording. The MUAP sound should be crisp and loud; otherwise, error may be introduced in measuring the amplitude, duration, and phases.

Polyphasia

Polyphasic potentials are only of diagnostic value when quantified with a trigger line by examining at least 20 individual MUAPs, and then calculating the percent of polyphasic potentials. An increase in polyphasic potentials only implies that at some point the motor unit has undergone remodeling. This is not by itself diagnostic of any specific disease or time of occurrence. All persons have some degree of polyphasic potentials.

Recruitment

Recruitment abnormalities are not especially sensitive and rarely aid in the diagnosis unless accompanied by fibrillation potentials, PSWs, and MUAP duration changes. It can be difficult for some patients to recruit only a single motor unit even during minimal voluntary contraction. Distal muscles are more prone to false-positive results.

Interference Pattern

An interference pattern is not equivalent to recruitment. It rarely provides any information and can be the subject of false-positive results due to lack of patient cooperation or pain, or needle placement too distant from the muscle tissue.

Age

It is believed that with age, there is a gradual loss of anterior horn cells.[121] This subclinical muscle denervation induces collateral sprouting to remodel the remaining motor units. The increase in the number of muscle fibers per motor unit results in an increase of the MUAP duration and amplitude with age, which can be falsely interpreted as a neurogenic lesion.

SUMMARY

Combined with a detailed medical history and a thorough upper extremity examination, the nerve conduction test can yield useful information. The test results, however, cannot be taken out of context. It is not uncommon for a patient to be totally asymptomatic yet a nerve conduction study is reported as showing mild slowing of the conduction velocities and latencies if the hand is cold, or if the electrode is making poor contact. The NCS findings may be of subclinical or no clinical significance. More so than nerve conduction studies, EMG is an art form honed through practice and experience. The EMG exam can provide useful information as to the normal and abnormal electrophysiology of muscle and its nerve. The various potentials described, however, do not point to a specific diagnosis.

Most hand surgeons intuitively understand that the indication for surgery still hinges on reproducible physical findings combined with the appropriate clinical symptoms rather than on a test abnormality. Through an understanding of the methodology and principles of testing the clinician will be better suited to recognizing when the report conclusions do not match the data, or when to request further testing in cases where insufficient data compromises one's ability to draw definitive conclusions.

REFERENCES

1. Slutsky D. Nerve conduction studies in hand surgery. J Am Soc Surg Hand 2002;3:1–18.
2. Slutsky DJ. Electrodiagnostic testing in hand surgery. Atlas of the Hand Clinics. Nerve Repair and Reconstruction: A Practical Guide, Vol. 10, No. 1. Philadelphia: W.B. Saunders, 2005: 33–63.
3. Slutsky D. Recurrent Carpal Tunnel Syndrome: Pathophysiology and Diagnosis. In: Programs and Abstracts of 59th annual meeting of the American Society for Surgery of the Hand, New York, September 11, 2004.
4. Slutsky D. Nerve Conduction Studies in the Office and Operating Room. Programs and Abstracts of the 57th annual meeting of the American Society for Surgery of the Hand, Phoenix, AZ, October 3, 2002.
5. Slutsky D. Electromyography in hand surgery. J Am Soc Surg Hand 2004;4:176–86.
6. Slutsky D. Electrophysiology in Nerve Injury. In: Programs and Abstracts of the 58th annual meeting of the American Society for Surgery of the Hand, Chicago, September 18, 2003.
7. Waxman SG. Determinants of conduction velocity in myelinated nerve fibers. Muscle Nerve 1980;3:141–50.
8. Dahlin LB, Shyu BC, Danielsen N, et al. Effects of nerve compression or ischaemia on conduction properties of myelinated and non-myelinated nerve fibres. An experimental study in the rabbit common peroneal nerve. Acta Physiol Scand 1989; 136:97–105.
9. Brumback RA, Bobele GB, Rayan GM. Electrodiagnosis of compressive nerve lesions. Hand Clin 1992;8:241–54.
10. Dellon A. Pitfalls in interpretation of electrophysiological testing. In: Gelberman RH, ed., Operative Nerve Repair and Reconstruction, vol. 1. Philadelphia: J.B. Lippincott, 1991:185–96.
11. Rydevik B, Lundborg G. Permeability of intraneural microvessels and perineurium following acute, graded experimental nerve compression. Scand J Plast Reconstr Surg 1977; 11:179–87.
12. Lundborg G, Dahlin LB. The pathophysiology of nerve compression. Hand Clin 1992;8:215–27.
13. Eversmann WW Jr, Ritsick JA. Intraoperative changes in motor nerve conduction latency in carpal tunnel syndrome. J Hand Surg Am 1978;3:77–81.
14. Felsenthal G. Median and ulnar distal motor and sensory latencies in the same normal subject. Arch Phys Med Rehabil 1977;58:297–302.
15. Johnson EW, Kukla RD, Wongsam PE, et al. Sensory latencies to the ring finger: normal values and relation to carpal tunnel syndrome. Arch Phys Med Rehabil 1981;62:206–8.
16. Wongsam PE, Johnson EW, Weinerman JD. Carpal tunnel syndrome: use of palmar stimulation of sensory fibers. Arch Phys Med Rehabil 1983;64:16–9.
17. Stevens JC. The electrodiagnosis of carpal tunnel syndrome. American Association of Electrodiagnostic Medicine. Muscle Nerve 1997;20:1477–86.
18. Kimura J. The carpal tunnel syndrome: localization of conduction abnormalities within the distal segment of the median nerve. Brain 1979;102:619–35.
19. Olney RK, Wilbourn AJ. Ulnar nerve conduction study of the first dorsal interosseous muscle. Arch Phys Med Rehabil 1985;66:16–8.
20. Eisen A. Early diagnosis of ulnar nerve palsy. An electrophysiologic study. Neurology 1974;24:256–62.
21. Buschbacher RM. Ulnar 14-cm and 7-cm antidromic sensory studies to the fifth digit: reference values derived from a large population of normal subjects. Am J Phys Med Rehabil 1999;78:S63–8.
22. Trojaborg W, Sindrup EH. Motor and sensory conduction in different segments of the radial nerve in normal subjects. J Neurol Neurosurg Psychiatry 1969;32:354–9.
23. Ma DM, Kim SH, Spielholz N, et al. Sensory conduction study of distal radial nerve. Arch Phys Med Rehabil 1981; 62:562–4.
24. Preston DC, Logigian EL. Lumbrical and interossei recording in carpal tunnel syndrome. Muscle Nerve 1992;15:1253–7.
25. Kothari MJ, Preston DC, Logigian EL. Lumbrical-interossei motor studies localize ulnar neuropathy at the wrist. Muscle Nerve 1996;19:170–4.
26. Nasr JT, Kaufman MA. Electrophysiologic findings in two patients with digital neuropathy of the thumb. Electromyogr Clin Neurophysiol 2001;41:353–6.
27. Spaans F. Neurographic assessment of lesions of single proper digital nerves. Clin Neurophysiol 2001;112:2113–7.
28. Terai Y, Senda M, Hashizume H, et al. Selective measurement of digital nerve conduction velocity. J Orthop Sci 2001; 6:123–7.
29. King JC, Dumitru D, Wertsch JJ. Digit distribution of proper digital nerve action potential. Muscle Nerve 2001;24:1489–95.
30. Dumitru D, eds. Electrodiagnostic Medicine. Philadelphia: Hanley and Belfus, 1995.
31. Buchthal F, Schmalbruch H. Motor unit of mammalian muscle. Physiol Rev 1980;60:90–142.
32. Buchthal F, Erminio F, Rosenfalck P. Motor unit territory in different human muscles. Acta Physiol Scand 1959;45:72–87.
33. Katz B, Miledi R. Propagation of electric activity in motor nerve terminals. Proc R Soc Lond B Biol Sci 1965;161:453–82.
34. Chu J, Bruyninckx F, Chan RC. Significance of motor unit action potential parameters in normal and neurogenic situations. Electromyogr Clin Neurophysiol 1986;26:465–79.

35. Thiele B, Bohle A. [Number of spike components contributing to the motor unit potential]. EEG EMG Z Elektroenzephalogr Elektromyogr Verwandte Geb 1978;9:125–30.

36. Miller RG. Injury to peripheral motor nerves. Muscle Nerve 1987;10:698–710.

37. Brown MC, Ironton R. Sprouting and regression of neuromuscular synapses in partially denervated mammalian muscles. J Physiol 1978;278:325–48.

38. Feinstein B, Lindegard B, Nyman E, et al. Morphologic studies of motor units in normal human muscles. Acta Anat (Basel) 1955;23:127–42.

39. Dumitru D, King JC, Stegeman DF. Endplate spike morphology: a clinical and simulation study. Arch Phys Med Rehabil 1998;79:634–40.

40. Buchthal F, Rosenfalck P. Spontaneous electrical activity of human muscle. Electroencephalogr Clin Neurophysiol 1966; 20:321–36.

41. Thesleff S, Ward MR. Studies on the mechanism of fibrillation potentials in denervated muscle. J Physiol 1975;244:313–23.

42. Partanen JV, Danner R. Fibrillation potentials after muscle injury in humans. Muscle Nerve 1982;5:S70–3.

43. Kraft GH. Are fibrillation potentials and positive sharp waves the same? No. Muscle Nerve 1996;19:216–20.

44. Daube JR. Needle examination in clinical electromyography. Muscle Nerve 1991;14:685–700.

45. Carter GT, Robinson LR, Chang VH, et al. Electrodiagnostic evaluation of traumatic nerve injuries. Hand Clin 2000;16: 1–12, vii.

46. Dorfman LJ. Quantitative clinical electrophysiology in the evaluation of nerve injury and regeneration. Muscle Nerve 1990;13:822–8.

47. Nandedkar SD, Barkhaus PE, Sanders DB, et al. Some observations on fibrillations and positive sharp waves. Muscle Nerve 2000;23:888–94.

48. Wiechers D, Stow R, Johnson EW. Electromyographic insertional activity mechanically provoked in the biceps brachii. Arch Phys Med Rehabil 1977;58:573–8.

49. Warmolts JR, Engel WK. Open-biopsy electromyography. I. Correlation of motor unit behavior with histochemical muscle fiber type in human limb muscle. Arch Neurol 1972;27:512–7.

50. Petajan JH. Motor unit recruitment. Muscle Nerve 1991;14: 489–502.

51. Dahlin LB, Lundborg G. The neurone and its response to peripheral nerve compression. J Hand Surg Br 1990;15:5–10.

52. Lundborg G. Ischemic nerve injury. Experimental studies on intraneural microvascular pathophysiology and nerve function in a limb subjected to temporary circulatory arrest. Scand J Plast Reconstr Surg Suppl 1970;6:3–113.

53. Trojaborg W. Early electrophysiologic changes in conduction block. Muscle Nerve 1978;1:400–3.

54. Kiraly JK, Krnjevic K. Some retrograde changes in function of nerves after peripheral section. Q J Exp Physiol Cogn Med Sci 1959;44:244–57.

55. Landau WM. The duration of neuromuscular function after nerve section in man. J Neurosurg 1953;10:64–8.

56. Chaudhry V, Cornblath DR. Wallerian degeneration in human nerves: serial electrophysiological studies. Muscle Nerve 1992; 15:687–93.

57. Kraft GH. Fibrillation potential amplitude and muscle atrophy following peripheral nerve injury. Muscle Nerve 1990;13: 814–21.

58. Kline DG. Surgical repair of peripheral nerve injury. Muscle Nerve 1990;13:843–52.

59. Trojaborg W, Sindrup E. Radial nerve palsies: clinical and electrophysiological aspects. Electroencephalogr Clin Neurophysiol 1969;26:342.

60. Terzis JK BM. Sensory receptors. In: Gelberman RH, ed., Operative Nerve Repair and Reconstruction. Philadelphia: J.B. Lippincott, 1991:85–105.

61. Kothari MJ, Rutkove SB, Caress JB, et al. Comparison of digital sensory studies in patients with carpal tunnel syndrome. Muscle Nerve 1995;18:1272–6.

62. Redmond MD, Rivner MH. False positive electrodiagnostic tests in carpal tunnel syndrome. Muscle Nerve 1988;11:511–8.

63. Robinson LR, Micklesen PJ, Wang L. Optimizing the number of tests for carpal tunnel syndrome. Muscle Nerve 2000; 23:1880–2.

64. Robinson LR, Micklesen PJ, Wang L. Strategies for analyzing nerve conduction data: superiority of a summary index over single tests. Muscle Nerve 1998;21:1166–71.

65. Lundborg G, Gelberman RH, Minteer-Convery M, et al. Median nerve compression in the carpal tunnel—functional response to experimentally induced controlled pressure. J Hand Surg Am 1982;7:252–9.

66. Bennett JB, Crouch CC. Compression syndrome of the recurrent motor branch of the median nerve. J Hand Surg Am 1982;7:407–9.

67. Mackinnon SE, Dellon AL. Experimental study of chronic nerve compression. Clinical implications. Hand Clin 1986;2:639–50.

68. al-Qattan MM, Bowen V, Manktelow RT. Factors associated with poor outcome following primary carpal tunnel release in nondiabetic patients. J Hand Surg Br 1994;19:622–5.

69. Braun RM, Jackson WJ. Electrical studies as a prognostic factor in the surgical treatment of carpal tunnel syndrome. J Hand Surg Am 1994;19:893–900.

70. Glowacki KA, Breen CJ, Sachar K, et al. Electrodiagnostic testing and carpal tunnel release outcome. J Hand Surg Am 1996;21:117–21.

71. Steyers CM. Recurrent carpal tunnel syndrome. Hand Clin 2002;18:339–45.

72. Hunter JM. Recurrent carpal tunnel syndrome, epineural fibrous fixation, and traction neuropathy. Hand Clin 1991;7: 491–504.

73. Bronson J, Beck J, Gillet J. Provocative motor nerve conduction testing in presumptive carpal tunnel syndrome unconfirmed by traditional electrodiagnostic testing. J Hand Surg Am 1997;22:1041–6.

74. Read RL. Stress testing in nerve compression. Hand Clin 1991;7:521–6.

75. Ekman-Ordeberg G, Salgeback S, Ordeberg G. Carpal tunnel syndrome in pregnancy. A prospective study. Acta Obstet Gynecol Scand 1987;66:233–5.

76. Seror P. [Carpal tunnel syndrome in pregnancy]. J Gynecol Obstet Biol Reprod (Paris) 1997;26:148–53.

77. Stolp-Smith KA, Pascoe MK, Ogburn PL Jr. Carpal tunnel syndrome in pregnancy: frequency, severity, and prognosis. Arch Phys Med Rehabil 1998;79:1285–7.

78. Weimer LH, Yin J, Lovelace RE, et al. Serial studies of carpal tunnel syndrome during and after pregnancy. Muscle Nerve 2002;25:914–7.

79. al Qattan MM, Manktelow RT, Bowen CV. Pregnancy-induced carpal tunnel syndrome requiring surgical release longer than 2 years after delivery. Obstet Gynecol 1994;84: 249–51.

80. Wand JS. Carpal tunnel syndrome in pregnancy and lactation. J Hand Surg Br 1990;15:93–5.

81. Wand JS. The natural history of carpal tunnel syndrome in lactation. J R Soc Med 1989;82:349–50.

82. Eversmann WW. Proximal median nerve compression. Hand Clin 1992;8:307–15.

83. Werner CO, Rosen I, Thorngren KG. Clinical and neurophysiologic characteristics of the pronator syndrome. Clin Orthop 1985;231–6.

84. Hartz CR, Linscheid RL, Gramse RR, et al. The pronator teres syndrome: compressive neuropathy of the median nerve. J Bone Joint Surg Am 1981;63:885–90.

85. Johnson RK, Spinner M, Shrewsbury MM. Median nerve entrapment syndrome in the proximal forearm. J Hand Surg Am 1979;4:48–51.

86. Buchthal F, Rosenfalck A, Trojaborg W. Electrophysiological findings in entrapment of the median nerve at wrist and elbow. J Neurol Neurosurg Psychiatry 1974;37:340–60.

87. Mysiew WJ, Colachis SC 3rd. The pronator syndrome. An evaluation of dynamic maneuvers for improving electrodiagnostic sensitivity. Am J Phys Med Rehabil 1991;70:274–7.

88. Olehnik WK, Manske PR, Szerzinski J. Median nerve compression in the proximal forearm. J Hand Surg Am 1994; 19:121–6.

89. Gross PT, Jones HR Jr. Proximal median neuropathies: electromyographic and clinical correlation. Muscle Nerve 1992; 15:390–5.

90. Mysiew WJ, Coalchis SC. Electrophysiologic study of the anterior interosseous nerve. Am J Phys Med Rehabil 1988;50–54.

91. Srinivasan R, Rhodes J. The median-ulnar anastomosis (Martin-Gruber) in normal and congenitally abnormal fetuses. Arch Neurol 1981;38:418–9.

92. Wong L, Dellon AL. Brachial neuritis presenting as anterior interosseous nerve compression—implications for diagnosis and treatment: a case report. J Hand Surg Am 1997;22:536–9.

93. Shea JD, McClain EJ. Ulnar-nerve compression syndromes at and below the wrist. J Bone Joint Surg Am 1969;51:1095–103.

94. Wu JS, Morris JD, Hogan GR. Ulnar neuropathy at the wrist: case report and review of literature. Arch Phys Med Rehabil 1985;66:785–8.

95. McIntosh KA, Preston DC, Logigian EL. Short-segment incremental studies to localize ulnar nerve entrapment at the wrist. Neurology 1998;50:303–6.

96. Spinner M, Spencer PS. Nerve compression lesions of the upper extremity. A clinical and experimental review. Clin Orthop 1974;46–67.

97. Campbell WW, Pridgeon RM, Riaz G, et al. Sparing of the flexor carpi ulnaris in ulnar neuropathy at the elbow. Muscle Nerve 1989;12:965–7.

98. Dellon AL, Schlegel RW, Mackinnon SE. Validity of nerve conduction velocity studies after anterior transposition of the ulnar nerve. J Hand Surg Am 1987;12:700–3.

99. Campbell WW, Pridgeon RM, Sahni KS. Short segment incremental studies in the evaluation of ulnar neuropathy at the elbow. Muscle Nerve 1992;15:1050–4.

100. Azrieli Y, Weimer L, Lovelace R, et al. The utility of segmental nerve conduction studies in ulnar mononeuropathy at the elbow. Muscle Nerve 2003;27:46–50.

101. Campbell WW, Sahni SK, Pridgeon RM, et al. Intraoperative electroneurography: management of ulnar neuropathy at the elbow. Muscle Nerve 1988;11:75–81.

102. Felsenthal G, Freed MJ, Kalafut R, et al. Across-elbow ulnar nerve sensory conduction technique. Arch Phys Med Rehabil 1989;70:668–72.

103. Jabre JF. Ulnar nerve lesions at the wrist: new technique for recording from the sensory dorsal branch of the ulnar nerve. Neurology 1980;30:873–6.

104. Venkatesh S, Kothari MJ, Preston DC. The limitations of the dorsal ulnar cutaneous sensory response in patients with ulnar neuropathy at the elbow. Muscle Nerve 1995;18:345–7.

105. Tomaino MM, Brach PJ, Vansickle DP. The rationale for and efficacy of surgical intervention for electrodiagnostic-negative cubital tunnel syndrome. J Hand Surg Am 2001;26:1077–81.

106. Spinner RJ, Poliakoff MB, Tiel RL. The origin of "Saturday night palsy"? Neurosurgery 2002;51:737–41, discussion 741.

107. Seror P. Posterior interosseous nerve conduction. A new method of evaluation. Am J Phys Med Rehabil 1996;75:35–9.

108. Eaton CJ, Lister GD. Radial nerve compression. Hand Clin 1992;8:345–57.

109. Kupfer DM, Bronson J, Lee GW, et al. Differential latency testing: a more sensitive test for radial tunnel syndrome. J Hand Surg Am 1998;23:859–64.

110. Dellon AL, Mackinnon SE. Radial sensory nerve entrapment in the forearm. J Hand Surg Am 1986;11:199–205.

111. Mackinnon SE, Dellon AL. The overlap pattern of the lateral antebrachial cutaneous nerve and the superficial branch of the radial nerve. J Hand Surg Am 1985;10:522–6.

112. Spindler HA, Dellon AL. Nerve conduction studies in the superficial radial nerve entrapment syndrome. Muscle Nerve 1990;13:1–5.

113. Dellon AL. Radial sensory nerve entrapment. In: Gelberman RH, ed., Operative Nerve Repair and Reconstruction. Philadelphia: J.B. Lippincott, 1991:1039–51.

114. Johnson EW, Melvin JL. Value of electromyography in lumbar radiculopathy. Arch Phys Med Rehabil 1971;52:239–43.

115. Marra TR. The clinical and electrodiagnostic features of idiopathic lumbo-sacral and brachial plexus neuropathy: a review of 20 cases. Electromyogr Clin Neurophysiol 1987;27:305–15.

116. Corwin HM, Kasdan ML. Electrodiagnostic reports of median neuropathy at the wrist. J Hand Surg Am 1998;23:55–7.

117. Krarup C. Compound sensory action potential in normal and pathological human nerves. Muscle Nerve 2004;29:465–83.

118. Halar EM, DeLisa JA, Soine TL. Nerve conduction studies in upper extremities: skin temperature corrections. Arch Phys Med Rehabil 1983;64:412–6.

119. Denys EH. The influence of temperature in clinical neurophysiology. Muscle Nerve 1991;14:795–811.

120. Wiechers DO. Mechanically provoked insertional activity before and after nerve section in rats. Arch Phys Med Rehabil 1977;58:402–5.

121. Brown WF. Functional compensation of human motor units in health and disease. J Neurol Sci 1973;20:199–209.

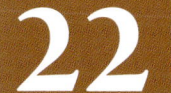

22 Intraoperative Nerve Recordings in the Management of Peripheral Nerve Injuries

Tuna Ozyurekoglu and Warren C. Breidenbach

In the management of peripheral nerve injuries, it is crucial to determine the level and the extent of a lesion. An accurate history and a detailed clinical examination are the first step. The exact location of a lesion can further be confirmed by electrodiagnostic studies and imaging studies. Recent technical advances in magnetic resonance imaging (MRI) have made it a valuable modality for visualization of peripheral nerve injuries.[1] Despite the increasing quality of imaging studies, however, the ability to comprehensively evaluate a nerve lesion from a prognostic point of view is lacking. This is because anatomic continuity does not always equate with functional continuity.

The gross appearance of a lesion during surgery does not provide conclusive information about the internal arrangement or functional status of the nerve.[2] Similarly, in brachial plexus lesions, surgical exploration alone cannot determine whether there is a connection between the peripheral nerve and the brain. For these reasons, intraoperative electrodiagnostic tests have been developed to help delineate the extent of a nerve lesion as well as the functional status of a peripheral nerve. In this chapter, we will first introduce the available electrodiagnostic techniques and then discuss clinical applications.

INTRAOPERATIVE ELECTRODIAGNOSTIC TECHNIQUES

Several electrodiagnostic techniques have been successfully applied during surgery to monitor nerve function, guide dissection, identify and localize neural elements, and to assess nerve function.[2–8] Du Bois-Reymond was the first to demonstrate the action potential of nerves in 1848.[5] He also is credited with describing the electrical activity of muscle (the first electromyogram). Dawson recorded the first somatosensory evoked potentials (SEPs) in 1947.[9] An understanding of other evoked potentials, including those produced by motor activity and by visual and auditory stimulation, followed. Hakstian, in 1968, used a nerve stimulator to map the fascicular topography of the proximal end of peripheral nerves.[10] He then mapped the distal stump by direct fascicular dissection. Kline used intraoperative nerve recordings in the treatment of peripheral nerve injuries and neuromas.[3,11,12] Later he recorded evoked potentials from the surface of nerves. In 1976, Williams and Terzis developed a technique for single fascicular recordings.[2] Around the same period various investigators were studying SEPs recorded from the sensory cortex or cervical spine.[4,13] Jones used sensory nerve action potentials and SEPs in the diagnosis of brachial plexus lesions.[7] In 1980, he introduced a technique for direct root stimulation while recording over the contralateral parietal zone. Celli et al.[14] introduced a method for using intraoperative paravertebral muscular evoked potentials to evaluate the functional continuity of the anterior motor root. Later, motor evoked potential recordings were described to verify the function of anterior spinal roots.[15] Van Beek in 1983 and 1986 used signal-averaging software to minimize technical errors.[5,15,16] Recently, Oberle et al.[17] described their technique for using intraoperative evoked muscle action potentials and SEP recordings to selectively assess partial and/or complete anterior and posterior root disruption.

Whichever technique is used, the success of intraoperative electrodiagnostic studies is highly dependent on the interactions among the surgeon, neurophysiologist, and anesthesiologist. The clinical examination, the preoperative test results, and the operative procedure should be discussed with the neurophysiologist. The surgeon should be familiar with the various electrodiagnostic techniques in order to tailor the choice of technique to provide the most relevant information at any point during the surgery.

The anesthesiologist plays an important role during the intraoperative nerve recording. A deeply anesthetized patient will have no recordable muscular electrical activity in response to peripheral nerve stimulation. The level of anesthesia should be lightened in order to allow the surgeon to elicit and record an evoked potential. The choice of anesthetic agent is critical. The halogenated anesthetics and nitrous oxide depress the appearance of the evoked potentials and prolong the latency of onset.[18,19] These effects are dose dependent. They affect cortically evoked responses more than subcortical, spinal, or peripherally evoked responses. The benzodiazepines, barbiturates, and propofol produce a smaller dose-related depression than the inhalational agents. Ketamine and the opioids have less of an effect on the evoked responses. The use of ketamine, however, does result in some increase in the amplitude of cortically generated SEPs. Muscle relaxants have a minimal effect on nerve recordings.[18–20]

Nerve Conduction Studies

Nerve conduction studies are an important means for evaluating the functional integrity of peripheral nerves.

In a nerve conduction study, the nerve is artificially depolarized with a stimulating electrode. The stimulating electrodes can be unipolar or bipolar. The type of unipolar electrode may include a flush tip probe, a ball tip probe, or a hook electrode. Due to current spread, the use of a unipolar electrode results in co-stimulation of adjacent nerves more commonly than with a bipolar electrode. There is less current dispersal with bipolar electrodes, which restricts the stimulation to a very localized region of the nerve. This allows for single fascicle stimulation. The magnitude of an action potential is directly related to the number of fibers, the synchrony of firing and the fiber diameter.[5,21] In order to minimize error, it is important to maximally stimulate the nerve so that all of the fibers that are capable of conducting current are depolarized. This is accomplished by gradually increasing the stimulus until the nerve amplitude is maximized. The depolarizing current is recorded by surface or needle electrodes placed over the course of the nerve at a measured distance. The depolarizing current travels both in both a physiologic (orthodromic) and nonphysiologic (antidromic) direction. A compound motor or sensory nerve action potential (CMAP/SNAP) can therefore be recorded proximally and distally along the nerve. These potentials provide a direct assessment of the nerve's ability to conduct.

Recorded action potentials are very small and must be amplified a thousand-fold. The electrical noise that is present in the environment should be filtered to eliminate various non-neurogenic high and low frequency waveforms that may obscure the action potential. The nerve is stimulated several hundred times. The resultant potentials are amplified, summated, and averaged by signal averaging computer software, and then displayed on an oscilloscope and broadcast over a loudspeaker.[5] The measurable parameters of an evoked potential include its latency, amplitude, and conduction velocity (Fig. 22–1). The latency is defined as the time between the nerve stimulation and the appearance of the action potential, both for sensory and motor fibers. The amplitude is represented by the area under the curve. It corresponds to the number of conducting nerve fibers, and provides some estimate as to the number of functionally conducting axons in the nerve. The sharper the waveform, the more synchronous the firing of the individual nerve fibers. The nerve conduction velocity (NCV) provides some information regarding the integrity of the myelin sheath. It is calculated by subtracting the latencies between two points along the nerve and then dividing by the distance between them.[21] The NCV is directly related to body temperature, myelin thickness, and internode distance.[5] The patient's body temperature, as well as the room temperature, should be controlled at all times. All electrophysiologic measurement should be done at an arm temperature of 32° to 34°C.

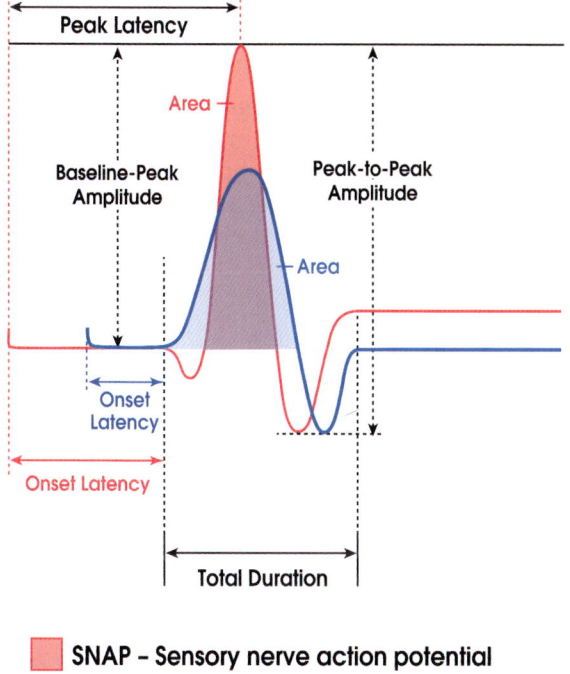

Peak Latency

Area

Baseline-Peak Amplitude

Peak-to-Peak Amplitude

Area

Onset Latency

Onset Latency

Total Duration

SNAP – Sensory nerve action potential

CMAP – Compound motor action potential

Figure 22–1   The measurable parameters of sensory nerve action potential and compound motor action potential. (Courtesy of The Christine M. Kleinert Institute for Hand and Microsurgery, Inc.)

The size and shape of the action potential can lead to the recognition of a partial or complete conduction block. A focal nerve injury results in diminished amplitudes and abnormal morphology of the motor and/or sensory potential. The NCV may also be slowed. With a complete lesion no CMAPs can be recorded distal to the zone of injury with proximal nerve stimulation. Nerve stimulation distal to a complete lesion may continue to elicit a response until Wallerian degeneration is complete. With a partial injury, stimulation proximal to the lesion would elicit a smaller response than normal. During surgery, the nerve can be stimulated directly within the operative site or percutaneously, distal to the wound margins. The nerve action potentials (NAPs) are recorded at a measured distance from the stimulus site (usually within the surgical field), which allows calculation of the nerve conduction velocity. An area of conduction block results in a decreased NCV. With a neuroma-in-continuity, the degree of conduction across the lesion and the amplitude of the recorded action potential may provide an estimate of the number of functional fibers.

Electromyography

Electromyography (EMG) is the method for recording electrical activity in the nerve muscle unit. The EMG study involves the insertion of a recording needle elec-

trode directly into the muscle. The electrical signal is amplified, processed, and displayed on an oscilloscope or a video monitor for visual analysis and broadcast over a loudspeaker for auditory analysis. In a normal muscle, the motor unit action potentials (MUAPs) are bi- or triphasic with duration of 7 to 15 milliseconds and amplitude of 200 microvolts (μV) to 3 millivolts (mV). The MUAP represents the combined electrical activity of all the muscle fibers innervated by a single motor neuron. A decrease in the MUAP amplitude would be suggestive of axonal loss. MUAPs are absent if the muscle is totally denervated. Increased insertional activity and the presence of abnormal spontaneous activity in the resting muscle (i.e., fibrillation potentials or positive sharp waves) are suggestive of denervation. Long-duration, high-amplitude, polyphasic motor unit potentials are characteristic of muscle reinnervation.

There are two types of intraoperative EMG studies: spontaneous and triggered.

During a spontaneous EMG study, the electrical muscle activity is continuously monitored. At rest the muscle should be electrically silent. If mechanical stimulation depolarizes the nerve under examination, it will be detected and recorded by the EMG electrodes in the muscle. This type of study may minimize injury to the nerve fibers during nerve dissection and manipulation. A triggered EMG study involves recording the electrical activity in a nerve muscle unit after nerve stimulation with an electrode. The nerve is stimulated in the operative field and the activity is recorded in the target muscles. By recording the activity in certain muscle groups specific motor fibers can be identified. When a nerve innervates a single muscle, identification is straightforward. When a nerve or a portion of the plexus innervates several muscles, however, the analysis is more complex.[21] Due to the complexity associated with examining nerves at a proximal level, the recording electrodes should be placed in a number of muscles prior to the start of the operation. Changes in the MUAP morphology, duration, amplitude, or firing frequency provide information as to the integrity of the nerve supplying that muscle.

Somatosensory-Evoked Potentials

Somatosensory-evoked potentials (SEPs) involve the recording of the electrical activity of a peripheral nerve at a central (cortical or brainstem) level or proximal (nerve root) level after stimulation of the distal nerve.[22] The nerve under examination is typically stimulated at the hand or wrist. Cortical-evoked responses are then recorded by means of a scalp lead. Brainstem responses are recorded with a mastoid lead, and spinal cord responses are recorded with a cervical spine lead. These potentials can also be recorded within the surgical field. In an anesthetized patient, the stimulation intensity is not limited by the patient's pain tolerance. The stimulus typically consists of a single square impulse of 0.1 to 0.2 milliseconds in duration, at a frequency of 10 per second, and an intensity of 40 to 60 volts (V). Recording is achieved with the aid of a preamplifier connected to surface electrodes over the parietal hemisphere.

SEPs recorded at the different levels can yield information regarding conduction along the length of a nerve. Central recordings serve to monitor or assess the function of afferent nerve fibers, which helps to localize and evaluate the extent of a nerve lesion. When recorded over the surgical site, SEPs may aid in the identification of nerve fibers. SEPs can also be used to determine the state of conduction along the proximal segments of a nerve or nerve roots.[21] These central recordings can reflect the continuity between the brain and a proximal nerve or a nerve root.[21,23,24] This information is particularly important for identifying a root avulsion or for detecting a second nerve lesion at a more proximal site. Intraoperative SEP recordings allow one to evaluate the integrity of the intraforaminal part of the dorsal sensory tracts. Unfortunately, no direct or indirect information can be obtained as to the condition of the anterior motor roots.[14,17] This limitation is important to understand, since some dissociative lesions may be restricted to only to a motor or sensory root. Paravertebral motor evoked potential recordings may remedy this deficiency.[17,25,26]

Motor Evoked Potentials

Motor evoked potentials (MEPs) can be of value in assessing the motor components of nerves.[27,28] These potentials are elicited by transcranial electrical stimulation of the motor cortex and are then recorded over nerves (neurogenic potentials) or over muscle (myogenic potentials). MEPs are one means to demonstrate the continuity of the motor pathways from the brain to the muscle. Anesthetics and neuromuscular blockers can dampen these potentials. The optimal use of this technique has yet to be determined.

CLINICAL APPLICATIONS

We have identified four main clinical situations in which to apply intraoperative nerve recordings: (1) intraoperative nerve monitoring, (2) brachial plexus injuries, (3) nerve mapping, and (4) neuroma-in-continuity.

Intraoperative Nerve Monitoring

Intraoperative nerve recordings can facilitate nerve identification during the surgical approach.[21,23,25,29–32] When the identity of tissues is uncertain, such as in patients with a previous surgery or heavy scarring,

stimulating the scar tissue while recording the muscle response allows one to identify and preserve any functioning nerves. Mechanical stimulation of a viable nerve typically causes a brief burst of motor unit potentials, which can be detected in the muscle(s) that are innervated by that nerve. This technique can help prevent nerve fiber damage during nerve elevation or retraction, during tumor excision, or during internal fixation of fractures.[29–32] Preserving viable nerve fibers is particularly important when approaching lesions where partial function has remained despite the heavy scarring.

SEPs have been the standard monitoring technique for spinal surgery whereas EMG has been widely used during nerve root surgery. Continuous EMG and/or SEP can also be used to monitor peripheral nerves. The advent of equipment that is capable of performing simultaneous SEPs, MEPs, and EMG has added a new dimension to nerve monitoring. The question of whether or not this more comprehensive monitoring results in greater protection of the nervous system awaits future analysis.

Technique

At the start of the operation, the EMG recording electrodes are inserted into the appropriate muscles. With the median nerve, the electrical activity is recorded from the abductor pollicis brevis muscle. In the case of the ulnar nerve, the first dorsal interosseous muscle is monitored. For the radial nerve, electrodes are inserted into the extensor pollicis brevis and the abductor pollicis longus muscles. The surface electrodes for SEP recordings are placed on the cervical, mastoid and scalp areas using colloid and adhesive plasters. The somesthetic cortex area of the hand corresponds to a point that is 2 cm posterior and 7 cm lateral to the vertex, on the parietal lobe. The passive electrode is placed on the frontal zone. The ground electrode is placed over the occiput or contralateral arm. The neurophysiologist monitors the nerves during the dissection and keeps the surgeon apprised of any abnormal potentials.

Triggered EMG or SEP can be used to identify the location and the nature of a nerve. It is especially difficult to identify the neural elements in situations with dense scarring. In these instances bipolar electrodes are used to stimulate the nerve directly, typically at a frequency of 2 per second and a duration of 0.1 ms. The voltage can be increased from 5 to 60 V without fear of inducing electrical burns in the nerve. Recordings are taken from individual muscles or muscle groups, which then aids in the identification of the particular neural element (i.e., nerve, cord, trunk, or root).

Brachial Plexus Injuries

Accurate evaluation of the type, level, and extent of a brachial plexus lesion is crucial.[2,4,6–8,17,24,33–36] Both the management of and the prognosis for this injury are largely determined by the location of the lesion i.e., intraforaminal (preganglionic) or extraforaminal (postganglionic). Traction injuries are frequently preganglionic, which often have a poor prognosis. Anatomically, the angle formed by the roots on the edge of the transverse groove progressively flattens from C5 to T1. As a consequence, extraforaminal lesions are more commonly observed at the C5, C6 level with a lesser incidence at the C7 root level and the C8, T1 level.[34,36] In postganglionic lesions the nerve roots are in continuity with the spinal cord and are amenable to neurolysis, neuroraphy or nerve grafts. In preganglionic lesions, the connection to the spinal cord has been disrupted; hence, neurotization, and tendon or muscle transfers are needed to restore motor function.[4,6,7,12,14,17,36–40]

The clinical evaluation is the first step in determining the type of the lesion. The absence of a Tinel's sign and the presence of a Horner's syndrome or hemidiaphragm paralysis may indicate root avulsion. EMG evidence of denervation of the paravertebral muscles or normal sensory nerve conduction velocities in an anesthetic area may denote a preganglionic lesion.[14,17] Imaging studies such as computed tomography myelography and MRI are quite helpful.[1,7,8,35] Anatomic continuity, though, as demonstrated by imaging studies or by direct observation, does not necessarily guarantee the presence of functional continuity.[2]

Intraoperative nerve recordings (IONR) are especially useful in the management of brachial plexus injuries.[7,8,12,21,38] These techniques included the use of SEPs, nerve conduction studies, and nerve root potential recordings. Nerve action potentials (NAPs) are recorded directly from the nerve using bipolar electrodes. They are valuable for evaluating the functional status of mixed peripheral nerves as well as for localizing a lesion in the nerve branches distal to the dorsal root ganglion. Any neuromas that are identified during the surgical exploration can further be investigated with nerve conduction studies or by triggered EMG.

NAPs may be useful if there are any visible gaps or palpable neuromas once the plexus has been dissected.[39–41] If a gap is observed the corresponding root is stimulated and recordings are taken from nerve branches proximal to the lesion. When a neuroma is observed or palpated, the nerve is stimulated proximal to the site while recordings are taken from the nerve distal to the lesion. The presence of NAPs distal to the site 3 or more weeks after the injury is indicative of functional continuity of the nerve fibers. A postganglionic lesion will yield a flat trace. In cases where the injury to a specific region of the plexus appears complete on clinical exam, the presence of a small and slowly conducting NAP is indicative of either nerve regeneration or significant partial sparing. Low-

amplitude polyphasic potentials may be recorded following nerve regeneration across a lesion as early as 6 to 8 weeks postinjury.[12] The amplitude of the potential gives some indication of the number of viable axons that are still capable of conducting, but controversy exists with regards to the cut-off point for resection and grafting the neuroma. Unless contraindicated by the clinical findings, the general consensus is to recommend resection and repair of the damaged segment when the NCV across a lesion is less than 10 m/s, and the amplitude is less than 25% to 30% of normal. These studies may help differentiate the functional cords from nonfunctional ones. In some instances, there may be a second lesion that is proximal or distal to the neuroma. The presence or absence of a proximal nerve root injury has important prognostic implications, and serves to guide the subsequent surgical treatment.

SEPs may help to evaluate the functional continuity between a cord or nerve root and the brain, as well as between the dorsal root sensory fibers and the spinal cord. As many as 11% of patients with brachial plexus avulsions however, have been reported to have partial root avulsions such as intact ventral rootlets and avulsed dorsal rootlets or vice versa.[35]

The spinal nerve, which is formed by the intradural union of the anterior and posterior rootlets, divides into a large anterior ramus and a smaller posterior ramus immediately after leaving the intervertebral foramen. The posterior ramus innervates the skin and paravertebral muscles of the neck. The anterior ramus, which is now called a root, joins the other roots and divides and unites to form the brachial plexus.[17,24,40,42,43] Intraoperative SEP recordings can be used to evaluate the afferent sensory tracts, but no information can be obtained regarding the condition of the anterior rootlets. This limitation may lead to a false-positive or false-negative SEP recording. Potentials may still be recorded when the posterior rootlet is intact but the anterior rootlet is disrupted. Conversely, the SEP may be absent when the posterior rootlet is interrupted, despite an intact anterior rootlet.[14,17]

Direct intradural inspection can provide additional information about the integrity of the anterior and posterior rootlets, but it requires additional surgery through a different surgical approach (i.e., a cervical hemilaminectomy).[12,14,17] Moreover, the anatomic continuity of the rootlets does not necessarily reflect their functional status. To remedy this problem Celli et al.[14] developed a method for stimulating the nerve root as it exited from the neural foramen with a bipolar electrode, while recording the paravertebral muscle response with EMG needles. Later, Oberle et al.[17] recorded evoked muscle action potentials from neck muscles in a similar fashion. Their technique involved the simultaneous recording of the cortical SEP recordings and evoked muscle action potentials (EMAPs) while stimulating the nerve root at the vertebral foramen. This technique is initially performed without muscle relaxants. In the case of a functionally intact anterior rootlet, the dorsal ramus, which is located a short distance proximal to the stimulation site, is also depolarized by the upward-spreading current. EMAPs can therefore be recorded in the paravertebral muscles. If a cortical SEP is recorded at the same time, the posterior rootlet is functionally intact. In the case of anterior rootlet avulsion, the neck muscles are denervated and EMAPs are absent. Muscle relaxants are then administered until full muscle relaxation is achieved and the stimulation is repeated.[17] The EMAPs are lost at that time, but the SEPs can still be recorded.

An alternative approach is to record the motor evoked potentials. Turkof et al.[24] introduced a method for recording transcranial electrical motor–evoked potentials to evaluate the functional status of the anterior spinal roots and spinal nerves during brachial surgery. The patients were anesthetized with propofol and 0.4% nitrous oxide. The motor cortex was stimulated transcranially with single pulses of 100 microseconds in duration and 750 mV in amplitude. After the initial testing, the patients were paralyzed with pancuronium to avoid any muscle action potentials. Action potentials were then recorded directly from the spinal nerve or nerve stump. These investigators were able to record nerve action potentials from 32 of the 38 nerves that were in continuity and from 21 of 25 nerve stumps. Although this method has found several clinical applications, experience is limited and the reliability and sensitivity of the method still needs to be determined.

Technique

At the start of the operation, EMG recording electrodes are inserted into the muscles that will be monitored. The surface electrodes for SEP recordings are placed on the cervical, mastoid, and scalp areas using colloid and adhesive plasters. A needle electrode is inserted in the paravertebral muscles. The brachial plexus is exposed via an anterior scalenectomy, and then explored for any gaps or thickened and firm segments. Ideally, the roots are exposed as far proximally as the vertebral foramen. This provides enough space to allow for 4 to 6 cm of separation between the stimulating and recording electrodes. All halogenated agents are discontinued. Anesthesia is maintained by a mixture of propofol at a dose of 2 to 4 mg/kg/hr and 0.5% or less nitrous oxide. Bipolar electrodes are used to stimulate the nerve roots close to the neural foramen using a stimulus intensity of 0.1 to 0.2 milliseconds and a constant current of 10 to 25 mA. To test the equipment setup the recording electrode is first situated proximal to the lesion and at least 3 to 4 cm away from the stimulating electrode. The stimulus intensity is increased until a NAP is evoked. The filter and amplifier settings are optimized. The

recording electrode is then placed distal to the site of injury and the root stimulation is repeated. This allows an evaluation of any evoked potentials across the lesion. The recording electrode is moved farther down the nerve to determine at what point a NAP can no longer be recorded.

Electrodiagnostic studies are very useful for evaluating the plexus for the presence of a neuroma-in-continuity. They also aid in the decision making as to whether to preserve or excise and graft the neuroma (see neuroma-in-continuity below). The brachial plexus is stimulated distal to the lesion or in the fingers. EMG and SEP recordings are simultaneously performed during stimulation of the root. Sensory nerve action potentials (SNAPs) are recorded proximal to the lesion. Preserved SNAPs combined with an absent SEP is presumptive evidence of a preganglionic lesion. This is because the sensory fibers which remain in continuity with the dorsal root ganglion do not degenerate and can still conduct. If there are intact fibers crossing the lesion, electrical activity will also be observed on the EMG tracings in the muscles innervated by their corresponding roots. Similarly, cortical SEPs can be recorded if there is a connection between the roots and the brain. When SNAPs are absent, a postganglionic lesion is suspected. The absence of SNAPs, however, does not necessarily exclude a preganglionic lesion. Often there is combination of different types of lesions. The electrodiagnostic findings should be considered in the context of the clinical examination in addition to the surgical and radiological findings. This in turn will dictate the type of procedure (Fig. 22–2).

We have examined 85 roots with intraoperative nerve recordings in 23 brachial plexus patients. Forty-eight roots were shown to be in continuity with the brain. Nerve grafting was performed in 23 roots and neurolysis in 15 roots. Neurotization was performed using intercostal nerves in three patients. The hemicontralateral C7 root was used in four patients, the spinal accessory nerve in seven patients, and the phrenic nerve in two patients. In eight patients, muscle and tendon transfers were required to improve the final functional result. Of the 23 grafted roots, 14 (61%) nerves showed functional clinical recovery (≥M3). Of the 15 neurolyzed roots, 10 (66%) roots showed functional recovery of M3 or more. After neurotization, functional recovery was obtained in eight of 16 patients (50%). Free gracilis muscle transfers were performed in 2 patients to improve their overall function. Preoperatively, it was presumed that all of the roots were in continuity with CNS. Thirty-seven roots were shown to have no continuity with brain however, which changed the diagnosis in 43% of the cases. IONR was a invaluable for identifying those roots without a connection to the brain, and in differentiating those neuromas that should be resected from those that could be neurolyzed.

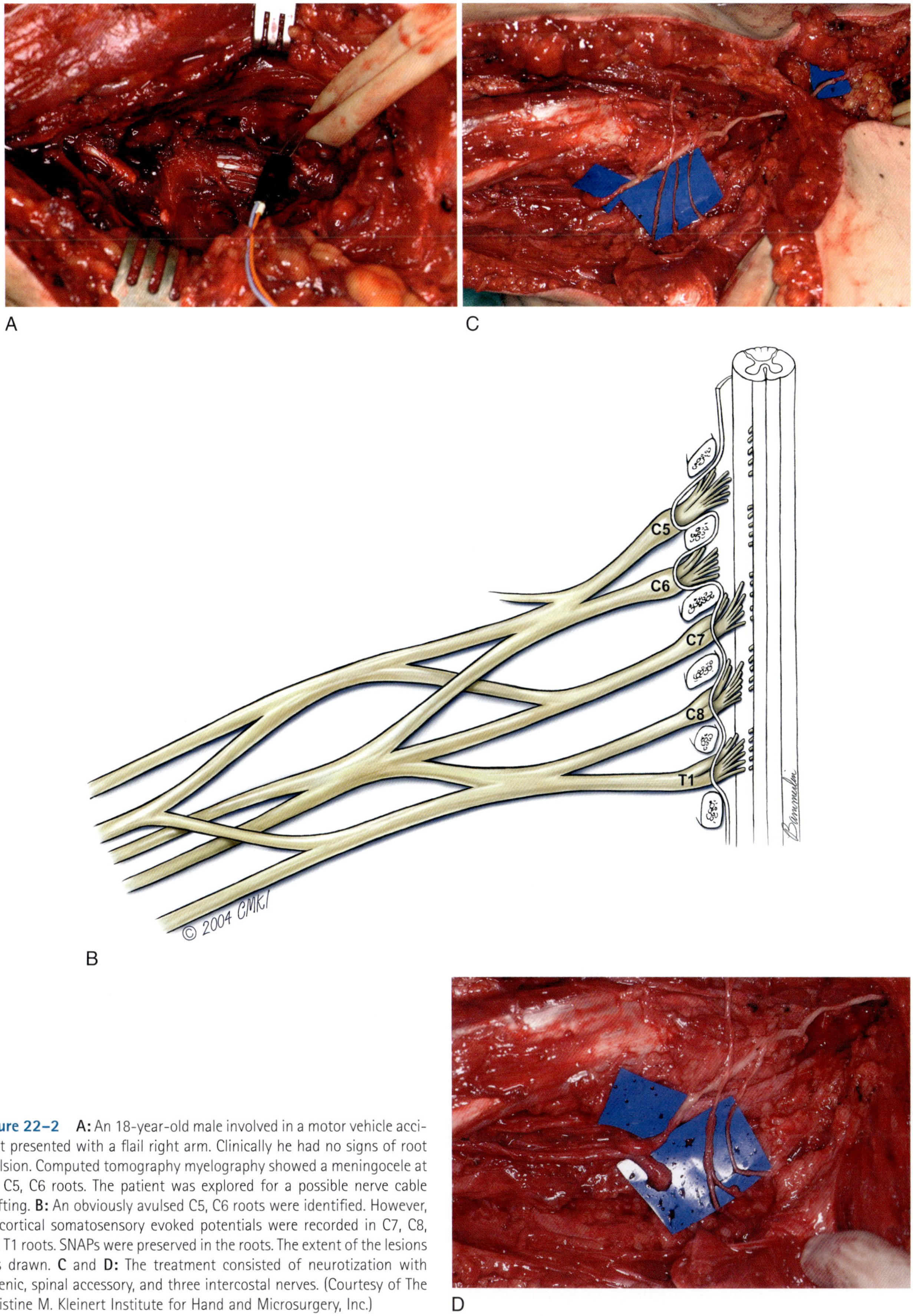

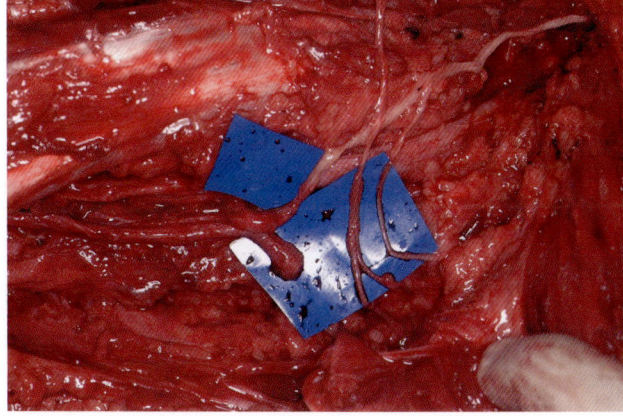

A

C

B

© 2004 CMKI

C5

C6

C7

C8

T1

D

Figure 22–2 **A:** An 18-year-old male involved in a motor vehicle accident presented with a flail right arm. Clinically he had no signs of root avulsion. Computed tomography myelography showed a meningocele at the C5, C6 roots. The patient was explored for a possible nerve cable grafting. **B:** An obviously avulsed C5, C6 roots were identified. However, no cortical somatosensory evoked potentials were recorded in C7, C8, and T1 roots. SNAPs were preserved in the roots. The extent of the lesions was drawn. **C** and **D:** The treatment consisted of neurotization with phrenic, spinal accessory, and three intercostal nerves. (Courtesy of The Christine M. Kleinert Institute for Hand and Microsurgery, Inc.)

Nerve Mapping

Intraoperative electrodiagnosis can be helpful in the repair of acutely transected nerves by aiding in the differentiation of motor and sensory fibers. In the acute phase of nerve transection, the distal motor fibers can be identified by electrical stimulation. Stimulation of the proximal stump is performed using awake stimulation. If the transection is subacute and Wallerian degeneration has already occurred, the distal motor fibers will not conduct. In this instance, the motor fascicles can be identified by direct dissection in those nerves where the motor and sensory fascicles are not intermingled and run in fascicular groups (i.e., deep motor branch of the ulnar nerve, thenar motor branch of the median nerve).

Technique

Nerve mapping with awake stimulation requires the cooperation of the patient. The patient should be instructed and rehearsed in localizing the stimulus and differentiating sharp and dull sensation prior to the surgery. The patient is then started on a short-acting anesthetic and the wound is explored. The nerve stumps are identified and an internal neurolysis is performed prior to stimulation. The tourniquet is then deflated for at least 15 minutes to allow the reperfusion of the nerve and reversal of any ischemic conduction block. When the patient becomes cooperative, the fascicles in the proximal stump are stimulated at a frequency of two per second, with an intensity of 2 to 20 mA and a duration of 0.2 milliseconds. The patient is asked to report where they feel the stimulus, and whether it is dull or sharp. A dull aching sensation is typical of motor fiber stimulation, whereas a sharp painful sensation is usually associated with sensory fascicles.

In delayed repairs when the distal fascicles will no longer conduct, the motor branch of the ulnar or median nerve is identified. The motor fascicles are then followed proximally to the cut nerve end and tagged with 10-0 nylon. The remaining fibers are assumed to be sensory. The proximal stump is mapped using awake stimulation as described. If there is no response at the cut surface, the proximal nerve is stimulated higher up. After the fascicular topography has been mapped, the motor and sensory fascicles in the proximal and distal stumps are matched and repaired in a grouped fascicular fashion.

Neuroma-in-Continuity

A partial laceration, crush, contusion, stretch, or thermal damage to a nerve will often result in a partial nerve injury.[3,10–12,29,30,44,45] Partial lesions constitute approximately 60% of all peripheral nerve injuries.[11,31] There is a broad range of outcomes in lesions where there is some degree of anatomic continuity. Some nerves will recover completely, while others show no improvement. Partial nerve lesions and failed repairs of a complete transection will often result in a neuroma-in-continuity.

Sunderland's grading scale for nerve lesions-in-continuity ranges from mild internal derangement (Grade 1) to severe derangements that profoundly affect all aspects of the nerve (Grade 4). Between these extremes is a spectrum of changes that comprise the partial injuries.[10–12,31] Histopathologic examination of the neuroma-in-continuity reveals a mixture of intact nerve fibers crossing the lesion intermingled with randomly oriented regenerating nerve fibers embedded in a collagenous scar.[31,45]

IONRs play an important role in the management of a neuroma-in-continuity, which have been popularized by Kline.[3,11] Williams and Terzis[45] have devised a technique for single fascicle recordings.[2] Mackinnon et al. used intraoperative electrical stimulation to identify and preserve the motor fascicles within the neuroma itself, which avoids the need for a tedious dissection.

A neuroma-in-continuity may present in a variety of ways, ranging from total motor and sensory loss to a significant preservation of motor and sensory function (Table 22–1). Pain is often a prominent feature of this lesion. Timing is critical in the management of partial nerve lesions. Clinically it is not possible to accurately determine the grade of nerve injury nor to predict which ones will improve versus those that will worsen over time. This is especially so with proximal injuries such as a brachial plexus lesion, which may have to followed for more than a year before the clinical outcome can be determined. There is a high price to pay for an inordinate delay in exploring these injuries due to the diminished potential for nerve regeneration. Premature exploration of the neuroma, however, may lead to an erroneous impression of the potential for recovery.

It is our practice to manage partial nerve injuries caused by penetration from sharp objects with early surgical exploration. In closed injuries or high velocity injuries such as gunshot wounds, we prefer to wait 3

TABLE 22–1

Clinical Classification of Neuroma-in-Continuity

Type	Description
Type A	Poor or no clinical function
Type B	Partial preservation of motor or sensory function
	B1 Preserved motor function with absent or very poor sensory function
	B2 Preserved sensory function with absent or very poor motor function
Type C	Significant preservation of both motor and sensory function
(p)	Added if pain is present

months in order to observe for signs of regeneration in the muscle(s) closest to the lesion and the distal nerve by clinical exam, EMG, and nerve conduction studies. A prolonged polyphasic potential is a sign of regenerating fibers. The conduction velocity across the lesion is initially prolonged, but becomes faster over time as the regenerating fibers mature. Partial reinnervation may be indicative of a neuroma-in-continuity. If there are no clinical and electrodiagnostic signs of progressive regeneration over time, surgical exploration is indicated.

A neuroma-in-continuity may be present, even though the nerve appears grossly intact. The nerve may be partially or completely scarred with a loss of the fascicular pattern, and it is often firm to palpation. In some cases, the neuroma may seem small even though the intraneural derangement is severe. The outward appearance of the damaged segment, however, provides no information as to the nerve function itself. The onus lies with the surgeon to determine whether any useful nerve function remains and whether a neuroma resection is indicated. There are two important determinants in the decision making. The first is a detailed preoperative clinical examination, which provides information regarding the sensory or motor function in each fascicular group. The second is the data obtained from intraoperative nerve recordings. The application of intraoperative electrodiagnostic techniques is especially valuable in those challenging patients who have some partial preservation of nerve function.

Technique

The nerve lesion is widely exposed under tourniquet control. The dissection proceeds from proximal to distal, starting from healthy looking neural tissue and moving towards the scarred neuroma-in-continuity. An external neurolysis is performed and the nerve is gently elevated. The halogenated agents are then stopped and anesthesia is maintained with propofol at a rate of 2 to 4 mg/kg/hr. The tourniquet is released, and hemostasis is obtained. It is particularly important to obtain a bloodless field for nerve recordings. At least 15 minutes should pass before nerve stimulation is performed. The nerve is first stimulated proximal to the lesion with bipolar electrodes that are separated from the recording electrodes by at least 4 to 6 cm. A narrow pulse width of 0.01 to 0.02 milliseconds is necessary when recording over short nerve segments, with a gain of 10 mA. The filter and amplifier settings are optimized once a normal nerve action potential is identified. The nerve conduction velocity and the amplitude of the nerve action potential are measured across the lesion and compared to the normal segment. It is our preference to resect the neuroma and graft the defect when the amplitude of the action potential is 25% to 30% of normal or

less, and the nerve conduction velocity across the neuroma is less than 10 m/s.

We have classified the neuroma-in-continuity into three types (Table 22–1). In a Type A neuroma-in-continuity, there is no clinically important sensory or motor function. If poor nerve action potentials are obtained, the neuroma is resected and grafted.

In a Type B neuroma-in-continuity where there is partial preservation of either sensory or motor function, an internal neurolysis is performed proximal and distal to the lesion without dissecting the neuroma itself. The individual nerve fascicles are then stimulated proximal to the neuroma-in-continuity while recording directly from the nerve distal to the lesion. This permits the identification of any functional fascicular groups proximal to the lesion, which are then matched with the corresponding fascicles distal to the lesion. The functional fibers coursing through the neuroma are left intact; the nonfunctional ones are resected and grafted. In a Type C neuroma-in-continuity, good-quality nerve action potentials are usually seen and an external neurolysis suffices (Fig. 22–3).

We have identified 38 patients with 47 neuromas-in-continuity that were managed with the aid of IONR. There were 16 patients with 19 brachial plexus level neuromas and 22 patients with 28 peripheral neuromas. The timing of nerve exploration varied between 2 and 38 months. There were 37 Type A, 7 Type B (four Type B1 with preserved motor function and three Type B2 with sensory function preserved and motor function lost), and 3 Type C neuromas-in-continuity. Overall, 26 neuromas were excised and grafted, while a neurolysis was performed in 21. Fourteen of these neuromas were examined histologically.

In 20 of the 37 Type A lesions, the amplitude of the nerve compound action potential (NCAP) was less than 30% of normal. In those cases, neuroma resection and sural nerve grafting was performed. IONR influenced the treatment method in 17 of the Type A neuromas, which were managed by a neurolysis rather than resection. The gain in information was 46%. In Type B neuromas, IONR helped to correctly identify the functional fascicles. In six of the seven neuromas, resection and grafting were performed; one was treated with neurolysis alone (Fig. 22–4). In the three Type C neuromas, good-quality potentials were recorded across the neuroma; hence, neurolysis alone was performed. In our series, no functional loss was observed after surgery. There was a good correlation between the percentage of myelinated fibers in the histologic sections and the amplitude of NCAPs.

In summary, adjunctive intraoperative electrodiagnostic technique can provide valuable information as to the physiology of the injured nerve, which in turn can aid the surgeon in the decision-making process during management of these complex injuries.

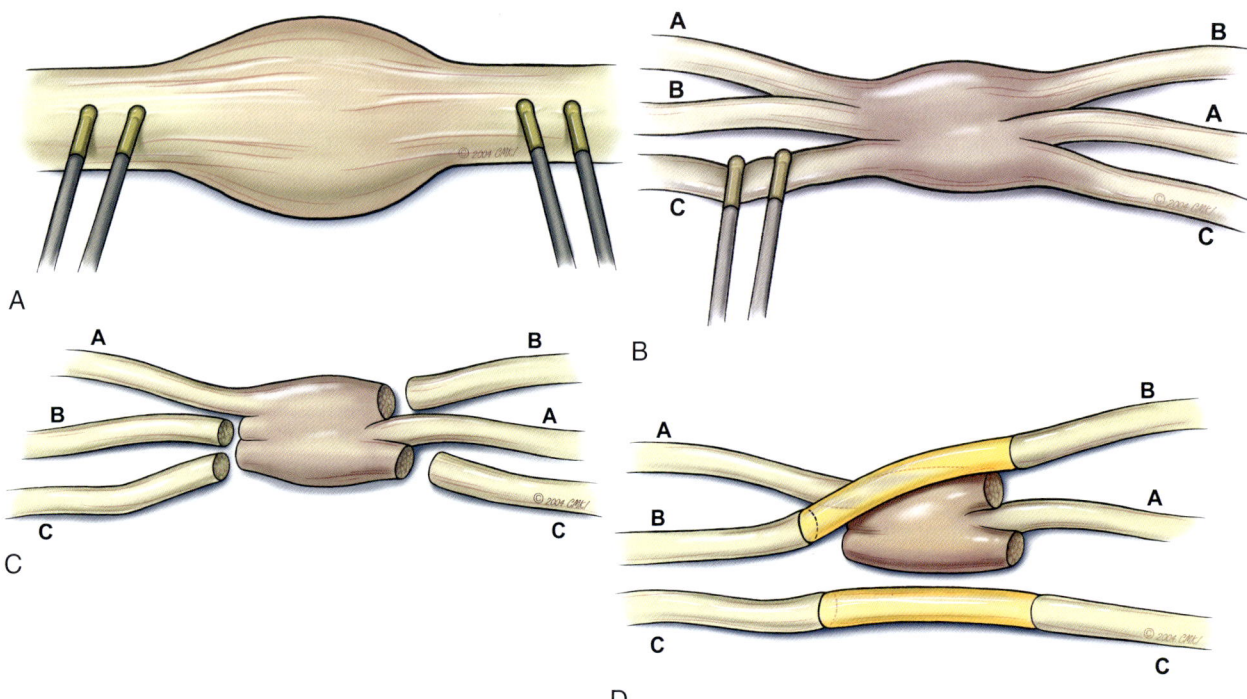

Figure 22–3 **A:** Type B neuroma-in-continuity with partially preserved sensory or motor function. **B:** Internal neurolysis is performed outside the neuroma-in-continuity, and each fascicular group is stimulated proximally, and the corresponding distal fascicle is identified. **C:** The fascicles that respond to stimulation are preserved with the neuroma. **D:** The fascicles that do not respond to stimulation are resected and grafted. (Courtesy of The Christine M. Kleinert Institute for Hand and Microsurgery, Inc.)

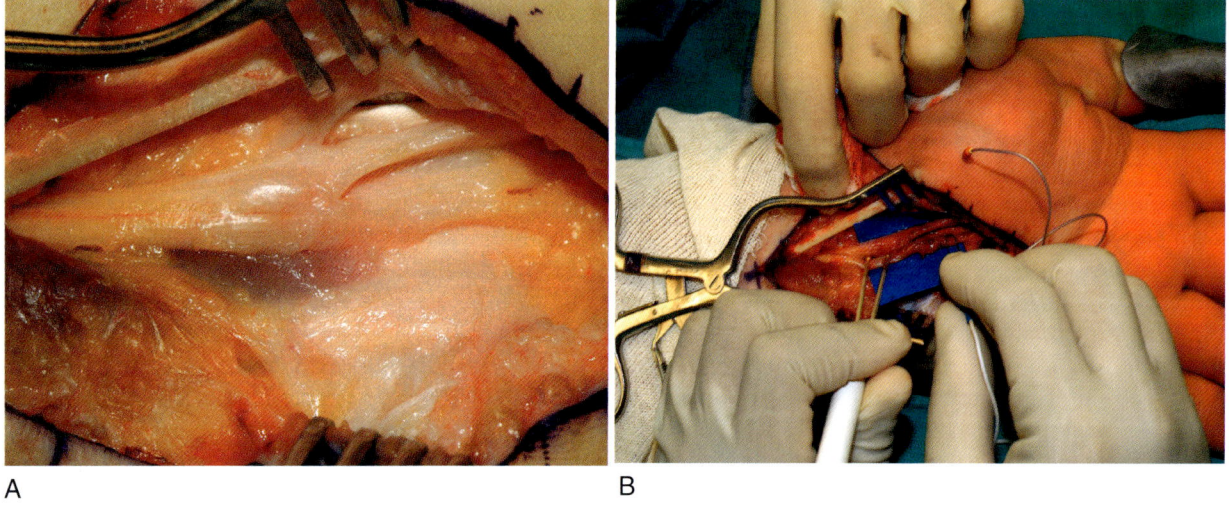

Figure 22–4 A 38-year-old female with a nerve lesion after endoscopic carpal tunnel release. She had good motor function in thenar muscles, diminished sensation in the thumb, and no sensation in the index, middle, and ring fingers. **A:** Surgical exploration revealed a neuroma-in-continuity Type B1. **B:** Stimulation of the fascicle groups showed good motor compound action potentials to the thenar muscles. Sensory nerve action potentials were recorded on thumb and index finger stimulation. No potentials were recorded on second and third common digital nerves. These fascicles were resected and grafted. The patient achieved good sensation in the thumb and index finger and diminished sensation in the middle and ring fingers. (Courtesy of The Christine M. Kleinert Institute for Hand and Microsurgery, Inc.)

Acknowledgments

The authors thank Dr. David J. Slutsky for his review and edit of the manuscript, and Elaine Bammerlin for the illustrations.

REFERENCES

1. Jarvik JG, Kliot M, Maravilla KR. MR nerve imaging of the wrist and hand. Hand Clin 2000;16:25–36.
2. Williams HB, Terzis JK. Single fascicular recordings: an intraoperative diagnostic tool for the management of peripheral nerve lesions. Plast Reconstr Surg 1976;57:562–9.
3. Kline DG. Early evaluation of peripheral nerve lesions in continuity with a note on nerve recording. Am Surg 1968;34:77–81.
4. Zverina E, Kredba J. Somatosensory cerebral evoked potentials in diagnosis of brachial plexus injury. Scand J Rehabil Med 1977;9:47–54.
5. Van Beek AL, Massac E Jr, Smith DO. The use of the signal averaging computer for evaluation of peripheral nerve problems. Clin Plast Surg 1986;13:407–18.
6. Landi A, Copeland SA, Wynn CB, et al. The role of somatosensory evoked potentials and nerve conduction studies in the surgical management of brachial plexus injuries. J Bone Joint Surg Br 1980;62:492–6.
7. Jones SJ. Investigation of brachial plexus traction lesions by peripheral and somatosensory evoked potentials. J Neurol Neurosurg Psychiatry 1979;42:107.
8. Sugioka H, Tsuyama N, Hara T, et al. Investigation of brachial plexus injuries by intraoperative cortical somatosensory evoked potentials. Arch Orthop Trauma Surg 1982;99:143–51.
9. Dawson GD. Cerebral response to electrical stimulation of peripheral nerves in man. J Neurol Neurosurg Psychiatry 1947;10:134–40.
10. Hakstian RW. Funicular orientation to direct stimulation. An aid to peripheral nerve repair. J Bone Joint Surg Am 1968;50:1178–86.
11. Kline DG, Nulsen FE. The neuroma in continuity: its preoperative and operative management. Surg Clin North Am 1972;52:1189–209.
12. Spinner RJ, Klein DG. Surgery for peripheral nerve and brachial plexus injuries or other nerve lesions. Muscle Nerve 2000;23:680–95.
13. Rosen I, Sornas R, Elmqvist D. Cervical root avulsion. Scand J Plast Reconstr Surg 1977;11:247.
14. Celli L, Rovesta C, de Luise G. Intraoperative paravertebral muscular evoked potentials (PMEP) in treatment of traumatic root lesions of the brachial plexus. Acta Orthop Belg 1983;49:564–70.
15. Merton PA, Morton HB. Stimulation of the cerebral cortex in the intact human subject. Nature 1980;285:227.
16. Van Beek AL. Electrodiagnostic evaluation of peripheral nerve injuries. Hand Clin 1986;2:747–60.
17. Oberle J, Antoniadis G, Kast E, et al. Evaluation of traumatic cervical nerve root injuries by intraoperative evoked potentials. Neurosurgery 2002;51:1182–90.
18. McPherson RW, Mahla M, Johnson R, et al. Effects of enflurane, isoflurane, and nitrous oxide on somatosensory evoked potentials during fentanyl anesthesia. Anesthesiology 1985;62:626–33.
19. Peterson DO, Drummond JC, Todd MM. Effects of halothane, enflurane, isoflurane, and nitrous oxide on somatosensory evoked potentials in humans. Anesthesiology 1986;65:35–40.
20. Aminoff MJ. Electrophysiologic testing for the diagnosis of peripheral nerve injuries. Anesthesiology 2004;100:1298–303.
21. Slimp JC. Intraoperative monitoring of nerve repairs. Hand Clin 2000;16:25–36.
22. Alon M, Rochkind S. Pre-, intra, and postoperative electrophysiologic analysis of the recovery of old injuries of the peripheral nerve and brachial plexus after microsurgical management. J Reconstr Microsurg 2002;18:77–82.
23. Liberson WT, Terzis JK. Some novel techniques of clinical electrophysiology applied to the management of brachial plexus palsy. Electromyogr Clin Neurophysiol 1987;27:371–83.
24. Turkof E, Monsivas J, Dechtyar I, et al. Motor evoked potential as a reliable method to verify the conductivity of anterior spinal roots in brachial plexus surgery: an experimental study on goats. J Reconstr Microsurg 1995;11:357–62.
25. Van Beek A, Hubble B, Kinkead L, et al. Clinical use of nerve stimulation and recording techniques. Plast Reconstr Surg 1983;71:225–40.
26. Oberle J, Antoniadis G, Rath SA, et al. Intra-operative electrophysiological diagnosis of spinal root avulsion during surgical repair of brachial plexus stretch injuries. Acta Neurochirurgie 1997;139:238–9.
27. Abbruzzese G, Morena M, Caponnetto C, et al. Motor evoked potentials following cervical electrical stimulation in brachial plexus lesions. J Neurol 1993;241:63–7.
28. Burkholder LM, Houlden DA, Midha R, et al. Neurogenic motor evoked potentials: role in brachial plexus surgery (case report). J Neurosurg 2003;98:607–10.
29. Kline DG, Hackett ER, LeBanc HJ. The value of primary repair for bluntly transected nerve injuries: physiological documentation. Surg Forum 1974;25:436–8.
30. Kline DG. Timing for exploration of nerve lesions and evaluation of the neuroma-in-continuity. Clin Orthop 1982;163:42–9.
31. Kline DG, Hackett ER. Reappraisal of timing for exploration of civilian peripheral nerve injuries. Surgery 1975;78:54–65.
32. Kline DG, Kott J, Barnes G, et al. Exploration of selected brachial plexus lesions by the posterior subscapular approach. J Neurosurg 1978;49:872–80.
33. Jones SJ, Parry CB, Landi A. Diagnosis of brachial plexus traction lesions by sensory nerve action potentials and somatosensory evoked potentials. Injury 1981;12:376–82.
34. Sugioka H. Evoked potentials in the investigation of traumatic lesions of the peripheral nerve and the brachial plexus. Clin Orthop 1984;184:85–92.
35. Carvalho GA, Nikkhah G, Cordula M, et al. Diagnosis of root avulsions in traumatic brachial plexus injuries: value of computerized tomography myelography and magnetic resonance imaging. J Neurosurg 1997;86:69–76.
36. Carvalho GA, Nikkhah G, Samii M. Diagnosis and surgical indications of traumatic brachial plexus lesions from the neurosurgery viewpoint. Orthopade 1997;26:599–605.
37. Alnot JY, Jolly A, Frot B. Direct treatment of nerve lesions in brachial plexus injuries in adults: a series of 100 operated cases. Int Orthop 1981;5:151–68.
38. Millesi H. Surgery of post-traumatic brachial plexus lesions (personal approach in 2003). Handchir Mikrochir Plast Chir 2004;36:29–36.
39. Dubuisson A, Kline DG. Indications for peripheral nerve and brachial plexus surgery. Neurol Clin 1992;10:935–51.
40. Penkert G, Carvalho GA, Nikkhah G, et al. Diagnosis and surgery of brachial plexus injuries. J Reconstr Microsurg 1999;15:3–8.
41. Murase T, Kawai H, Masotomi T, et al. Evoked spinal cord potentials for diagnosis during brachial plexus surgery. J Bone Joint Surg Br 1993;75:775–81.
42. Orlandini A, Gualandi GF, Tansini A, et al. Traumatic lesions of the brachial plexus. Evaluation of 144 cases studied using direct

cervical myelography and non-ionic contrast media. Radiol Med (Torino) 1988;75:15–9.

43. Tonkin MA, Eckersley JR, Gschwind CR. The surgical treatment of brachial plexus injuries. Aust N Z J Surg 1996;66:29–33.

44. Hurst LC, Dowd A, Sampson SP, et al. Partial lacerations of median and ulnar nerves. J Hand Surg Am 1991;16:207–10.

45. Mackinnon SE, Glickman LT, Dagum A. A technique for the treatment of neuroma incontinuity. J Reconstr Microsurg 1992;8:379–83.

Numbers followed by *f* indicate figures; those followed by *t* indicate tabular material.